Chemotherapy and Radiotherapy

Chemotherapy and Radiotherapy

Edited by Brielle Pittman

hayle
medical

New York

Hayle Medical,
750 Third Avenue, 9th Floor,
New York, NY 10017, USA

Visit us on the World Wide Web at:
www.haylemedical.com

ISBN: 978-1-63241-691-9

The publisher's policy is to use permanent paper from mills that operate a sustainable forestry policy. Furthermore, the publisher ensures that the text paper and cover boards used have met acceptable environmental accreditation standards.

Printed in China.

Cataloging-in-Publication Data

Chemotherapy and radiotherapy / edited by Brielle Pittman.
p. cm.
Includes bibliographical references and index.
ISBN 978-1-63241-691-9
1. Chemotherapy. 2. Radiotherapy. 3. Oncology. I. Pittman, Brielle.
RM262 .C44 2019
615.58--dc23

Table of Contents

Preface

Over the recent decade, advancements and applications have progressed exponentially. This has led to the increased interest in this field and projects are being conducted to enhance knowledge. The main objective of this book is to present some of the critical challenges and provide insights into possible solutions. This book will answer the varied questions that arise in the field and also provide an increased scope for furthering studies.

Chemotherapy is a form of cancer treatment which uses anti-cancer drugs as part of a cancer treatment regimen. It may be administered with a curative intent or as a palliative therapy for prolonging life and managing symptoms. Chemotherapy drugs directly affect the immune system. They are applied to target the overactivity of the immune system as in the case of diseases such as multiple sclerosis, rheumatoid arthritis, vasculitis and systemic lupus erythematosus, among others. Radiation therapy or radiotherapy (RT) is a cancer therapy that uses ionizing radiation to kill or control malignant cells. It is used to target cancer that is localized to a certain area of the body, or to prevent tumor recurrence after surgery. It can be used in combination with chemotherapy. Like chemotherapy, radiotherapy administration also varies for curative, palliative, adjuvant or neoadjuvant therapeutic intent. This book covers in detail some existing theories and innovative concepts revolving around chemotherapy and radiotherapy. It is a valuable compilation of topics, ranging from the basic to the most complex advancements in these fields. For all readers who are interested in oncology and cancer care, the case studies included in this book will serve as excellent guide to develop a comprehensive understanding.

I hope that this book, with its visionary approach, will be a valuable addition and will promote interest among readers. Each of the authors has provided their extraordinary competence in their specific fields by providing different perspectives as they come from diverse nations and regions. I thank them for their contributions.

Editor

1

Clinical Outcomes for Gastric Cancer following Adjuvant Chemoradiation Utilizing Intensity Modulated versus Three-Dimensional Conformal Radiotherapy

Gene-Fu F. Liu[1], Ryan J. Bair[1], Eric Bair[2], Stanley L. Liauw[1], Matthew Koshy[1,3]*

1 Department of Radiation and Cellular Oncology, University of Chicago Medical Center, Chicago, Illinois, United States of America, **2** Departments of Endodontics and Biostatistics, University of North Carolina-Chapel Hill, Chapel Hill, North Carolina, United States of America, **3** Department of Radiation Oncology, University of Illinois Hospital, Chicago, Illinois, United States of America

Abstract

Purpose/Objective(s): To determine if intensity modulated radiation therapy (IMRT) in the post-operative setting for gastric cancer was associated with reduced toxicity compared to 3D conformal radiation therapy (3DCRT).

Materials/Methods: This retrospective study includes 24 patients with stage IB-IIIB gastric cancer consecutively treated from 2001–2010. All underwent surgery followed by adjuvant chemoradiation. Concurrent chemotherapy consisted of 5-FU/leucovorin (n = 21), epirubicin/cisplatin/5FU (n = 1), or none (n = 2). IMRT was utilized in 12 patients and 3DCRT in 12 patients. For both groups, the target volume included the tumor bed, anastomosis, gastric stump, and regional lymphatics.

Results: Median follow-up for the entire cohort was 19 months (range 0.4–8.5 years), and 49 months (0.5–8.5 years) in surviving patients. The 3DCRT group received a median dose of 45 Gy, and the IMRT group received a median dose of 50.4 Gy ($p = 0.0004$). For the entire cohort, 3-year overall survival (OS) was 40% and 3-year disease free survival (DFS) was 41%. OS and DFS did not differ significantly between the groups. Acute toxicity was similar. Between 3DCRT and IMRT groups, during radiotherapy, median weight lost (3.2 vs. 3.3 kg, respectively; $p = 0.47$) and median percent weight loss were similar (5.0% vs. 4.3%, respectively; $p = 0.43$). Acute grade 2 toxicity was experienced by 8 patients receiving 3DCRT and 11 receiving IMRT ($p = 0.32$); acute grade 3 toxicity occurred in 1 patient receiving 3DCRT and none receiving IMRT ($p = 1.0$). No patients in either cohort experienced late grade 3 toxicity, including renal or gastrointestinal toxicity. At last follow up, the median increase in creatinine was 0.1 mg/dL in the IMRT group and 0.1 mg/dL in the 3DCRT group ($p = 0.78$).

Conclusion: This study demonstrates that adjuvant chemoradiation for gastric cancer with IMRT to 50.4 Gy was well-tolerated and compared similarly in toxicity with 3DCRT to 45 Gy.

Editor: Ramon Andrade de Mello, University of Algarve, Portugal

Funding: The authors have no support or funding to report.

Competing Interests: The authors have declared that no competing interests exist.

* E-mail: mkoshy@radonc.uchicago.edu

Introduction

Gastric cancer (GC) accounts for 738,000 deaths worldwide and 10% of total annual cancer deaths [1]. Approximately 20,000 Americans will be diagnosed with GC this year, half of whom are expected to die from the disease [2]. Thus, the development of effective treatments with limited toxicity remains an area of active interest.

In 2001, the Intergroup 0116 randomized trial demonstrated both a relapse-free and overall survival (OS) benefit for the addition of postoperative chemoradiotherapy over surgery alone [3]. However, the benefit of radiotherapy (RT) is tempered by its acute and late effects on adjacent vital organs, highlighting the importance of developing techniques able to spare normal tissues [4].

One such technique is Intensity Modulated Radiation Therapy (IMRT), which utilizes intensity-modulated "beamlets" to conform dose away from vital organs and more closely towards tumor. In comparison, three-dimensional conformal radiotherapy (3DCRT) uses beams of uniform intensity, offering less freedom in sculpting dose around the tumor. Prior dosimetric studies in GC suggest the superior conformality of IMRT may reduce liver and kidney radiation doses [5,6]. However, whether these dosimetric advantages translate into meaningful clinical improvement is an area of ongoing research.

The purpose of this study is to identify patients with GC who underwent adjuvant chemoradiotherapy and report the comparative outcomes of those treated with IMRT versus 3DCRT.

Materials and Methods

Our study was approved by the institutional review boards of the University of Chicago Medical Center, University of Illinois at Chicago Medical Center, and the Unversity of Illinois at Chicago Cancer Center. All data was anonymized and individual patient consent was not required as a waiver for the need for written informed consent was approved by the institutional review board of each participating institution.

Patients

From October 2001 to January 2011, 24 consecutive patients with Stage IB-IIIC GC or gastroesophageal junction cancer were treated with adjuvant RT at the University of Chicago (UCMC) and University of Illinois at Chicago Medical Center (UIMC).

Treatment

All patients underwent surgical resection. Surgery consisted of subtotal gastrectomy in 12 patients, total gastrectomy in 10 patients, and esophagogastrectomy in 2 patients. The majority of patients received 1 cycle of 5-fluorouracil (5FU) and leucovorin followed by concurrent 5FU/leucovorin with radiation.

Radiation was delivered utilizing IMRT in 12 patients and 3DCRT in 12 patients. For both groups, the planning target volume (PTV) included the tumor bed, anastomosis, gastric stump, and regional lymphatics. In patients who received 3DCRT, the total dose prescribed was 45 Gy in 1.8 Gy daily fractions. In patients who underwent IMRT, four patients received a dose of 45 Gy, seven patients received 50.4 Gy and one patient received 54 Gy due to the presence of a positive surgical margin. Radiation plans were developed on Eclipse (Varian, Palo Alto, U.S.A.) for 14 patients, Pinnacle (Philips, Amsterdam, Netherlands) for 5 patients, and CORVUS (Nomos, Pittsburgh, U.S.A.) for 5 patients. 3DCRT plans were delivered using 3 or more fields. Patients were staged according to American Joint Committee on Cancer (AJCC) 7th Edition 2010 tumor-node-metastasis (TNM) Classification [7].

Data Collection

Maximal acute and late toxicity grade was scored according to RTOG Acute Morbidity Scoring Criteria and Toxicity Criteria and RTOG/EORTC Late Radiation Morbidity Scoring Schema, respectively, with late toxicity defined as any toxicity occurring greater than 3 months after treatment completion [8]. Acute toxicities were recorded primarily from on-treatment visit notes, while late toxicities were collected across departmental follow-up notes.

Patients were seen at least once weekly while receiving RT, at which point they were evaluated for acute toxicities. Patients were then seen 4–6 weeks following treatment completion. Afterwards, they were followed every 3–6 months for the first 2 years, and every 6–12 months for the next 3 years. Imaging and bloodwork were drawn at similar intervals.

Statistics

Clinical-pathologic variables of the 2 cohorts were statistically analyzed using JMP version 9 (SAS Institute). All tests of statistical significance were two-sided, and significance was defined as a value of $p<0.05$. The log rank test was used to compare toxicities between IMRT and 3DCRT. Survival estimates were obtained using the Kaplan-Meier method. Outcome parameters were defined as: OS: time of surgery to time of death or last known follow-up; disease free survival (DFS). All events were calculated using standard life table methods, and the differences were compared using Cox regression models.

To estimate the power to detect an association using a Cox proportional hazards model, two simulated data sets of size 12 were generated. The first simulated data set was exponentially distributed with rate parameter 1, and the second simulated data set was exponentially distributed with rate parameter log(HR), where HR is the target hazard ratio. Censoring times were also generated as exponential random variables such that approximately 50% of the data points were censored. This process was repeated 10,000 times for each target hazard ratio. For each of the 10,000 simulated data sets, a Cox proportional hazards model was used to test the null hypothesis of no difference between the two groups. The power was estimated to be the number of times the p-value associated with this null hypothesis was less than 0.05.

Results

Median follow up for the entire cohort was 19 months (range 0.4–8.5 years), and 49 months (0.5–8.5 years) in surviving patients. Median follow up was similar in those receiving IMRT vs. 3DCRT (24.3 vs. 16.0 months, p = 0.63).

Table 1 describes patient and tumor characteristics. There were no statistically significant differences in mean age, gender distribution, tumor grade, and TNM or overall AJCC stage.

Table 2 describes treatment characteristics. The 3DCRT group received a median dose of 45 Gy, and the IMRT group received a median dose of 50.4 Gy (p = 0.0004). Otherwise, both groups shared a statistically similar distribution of type of surgery

Table 1. Patient Characteristics.

	3DCRT (n = 12)	IMRT (n = 12)	*p*-value
Mean age (years)	64	56	0.23
Gender			0.64
Male	10	8	
Female	2	4	
Tumor grade*			0.59
Grade 1	1	2	
Grade 2	5	2	
Grade 3	6	6	
T stage			0.90
1	1	1	
2	7	5	
3	3	5	
4	1	1	
N stage			0.23
0	2	0	
1	1	5	
2	4	3	
3	4	4	
4	1	0	
AJCC stage			0.53
IB	3	1	
IIA	0	1	
IIB	2	4	
IIIA	5	4	
IIIB	1	2	
IIIC	1	0	

AJCC = American Joint Committee on Cancer; 3DCRT = 3-dimensional conformal radiotherapy; IMRT = intensity modulated radiotherapy.
*Two patients in the IMRT group did not have tumor grade documented in pathology report.

Table 2. Treatment Characteristics.

		3DCRT (n = 12)	IMRT (n = 12)	*p*-value
Surgery Type	Esophagogastrectomy	2	0	0.58
	Total gastrectomy	5	5	
	Subtotal gastrectomy	5	7	
Margin Status	Negative	6	7	0.30
	<3 mm	3	0	
	Positive	3	4	
	Not recorded	0	1	
Extent of node dissection	D1	3	3	0.63
	D2	8	4	
	Not recorded	1	5	
Concurrent chemotherapy	None	1	1	1.00
	5FU/leucovorin	10	11	
	ECF	1	0	
Radiotherapy dose				0.0004[¥]
	45 Gy	12	4	
	≥50.4 Gy	0	8	

3DCRT = 3-dimensional conformal radiotherapy; IMRT = intensity modulated radiotherapy; ECF = epirubicin, cisplatin, 5FU.
[¥]Difference between median dose.

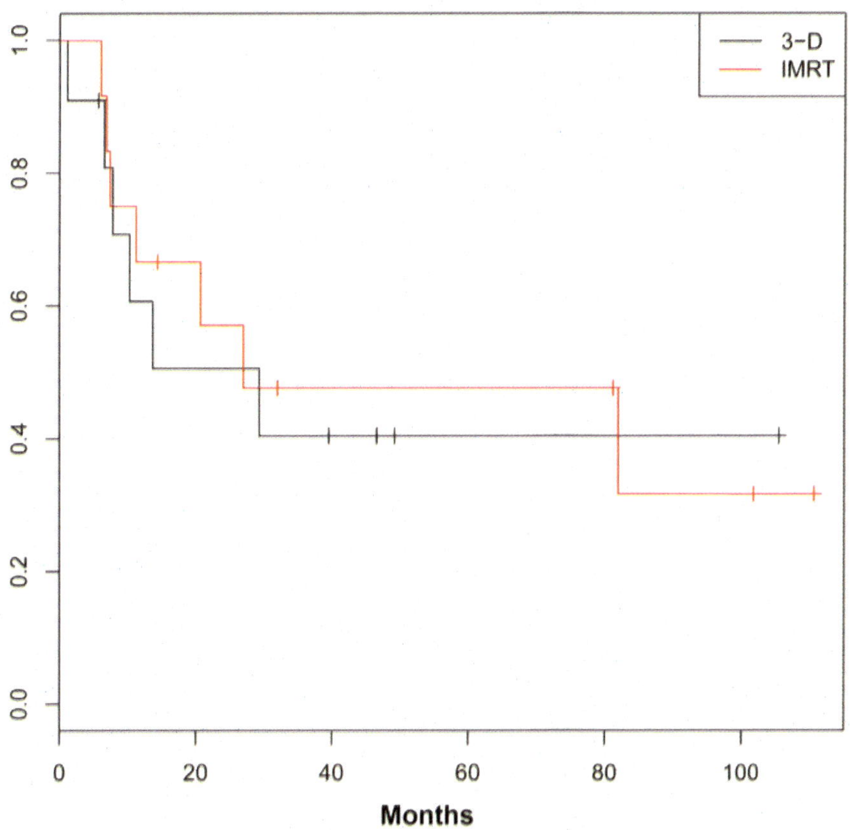

Figure 1. Disease-Free Survival.

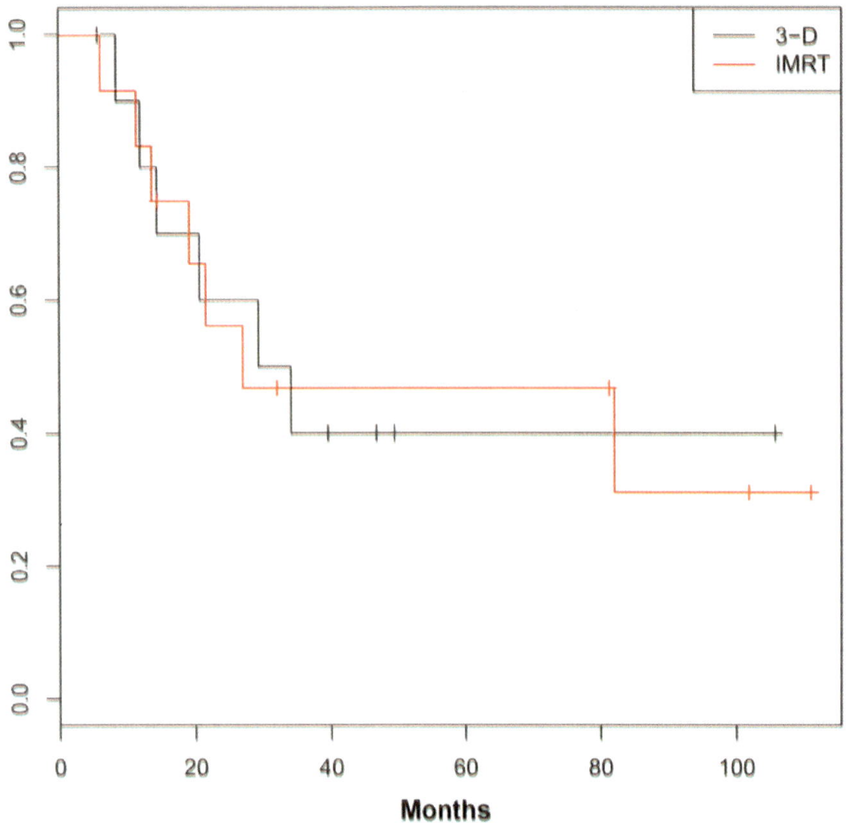

Figure 2. Overall Survival.

received, surgical margin status, extent of node dissection, type of concurrent chemotherapy.

For the entire cohort, 3-year DFS was 40.6% (Figure 1) and 3-year OS was 40.0% (Figure 2). OS and DFS were similar between the IMRT and 3DCRT groups.

Table 3 describes RT-related acute and late toxicity. Regarding acute toxicities, median weight lost from the first to last week of RT was 3.2 kg in the 3DCRT group and 3.3 kg in the IMRT group (p = 0.47). The median percent weight loss over the same period was also similar (5.0% in the 3DCRT group and 4.3% in the IMRT group, p = 0.43). There were two acute grade 3 toxicities. One patient who received 3DCRT became feeding-tube dependent, and one patient who received IMRT required esophageal dilatation 1 month after completing RT. Acute normal tissue toxicities are detailed in Table 4.

Regarding long term toxicities, there were no patients in either cohort, who experienced grade 3 long term renal toxicity. At last follow up, the median increase in serum Cr was 0.1 mg/dL in the IMRT group and 0.1 mg/dL in the 3DCRT group (p = 0.78). There were no late grade 3 gastrointestinal toxicities in either group. Late normal tissue toxicities are detailed in Table 5.

Discussion

This study compares the outcomes of patients with GC treated with postoperative IMRT versus a similar cohort treated with postoperative 3DCRT. Overall, toxicity rates were comparable between cohorts, though patients receiving IMRT received a higher median dose. There were no differences between cohorts in regards to OS or DFS.

Table 3. Acute Radiation Morbidity.

	3DCRT (n = 12)	IMRT (n = 12)	*p*-value
Median weight loss through radiotherapy (kg)	3.2	3.3	0.47
Median percent body weight loss through radiotherapy	5.0%	4.3%	0.43
No. patients with acute grade 2 toxicities	8	11	0.32
No. patients with acute grade 3 toxicities	1	0	1.00
No. patients with late grade 2 toxicities	1	3	0.59
No. patients with late grade 3 toxicities	0	0	NS
Median serum creatinine increase (mg/dL)	0.1	0.1	0.78

Table 4. RTOG Acute Radiation Morbidity Grade Detail.

		Grade 2	Grade 3	Total grade ≥2
		(No. patients)	(No. patients)	(No. patients)
Pharynx and esophagus	IMRT	3	1	4
	3DCRT	4	1	5
Upper gastrointestinal	IMRT	9	0	9
	3DCRT	4	0	4

Table 5. EORTC/RTOG Late Effects Grade Detail.

		Grade 2	Grade 3	Total grade ≥2
		(No. patients)	(No. patients)	(No. patients)
Esophagus	IMRT	1	0	1
	3DCRT	0	0	0
Small/Large Intestine	IMRT	0	0	0
	3DCRT	1	0	1
Kidney	IMRT	3	0	3
	3DCRT	1	0	1
Liver	IMRT	0	0	0
	3DCRT	0	0	0

Prior series have suggested a potential role for IMRT in the adjuvant treatment of GC. In 2009, investigators from Germany reported the outcomes of two sequentially treated GC cohorts, with 27 patients treated with 3DCRT from 2001–2005, and 33 patients treated with IMRT from 2002–2007; the majority of both the 3DCRT and IMRT groups received 45 Gy (68% vs. 91%, respectively, p = NS) [9]. Median OS (18 months vs. not reached, $p = 0.0492$) and DFS (13 months vs. not reached, $p = 0.0216$) favored the IMRT cohort. Actuarial 2-year OS also statistically favored the IMRT group (67% vs. 37%, $p = 0.0492$). Dosimetric parameters suggested that this benefit may be attributed to IMRT allowing for larger PTVs (mean 1,397 vs. 1,768 cm^3, $p = 0.0368$), while maintaining lower V30 parameters for the left (mean 26.8% vs. 19.5%, $p = 0.0015$) and right kidneys (mean 11.6 vs. 15.6%, $p = 0.0170$). Reduced renal irradiation was associated with statistically lower creatinine 6 weeks post-RT for the IMRT group (mean 0.71 vs. 0.84 µmol/L, $p = 0.0210$). However, creatinine values were similar at last follow-up and no late renal toxicity grade 3–4 (LENT-SOMA scale) was observed in either cohort. Of note, the results of this study are complicated by the two groups having received varied chemotherapy regimens, with 96% of the 3DCRT group receiving 5FU/folinic acid and 70% of the IMRT group receiving oxaliplatin/capecitabine ($p < 0.0001$).

A more recent series from Stanford University also demonstrated IMRT to have a more favorable toxicity profile [10]. In 26 patients who received 3DCRT versus 31 patients who received IMRT, more patients receiving 3DCRT required a treatment break (3 days vs. 0, no p-value reported). Regarding late toxicity, at a median follow-up of 1.4 years, the median serum creatinine was unchanged for patients treated with IMRT (0.80 mg/dL), whereas it had increased 0.20 mg/dL in those receiving 3DCRT (0.80 to 1.0 mg/dL, $p = 0.02$). However, IMRT was not associated with a clear dosimetric advantage, as the median kidney V20 was statistically similar between the IMRT and 3D CRT groups (17.5% vs. 22%, respectively, $p = 0.17$). As in our series, differences in hepatotoxicity between those receiving 3DCRT versus IMRT were not detected, though median liver V30 was reduced in the IMRT group (16.1 and 28%, $p < 0.001$). In contrast to the previously discussed series from Germany, disease outcomes between the 3DCRT and IMRT groups were similar; 2-year OS (51 vs. 65%, $p = 0.5$), DFS (60% vs. 54%, $p = 0.8$), and local control (83% vs. 81%, $p = 0.9$), respectively.

In this study, there were no detected differences in toxicity or disease control despite the IMRT cohort having received a higher median dose (50.4 Gy vs. 45 Gy, $p = 0.0004$) than the 3DCRT cohort. This dose is also higher than that received by the IMRT cohorts of the two previously discussed studies. Potentially, if our entire 3DCRT cohort was prescribed 50.4 Gy, then indeed toxicity rates may have been different. This is suggested by our prior dosimetric analysis, in which patients were planned to receive 50.4 Gy using either two- or three-field 3DCRT versus IMRT [6]. Compared with the three-field plan, IMRT significantly reduced liver V30 dose (63.6% vs. 18.9%, $p = 0.010$), as well as right kidney V20 dose (20.9% vs. 11.6%, $p = 0.027$).

Dosimetric studies analyzing the feasibility of IMRT vs. 3DCRT in GC suggest that neither modality is categorically superior, but that individual patient anatomy should dictate the choice. In a study from the University of Toronto where both 5-field 3DCRT and IMRT plans were created and evaluated by gastrointestinal radiation oncologists, IMRT was preferred in 17 of 19 cases (89%) [11]. Similarly while IMRT was dosimetrically rated higher for kidney sparing in 69% of the reviewers' ratings, conversely 31% considered 3DCRT better able to spare the kidneys. Therefore, it stands to reason that the decision between the two modalities should likely be individualized. Figures 3A and 3B pictorially highlight the dosimetric characteristics of 3DCRT and IMRT, respectively, in two patients treated adjuvantly for GC. While 3DCRT generally spreads low-dose radiation across a smaller body volume, IMRT better conforms high-dose radiation towards tumor and away from normal tissues.

When neither modality is dosimetrically superior, 3DCRT should be encouraged, as it holds other advantages over IMRT. 3DCRT typically irradiates a smaller volume of normal tissue by distributing its dose through fewer beams, has less interleaf scatter dose, and utilizes fewer monitored units. In addition, 3DCRT may also better treat tumors subject to intrafraction motion. The sub-diaphragmatic location of the gastric bed subjects it to respiratory motion, and investigators from Fudan University recently reported a mean superior-inferior intrafraction respiratory motion of 11.1 mm in 22 patients treated with postoperative RT for GC [12]. Because IMRT delivers dose through smaller beam apertures, there is an increased risk of intrafraction miss for patients whose tumors move significantly. Finally, there are substantial medical cost savings when using 3DCRT over IMRT. These differences should encourage the individualized evaluation of both modalities.

Our study is limited by biases inherent in any retrospective review. However, in contrast to prior series, our study population was not preferentially treated with IMRT despite its availability. Rather, patients were treated with IMRT and 3DCRT contemporaneously, with 8 of 12 patients treated with 3DCRT after 2006, potentially eliminating bias associated with treating across different

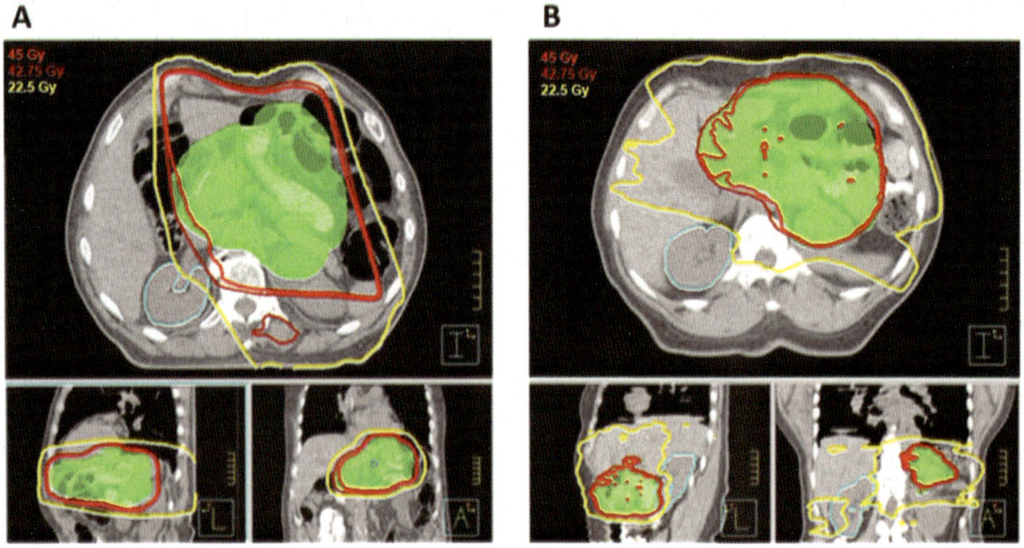

Figure 3. A. 79 year-old gentleman with gastric adenocarcinoma, T1N1M0, who underwent subtotal gastrectomy with D2 nodal dissection and adjuvant chemoradiotherapy with 3DCRT to a dose of 45 Gy. Figure 3B. 64 year-old woman with gastric adenocarcinoma, T2bN2M0, who underwent gastrectomy with D2 nodal dissection. Ten of 14 nodes were positive and she had positive proximal and distal surgical margins. She then received adjuvant chemoradiotherapy with IMRT to a dose of 45 Gy, with a 5.4 Gy boost to the anastomosis.

eras. Another study limitation is that a range of tumor stages/grades were included in our patient population, though there was no statistical difference between groups.

Furthermore, we performed a retrospective power analysis, determining our study size has a power of 0.12 to detect a hazard ratio of at least 1.5 in regards to overall survival. Thus, our study is not powered to reveal significant differences between the groups regarding disease outcomes. However, we believe our results remain worthwhile, as they further quantify the clinical magnitude of nephrotoxicity post-RT, agreeing with prior series that median creatinine increases are small, an important consideration for a patient population that may require systemic therapy in the future. Additionally, our results reiterate that should IMRT reduce nephrotoxicity, this advantage may also be small; in the series from Stanford, creatinine increased by 0.0 mg/dL for IMRT vs. 0.2 mg/dL for 3DCRT ($p = 0.02$), and in the series from Germany, there was no statistical difference in creatinine at 1 year or at last follow-up between RT modalities. In our series, both groups experienced a median creatinine increase of 0.1 mg/dL ($p = 0.78$). Furthermore, while kidneys do not respond acutely to radiation, we believe our median follow-up of 19 months should capture radiation nephropathy, as such changes have been detected at 6 months [4]. Finally, we believe our results are noteworthy, as they agree with available dosimetric studies. As noted in the series from Stanford reporting reduced creatinine levels with IMRT, V20 and mean kidney radiation doses were not statistically lowered with IMRT. Instead, IMRT was associated with a significant increase in right mean kidney dose (11.9 Gy vs 10.54 Gy, $p = 0.04$). Finally, given the decline of GC incidence and that less than half of patients eligible are currently referred for adjuvant RT [13], future retrospective series on this topic will likely feature small numbers of patients as well.

In conclusion, this analysis revealed that patients treated with IMRT to a total dose of 50.4 Gy tolerated their treatment well and had long term outcomes similar to a cohort treated with 3DCRT to 45 Gy. The decision between IMRT and 3DCRT will vary by patient anatomy, for which individual comparison plans should be considered.

Author Contributions

Conceived and designed the experiments: GFL RJB EB SLL MK. Performed the experiments: GFL RJB EB SLL MK. Analyzed the data: GFL RJB EB SLL MK. Wrote the paper: GFL RJB EB SLL MK.

References

1. Jemal A, Bray F, Center MM, Ferlay J, Ward E, et al. (2011) Global cancer statistics. CA Cancer J Clin 61: 69–90.
2. Siegel R, Ward E, Brawley O, Jemal A (2011) Cancer statistics, 2011: the impact of eliminating socioeconomic and racial disparities on premature cancer deaths. CA Cancer J Clin 61: 212–236.
3. Macdonald JS, Smalley SR, Benedetti J, Hundahl SA, Estes NC, et al. (2001) Chemoradiotherapy after surgery compared with surgery alone for adenocarcinoma of the stomach or gastroesophageal junction. N Engl J Med 345: 725–730.
4. Jansen EP, Saunders MP, Boot H, Oppedijk V, Dubbelman R, et al. (2007) Prospective study on late renal toxicity following postoperative chemoradiotherapy in gastric cancer. Int J Radiat Oncol Biol Phys 67: 781–785.
5. Ringash J (2001) Preventive health care, 2001 update: screening mammography among women aged 40–49 years at average risk of breast cancer. CMAJ 164: 469–476.
6. Milano MT, Garofalo MC, Chmura SJ, Farrey K, Rash C, et al. (2006) Intensity-modulated radiation therapy in the treatment of gastric cancer: early clinical outcome and dosimetric comparison with conventional techniques. Br J Radiol 79: 497–503.
7. Edge SB BD, Compton CC, Fritz AG, Greene FL, Trotti A (2010) AJCC Cancer Staging Manual. New York City: Springer.
8. Cox JD, Stetz J, Pajak TF (1995) Toxicity criteria of the Radiation Therapy Oncology Group (RTOG) and the European Organization for Research and Treatment of Cancer (EORTC). Int J Radiat Oncol Biol Phys 31: 1341–1346.
9. Boda-Heggemann J, Hofheinz RD, Weiss C, Mennemeyer P, Mai SK, et al. (2009) Combined adjuvant radiochemotherapy with IMRT/XELOX improves outcome with low renal toxicity in gastric cancer. Int J Radiat Oncol Biol Phys 75: 1187–1195.
10. Minn AY, Hsu A, La T, Kunz P, Fisher GA, et al. (2010) Comparison of intensity-modulated radiotherapy and 3-dimensional conformal radiotherapy as adjuvant therapy for gastric cancer. Cancer 116: 3943–3952.
11. Ringash J, Perkins G, Brierley J, Lockwood G, Islam M, et al. (2005) IMRT for adjuvant radiation in gastric cancer: a preferred plan? Int J Radiat Oncol Biol Phys 63: 732–738.

2

BRCA1 mRNA Expression as a Predictive and Prognostic Marker in Advanced Esophageal Squamous Cell Carcinoma Treated with Cisplatin- or Docetaxel-Based Chemotherapy/Chemoradiotherapy

Yong Gao[1], Jing Zhu[1], Xiaohui Zhang[1], Qingquan Wu[2], Shaoning Jiang[3], Yangqing Liu[1], Zhibin Hu[4], Baorui Liu[5]*, Xiaofei Chen[1]*

1 Department of Medical Oncology, Huai'an First People's Hospital, Nanjing Medical University, Huai'an, China, **2** Department of Thoracic Surgery, Huai'an First People's Hospital, Nanjing Medical University, Huai'an, China, **3** Department of Medicine, University of Alabama at Birmingham, Birmingham, Alabama, United States of America, **4** Department of Epidemiology and Biostatistics, Nanjing Medical University, Nanjing, China, **5** The Comprehensive Cancer Center, Gulou School of Clinical Medicine, Nanjing Medical University, Nanjing, China

Abstract

Background: The molecular backgrounds that determine therapeutic effectiveness in esophageal cancer remain largely unknown. Breast cancer susceptibility gene 1 (BRCA1) expression has been found to switch the response to cisplatin- or paclitaxel-based chemotherapy. It remains unclear how variations in BRCA1 expression influence clinical outcomes in esophageal cancer.

Patients and Methods: Quantitative real-time polymerase chain reaction (qPCR) was performed to examine BRCA1 mRNA expressions in paraffin-embedded specimens from 144 patients with advanced or metastatic esophageal squamous cell carcinoma who received cisplatin- or docetaxel-based first-line treatments.

Results: Low BRCA1 mRNA expression correlated with increased response rate (RR; $P = 0.025$ and 0.017, respectively) and median overall survival (mOS; $P = 0.002$ and $P < 0.001$, respectively) in cisplatin-based chemotherapy or chemoradiotherapy group and also correlated with decreased RR ($P = 0.017$ and 0.024, respectively) and mOS (both $P < 0.001$) in docetaxel-based chemotherapy or chemoradiotherapy group. Multivariate analysis revealed that low BRCA1 expression was an independent prognostic factor in cisplatin-based chemotherapy (HR 0.29; 95%CI 0.12–0.71; $P = 0.007$) or chemoradiotherapy (HR 0.12; 95%CI 0.04–0.37; $P < 0.001$) group and higher risk for mortality in docetaxel-based chemotherapy (HR 5.02; 95%CI 2.05–12.28; $P < 0.001$) or chemoradiotherapy (HR 7.02; 95%CI 2.37–27.77; $P < 0.001$) group.

Conclusions: BRCA1 mRNA expression could be used as a predictive and prognostic marker in esophageal cancer who underwent first-line cisplatin- or docetaxel-based treatments.

Editor: Goli Samimi, Kinghorn Cancer Centre, Garvan Institute of Medical Research, Australia

Funding: This work was supported in part by Science Developing Foundation of Nanjing Medical University (09NJMUM063 to Y.G.) and Science Developing Foundation of Huaian Government (HAS2011028 to X.F.C.). The funders had no role in study design, data collection and analysis.

Competing Interests: The authors have declared that no competing interests exist.

* E-mail: hayycxf@163.com (XC); baoruiliu@hotmail.com (BL)

Introduction

Esophageal cancer, as the sixth most common cause of cancer death in the world, lead to 407,000 deaths estimated in 2008 [1]. Patients with such an aggressive tumor have a poor 5-year survival rate less than 20%, which is most likely attributed to the presence of locally advanced and undetected metastatic disease at the time of diagnosis [2]. Chemotherapy has been playing important roles in improving survivals of esophageal cancer patients as part of multimodal therapy. Several chemotherapeutic agents commonly used in esophageal cancer have been investigated as single agent therapies with limited response rates as follows: 20% to 26% with cisplatin [3], 28% to 34% with paclitaxel [4] and 15% with 5-fluorouracil [5]. Combination chemotherapies with these chemotherapeutic agents appeared to be superior to single agent treatment with increased toxicity. Responsiveness to these chemotherapeutic agents and modalities varies among patients owing to genetic variations in pharmacokinetic and pharmacodynamic action [6]. The molecular backgrounds that determine therapeutic effectiveness in esophageal cancer still remain largely unknown. Some molecular markers have been identified for tailored treatment of esophageal cancer, including platinum related markers [glutathione S-transferase π (GST-π), excision repair cross-complementing 1 (ERCC1) and p-glycoprotein (P-gp)], 5-FU related markers [thymidylate synthase (TS) and dihydropyrimidine dehydrogenase (DPD)] and some proteins in various DNA repair pathways [7–9]. However, these studies mostly focused on the personalized therapies of 5-Fu or/and cisplatin-based treatments.

Breast cancer susceptibility gene 1 (BRCA1) was firstly identified as one of the genes that conferred genetic predisposition to early-onset breast and ovarian cancer [10]. However, due to its central component involved in multiple aspects of DNA damage responses and pivotal roles in the DNA repair pathway [10–13], increasing number of experimental and clinical investigations on BRCA1 as a regulator of chemotherapy-induced DNA damage have been performed [14]. The vast majority of cellular models have shown that BRCA1 upregulaion is notably associated with DNA repair mediated resistance to the DNA-damaging agent cisplatin through regulation of interstrand cross-link-induced premature senescence [15], nucleotide excision repair (NER) [16] and DNA double-strand-break homologous recombination (HR) repair pathway [17,18]. Conversely, downregulation of BRCA1 confers resistance to antimicrotubule agent taxane through precocious inactivation of the spindle checkpoint [19], regulation of apoptotic pathways [20,21] and transcriptional modifications of JNK signaling pathway [22]. It was also confirmed in clinic that BRCA1 mutations or alterations in BRCA1 mRNA and protein expression switch the response to cisplatin- or paclitaxel-based chemotherapy as well as influence the survivals in a number of malignancies, including breast cancer [23,24], ovarian cancer [25–27], gastric cancer [28–30] and lung cancer [16,31]. In our previous studies [29,30], high levels of BRCA1 mRNA were negatively associated with cisplatin sensitivity but positively associated with docetaxel sensitivity in gastric cancer patients. Those advanced gastric carcinoma patients with high BRCA1 expression had significantly longer overall survivals compared to those with low expression (25.8 *vs* 9.5 months, $P = 0.006$) who received second-line docetaxel-based chemotherapy after first-line FOLFOX chemotherapy [29].

Cisplatin or docetaxel have been showed the most commonly and effectively utilized chemotherapeutic agents in clinic for patients with esophageal cancer [32–34]. However, no studies have addressed how variations in BRCA1 expressions influence clinical outcomes in patients with esophageal cancer treated with these chemotherapeutic agents. In this study, we firstly determined whether the levels of BRCA1 mRNA expression as predictive and prognostic biomarker were associated with clinical outcomes in esophageal cancer patients who received cisplatin- or docetaxel-based treatments.

Patients and Methods

Patients

A total of 155 patients with histologically confirmed locally advanced or metastatic esophageal squamous cell carcinoma (stage II-IV) and available paraffin-embedded tumor material for molecular analysis were enrolled in the study. They all had a better Eastern Cooperative Oncology Group performance status (PS; 0 to 2) and had measurable lesions. Among them 79 patients with surgically unresectable or metastatic disease received cisplatin- or docetaxel-based chemotherapy as the first-line treatment. The chemotherapy regimens comprised cisplatin-based regimens (cisplatin 25 mg/m2 on day 1–3 plus 5-fluorouracil 500 mg/m2 on day 1–5), docetaxel-based regimens (docetaxel 60–75 mg/m2 plus 5-fluorouracil 500 mg/m2 on day 1–5) and the combination with both (cisplatin 25 mg/m2 on day 1–3 plus docetaxel 60–75 mg/m2 on day 1). All chemotherapies were repeated every 3–4 weeks for a maximum of six cycles unless there was earlier evidence of disease progression or intolerable adverse effects. The other 76 patients with locally advanced disease received cisplatin or docetaxel-based concurrent chemoradiotherapy (CCRT) or radiotherapy alone as the first-line treatment. CCRT included chemotherapy and concurrent thoracic radiotherapy. The chemotherapy regimens consisted of weekly docetaxel (25 mg/m2 on day 1 per week) plus 5-fluorouracil (300 mg/m2 on day 1–3 per week) or cisplatin (25 mg/m2 on day 1 per week) plus 5-fluorouracil (300 mg/m2 on day 1–3 per week) for 5 weeks. The radiation dose was 50–60 grays (Gy) over 5 weeks (2 Gy/fraction per day, 5 fractions per week) with the use of CT simulation and 3 D treatment planning. Baseline and restaging assessment of measurable lesions were assessed by barium swallow and computed tomography scans, which was repeated every 2 cycle of chemotherapy or 4 weeks after radiotherapy.

The study was approved by the institutional ethics committee of Huai'an first people's hospital of Nanjing medical university and all patients gave their signed informed consent for the use of the tissue material in translational research.

qPCR analysis for BRCA1 mRNA expression

We examined BRCA1 gene expression in paraffin-embedded specimens by biopsy under endoscope from the 155 patients as previously described [29]. Briefly, serial sections of 7-μm thickness with more than 80% tumor cells were prepared from primary tumor blocks by microdissection. Samples were lysed in a proteinase K-containing buffer after paraffin was removed by xylene. RNA was then extracted with phenol-chloroform-isoamyl alcohol followed by precipitation with isopropanol in the presence of glycogen and sodium acetate. RNA was resuspended in water and treated with DNAse I to avoid DNA contamination. cDNA was synthesized by using M-MLV retrotranscriptase enzyme. Template cDNA was amplified with specific primers and probes for BRCA1 and β-actin with using Taqman Universal Master Mix (Applied Biosystems, Foster City, CA). The primer and probe sets as reported in our previous study [29] were designed using Primer Express 2.0 Software (AB, Foster City, CA, USA). All primers and probes sequence were as follows: β-actin (NM_001101.3) forward 5′ TGAGCGCGGCTACAGCTT 3′, reverse 5′ TCCTTAATGTCACGCACGATTT 3′, and probe 6FAM - 5′ACCACCA CGGCCGAGCGG 3′ TAMRA; BRCA1 (NM_007294) forward 5′GGCTATCCTCTCAGAGTGA-CATTTTA 3′, reverse 5′GCTTTATCAGGTTATGTTG-CATGGT 3′, and probe 6FAM -5′CCACTCAGCAGAGGG 3′ MGB.

Quantitative real-time polymerase chain reaction (qPCR) was performed to quantify gene expression using the ABI Prism 7900HT Sequence Detection System (Applied Biosystems), which is more quantitative and accurate than immunohistochemistry used to assess protein expression as biomarker in clinical studies. The PCR conditions were 50°C for 2 minutes, 95°C for 10 minutes, followed by total 45 cycles at 95°C for 15 seconds and 60°C for 1 minute. Each sample was assayed in triplicate with commercial RNA as positive control and RNase-free water as negative control. In all quantitative experiments, only triplicates with a standard deviation (SD) of the quantification cycle (Cq) values of target genes less than 0.30 were accepted. Quantification of relative gene expression was performed according to the comparative Cq method using β-actin as an endogenous control. Gene expression analyses were conducted with the same calibrators throughout, specifically commercial human lung and liver RNA (Stratagene, La Jolla, CA, USA), to compare gene expression levels between different tumor types and between different cohorts of patients. Final values were determined by the formula $2^{-\Delta\Delta Cq}$ [$= 2^{-(Cq\ sample\ -\ Cq\ calibrator)}$] [29]. All analyses

Table 1. Patient characteristics of advanced (stage II–IV) esophageal cancer patients.

		Chemotherapy 72			Chemoradiotherapy 72		
Characteristic	**All patients**	**Cis/5-Fu**	**Doc/5-Fu**	**Cis/Doc**	**Radiotherapy alone**	**Radiotherapy+Cis/5-Fu**	**Radiotherapy+Doc/5-Fu**
Patients, No. (%)	144 (100)	27 (18.8)	29 (20.1)	16 (11.1)	16 (11.1)	29 (20.1)	27 (18.8)
Age, y median (range)	63 (44–79)	60 (51–79)	62 (50–78)	61 (45–70)	69 (44–79)	63 (45–77)	64 (52–78)
Sex, No. (%)							
Male	90 (62.5)	17 (63.0)	16 (55.2)	12 (75.0)	8 (50.0)	19 (65.5)	18 (66.7)
Female	54 (37.5)	10 (37.0)	13 (44.8)	4 (25.0)	8 (50.0)	10 (34.5)	9 (33.3)
ECOG PS, No. (%)							
0–1	134 (93.1)	24 (88.9)	26 (89.7)	13 (81.2)	16 (100.0)	28 (96.6)	27 (100.0)
2	10 (6.9)	3 (11.1)	3 (10.3)	3 (18.8)	0 (0.0)	1 (3.4)	0 (0.0)
Stage, No. (%)							
II	31 (21.5)	0 (0.0)	0 (0.0)	0 (0.0)	9 (56.3)	14 (48.3)	8 (29.6)
III	45 (31.3)	2 (7.4)	1 (3.4)	1 (6.3)	7 (43.7)	15 (51.7)	19 (70.4)
IV	68 (47.2)	25 (92.6)	28 (96.6)	15 (93.7)	0 (0.0)	0 (0.0)	0 (0.0)
Site of tumor, No. (%)							
Upper	20 (13.9)	2 (7.4)	3 (10.3)	2 (12.5)	3 (18.8)	6 (20.7)	4 (14.8)
Middle	93 (64.6)	17 (63.0)	17 (58.6)	11 (68.8)	10 (62.5)	20 (70.0)	18 (66.7)
Lower	31 (21.5)	8 (29.6)	9 (31.0)	3 (18.8)	3 (18.8)	3 (10.3)	5 (18.5)
BRCA1 median (range)	11.96 (0.39–70.03)	10.63 (0.39–70.03)	8.69 (0.56–44.94)	13.58 (4.56–41.93)	10.23 (0.43–44.17)	11.39 (1.16–32.45)	14.37 (2.03–62.90)
Response rate (CR+PR), No. (%)		28 (38.9)			52 (72.2)		
Median OS (months, 95% CI)		11.3 (9.0–13.6)			15.0 (12.4–17.6)		

BRCA1, breast cancer susceptibility gene 1; Cis, cisplatin; 5-Fu, 5-fluorouracil; Doc, docetaxel; CR, complete response; PR, partial response; OS, overall survival; CI, confidence interval; ECOG, Eastern Cooperative Oncology Group; PS, performance status; y, years.

Table 2. Clinical factors associated with BRCA1 mRNA expression levels.

	BRCA1 expression levels			Overall survival	
Characteristic	**low**	**high**	***P* value**	**MST (Months, 95% CI)**	***P* Log-rank test**
Age, No. (%)					
≤63	34	40		12.0 (10.0–14.0)	
>63	38	32	0.317	14.5 (12.8–16.2)	0.135
Sex, No. (%)					
Male	48	43		12.0 (10.0–14.0)	
Female	24	29	0.388	16.0 (13.2–18.8)	0.182
ECOG PS, No. (%)					
0–1	67	67		14.0 (12.5–15.5)	
2	5	5	1.000	6.1 (5.0–7.2)	<0.001
Stage, No. (%)					
II	15	17		16.0 (13.1–18.9)	
III	21	23		13.0 (11.1–14.9)	
IV	36	32	0.798	11.3 (9.6–13.0)	0.002
Grade, No. (%)					
G1	11	7		18.0 (11.1–24.9)	
G2	40	44		12.0 (9.8–14.2)	
G3	21	21	0.583	14.0 (11.0–17.0)	0.077
Site of tumor, No. (%)					
Upper	9	11		12.8 (6.8–18.8)	
Middle	46	47		13.5 (11.4–15.6)	
Lower	17	14	0.778	13.5 (10.4–16.6)	0.763

BRCA1, breast cancer susceptibility gene 1; CI, confidence interval; MST, median survival time, ECOG, Eastern Cooperative Oncology Group; PS, Performance status;

were performed at the molecular biology laboratory of Clinical Cancer Institute of Nanjing University (Nanjing, China).

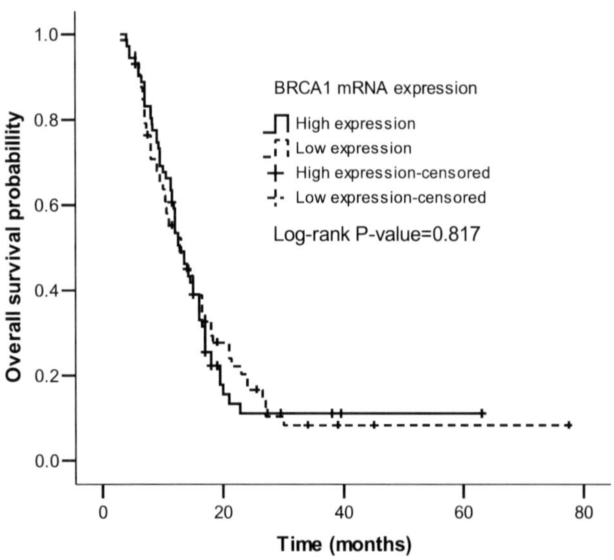

Figure 1. Median overall survival (mOS) in total 144 advanced and metastasis (stage II–IV) esophageal cancer patients receiving cisplatin- or docetaxel-based first-line treatments according to BRCA1 mRNA levels (for more details see Table 1).

Study design and statistical analysis

The primary endpoint of the study was to examine the potential effects of BRCA1 mRNA expression levels on clinical responses and overall survival in esophageal cancer patients treated with cisplatin- or docetaxel-based chemotherapy or chemoradiotherapy in the first-line. Clinical responses were evaluated according to the Response Evaluation Criteria in Solid Tumors (RECIST) [35]. Overall survival was calculated from the date of diagnosis to the date of last follow-up or death from any cause. Progression-free survival was not examined because part of patients did not receive further assessments of disease after fist-line treatment and we could not get exact time of progress-free survival of these patients in the present retrospective study. Qualitative variables were summarized by absolute frequencies and percentages and quantitative variables were calculated in median values and ranges. BRCA1 expression values were divided into terciles and cutoff points were calculated according to the median value for the mRNA expression of BRCA1 [36–38]. The normality of quantitative variables was analyzed by the Kolmogorov-Smirnov test and compared with the Mann-Whitney U test. All statistical tests were two-sided. In order to correlate gene expression levels with clinical characteristics and compare categorical variables and response percentages, the two-sided chi-square test or Fisher's exact test was used for qualitative variables. The distributions of survival were obtained by the Kaplan-Meier method and compared with the two-sided log-rank test. A multivariate Cox proportional hazards regression model was performed to assess the association between each potential prognostic factor and survival.

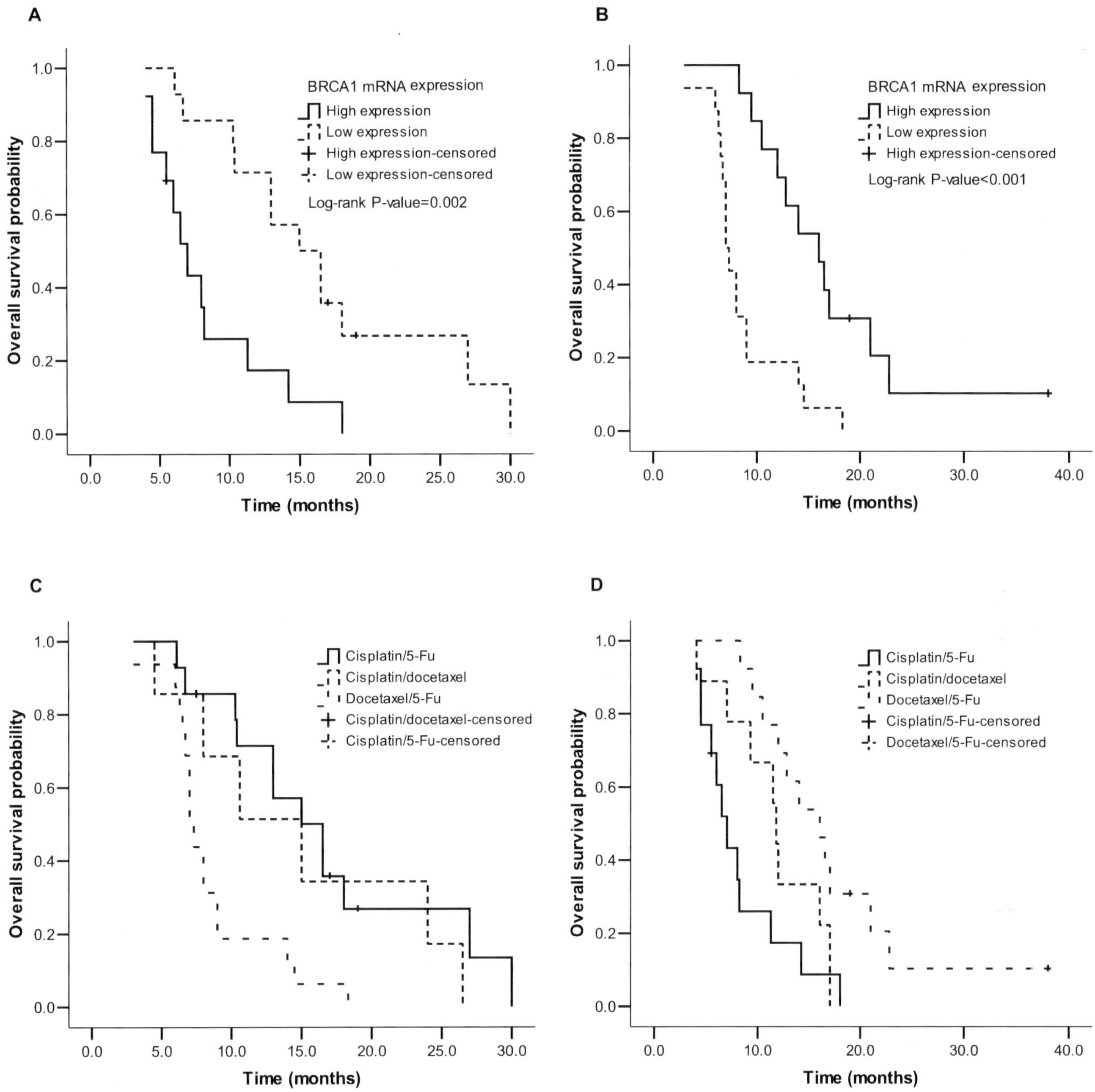

Figure 2. Median overall survival (mOS) in chemotherapy group: mOS in cisplatin/5-Fu (A) and docetaxel/5-Fu (B) subgroup according to BRCA1 mRNA levels (for more details see Table 3); mOS in low (C) and high (D) BRCA1 mRNA levels according to regimens of chemotherapy (for more details see Table 4).

All statistical analyses were performed with a power of 80% and at a 5% level of significance using the Statistical Package for the Social Sciences (SPSS) for Windows version 16 (SPSS Inc, Chicago, IL).

Results

Patients' characteristics

Clinical data and paraffin-embedded samples from the primary tumors were collected from 155 esophageal squamous cell carcinoma patients treated with cisplatin- or docetaxel-based chemotherapy/chemoradiotherapy in our centre. Successful amplification of BRCA1 gene was achieved in 144 specimens. The median age was 64; 90 patients were male and the majority of patients had PS 0-1. Among them, 72 patients treated with chemotherapy had stage III–IV and other 72 patients treated with chemoradiotherapy or radiotherapy alone had stage II–III at the time of diagnosis. In the chemotherapy group, the overall response rate (RR) was 38.9% and the median overall survival (mOS) was 11.3 months (95% CI, 9.0 to 13.6 months) after a median follow-up period of 10.6 months (range 3.0–30.0); while in the chemoradiotheapy group including those with radiotherapy alone, RR was 72.2% and mOS was 15.0 months (95% CI, 12.4 to 17.6

Table 3. Outcomes in different treatment groups according to BRCA1 expression levels.

		RR, *N* (%)			OS (months)		
Treatment	**BRCA1**	**CR+PR (%)**	**SD+PD (%)**	***P*-value**	**No. of patients**	**Median (95% CI)**	***P*-value**
Cis/5-Fu	Low	57.1	42.9	0.025	14	15.0 (10.7–19.3)	0.002
	High	15.4	84.6		13	7.0 (5.4–8.6)	
Doc/5-Fu	Low	25.0	75.0	0.017	16	7.0 (6.4–7.6)	<0.001
	High	69.2	30.8		13	16.0 (11.7–20.3)	
Cis/Doc	Low	28.6	71.4	0.635	7	15.0 (7.2–22.8)	0.220
	High	33.3	66.7		9	11.8 (10.1–13.5)	
Radiotherapy alone	Low	72.7	27.3	0.516	11	15.0 (9.2–20.8)	0.839
	High	60.0	40.0		5	12.5 (2.8–22.2)	
Radiotherapy+Cis/5-Fu	Low	87.5	12.5	0.017	16	24.0 (13.0–35.0)	<0.001
	High	46.2	53.8		13	11.3 (9.1–13.5)	
Radiotherapy+Doc/5-Fu	Low	50.0	50.0	0.024	8	7.5 (6.1–8.9)	<0.001
	High	89.5	10.5		19	19.5 (13.9–25.1)	

BRCA1, breast cancer susceptibility gene 1; Cis, cisplatin; 5-Fu, 5-fluorouracil; Doc, docetaxel; CR, complete response; PR, partial response; SD, stable disease; PD, progress disease; RR, response rate; OS, overall survival; CI, confidence interval; ECOG, Eastern Cooperative Oncology Group; PS, performance status;

months) after a median follow-up period of 15.0 months (range 4.0–77.5). Patient characteristics are summarized in Table 1.

BRCA1 mRNA expression levels

BRCA1 mRNA expressions were detected successfully in total 144 tumor samples by using quantitative real-time PCR and the median mRNA expression levels of BRCA1 relative to reference gene of β-actin were 11.96 (range 0.39–70.03). Patients were subdivided into two groups based on low (0.39–11.75; mean, 6.60) and high (12.17–70.03; mean, 23.90) levels of BRCA1 mRNA expression using a cutoff value of 11.96. The number of patients with low or high expression levels of BRCA1 was 72 in each cohort. There were no significant correlations between BRCA1 expression levels and clinical characteristics, including age ($P=0.317$), gender ($P=0.388$), performance status ($P=1.0$), stage ($P=0.798$), grade ($P=0.583$) or site of tumor ($P=0.778$) (Table 2).

In the whole cohort, 144 esophageal cancer patients had a mOS of 13.0 months (95% CI: 11.5–14.5 months), without statistical significance between the high and low expression of BRCA1 (13.0 *vs* 12.8, $P=0.817$) (Figure 1).

BRCA1 mRNA expression and treatment outcomes in chemotherapy group

In the chemotherapy group, patients with low BRCA1 expression had increased RR (57.1 *vs* 15.4%, $P=0.025$) and mOS (15.0 *vs* 7.0, $P=0.002$; Figure 2A) compared to those with

Table 4. Outcomes in low or high BRCA1 expression levels according to regimens.

		RR, N (%)			OS (months)		
BRCA1	**Treatment**	**CR+PR (%)**	**SD+PD (%)**	***P*-value**	**No. of patients**	**Median (95% CI)**	***P*-value**
Low	Cis/5-Fu	57.1	42.9	1.000	14	15.0 (10.7–19.3)	1.000
	Doc/5-Fu	25.0	75.0	0.073	16	7.0 (6.4–7.6)	0.002
	Cis/Doc	28.6	71.4	0.217	7	15.0 (7.2–22.8)	0.450
High	Doc/5-Fu	69.2	30.8	1.000	13	16.0 (11.7–20.3)	1.000
	Cis/5-Fu	15.4	84.6	0.024	13	7.0 (5.4–8.6)	0.001
	Cis/Doc	33.3	66.7	0.096	9	11.8 (10.1–13.5)	0.081
Low	Radiotherapy+Cis/5-Fu	87.5	12.5	1.000	16	24.0 (13.0–35.0)	1.000
	Radiotherapy+Doc/5-Fu	50.0	50.0	0.046	8	7.5 (6.1–8.9)	<0.001
	Radiotherapy alone	72.7	27.3	0.332	11	15.0 (9.2–20.8)	0.070
High	Radiotherapy+Doc/5-Fu	89.5	10.5	1.000	19	19.5 (13.9–25.1)	1.000
	Radiotherapy+Cis/5-Fu	46.2	53.8	0.007	13	11.3 (9.1–13.5)	<0.001
	Radiotherapy alone	60.0	40.0	0.116	5	12.5 (2.8–22.2)	0.179

BRCA1, breast cancer susceptibility gene 1; Cis, cisplatin; 5-Fu, 5-fluorouracil; Doc, docetaxel; CR, complete response; PR, partial response; SD, stable disease; PD, progress disease; RR, response rate; OS, overall survival; CI, confidence interval; ECOG, Eastern Cooperative Oncology Group; PS, performance status;

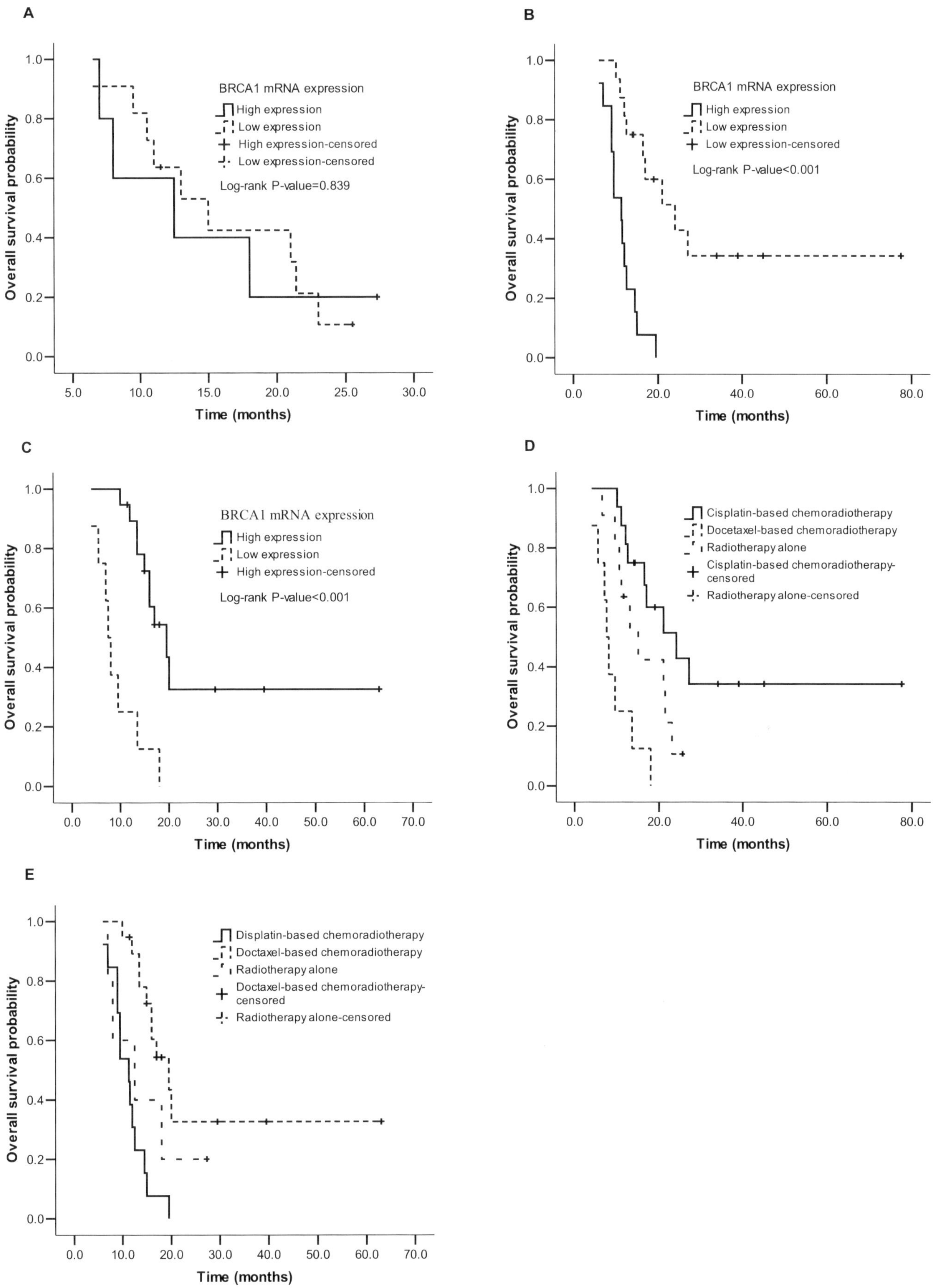
A
Overall survival probability
Time (months)
BRCA1 mRNA expression
High expression
Low expression
High expression-censored
Low expression-censored
Log-rank P-value=0.839
B
Overall survival probability
Time (months)
BRCA1 mRNA expression
High expression
Low expression
Low expression-censored
Log-rank P-value<0.001
C
Overall survival probability
Time (months)
BRCA1 mRNA expression
High expression
Low expression
High expression-censored
Log-rank P-value<0.001
D
Overall survival probability
Time (months)
Cisplatin-based chemoradiotherapy
Docetaxel-based chemoradiotherapy
Radiotherapy alone
Cisplatin-based chemoradiotherapy-censored
Radiotherapy alone-censored
E
Overall survival probability
Time (months)
Displatin-based chemoradiotherapy
Doctaxel-based chemoradiotherapy
Radiotherapy alone
Doctaxel-based chemoradiotherapy-censored
Radiotherapy alone-censored

Figure 3. Median overall survival (mOS) in chemoradiotherapy group: mOS in radiotherapy alone (A), cisplatin-based chemotherapy (B) and docetaxel-based chemotherapy (C) subgroup according to BRCA1 mRNA levels (for more details see Table 3); mOS in low (D) and high (E) BRCA1 mRNA levels according to regimens of chemoradiotherapy (for more details see Table 4).

high expression when treated with cisplatin-based chemotherapy; whereas when treated with docetaxel-based chemotherapy, patients with high BRCA1 mRNA expression had increased RR (69.2 *vs* 25.0%, $P=0.017$) and mOS (16.0 *vs* 7.0, $P<0.001$; Figure 2B) compared to those with low expression (Table 3). Then we further investigated correlations of BRCA1 mRNA expression to clinical outcomes in chemotherapy group stratified by BRCA1 levels. Patients with low BRCA1 expression had the best clinical results when treated with cisplatin/5-Fu compared to docetaxel/5-Fu or cisplatin/docetaxel regimens [RR were 57.1, 25.0 ($P=0.073$) and 28.6% ($P=0.217$), respectively; mOS were 15.0, 7.0 ($P=0.002$) and 15.0 months ($P=0.450$), respectively; Figure 2C]. For those patients with high BRCA1 expression levels, regimen of docetaxel/5-Fu became the optimization choice in comparison with cisplatin/5-Fu or cisplatin/docetaxel regimens [RR were 69.2, 15.4 ($P=0.024$) and 33.3% ($P=0.096$), respectively; mOS were 16.0, 7.0 ($P=0.001$) and11.8 months ($P=0.081$), respectively; Figure 2D] (Table 4).

BRCA1 mRNA expression and treatment outcome in chemoradiotherapy group

No significant differences were observed in RR (72.7 *vs* 60.0%, $P=0.516$) and mOS (15.0 *vs* 12.0 months, $P=0.839$; Figure 3A) between patients with low and high BRCA1 expression who were treated with radiotherapy alone. Nevertheless, when treated with concurrent chemoradiotherapy, patients with low BRCA1 expression had increased RR (87.5 *vs* 46.2%, $P=0.017$) and mOS (24.0 *vs* 11.3 months, $P<0.001$; Figure 3B) compared to those with high expressions in the cisplatin-based chemoradiotherapy subgroup; and those with high BRCA1 expression had increased RR (89.5 *vs* 50.0%, $P=0.024$) and mOS (19.5 *vs* 7.5 months, $P<0.001$; Figure 3C) compared to those with low expressions in the docetaxel-based chemoradiotherapy subgroup (Table 3). Further study on correlations of BRCA1 expression to clinical outcomes stratified by the BRCA1 expression suggested that cisplatin-based chemoradiotherapy was the best choice of treatment for patients with low BRCA1 expressions compared with treatment of docetaxel-based chemoradiotherapy or radiotherapy alone [RR were 87.5, 50.0 ($P=0.046$) and 72.7% ($P=0.332$), respectively; mOS were 24.0, 7.5 ($P<0.001$) and 15.0 months ($P=0.070$), respectively; Figure 3D]; whereas, docetaxel-based chemoradiotherapy was the best one for those with high BRCA1 expressions compared with cisplatin-based chemoradiotherapy or radiotherapy alone [RR were 89.5, 46.2 ($P=0.007$) and 60.0% ($P=0.116$), respectively; mOS were 19.5, 11.3 ($P<0.001$) and 12.5 months ($P=0.179$), respectively; Figure 3E] (Table 4).

Univariate and multivariate analyses

Univariate analysis demonstrated that a significant association was observed between mOS and PS ($P<0.001$) or stage of disease ($P=0.002$) in the whole cohort. No other association between clinical characteristics and survival was found (Table 2).

Cox proportional hazard analysis revealed that low BRCA1 expression as an independent prognostic factor was significant associated with increased mOS in cisplatin-based chemotherapy (HR 0.29; 95%CI 0.12–0.71; $P=0.007$) or chemoradiotherapy (HR 0.12; 95%CI 0.04–0.37; $P<0.001$) group, whereas low BRCA1 expression emerged conversely as higher risk for mortality associated with decreased mOS in docetaxel-based chemotherapy (HR 5.02; 95%CI 2.05–12.28; $P<0.001$) or chemoradiotherapy (HR 7.02; 95%CI 2.37–27.77; $P<0.001$) group (Table 5).

Discussion

In present study, we firstly applied qPCR analysis of BRCA1 mRNA expression in formalin-fixed paraffin-embedded tumor tissue in advanced and metastasis esophageal cancer and evaluated the relationship between BRCA1 mRNA expression levels and cisplatin- or docetaxel-based treatments. The antimetabolite 5-fluorouracil was used as combination agent in cisplatin- or docetaxel-based treatment because BRCA1 failed to modulate resistance or sensitivity to it [21]. BRCA1 was discovered to be involved in the inverse resistance relationship between cisplatin- and docetaxel-based treatments in esophageal cancer patients. Over expression of BRCA1 mRNA was negatively associated with RR and mOS in patients treated with cisplatin-based chemotherapy or chemoradiotherapy; whereas conversely, over expression of BRCA1 was positively associated with clinical outcomes in those patients who received docetaxel-based treatments. Multivariate analysis revealed that low BRCA1 expression was an independent prognostic factor for patients with cisplatin-based treatment and conversely higher risk for mortality for patients with docetaxel-based treatment. These findings support the hypothesis that BRCA1 mRNA expression levels could be a valid indicator of differential sensitivity to cisplatin or docetaxel in esophageal cancer, which is consistent with findings in previous clinical studies on other malignancies [23–31]. As a predictive marker in previous studies, overexpression of BRCA1 was significantly correlated with higher RR and progression-free survival (PFS) but not with mOS

Table 5. Multivariate analysis of factors associated with overall survival of esophageal cancer according to regimens.

	Cis/5-Fu			Doc/5-Fu			Radiotherapy+Cis/5-Fu			Radiotherapy+Doc/5-Fu		
	HR.	**CI,**	***P***	**HR.**	**CI,**	***P***	**HR.**	**CI**	***P***	**HR.**	**CI,**	***P***
BRCA1 (low *vs* high)	0.29	0.12–0.71	0.007	5.02	2.05–12.28	<0.001	0.12	0.04–0.37	<0.001	7.02	2.37–27.77	<0.001
Stage (II vs III or III vs IV)	0.23	0.03–1.76	0.156	4.39	0.51–38.03	0.179	1.72	0.71–4.18	0.232	1.14	0.37–3.45	0.823
PS (0–1 *vs* 2)	0.33	0.08–1.37	0.127	0.13	0.03–0.54	0.005	0.47	0.004–0.51	0.012	-	-	-

BRCA1, breast cancer susceptibility gene 1; HR, hazard ratio; CI, confidence interval; *P*, *P*-value.

in non-small-cell lung cancer (NSCLC) treated with docetaxel-gemcitabine as first-line chemotherapy [36]; BRCA1 mutation appeared to be related with high pathologic complete response in breast cancer treated with platinum-based neoadjuvant therapy [23,24]. Meanwhile, as a prognostic marker, low BRCA1 expression correlated with improved survival in advanced ovarian cancer who received platinum-based chemotherapy [27] and high BRCA1 expression correlated with longer mOS in gastric cancer patients treated with second-line docetaxel-based chemotherapy after first-line FOLFOX chemotherapy [29]. As both predictive and prognostic marker, low BRCA1 protein expression correlated with better clinical outcome in terms of both PFS and OS in patients with epithelial ovarian cancer treated with platinum [25,26]. In the present study, BRCA1 mRNA determined by qPCR with merits of better quantitative and accurate measurement compared to protein expression determined by immunohistochemistry, was found to be both predictive marker associated with RR and prognostic marker associated with mOS in esophageal cancer patients treated with docetaxel- or cisplatin-based treatments.

These results are also in line with findings in the pre-clinical cell line model, which indicated that reconstitution of wild-type BRCA1 function into human breast cancer HCC1937 cell line caused a 1000-fold increase in sensitivity to taxane and a 20-fold increase in resistance to cisplatin [21]. Several mechanisms were involved in the resistance of DNA-damaging agent cisplatin [15–18] as mentioned previously. Among them, NER is considered as the main mechanism for the resistance of cisplatin through removal of the cisplatin-DNA adducts that mainly cause cellular death and tumor response [38]. ERCC1 involved in GG-NER pathway has been proved an effective predictive marker of cisplatin response [39]. By contrast, BRCA1 may be a better predictive marker of cisplatin response owing to its involvement in TC-NER that is relevant for the antiproliferative activity of cisplatin [16]. Meanwhile, downregulation of BRCA1 confers resistance to taxane through inactivation of the spindle checkpoint, regulation of apoptotic and JNK signaling pathways [19–22].

Cisplatin- and docetaxel-based treatments were found to be the optimized choices for patients with low and high expression of BRCA1 to get more clinical benefits in the present study, respectively. Survival benefits can be brought to esophageal caner patients by appropriate treatments based on BRCA1 expression. In this retrospective study, patients with stage III–IV had longer mOS of 15.0 months (95% CI: 10.7–19.3) when treated with cisplatin-based chemotherapy for low BRCA1 expression and 16.0 months (95% CI: 11.7–20.3) when treated with docetaxel-based chemotherapy for high BRCA1 expression. By contrast, previous phase II clinical trial indicated that esophageal cancer patients with similar stages only had mOS of 10.8 months when treated with a combination therapy of three chemotherapeutic agents including paclitaxel, cisplatin and 5-FU [33]. Meanwhile, no clinical benefits were observed in patients with low BRCA1 expression who received docetaxel-based treatments and patients with high BRCA1 expression who received cisplatin-based treatments (Table 4). Patients with low BRCA1 expression treated with cisplatin/docetaxel chemotherapy had similar OS (15.0 *vs* 15.0 months, $P=0.450$, Figure 2C) compared to cispalin/5-Fu chemotherapy and patients with high BRCA1 expression treated with cisplatin/docetaxel chemotherapy also had no better OS (11.8 vs 16.0 months, $P=0.081$, Figure 2D) compared to docetaxel/5-Fu chemotherapy (Table 4). These results were consistent with findings in previous study on NSCLC that overexpression of BRCA1 was significantly correlated with better clinical outcomes in patients treated with docetaxel/gemcitabine but not in those treated with cisplatin/docetaxel regimen [36].

Radiotherapy is considered extremely effective in local control of cancer, but its curative potential is often limited by intrinsic radioresistance of the tumor cells. BRCA1 is involved in HR repair of double strands break with relation to radiation resistance and considered important in maintenance of genomic stability through DNA repair while cell DNA-damage takes place due to radiation [17], which is supported by the observation that cells deficient in BRCA1 are highly sensitive to radiation [40]. Nevertheless, we didn't observe the effect of BRCA1 on resistance of radiotherapy for patients with esophageal cancer. In present study, there was no significant difference in clinical outcomes between patients with low and high BRCA1 expression when treated with radiotherapy alone. This result was in agreement to the previous study of breast cancer, which showed no evidence of increased radiation sensitivity in breast tissue heterozygous for a BRCA1/2 germline mutation [23]. This finding might also explain why BRCA1 mRNA expression was significantly associated to cisplatin- or docetaxel-based concurrent chemoradiotherapy in the same trend that existed in chemotherapy group.

Several limitations exist in this study which is based on an unplanned and retrospective analysis, lack of validation group and has relatively small number of patients in treatment subgroups. However, we provide the first evidence to support the tumor mRNA expression levels of BRCA1 as predictive and prognostic marker in esophageal cancer with cisplatin- or docetaxel-based treatments and indicated the need to further validate in a large number of patients prospectively.

Acknowledgments

We are grateful for the assistance of L. X. Yu and J Wei in facilitating this project.

Author Contributions

Conceived and designed the experiments: YG BL XC. Performed the experiments: JZ XZ QW. Analyzed the data: SJ YL ZH. Wrote the paper: YG XC.

References

1. Jemal A, Bray F, Center MM, Ferlay J, Ward E, et al. (2011) Global cancer statistics. CA Cancer J Clin 61: 69–90.
2. Shibata T, Kokubu A, Saito S, Narisawa-Saito M, Sasaki H, et al. (2011) NRF2 mutation confers malignant potential and resistance to chemoradiation therapy in advanced esophageal squamous cancer. Neoplasia 13: 864–873.
3. Panettiere FJ, Leichman LP, Tilchen EJ, Chen TT (1984) Chemotherapy for advanced epidermoid carcinoma of the esophagus with single-agent cisplatin: final report on a Southwest Oncology Group study. Cancer Treat Rep 68: 1023–1024.
4. Ajani JA, Ilson DH, Daugherty K, Pazdur R, Lynch PM, et al. (1994) Activity of taxol in patients with squamous cell carcinoma and adenocarcinoma of the esophagus. J Natl Cancer Inst 86: 1086–1091.
5. Ezdinli EZ, Gelber R, Desai DV, Falkson G, Moertel CG, et al. (1980) Chemotherapy of advanced esophageal carcinoma: Eastern Cooperative Oncology Group experience. Cancer 46: 2149–2153.
6. Evans WE, Relling MV (1999) Pharmacogenomics: translating functional genomics into rational therapeutics. Science 286: 487–491.
7. Alexander BM, Wang XZ, Niemierko A, Weaver DT, Mak RH, et al. (2012) DNA repair biomarkers predict response to neoadjuvant chemoradiotherapy in esophageal cancer. Int J Radiat Oncol Biol Phys 83: 164–171.
8. Harpole DH Jr, Moore MB, Herndon JE 2nd, Aloia T, D'Amico TA, et al. (2001) The prognostic value of molecular marker analysis in patients treated with trimodality therapy for esophageal cancer. Clin Cancer Res 7: 562–569.
9. Joshi MB, Shirota Y, Danenberg KD, Conlon DH, Salonga DS, et al. (2005) High gene expression of TS1, GSTP1, and ERCC1 are risk factors for survival

in patients treated with trimodality therapy for esophageal cancer. Clin Cancer Res 11: 2215–2221.
10. Kennedy RD, Quinn JE, Johnston PG, Harkin DP (2002) BRCA1: mechanisms of inactivation and implications for management of patients. Lancet 360: 1007–1014.
11. Roy R, Chun J, Powell SN (2012) BRCA1 and BRCA2: different roles in a common pathway of genome protection. Nat Rev Cancer 12: 68–78.
12. Matsuoka S, Ballif BA, Smogorzewska A, McDonald ER 3rd, Hurov KE, et al. (2007) ATM and ATR substrate analysis reveals extensive protein networks responsive to DNA damage. Science 316: 1160–1166.
13. Huen MS, Sy SM, Chen J. (2010) BRCA1 and its toolbox for the maintenance of genome integrity. Nat Rev Mol Cell Biol 11: 138–148.
14. Tassone P, Tagliaferri P, Perricelli A, Blotta S, Quaresima B, et al. (2003) BRCA1 expression modulates chemosensitivity of BRCA1-defective HCC1937 human breast cancer cells. Br J Cancer 88: 1285–1291.
15. Santarosa M, Del CL, Tonin E, Caragnano A, Viel A, et al. (2009) Premature senescence is a major response to DNA cross-linking agents in BRCA1-defective cells: implication for tailored treatments of BRCA1 mutation carriers. Mol Cancer Ther 8: 844–854.
16. Taron M, Rosell R, Felip E, Mendez P, Souglakos J, et al. (2004) BRCA1 mRNA expression levels as an indicator of chemoresistance in lung cancer. Hum Mol Genet 13: 2443–2449.
17. Yun MH, Hiom K. (2009) CtIP-BRCA1 modulates the choice of DNA double-strand-break repair pathway throughout the cell cycle. Nature 459: 460–463.
18. Husain A, He G, Venkatraman ES, Spriggs DR (1998) BRCA1 up-regulation is associated with repair-mediated resistance to cis-diamminedichloroplatinum(II). Cancer Res 58: 1120–1123.
19. Chabalier C, Lamare C, Racca C, Privat M, Valette A, et al. (2006) BRCA1 downregulation leads to premature inactivation of spindle checkpoint and confers paclitaxel resistance. Cell Cycle 5: 1001–1007.
20. Mullan PB, Quinn JE, Gilmore PM, McWilliams S, Andrews H, et al. (2001) BRCA1 and GADD45 mediated G2/M cell cycle arrest in response to antimicrotubule agents. Oncogene 20: 6123–6131.
21. Quinn JE, Kennedy RD, Mullan PB, Gilmore PM, Carty M, et al. (2003) BRCA1 functions as a differential modulator of chemotherapy-induced apoptosis. Cancer Res 63: 6221–6228.
22. Lafarge S, Sylvain V, Ferrara M, Bignon YJ (2001) Inhibition of BRCA1 leads to increased chemoresistance to microtubule-interfering agents, an effect that involves the JNK pathway. Oncogene 20: 6597–6606.
23. Byrski T, Gronwald J, Huzarski T, Grzybowska E, Budryk M, et al. (2010) Pathologic complete response rates in young women with BRCA1-positive breast cancers after neoadjuvant chemotherapy. J Clin Oncol 28: 375–379.
24. Byrski T, Huzarski T, Dent R, Gronwald J, Zuziak D, et al. (2009) Response to neoadjuvant therapy with cisplatin in BRCA1-positive breast cancer patients. Breast Cancer Res Treat 115: 359–363.
25. Weberpals JI, Tu D, Squire JA, Amin MS, Islam S, et al. (2011) Breast cancer 1 (BRCA1) protein expression as a prognostic marker in sporadic epithelial ovarian carcinoma: an NCIC CTG OV.16 correlative study. Ann Oncol 22: 2403–2410.
26. Carser JE, Quinn JE, Michie CO, O'Brien EJ, McCluggage WG, et al. (2011) BRCA1 is both a prognostic and predictive biomarker of response to chemotherapy in sporadic epithelial ovarian cancer. Gynecol Oncol 123: 492–498.
27. Weberpals J, Garbuio K, O'Brien A, Clark-Knowles K, Doucette S, et al. (2009) The DNA repair proteins BRCA1 and ERCC1 as predictive markers in sporadic ovarian cancer. Int J Cancer 124: 806–815.
28. Shim HJ, Yun JY, Hwang JE, Bae WK, Cho SH, et al. (2010) BRCA1 and XRCC1 polymorphisms associated with survival in advanced gastric cancer treated with taxane and cisplatin. Cancer Sci 101: 1247–1254.
29. Wei J, Costa C, Ding Y, Zou Z, Yu L, et al. (2011) mRNA expression of BRCA1, PIAS1, and PIAS4 and survival after second-line docetaxel in advanced gastric cancer. J Natl Cancer Inst 103: 1552–1556.
30. Wang L, Wei J, Qian X, Yin H, Zhao Y, et al. (2008) ERCC1 and BRCA1 mRNA expression levels in metastatic malignant effusions is associated with chemosensitivity to cisplatin and/or docetaxel. BMC Cancer 8: 97.
31. Rosell R, Perez-Roca L, Sanchez JJ, Cobo M, Moran T, et al. (2009) Customized treatment in non-small-cell lung cancer based on EGFR mutations and BRCA1 mRNA expression. PLoS One 4: e5133.
32. Leichman L, Berry BT (1991) Experience with cisplatin in treatment regimens for esophageal cancer. Semin Oncol 18: 64–72.
33. Ilson DH, Ajani J, Bhalla K, Forastiere A, Huang Y, et al. (1998) Phase II trial of paclitaxel, fluorouracil, and cisplatin in patients with advanced carcinoma of the esophagus. J Clin Oncol 16: 1826–1834.
34. Muro K, Hamaguchi T, Ohtsu A, Boku N, Chin K, et al. (2004) A phase II study of single-agent docetaxel in patients with metastatic esophageal cancer. Ann Oncol 15: 955–959.
35. Therasse P, Arbuck SG, Eisenhauer EA, Wanders J, Kaplan RS, et al. (2000) New guidelines to evaluate the response to treatment in solid tumors. European Organization for Research and Treatment of Cancer, National Cancer Institute of the United States, National Cancer Institute of Canada. J Natl Cancer Inst 92: 205–216.
36. Papadaki C, Tsaroucha E, Kaklamanis L, Lagoudaki E, Trypaki M, et al. (2011) Correlation of BRCA1, TXR1 and TSP1 mRNA expression with treatment outcome to docetaxel-based first-line chemotherapy in patients with advanced/metastatic non-small-cell lung cancer. Br J Cancer 104: 316–323.
37. Rosell R, Scagliotti G, Danenberg KD, Lord RV, Bepler G, et al. (2003) Transcripts in pretreatment biopsies from a three-arm randomized trial in metastatic non-small-cell lung cancer. Oncogene 22: 3548–3553.
38. Olaussen KA, Dunant A, Fouret P, Brambilla E, André F, et al. (2006) DNA repair by ERCC1 in non-small-cell lung cancer and cisplatin-based adjuvant chemotherapy. N Engl J Med 355: 983–991.
39. Furuta T, Ueda T, Aune G, Sarasin A, Kraemer KH, et al. (2002) Transcription-coupled nucleotide excision repair as a determinant of cisplatin sensitivity of human cells. Cancer Res 62: 4899–4902.
40. Shen SX, Weaver Z, Xu X, Li C, Weinstein M, et al. (1998) A targeted disruption of the murine Brca1 gene causes gamma-irradiation hypersensitivity and genetic instability. Oncogene 17: 3115–3124.

3

Feasibility of Tomotherapy-Based Image-Guided Radiotherapy to Reduce Aspiration Risk in Patients with Non-Laryngeal and Non-Pharyngeal Head and Neck Cancer

Nam P. Nguyen[1]*, Lexie Smith-Raymond[1], Vincent Vinh-Hung[2], Paul Vos[3], Rick Davis[1], Anand Desai[4], Thomas Sroka[5], Dave Abraham[1], Shane P. Krafft[4], Michelle Stevie[1], Homayoun Modarresifar[6], Beng-Hoey Jo[1], Misty Ceizyk[1]

1 Department of Radiation Oncology, University of Arizona, Tucson, Arizona, United States of America, **2** Department of Radiation Oncology, University Hospitals of Geneva, Geneva, Switzerland, **3** Biostatistics, East Carolina University, Greenville, North Carolina, United States of America, **4** Department of Radiation Oncology, University of Texas at M. D. Anderson, Houston, Texas, United States of America, **5** Department of Radiation Oncology, Darmouth College, Hanover, New Hampshire, United States of America, **6** Department of Radiology University of Arizona, Tucson, Arizona, United States of America

Abstract

Purpose: The study aims to assess the feasibility of Tomotherapy-based image-guided radiotherapy (IGRT) to reduce the aspiration risk in patients with non-laryngeal and non-hypopharyngeal cancer. A retrospective review of 48 patients undergoing radiation for non-laryngeal and non-hypopharyngeal head and neck cancers was conducted. All patients had a modified barium swallow (MBS) prior to treatment, which was repeated one month following radiotherapy. Mean middle and inferior pharyngeal dose was recorded and correlated with the MBS results to determine aspiration risk.

Results: Mean pharyngeal dose was 23.2 Gy for the whole group. Two patients (4.2%) developed trace aspiration following radiotherapy which resolved with swallowing therapy. At a median follow-up of 19 months (1–48 months), all patients were able to resume normal oral feeding without aspiration.

Conclusion and Clinical Relevance: IGRT may reduce the aspiration risk by decreasing the mean pharyngeal dose in the presence of large cervical lymph nodes. Further prospective studies with IGRT should be performed in patients with non-laryngeal and non-hypopharyngeal head and neck cancers to verify this hypothesis.

Editor: Chin-Tu Chen, The University of Chicago, United States of America

Funding: The authors have no support or funding to report.

Competing Interests: The authors have declared that no competing interests exist.

* E-mail: NamPhong.Nguyen@yahoo.com

Introduction

Dysphagia and aspiration are common following radiotherapy for head and neck cancer [1]. Aspiration is potentially life-threatening as the cough reflex may be absent or ineffective following head and neck cancer radiotherapy. Head and neck cancer survivors with chronic aspiration following treatment may develop anxiety and depression because of social isolation, which may severely impact on their quality of life. Recent studies suggest a correlation between radiation dose to the pharyngeal constrictor muscles and the risk of tube feeding dependence following head and neck radiotherapy [2,3]. New radiotherapy techniques such as intensity-modulated radiotherapy (IMRT) may decrease dysphagia severity and the need for gastrostomy tubes because of decreased radiation dose to critical structures for swallowing. Some institutions advocate shielding the larynx separately with a midline block in the split-field (SF) IMRT technique to reduce radiation dose to the larynx and the middle and inferior constrictor muscles [4]. Since aspiration risk increases with pharyngeal dose, the prevalence of aspiration should be reduced following head and neck cancer treatment in those that have a decreased dose to this region. However, in the presence of cervical lymph nodes, a mid-line laryngeal block can under-dose the cervical lymph nodes in close proximity to the larynx, leading to regional recurrences [5]. Whole-field (WF) IMRT is often advocated in the presence of cervical lymph nodes to ensure adequate target coverage [6]. However, studies have demonstrated WF-IMRT to deliver higher laryngeal and pharyngeal radiation dose, leading to unnecessary complications such as laryngeal edema and aspiration. In a previous dosimetric study comparing WF-IMRT to Tomotherapy-based image-guided radiotherapy (IGRT), we had demonstrated that IGRT may significantly reduce the larynx, middle and inferior pharyngeal doses in non-laryngeal and non-hypopharyngeal cancer without compromising target coverage [7]. The dosimetric advantage of IGRT to spare laryngeal edema correlated with a significant reduction in the rate of severe laryngeal edema and improvement in the quality of the voice in patients treated with IGRT [8]. The current retrospective study was performed to determine if low radiation doses to these swallowing structures could decrease the aspiration rate in this subset of head and neck cancer patients as well.

Materials and Methods

The medical records of 48 patients undergoing helical Tomotherapy-based IGRT for head and neck cancer in non-laryngeal and non-hypopharyngeal sites at the University of Arizona Department of Radiation Oncology were retrospectively reviewed following institutional review board (IRB) approval. The University of Arizona IRB waived the patient consent requirement because of the retrospective nature of this study, which was limited to patient chart reviews. Laryngeal and hypopharyngeal cancers were excluded from the study because they are associated with a high rate of aspiration at diagnosis [9]. Prior to treatment, each patient was simulated in a supine position with a head and neck Aquaplast mask for treatment immobilization. A computed tomography (CT) scan with and without intravenous (IV) contrast for treatment planning was performed in the treatment position. The head and neck areas from the vertex to the mid thorax were outlined with a slice thickness of 3 mm. CT scan with IV contrast was employed to enhance target volume delineation. Radiotherapy planning was performed on the CT scan without contrast to avoid possible interference of contrast density on radiotherapy isodose distributions. Diagnostic positron emitting tomography (PET)-CT scan imaging was also incorporated with the CT planning when available. A 0.5 cm bolus was placed on any area of the skin involved by the tumor and on any palpable cervical lymph nodes. Normal organs at risk for complications were outlined for treatment planning, including the spinal cord, brain stem, cochlea, mandible, parotid glands, larynx, pharyngeal muscles, eyes, and oral cavity. The tumor and grossly enlarged lymph nodes on CT scan (CTV1) with a margin (PTV1) were treated to 70 Gy in 35 fractions (2 Gy/fraction). The margins were 0.5–1 cm circumferentially around CTV1 depending on the anatomic location. The areas at high risk (PTV2) were defined as at least 1 cm around the gross tumor and pathologic cervical lymph nodes. The areas at low risk (PTV3) were defined as the subclinical regional lymph nodes with 0.5 cm margins circumferentially. PTV2 and PTV 3 were treated to 63 Gy and 56 Gy in 35 fractions respectively. Patients undergoing postoperative radiation were treated to 66 Gy, 59.4 Gy, and 54 Gy in 33 fractions to PTV1, PTV2, and PTV3, respectively. Minimal target coverage was 95% for all targets with at least 99% of the prescribed dose delivered to 100% of PTV1. The lymph nodes in the ipsilateral neck, including the retropharyngeal lymph nodes, were treated to the base of skull if there was any cervical lymph node enlargement or PET – positive lymph nodes. Contralateral uninvolved lymph nodes were treated prophylactically with the C1 vertebral body as the superior border of the radiation field.

In the case of bilateral cervical lymph node involvement, both necks were treated to the base of skull to avoid any marginal misses. Mean dose to the parotid was kept below 2600 cGy if there was no ipsilateral cervical lymph node enlargement. Dose constraints for other normal organs at risk (OAR) were: spinal cord (45 Gy), brain stem (50 Gy), optic chiasm (45 Gy), mandible (70 Gy to less than 30% of the mandible). Doses to larynx and pharyngeal muscles for non-laryngeal and non-hypopharyngeal cancers were kept between 20–40 Gy if feasible, as it is our strict policy that all PTV targets should be covered by at least the 95% target dose. The larynx and pharyngeal muscles were contoured from the hyoid bone (superior border) to the cricoid cartilage (inferior border) following consultation with a radiologist. The pharyngeal muscles outlined included the middle and inferior pharyngeal constrictors muscles according to the guidelines developed by Eisbruch et al [10].

The larynx and pharyngeal muscles would have been effectively shielded from radiation with a laryngeal block in the conventional supraclavicular field of the SF -IMRT technique [4].

It is our recommendation that all head and neck cancer patients in our institution have a modified barium swallow (MBS) immediately prior to radiotherapy to exclude silent aspiration. The MBS was performed in the Department of Speech Pathology by speech pathologists who were blinded to the patient's cancer stage. However, they were instructed that these patients were at risk of aspiration. Patients with demonstrated aspiration on MBS who were scheduled to undergo concurrent chemoradiation had percutaneous gastrostomy (PEG) tube placement in anticipation of severe weight loss from mucositis. Repeat MBS was performed four to six weeks after treatment completion to assess aspiration risk. Although some patients continued to experience mucositis at four weeks following chemoradiation, excessive fibrosis may decrease the effectiveness of swallowing therapy if MBS was delayed [11]. Swallowing therapy and PEG tube feedings were recommended for patients who developed aspiration after radiotherapy. Patients with severe weight loss during treatment also continued with PEG tube feedings. All patients had PET-CT scans four and ten months after completion of treatment in addition to regularly scheduled follow-up consisting of physical exam and nasopharyngoscopy if indicated. The PEG tube was removed if there was no evidence of aspiration on post-treatment MBS, no evidence of disease on PET-CT scan after treatment, and if the patient had recovered from any treatment-related weight loss.

Patients with loco-regional recurrence underwent surgical salvage, and the PEG tube was not removed in anticipation of severe dysphagia post -surgery. All patients were monitored by a team of experienced dietitians to assess their nutritional needsfollowing treatment. The presence or absence of dysphagia, continued weight loss, and other parameters such as total protein, albumin, and pre-albumin were taken into consideration before the decision to remove the PEG tube even in the absence of aspiration was made.

Results

Among 170 head and neck cancer patients treated at the University of Arizona Department of Radiation Oncology from 2007 to 2012, we identified 48 patients with non-laryngeal and non-hypopharyngeal cancers who had both MBS immediately prior to and following radiotherapy. The patients selected did not have aspiration observed on the MBS prior to radiotherapy, although they may have been experiencing abnormal swallowing because of the cancer and/or previous surgery. Median age at diagnosis was 57 years (range: 25–83 years). Forty-four were males and four were females. The disease site distribution was: oropharynx (24), oral cavity (12), parotid (4), unknown (2), nasopharynx (3), maxillary sinus (2) and neck recurrence (1). The two patients that had an unknown primary also had submental lymph node metastases, which were resected. In both cases, the primary was presumed to be an occult oral cavity lesion and the larynx was not included in the radiotherapy fields. The three patients that had a parotid primary also had cervical lymph node metastases requiring bilateral neck irradiation. One patient had locally advanced maxillary sinus cancer which invaded into the cheek and also required bilateral neck irradiation. Another patient had locally advanced maxillary sinus cancer and gross lymph nodes metastases in the left neck. Breakdown by stage demonstrated one stage I, six stage II, 13 stage III, 16 stage IVA, ten stage IVB, one stage IVC, and one patient with recurrence.

Definitive concurrent chemoradiation was delivered to twenty-eight patients. Thirteen patients received postoperative chemoradiation, four patients had postoperative radiotherapy alone, and three patients had definitive radiotherapy alone.

Indications for postoperative chemoradiation were positive or close margins after surgery or extracapsular lymph node extension. Table 1 summarizes the patient characteristics.

The mean pharyngeal dose was 23.2 Gy (15.4–54 Gy) for the whole group. The most common abnormalities observed on pre-treatment MBS were decreased transit in the oral phase (5 patients), pooling in the vallecula (9 patients) and decreased laryngeal elevation in the pharyngeal phase of swallowing (3 patients). Following radiotherapy, two patients (4.6%) developed trace aspiration which resolved with swallowing therapy. Mean pharyngeal dose was 17.8 Gy and 19.3 Gy for the two patients with aspiration. The most common abnormalities observed on post-treatment MBS were decreased transit or residue in the oral phase (9 patients), decreased laryngeal elevation (4 patients), reduced base of tongue contraction (8 patients), reduced epiglottic inversion (4 patients), and pooling in the vallecula (13 patients). No patient developed aspiration pneumonia following treatment.

At a median follow-up of 19 months (1–48 months), all patients were able to resume normal oral feedings without aspiration. Among the 38 patients who had prophylactic PEG tube placement for chemoradiation (three declined tube placement), three remained dependent on PEG tube feedings because of severe weight loss, two were able to resume oral feedings but their PEG tubes were kept because of the short follow-up (three months), and one patient had severe dysgueusia and continued tube feedings even though he had no dysphagia. The other 32 patients had their PEG tubes removed four to 10 months after treatment. The delay in removing the PEG tube was recommended by the dietitians to ensure that the patients achieved their ideal body weight because of the severe weight loss and/or chronic dysgueusia which prevented the patient from having adequate nutrition. The three patients who declined prophylactic PEG tube placement did not have to undergo tubes feedings during or after treatment.

Discussion

To our knowledge, despite the relatively small number of patients, this is the first study to report aspiration rate following a pharyngeal musculature-sparing IGRT technique. No patient in the study had aspiration at cancer diagnosis. Thus, the prevalence of aspiration following radiotherapy was dependent on radiation dose delivered to the swallowing structures. All patients had WF-IGRT with the goal to limit the pharyngeal dose. We used the WF-IGRT technique in the study to provide adequate dose delivery to the low neck in the presence of cervical node metastases and to reduce the risk of low neck recurrences associated with a split field technique [5]. Mutliple studies have correlated the radiation dose to the pharyngeal muscles to the presence of severe dysphagia and/or aspiration. Fua et al [12] used the Common Toxicity Criteria (CTC) scale to grade the severity of dysphagia following WF-IMRT and SF-IMRT for nasopharyngeal cancers. Patients who had CTC grade 3 required tube feedings. The WF-IMRT was associated with a higher dose to the pharyngeal muscles and severe dysphagia. Severe dysphagia and prolonged tube feedings were reported more often in the WF-IMRT cohort (mean pharyngeal dose 55.2 Gy) compared to the SF-IMRT group (mean pharyngeal dose 27.2 Gy). The corresponding median time to insertion of the feeding tube was 36 days and 38 days, respectively. The mean pharyngeal dose in our study was 23.2 Gy, similar to the SF-IMRT. In another study, Caglar et al [3] investigated the aspiration risk following WF-IMRT of 96 patients with head and neck cancer of all anatomic sites, including laryngeal and hypopharyngeal cancers (18%). MBS was performed four to six weeks following treatment. There was no pretreatment MBS. Thus, the prevalence of silent aspiration pre-treatment could not be assessed in a population of patients which might be at a high risk for aspiration because of the tumor subsites included in the study. Aspiration was assessed according to the Swallowing Performance Scale (minimal aspiration: grade 5, severe aspiration: grade 6–7). Following treatment, 32% of the patients developed grade 5–7 aspiration. It was unclear how many

Table 1. Patient characteristics.

Patient Number		48
Age	Median	57
	Range	25–83
Sex	Male	44
	Female	4
Squamous Histology		48
Tumor Sites	Oropharynx	24
	Oral cavity	12
	Parotid	4
	Unknown (submental metastases)	2
	Nasopharynx	3
	Paranasal sinus (maxillary)	2
	Neck recurrence	1
Stages	I	1
	II	6
	III	13
	IVA	16
	IVB	10
	IVC	1
	Recurrence	1
T stages	Tx	2
	T1	7
	T2	13
	T3	10
	T4	15
	Recurrence	1
Neck nodes	N0	13
	N1	15
	N2	14
	N3	6
Treatment	Postoperative radiation	4
	Radiotherapy alone	3
	Postoperative chemoradiation	13
	Chemoradiation	28
Follow-up (months)	Median	19
	Range	1–48

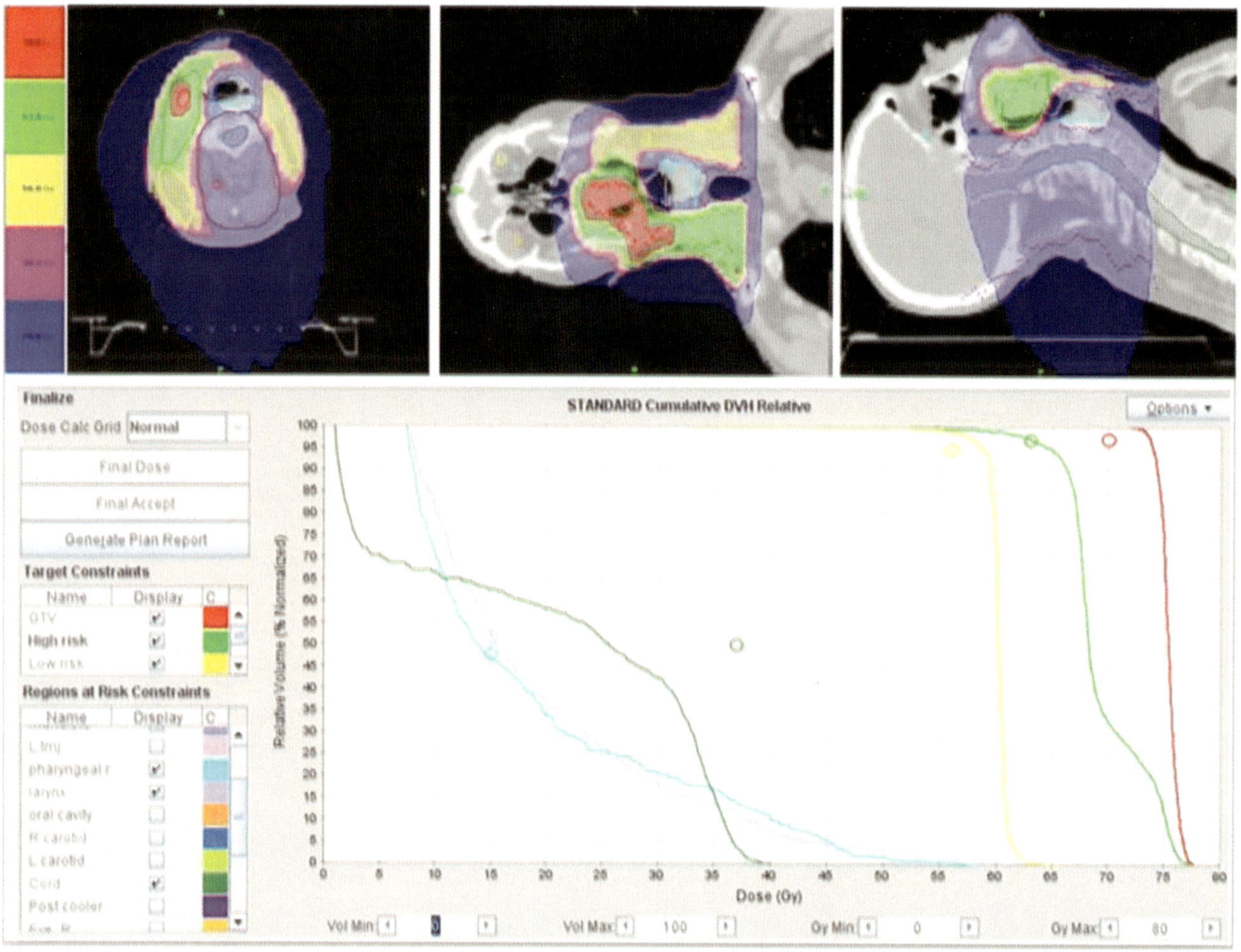

Figure 1. Illustration of the potential of Tomotherapy to spare the pharyngeal muscles in a patient with locally advanced base of tongue cancer and right neck nodal metastases treated with definitive concurrent chemoradiation. Despite the proximity of the gross tumor and neck nodes treated to 70 Gy, mean pharyngeal muscle radiation dose was 22.5 Gy. A split field intensity-modulated radiotherapy technique to shield the larynx and pharyngeal muscles would have underdosed the right neck nodes and gross tumor. The patient is in clinical remission two years following treatment and has no difficulty with swallowing except for xerostomia as the parotid gland could not be spared.

patients developed grade 5 aspiration. However, a high aspiration rate was observed when the radiation dose to the inferior pharyngeal muscles exceeded 52 Gy. High dose to the pharyngeal muscles was associated with WF-IMRT and the inclusion of patients with laryngeal and hypopharyngeal cancers. Thus, the methodology performed by Caglar et al was very similar to our study because the swallowing study was performed four to six weeks after treatment. We do not distinguish between minimal and severe aspiration because our aim was to correlate aspiration rate and radiation dose to the pharyngeal muscles. However, we demonstrated that IGRT by virtue of its rapid dose fall-off compared to WF-IMRT may significantly reduce pharyngeal muscle dose even in the presence of cervical lymph node involvement and can significantly reduce the aspiration risk. Figure 1 and 2 illustrated the ability of IGRT to spare the larynx and pharynx from a high radiation dose, though the involved adjacent cervical lymph nodes were treated to a curative dose of radiation. Nguyen et al [13] recently reported excellent regional control in head and neck cancer patients treated with WF-IGRT in the presence of cervical lymph nodes. Only one out of 76 patients with either unilateral or bilateral cervical lymph nodes developed regional recurrences. In another study correlating MBS before and three months after WF-IMRT for oropharyngeal (31) and nasopharyngeal (5) cancer, aspiration rate was 47% at three months after treatment [14]. Mean dose to the pharyngeal constrictors was 64 Gy. All patients who developed aspiration received more than 60 Gy to the pharyngeal constrictors. Two other studies also corroborated the correlation between high radiation dose to the pharyngeal muscles and dysphagia three months and 20 months after treatment [15,16]. Table 2 summarizes these studies correlating dysphagia and aspiration with pharyngeal muscle dose.

In studies reporting aspiration rates following either 3D-CRT, SF-IMRT, or WF-IMRT in patients with non-laryngeal and non-hypopharygeal cancers, the rates of aspiration ranged from 6.4–54% [17–21]. If we excluded the study of Schwartz et al [20] who used the SF-IMRT technique, aspiration rates ranged from 16–54%. Table 3 summarizes the reported aspiration rates in the literature for non-laryngeal and non-hypopharyngeal cancers.

Although controversy still exists about which swallowing structures are critical and need to be spared to prevent long-term dysphagia and aspiration, the studies that reported the least

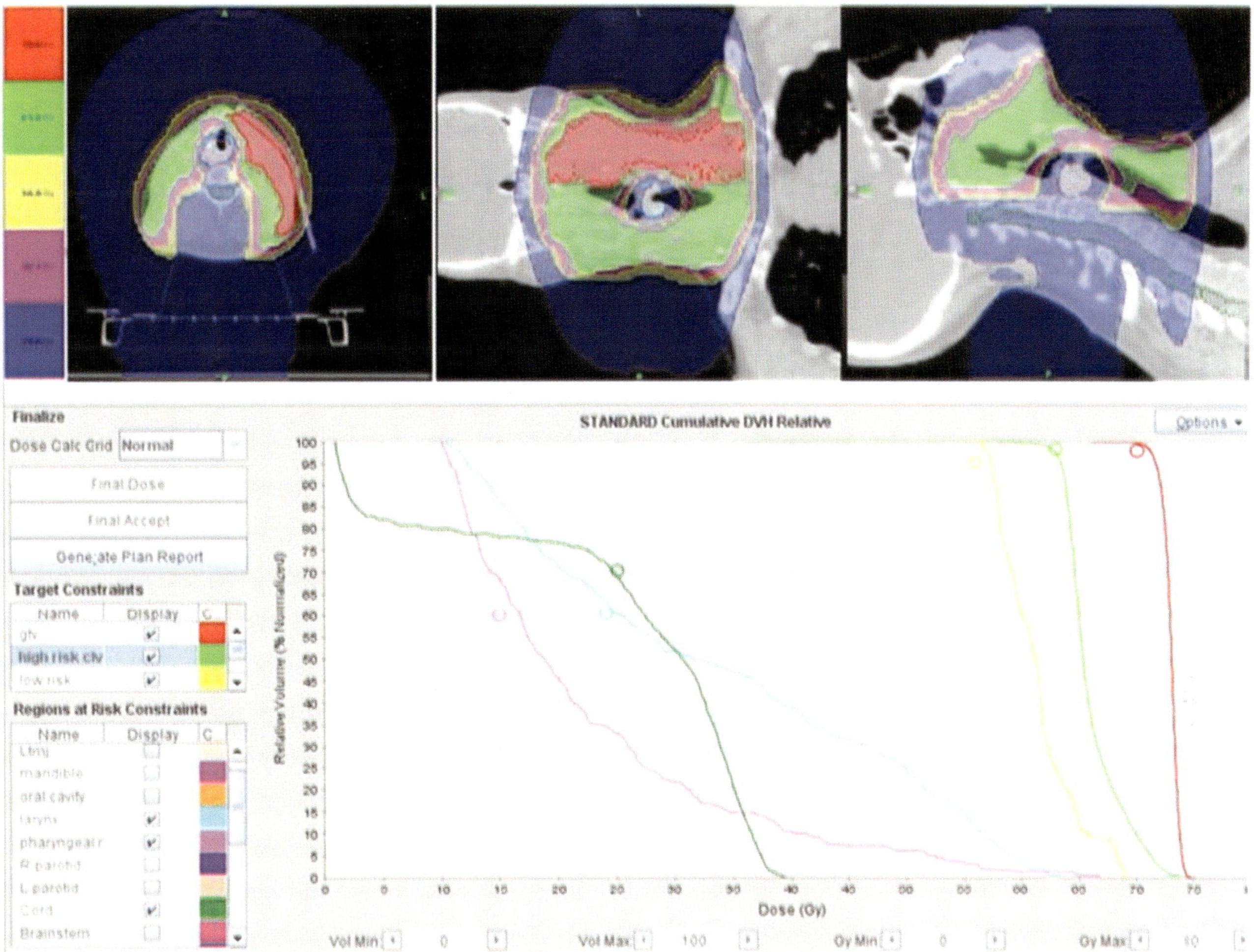

Figure 2. Illustrating the potential of Tomotherapy to spare the pharyngeal muscles in a patient who had postoperative chemoradiation for locally advanced base of tongue and bilateral neck metastases. Even though the right neck was dissected and required radiation of the surgical bed and scars to 63 Gy, the pharyngeal muscles can still be spared from excessive radiation dose. The midline laryngeal block with the split field intensity-modulated radiotherapy technique would have had underdosed the surgical scar and area of the surgical bed located in close proximity to the larynx and the gross lymph nodes on the left side. The patient is in remission 13 month after treatment.

amount of dysphagia and aspiration used techniques which effectively decreased radiation dose to the larynx, and middle and inferior pharyngeal constrictor muscles [12,20]. Thus, WF-IGRT, by virtue of its laryngeal and pharyngeal muscle sparing along with its decreased aspiration rate may be the technique of choice for non-hypopharyngeal and non-laryngeal head and neck cancer [8]. The additional advantage of WF-IGRT is the excellent regional control in the presence of cervical lymph nodes because of the delivery of high dose to these structures in the face of laryngeal and pharyngeal muscle sparing [13].

Table 2. Mean pharyngeal dose (Gy) correlation with dysphagia severity or aspiration reported in the literature.

Study	Mean pharyngeal dose (Gray)	Critical Structures implicated	Clinical endpoints	Time-frame following treatment
Caglar et al [3]	>52	Inferior constrictors larynx	Aspiration (32%)	4–8 weeks
Fua et al [12]	55.2	Middle constrictors Inferior constrictors	Prolonged tube feedings (median time: 38 days)	36–38 days
Feng et al [14]	>60	Superior constrictors Supraglottic larynz	Aspiration (47%)	3 months
Levendag et al [15]	48–51	Superior constrictors Middle constrictors	QOL questionnaires for dysphagia	3 months
Dirix et al [16]	50	Middle constrictors Inferior constrictors Supraglottic larynx	QOL questionnaires for dysphagia	20 months

NA: not assessed; QOL: quality of life.

Table 3. Aspiration rate reported in the literature following radiotherapy for non-laryngeal and non-hypopharyngeal head and neck cancer.

Study	Patient Number	Anatomic site	Treatment Modality	Technique	Aspiration rate
Nguyen et al [17]	46	oropharynx	chemoradiation	C	54%
Nguyen et al [18]	18	oropharynx	postoperative therapy	C	50%
Langerman et al [19]	13	oral cavity	chemoradiation	NS	23%
	18	oropharynx			44%
Feng et al [13]	36	oropharynx	chemoradiation	IMRT	44%
		oral cavity		WF	
Schwartz et al [14]	31	oropharynx	chemoradiation	IMRT	6.4%
				SF	
Feng et al [15]	73	oropharynx	chemoradiation	IMRT	16–26%
				WF	

C: conventional with two lateral and a supraclavicular field; NS: not specified; IMRT: intensity-modulated radiotherapy; WF: whole-field; SF: split-field; IGRT: image-guided radiotherapy.

We should point out that swallowing is a complex mechanism requiring a perfect coordination of multiple muscles within the tongue, pharynx, and larynx. Functional alteration of any of these structures may result in dysphagia and aspiration. Reduced tongue strength, tongue base retraction, and delayed laryngeal vestibule closure were commonly observed following chemoradiation for head and neck cancer [22]. Thus, shielding of the larynx and pharyngeal muscles may reduce the risk of aspiration but complete elimination of aspiration following radiotherapy may not be achieved because of high radiation dose to other swallowing structures such as the base of tongue. As an illustration, the two patients in our study who developed trace aspiration after radiotherapy both had mean pharyngeal dose less than 20 Gy. However, they did not require PEG tube feeding as their aspiration resolved with swallowing therapy. At a median follow-up of 19 months, all study patients were able to resume normal oral feeding without evidence of aspiration. Long-term PEG tube feeding was frequently linked to dysgueusia, which is commonly observed after chemoradiation for head and neck cancer [23].

The limitations of the present study include the retrospective nature of the study, the heterogeneity of the patient population and treatment modalities, the small number of patients, and the fact that we did not include patients with laryngeal or hypopharyngeal cancer. However, in such patients, it would not be feasible to spare the pharyngeal muscles from excessive radiation because of the close proximity of these tumor subsites, which often demonstrate invasion of the muscles in locally advanced stages. Nevertheless, despite these caveats, sparing of the pharyngeal musculature from excessive radiation may decrease aspiration rate, and merits further investigation. Prospective studies with large numbers of patients should be performed to assess the impact of WF-IGRT on dysphagia and aspiration in patients with head and neck cancer.

Conclusion

Tomotherapy-based IGRT may reduce the aspiration rate for non-laryngeal and non-hypopharyngeal head and neck cancer patients because of the decreased pharyngeal muscle dose. Prospective studies should be performed to assess the potential of IGRT to reduce treatment dysphagia and to possibly improve patient quality of life.

Author Contributions

Data collection and literature search: NPN MC MS HM BJ RD TS AD. Conceived and designed the experiments: NPN LS VV PV RD AD TS DA SPK MS HM BJ MC. Performed the experiments: LS PV VV DA MS HM MC. Analyzed the data: NPN LS VV PV RD AD TS DA SPK MS HM BJ MC. Contributed reagents/materials/analysis tools: RD BJ AD TS VH. Wrote the paper: NPN LS VV PV RD AD TS DA SPK MS HM BJ MC.

References

1. Nguyen NP, Frank C, Moltz CC, Vos P, Smith HJ, et al (2006). Aspiration rate following chemoradiation for head and neck cancer: an underreported occurrence. Radioth Oncol 80:302–306.
2. Gokhale AS, McLaughlin BT, Flickinger JC, Beriwal S, Heron DE, et al (2010). Clinical and dosimetry factors associated with a prolonged feeding tube requirement in patients treated with chemoradiotherapy for head and neck cancers. Ann Oncol 21:145–151.
3. Caglar HB, Tishler RB, Othus M, Burke E, Li Y, et al (2008). Dose to larynx predicts for swallowing complications after intensity-modulated radiotherapy. Int J Radiat Oncol Biol Phys 72:1110–1118.
4. Amdur Rj, Liu C, Li J, Hinerman R (2007) Matching intensity-modulated radiation therapy to an anterior low neck field. Int J Radiat Oncol Biol Phys 69:S46–S48.
5. Chao K, Ozyigit B, Tran B, Cengiz M, Dempsey JF, et al (2003). Patterns of failure in patients receiving definitive and postoperative IMRT for head and neck cancer. Int J Radiat Oncol Biol Phys 55:312–321.
6. Lee N, Mechalakos J, Puri DV, Hunt M (2007). Choosing an intensity-modulated radiation therapy technique in the treatment of head and neck cancer. Int J Radiat Oncol Biol Phys 68:1299–1309.
7. Nguyen NP, Ceizyk M, Vos P, Vinh-Hung V, Davis R, et al (2010). Effectiveness of image-guided radiotherapy for laryngeal sparing in head and neck cancer. Oral Oncol 46:283–286.
8. Nguyen NP, Abraham D, Desai A, Betz M, Davis R, et al (2011). Impact of image-guided radiotherapy to reduce laryngeal edema following treatment for non-laryngeal and non-hypopharyngeal head and neck cancers. Oral Oncology 47:900–904.
9. Eisbruch A, Schwartz M, Rasch C, Vineberg K, Damen E, et al (2004). Dysphagia and aspiration after chemoradiotherapy for head and neck cancer: which anatomic structures are affected and can they be spared by IMRT. Int J Radiat Oncol Biol Phys 60:1425–1439.
10. Nguyen NP, Vos P, Moltz CC, Frank C, Millar C, et al (2008). Analysis of the factors influencing dysphagia severity upon diagnosis of head and neck cancer. Br J Radiol 81:706–710

11. Nguyen NP, Moltz CC, Frank C, Vos P, Smith HJ, et al (2007). Impact of swallowing therapy on aspiration rate following treatment for locally advanced head and neck cancer. Oral Oncology 43:352–357.
12. Fua TF, Corry J, Milner AD, Cramb J, Walsham SF, et al (2007). Intensity-modulated radiotherapy for nasopharyngeal carcinoma: clinical correlation of dose to the pharyngo-esophageal axis and dysphagia. Int J Radiat Oncol Biol Phys 67:976–981.
13. Nguyen NP, Vock J, Vinh-Hung V, Almeida F, Ewell L, et al (2012). Effectiveness of prophylactic retropharyngeal lymph node irradiation in patients with locally advanced head and neck cancer. BMC Cancer 12:253.
14. Feng F, Kim H, Lyden T, Haxer MJ, Feng M, et al (2007). Intensity-modulated radiotherapy of head and neck cancer aiming to reduce dysphagia: Early dose-effect relationships for the swallowing structures. Int J Radiat Oncol Biol Phys 68:1289–1298.
15. Levendag PC, Teguh DN, Voet P, van der Est H, Noever I, et al (2007) Dysphagia disorders in patients with cancer of the oropharynx are significantly affected by the radiotherapy dose to the superior and middle constrictor muscles: a dose-effect relationship. Radiother Oncol 85:64–73.
16. Dirix P, Abbeel S, Vanstraelen B, Hermans R, Nuyts S (2009). Dysphagia after chemoradiotherapy for head and neck squamous cell carcinoma: Dose-effect relationship to the swallowing structures. Int J Radiat Oncol Biol Phys 78:1356–1365.
17. Nguyen NP, Frank C, Moltz CC, Vos P, Smith HJ, et al (2009) Analysis of factors influencing aspiration risks following chemoradiation for oropharyngeal cancer. Br J Radiol 82:675–680.
18. Nguyen NP, Frank C, Moltz CC, Vos P, Millard C, et al (2008). Dysphagia severity and aspiration following postoperative radiation for locally advanced oropharyngeal cancer. Anticancer Research 28:431–434.
19. Langerman A, MacCracken E, Kasza K, Haraf DJ, Voke EE, et al (2007). Aspiration in chemoradiated patients with head and neck cancer. Arch Otolaryngol Head Neck Surg 133:1289–1295.
20. Schwartz DL, Hutcheson K, Barringer D, Tucker SL, Kies M, et al (2010). Candidate dosimetric predictors of long-term swallowing dysfunction after oropharyngeal intensity-modulated radiotherapy. Int J Radiat Oncol Biol Phys 78:1356–1365.
21. Feng FY, Kim HM, Lyden TH, Haxer MJ, Worden FP, et al (2010). Intensity-modulated chemoradiotherapy aiming to reduce dysphagia in patients with oropharyngeal cancer. J Clin Oncol 28:27232–2738.
22. Logemann JA, Rademaker AW, Pauloski BR, Lazarus CL, Mittal BB, et al (2006). Site of disease and treatment protocol as correlates of swallowing function in head and neck cancer patients treated with chemoradiation. Head Neck 28:64–73.
23. Kamprad F, Ranft D, Weber A, Hilderbrandt G (2008). Functional changes of the gustatory organ caused by local radiation exposure during radiotherapy of the head and neck region. Strahlenther Onkol 184:157–162.

4

Quantitative Susceptibility Mapping Differentiates between Blood Depositions and Calcifications in Patients with Glioblastoma

Andreas Deistung[1], Ferdinand Schweser[1], Benedikt Wiestler[2], Mario Abello[6], Matthias Roethke[3], Felix Sahm[4], Wolfgang Wick[2], Armin Michael Nagel[5], Sabine Heiland[6], Heinz-Peter Schlemmer[3], Martin Bendszus[6], Jürgen Rainer Reichenbach[1], Alexander Radbruch[6,7]*

1 Medical Physics Group, Institute of Diagnostic and Interventional Radiology I, Jena University Hospital - Friedrich Schiller University Jena, Philosophenweg 3, Jena, Germany, **2** Department of Neurooncology, University of Heidelberg, INF 400, Heidelberg, Germany, **3** Department of Radiology, German Cancer Research Center (DKFZ), INF 280, Heidelberg, Germany, **4** Department of Neuropathology, University of Heidelberg, INF 220/221, Heidelberg, Germany, **5** Institute for Medical Physics, German Cancer Research Center (DKFZ), INF 280, Heidelberg, Germany, **6** Department of Neuroradiology, University of Heidelberg, INF 400, Heidelberg, Germany, **7** Section Neuro-oncologic Imaging (E 012), German Cancer Research Center, INF 280, Heidelberg, Germany

Abstract

Objectives: The application of susceptibility weighted imaging (SWI) in brain tumor imaging is mainly used to assess tumor-related "susceptibility based signals" (SBS). The origin of SBS in glioblastoma is still unknown, potentially representing calcifications or blood depositions. Reliable differentiation between both entities may be important to evaluate treatment response and to identify glioblastoma with oligodendroglial components that are supposed to present calcifications. Since calcifications and blood deposits are difficult to differentiate using conventional MRI, we investigated whether a new post-processing approach, quantitative susceptibility mapping (QSM), is able to distinguish between both entities reliably.

Materials and Methods: SWI, FLAIR, and T1-w images were acquired from 46 patients with glioblastoma (14 newly diagnosed, 24 treated with radiochemotherapy, 8 treated with radiochemotherapy and additional anti-angiogenic medication). Susceptibility maps were calculated from SWI data. All glioblastoma were evaluated for the appearance of hypointense or hyperintense correlates of SBS on the susceptibility maps.

Results: 43 of 46 glioblastoma presented only hyperintense intratumoral SBS on susceptibility maps, indicating blood deposits. Additional hypointense correlates of tumor-related SBS on susceptibility maps, indicating calcification, were identified in 2 patients being treated with radiochemotherapy and in one patient being treated with additional anti-angiogenic medication. Histopathologic reports revealed an oligodendroglial component in one patient that presented calcifications on susceptibility maps.

Conclusions: QSM provides a quantitative, local MRI contrast, which reliably differentiates between blood deposits and calcifications. Thus, quantitative susceptibility mapping appears promising to identify rare variants of glioblastoma with oligodendroglial components non-invasively and may allow monitoring the role of calcification in the context of different therapy regimes.

Editor: Christoph Kleinschnitz, Julius-Maximilians-Universität Würzburg, Germany

Funding: This research was funded by a Carl Zeiss Foundation dissertation fellowship for Ferdinand Schweser and a research grant by the German Research Foundation (DFG, RE 1123/9-2). The funders had no role in study design, data collection and analysis, decision to publish, or preparation of the manuscript.

Competing Interests: The authors have declared that no competing interests exist.

* E-mail: a.radbruch@dkfz.de

Introduction

Glioblastoma is the most frequently occurring intrinsic brain tumor, accounting for approximately 12–15% of all intracranial neoplasms [1]. Despite recent therapeutic advances, prognosis for patients suffering from glioblastoma remains dismal with a median overall survival period of 12 to 14 months for patients in study cohorts [2]. The suspected diagnosis of glioblastoma is usually based on contrast-enhanced T_1-weighted images and T2-weighted, FLAIR, diffusion weighted, and T_2^*-weighted images within clinical routine.

Recently, Susceptibility Weighted Imaging (SWI) has been suggested to potentially contribute to the differential diagnosis of enhancing brain lesions [3,4,5,6,7]. SWI is a non-quantitative technique that employs Gradient (Recalled) Echo (GRE) phase images to enhance smallest susceptibility variations on the corresponding magnitude images [8,9,10]. In brain tumors, SWI has been used to assess tumor visibility [5], small tumor vessels [11,12], contrast agent uptake [13], and tumor oxygenation

[14,15]. The basis for assessment of solitary enhancing brain lesions, such as high-grade glioma versus metastasis or lymphoma, on Susceptibility Weighted (SW) images are "susceptibility based signals" (SBS) within the tumor that are usually not seen on conventional MR images (T_1-w, T_2-w, T_2*-w, diffusion weighted, and contrast-enhanced T_1-w images) [3]. Park et al. defined intratumoral SBS as low signal intensity with a fine linear or dot-like structure, with or without conglomeration, seen within the tumor on SW images [16]. The authors also found that the frequency of intratumoral SBS is correlated with tumor malignancy and proved that the use of a semi-quantitative grading system of the intratumoral SBS can contribute to the grading of glioma. Furthermore, Radbruch et al. demonstrated that the appearance of SBS enables the differentiation between glioblastoma and primary CNS lymphoma with high sensitivity and specificity [17].

The underlying pathophysiology of tumor-related SBS, however, is not yet fully understood. It is supposed that susceptibility variations within glioblastoma are related to different forms of iron in blood products caused by extensive vascular proliferation, microhemorrhages, or small vessels [11]. The tumor-related susceptibility variations, however, may be also caused by calcifications [18,19].

Generally, calcification is supposed to appear rarely in glioblastoma. Presence of calcifications in glioblastoma, however, may be predictive for an oligodendroglial component. Initial results suggest that glioblastoma patients with oligodendroglial components have prolonged survival and show better response to temozolomide [20,21,22,23]. Furthermore, a recent report suggests that formation of calcifications in patients with glioblastoma after therapy with bevacizumab is associated with the response to therapy and improved outcome [24]. Therefore, the presence of calcifications in glioblastoma may represent an important biomarker for therapy decision, treatment response, and outcome.

Calcifications can, in general, be identified by using computed tomography (CT). However, since MRI has replaced CT for routine follow-up examinations, CT scans are usually not available. Reliable identification of calcifications by conventional MR imaging, however, is difficult, because their signal is variable on conventional T_1-w or T_2-w spin-echo images [25,26]. On SW images blood products and calcium both appear hypointense, thus impeding differentiation of these two biophysical sources of SBS. Consequently, an MRI approach for reliable identification of calcifications within the tumor is desirable.

Compared to healthy brain tissue, deoxyhemoglobin, methemoglobin, hemosiderin, and ferritin are more paramagnetic, whereas bone minerals, dystrophic and tumoral calcifications are usually more diamagnetic [27]. The presence of deoxyhemoglobin renders venous blood more paramagnetic, whereas fully oxygenated blood is slightly more diamagnetic than healthy brain tissue [28,29]. Recently, a novel post-processing technique was introduced that produces quantitative maps of tissue magnetic susceptibility using GRE phase data. This technique, called Quantitative Susceptibility Mapping (QSM), has been demonstrated to enable reliable identification of arbitrarily shaped brain lesions as being either blood products or calcium [30].

In the present study, QSM was applied to a cohort of patients with newly diagnosed glioblastoma to identify the origin of *de novo* SBS within the tumor. Furthermore, susceptibility maps of two cohorts of patients treated with radiochemotherapy either with or without additional anti-angiogenic medication with bevacizumab were evaluated to identify calcifications. Finally histopathological reports of the included patients were assessed to identify possible oligodendroglial components within the glioblastoma.

Materials and Methods

Patients and reference standards

All clinical investigations were conducted according to the principles expressed in the Declaration of Helsinki and all patients consented to the MRI examination according to German regulations. All patients provided written informed consent to the scientific analysis of the acquired MRI data including the performance of postprocessing procedures that do not require any additional scan time such as QSM. This consent procedure was approved by the ethics committee of the University of Heidelberg (approval number: S-096/2010).

Three cohorts of patients were investigated. Inclusion criteria for the first group were presence of a newly diagnosed glioblastoma prior to resection. Inclusion criteria for the second group were presence of a recurrent glioblastoma, treated with the temozolomid (Temodal, Essex Pharma GmbH, Munich, Germany) and concomitant radiation. Inclusion criteria for the third group were presence of a recurrent glioblastoma treated with standard radiochemotherapy and additional anti-angiogenic medication with bevacizumab (Avastin, F.Hoffmann-La Roche AG, Basel, Switzerland). The characteristics of the three patient cohorts are summarized in more detail in Table 1. All glioblastoma were assessed histopathologically using Hematoxylin-Eosin (H&E) staining after surgery.

MRI Data Acquisition

All MRI examinations were performed on a 3 T whole-body MR system (Magnetom Tim Trio, Siemens Healthcare, Erlangen, Germany) with a 12-channel head-matrix coil during routine clinical workup. SWI data were collected with a 3D, fully flow-compensated GRE sequence using the following parameters: echo time (TE) = 19.7 ms, repetition time (TR) = 27 ms, flip angle (FA) = 15°, bandwidth (BW) = 140 Hz/px, acquisition matrix = 320×240×52, and voxel size = 0.72 mm×0.72 mm×2.5 mm. Partial parallel imaging (generalized autocalibrating partially parallel acquisitions, GRAPPA [31]) with an acceleration factor (R) of 2, and 24 reference lines resulted in a total acquisition time of 3:20 min:sec.

Contrast-enhanced MP-RAGE and FLAIR images were used for morphological tumor assessment. The MP-RAGE data were acquired with inversion time (TI) = 1100 ms, TE = 4 ms, TR = 1710 ms, FA = 15°, BW = 130 Hz/px, acquisition matrix = 512×512×164, and voxel size = 0.5 mm×0.5 mm×1.3 mm. The parameters of the FLAIR scans included TI = 2400 ms, TE = 135 ms, TR = 8500 ms, FA = 170°, BW = 150 Hz/px, acquisition matrix = 256×192×26, and voxel size of 0.9 mm×0.9 mm×5 mm.

One patient with a newly diagnosed glioblastoma underwent additional scanning on an ultrahigh field 7 T MRI system (Magnetom 7T, Siemens Medical Solutions) with a 24-channel head coil (Nova Medical, Inc., Wilmington, USA) to assess intratumoral morphology in more detail. High-resolution SWI data were collected using the following parameters: TE = 15 ms, TR = 23 ms, FA = 20°, BW = 120 Hz/px, acquisition matrix = 512×416×104, and voxel size = 0.39 mm×0.39 mm×0.43 mm. Seventy-five percent partial Fourier along slice direction and partial parallel imaging [R = 2, 30 reference lines] was applied resulting in an acquisition time of 6:40 min:sec. For this patient, an axial post-contrast CT scan was available (Philips Brilliance 16 CT-slice, Best, The Netherlands). The parameters of the CT scan included voxel size = 0.43 mm×0.43 mm×1.5 mm, field-of-view = 220 mm, X-ray tube current = 300 mA, and peak voltage = 120 kV.

Table 1. Patients characteristics.

	cohort 1	cohort 2	cohort 3
inclusion criteria	- newly diagnosed glioblastoma prior to resection	- recurrent glioblastoma - initially treated with temozolomid and concomitant radiation	- recurrent glioblastoma - initially treated with temozolomid and concomitant radiation - in the course of the therapy additional treatment with anti-angiogenic medication
N (male/female)	14 (12/2)	24 (19/5)	8 (6/2)
age	41.4±9.2 (min 47, max 74)	59.8±12 (min 35, max 79)	55.75±11.6 (min 43, max 74)
surgery	1 patient: biopsy prior to MRI	17 patients: initially total resection; 5 patients: partial resection; 2 patients: biopsy without further resection	4 patients: initially total resection; 4 patients: partial resection

MRI Data Processing

Multi-channel GRE magnitude images were reconstructed using the sum-of-squares (SoS) method [32], whereas multi-channel GRE phase images were combined by taking into account the channel-dependent phase offset, which was estimated from the single channel images within the same homogenous region of interest [33]. The combined magnitude and phase images were then converted into SW images according to Reichenbach et al. [8].

For quantitative susceptibility mapping (QSM), remaining phase aliasing in the combined phase images was resolved by a 3D Laplacian-based phase unwrapping algorithm [34]. Background phase contributions were eliminated with sophisticated harmonic artifact reduction for phase data (SHARP) [35] with a spherical convolution kernel of radius 7.2 mm. In patients in whom the tumor tissue extended close to the brain boundary, a 3D discrete Laplacian operator was applied as SHARP convolution kernel to minimize the convolution edge artifact [36]. Back-

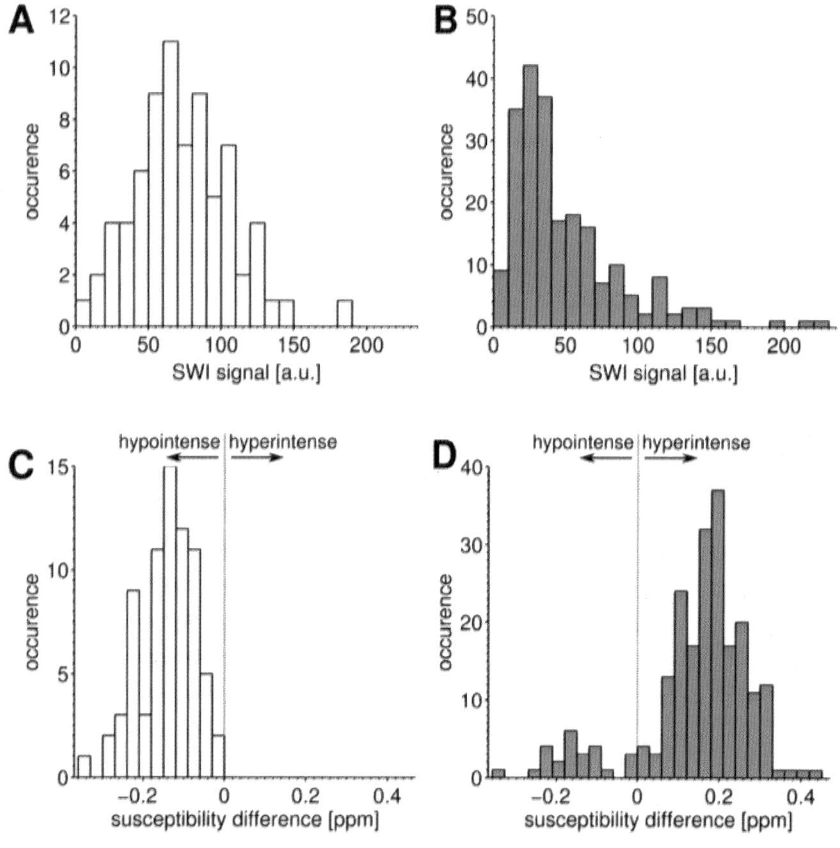

Figure 1. Results of VOI analysis. The signal intensity histograms (bin size = 10) of choroid plexus (n = 74) and SBS (n = 219) measured on susceptibility weighted images (SWI) in 46 GBM patients are shown in (a) and (b), respectively. The corresponding susceptibility differences of choroid plexus and SBS regions with respect to NAWM are shown in the histograms in (c) and (d), respectively, with a bin size of 0.03 ppm. (The white and grey bars indicate regions of the choroid plexus and SBS, respectively.)

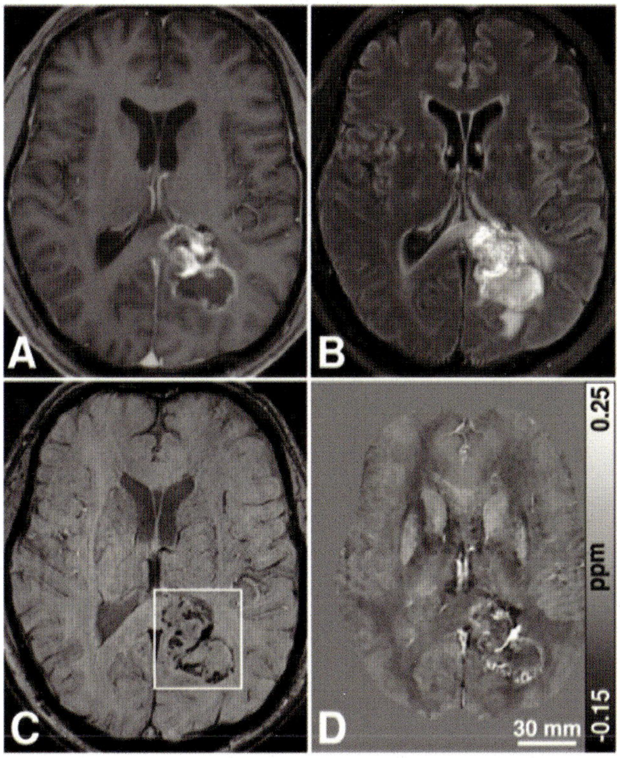

Figure 2. MR images of a 71-year-old man with a left occipital untreated glioblastoma. T1-w, FLAIR, SWI, and quantitative susceptibility map showing the same region are illustrated from (a) to (d), respectively.

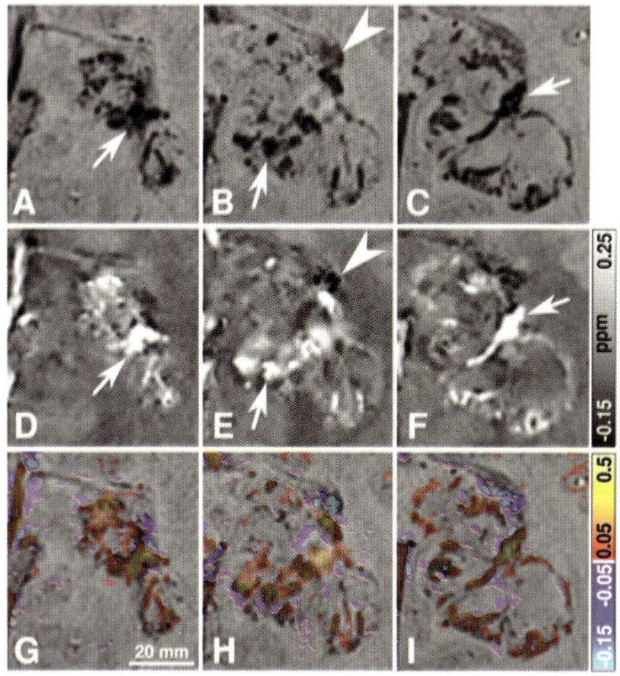

Figure 3. Sections of MR images of the glioblastoma presented in Figure 2. The top (a–c), middle (d–f), and bottom row (g–i) display sections of SW images, susceptibility maps, and overlays of the susceptibility maps onto the corresponding SW images, respectively. The columns from left to right sample the glioblastoma from inferior to superior direction with a slice distance of 2.5 mm. The location of these sections is indicated by the white rectangle in Figure 2c. The arrows and arrow heads indicate SBS and choroid plexus, respectively.

ground-corrected phase images were then supplied to a novel susceptibility mapping algorithm (homogeneity enabled dipole inversion, HEIDI) [37] to reconstruct quantitative susceptibility maps without streaking artifacts.

All data processing was carried out fully automatically in MATLAB (The Mathworks, Inc., Natick MA, USA) using the Medical Computation Server [38].

MRI Data Analysis

An experienced neuroradiologist (A.R.) assessed tumor-related SBS on both SW images and quantitative susceptibility maps. Volumes of interest (VOIs) were manually defined on SW images for tumor-related SBS and choroidal plexi in the lateral ventricle as a place of proven physiological calcifications. A VOI was defined for all choroidal plexi in the lateral ventricle that clearly delineated on SW images. All VOIs were then analyzed on both SW images and quantitative susceptibility maps. Furthermore VOIs were placed in normal appearing white matter (NAWM) on the susceptibility map. Since the calculated susceptibility values represent relative rather than absolute values [35], susceptibility differences were specified with respect to NAWM.

Results

Only 74 choroidal plexi in the lateral ventricles of all 92 plexi in 46 patients were clearly identified and appeared likewise uniformly hypointense on SW images. Forty-three of all 46 glioblastomas presented with multiple intratumoral SBS that appeared uniformly hypointense on SW images and uniformly hyperintense on susceptibility maps. None of the newly diagnosed glioblastoma but two patients of the cohort treated with radiochemotherapy and one patient who received additional medication with bevacizumab displayed hypointense correlates of SBS on susceptibility maps, indicating calcifications. Evaluation of the histopathologic reports revealed oligodendroglial components in only one patient out of the included 46 patients. All tumor-related SBS were clearly delineated on SWI, but did not show any correlates on contrast-enhanced T_1-weighted images.

VOI-based analysis of the choroid plexus and tumor-related SBS are summarized as histograms in Figure 1. SW image intensity was not able to discriminate between the hypointense choroid plexus and tumor-related SBS (Fig. 1a and 1b). In contrast, quantitative magnetic susceptibility differences were negative between the choroid plexus and NAWM, indicating calcium deposits. A mean susceptibility difference of -0.141 ± 0.07 ppm was measured in VOIs of the choroid plexus relative to NAWM. The majority of susceptibility differences between correlates of SBS and NAWM (Fig. 1d) were positive, indicating blood deposits that were clearly discriminable from the calcified choroid plexus (Fig. 1c). Twenty-five of 219 tumor-related SBS regions revealed negative susceptibility differences relative to NAWM, indicating calcifications.

Representative MR images of a patient with a newly diagnosed glioblastoma are demonstrated in Figure 2 and Figure 3. The intratumoral SBS clearly correspond to high signal regions on quantitative susceptibility maps, i.e., paramagnetic susceptibility variations, indicating the presence of blood products (arrows in Fig. 3). Low-susceptibility regions on the susceptibility maps with direct correspondence to hypointense areas on the SW image suggest diamagnetic susceptibility variations. This is evident for the

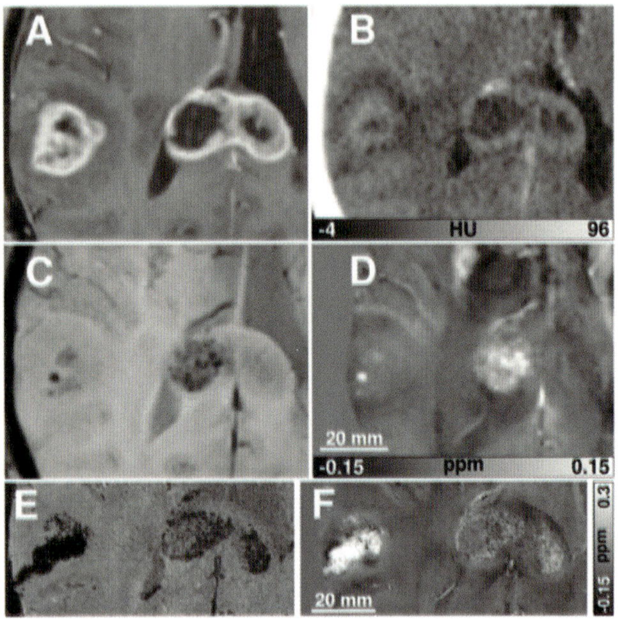

Figure 4. Imaging results of a 67-year-old female patient with a multilocular glioblastoma before radiochemotherapy. The contrast-enhanced T1-w image reveals the typical ring-enhancement (a), whereas the susceptibility weighted image shows intratumoral SBS in the temporal lesion and in the right part of the corpus callosum (c). Corresponding SBS on the susceptibility map (d) are hyperintense, indicating blood products as the biophysical source of the intratumoral SBS. The contrast-enhanced CT image (b), displaying a comparable section, proves these findings because no calcifications can be identified as possible sources of the tumor-related SBS. A single slice of the high-resolution 7 T GRE magnitude data and the corresponding susceptibility map are displayed in (e) and (f), respectively. Since the 7 T data were acquired 10 days after the routine MRI, biopsy of the right temporal lesion had been performed in the meantime.

calcification in the choroid plexus (arrow head in Fig. 3). Histological assessment of the newly diagnosed glioblastomas revealed prominent microvascular proliferation, blood products and necrosis in all 14 patients. Macroscopic calcifications and microcalcifications were not observed histopathologically in any of the newly diagnosed glioblastomas.

One case of a multilocular glioblastoma with lesions in the right temporal lobe and in the splenium of the corpus callosum is presented in Figure 4. Intratumoral SBS were clearly discernible in the right part of the lesion in the corpus callosum and in the temporal lobe lesion (Fig. 4c). Since these areas displayed hyperintensely on the susceptibility maps (Fig. 4d), they were identified as blood products. These findings were confirmed by CT (Fig. 4b). Although the high-resolution 7 T data revealed detailed variations within the tumor matrix, the susceptibility maps at 3 T were already able to characterize the tumor-related SBS unequivocally. Prior to the 7 T scan a biopsy of the temporal tumor lesion was performed, which manifests itself by the strong hypointensity on the magnitude image of the GRE scan (Fig. 4e) and the strong hyperintensity on the susceptibility map (Fig. 4f). This paramagnetic behavior was caused by hemorrhage and residual air inclusions close to the biopsy channel.

The patient diagnosed with an oligodendroglial component presented multiple hypointense correlates of SBS located within the recurrent tumor right temporal on susceptibility maps (Figure 5).

One of 8 patients treated with additional anti-angiogenic medication (bevacizumab) presented multiple punctuate hypointense signal regions on susceptibility maps within the border of the resection cavity (Figure 6j) while the remaining seven patients presented hyperintense correlates of SBS on susceptibility maps (Figure 6i).

Discussion

Hitherto, the diagnostic value of SWI in tumor imaging has mainly been investigated for visualizing signal intensity changes in GRE magnitude and SW images based on magnetic susceptibility variations and for differentiating tumors based on SBS. In this study, we have demonstrated for the first time that post-processing

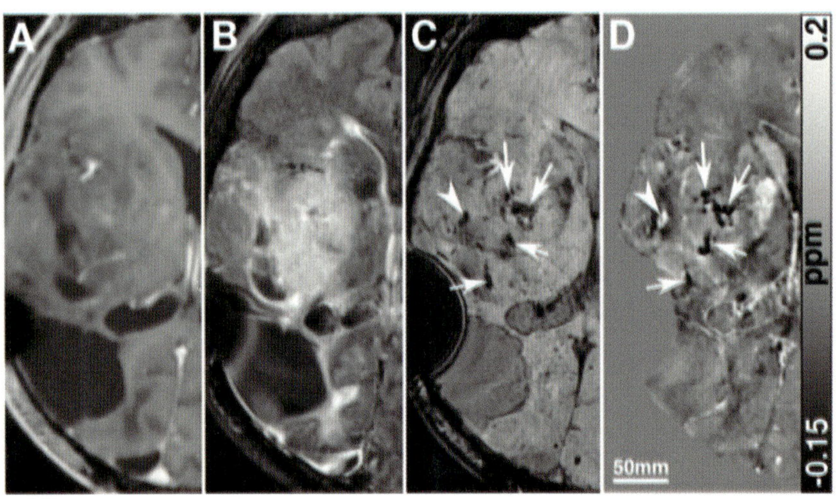

Figure 5. Images of a 49 year-old man with a glioblastoma with an oligodendroglial component after radiochemotherapy. The contrast-enhanced T1-w and FLAIR images are presented in (a) and (b), respectively. SBS, indicated by the arrow and arrow head, are discernable on the SW image (c). The corresponding susceptibility map in (d) clearly suggests that these SBS are likely produced by calcium deposits (arrow) and blood products (arrow head).

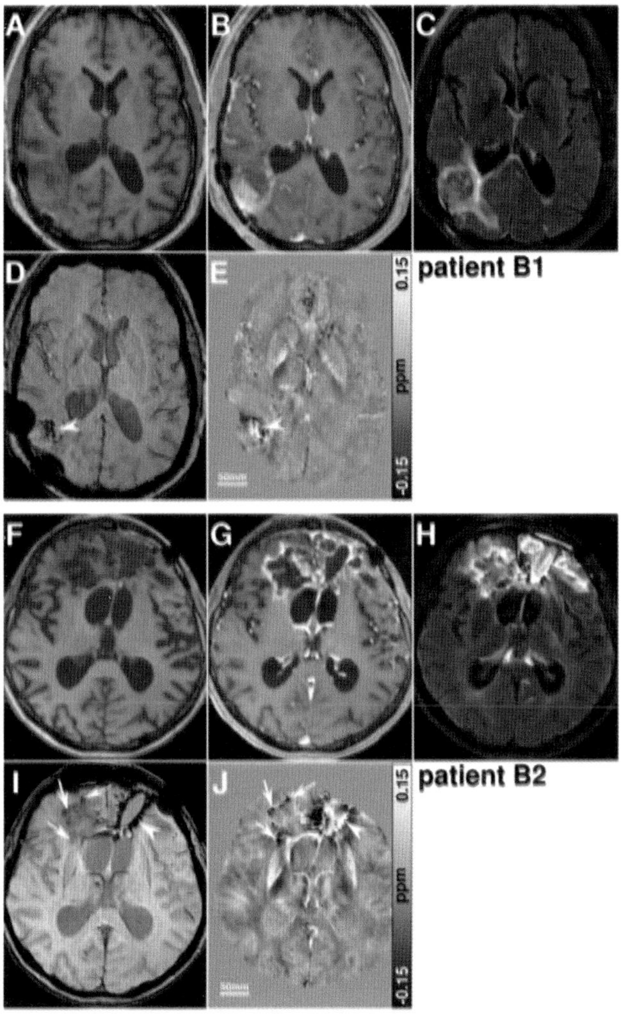

Figure 6. Images of two patients who were treated with bevacizumab after completion of radiochemotherapy. Images of a 42 year old man with a glioblastoma in the right occipital lobe (patient B1), who was treated with 12 cycles of bevacizumab after completion of radiochemotherapy are presented in the upper part (a–e). The lower part (f–j) reveals images of a 46 year old man with a glioblastoma in the frontal lobe (patient B2), who was treated with 5 cycles of bevacizumab. T1-weighted images before (a,f) and after contrast agent administration (b,g), FLAIR images (c,h), SW images (d,i) and susceptibility maps (e,j) are presented for each patient. The patient in the upper part represents SBS that only correlate with hyperintense areas on the susceptibility maps (arrow heads), whereas the patient in the lower part reveals additional calcifications indicated by hypointense correlates of SBS on susceptibility maps (arrows).

of GRE data using quantitative susceptibility mapping (QSM) enables unequivocal differentiation between paramagnetic blood deposits and diamagnetic calcifications in brain tumors and that intratumoral SBS in newly diagnosed glioblastoma originate from blood products. Furthermore, we demonstrated that calcifications may occur in recurrent glioblastoma.

Relative to normal white matter, paramagnetic structures are represented as hyperintense areas on these susceptibility maps, whereas diamagnetic structures are displayed as hypointense areas. This is in agreement with our previous findings that paramagnetic venous vessels displayed hyperintensely, and choroid plexus, representing physiologic calcification, appeared hypointensely on susceptibility maps [30,35].

The finding that tumor-related SBS in newly diagnosed glioblastoma represent blood products and/or microvascular proliferation is in accordance with the WHO classification for glioma that requires prominent microvascular proliferation as an essential diagnostic feature for the diagnosis of glioblastoma. We were unable to identify any hypointense SBS correlates on the susceptibility maps as an indication of calcification within the newly diagnosed glioblastoma. This finding is consistent with the histopathological literature about glioblastoma, as calcifications are not reported to be a common feature in glioblastoma [21].

Histopathological analysis revealed only one patient (49 year old, male) with an oligodendroglial component among all patients. Interestingly, this patient revealed areas of clear uniform hypointense SBS correlates on the susceptibility maps indicating calcification (Fig. 5d). This finding is in agreement with the known tendency of oligodendroglioma to present calcifications [21]. Typically, calcifications are detected by histopathological evaluation of the tumor. Calcifications, however, may be missed, if the histopathological evaluation does not reflect the entire tumor tissue or – in cases of biopsy – represent only very small portions of it. In these cases, additional identification of tumor-related hypointense SBS correlates on QSM may help to identify glioblastoma with an oligodendroglial component that potentially require a different therapy [39]. Further studies with larger patient cohorts and supplemental histopathological evaluation are needed to investigate the specificity of QSM for differentiating between glioblastoma and glioblastoma with oligodendroglial components.

Furthermore, we could identify calcifications in the resection cavity in one patient (47 years old, male) treated with bevacizumab. Bevacizumab is an antibody against the VEGF receptor, which is currently used in the treatment of recurrent glioblastoma [1]. Bähr et al. [24] recently reported a correlation between therapy-induced hyperintense lesions on pre-contrast T_1-weighted MR images and overall response to bevacizumab. Hypothesizing that the observed hyperintensities were bevacizumab-induced tumor calcifications, the authors concluded that these tumor calcifications may present a novel biomarker associated with response and improved outcome of therapy. Since no CT scans had been acquired on a regular basis, the authors were unable to definitely identify calcifications during follow-up examinations and argued that the identified hyperintensities could have also been caused by methemoglobin, cholesterol, fat, or proteinaceous material. Larger cohorts are certainly needed to correlate clinical parameters with calcification processes in future studies.

Finally, only one patient with glioblastoma (52 year old, female) treated with radiochemotherapy exclusively (besides the patient with the oligodendromal component) exhibited calcifications. The pathogenetic mechanisms of tumor-related calcifications during radiochemotherapy are currently unknown. It is, however, supposed that radiation induced vasculopathy may result in hypoxia-induced tissue damage that causes calcification [40]. Currently, only limited literature exists about calcification during the course of different therapy regimes. This may be explained with the low incidence of calcification processes and with the missing awareness of radiologists to reliably identify calcifications.

Traditionally, calcifications are diagnosed using CT. However, CT is usually not part of the routine follow-up examination to assess progression of a glioblastoma. An additional CT as a reference standard to detect calcifications would result in increased patient discomfort and stress and would increase the patient's examination times. Integrating the SWI sequence into the tumor

MR imaging protocol is significantly more convenient than applying an additional CT. QSM, which relies on the same GRE data as routine SWI, provides a unique and convenient method of differentiating between calcifications and blood deposits during follow-up examinations. The fact that QSM does not require additional scan time or co-registration is particularly important for patients suffering from glioblastoma, who are often already in dire physical condition and for whom lengthy imaging protocols can be extremely difficult.

Precise identification of calcification may be of major interest for understanding the histopathology of tumor growth and the impact of different therapies. The increasing use of bevacizumab for treatment of glioblastoma may underline this need. Consequently, QSM stands to improve the monitoring of therapy response during follow up examinations under different treatment regimes. Future studies, however, have to clarify if SWI and QSM can contribute to the therapy assessment of glioma patients by assessing SBS within the treatment course of different therapy regimes such as radiation or anti-angiogenic therapies.

Currently, QSM has several limitations that future research must overcome in order to fully integrate it into clinical routine. First, it is currently not possible to reliably calculate susceptibility values at the outer surface region of the cortex and the outer CSF spaces due to loss of information associated with the phase data pre-processing [35]. Second, voxels with unreliable GRE phase information, e.g., due to low signal-to-noise ratio (SNR) or partial volume effects may produce non-local artifacts in the resulting susceptibility maps. Partial volume effects of intratumoral susceptibility variations and cerebral veins may occur if spatial resolution is traded against acquisition time. Though QSM profits from higher spatial resolution [41], Figure 4 suggests that tumor-related SBS can obviously be reliably detected based on 3 T GRE data that is routinely acquired in the course of SWI. Furthermore, the applied QSM technique neglects effects of diffusion due to variations in magnetic susceptibility which have been shown to influence the gradient-echo MRI signal [42,43].

Analyzing the magnetic field variations induced by the magnetic susceptibility distribution on GRE phase images is another approach to classify isolated spherical susceptibility variations into diamagnetic or paramagnetic lesions, indicating blood deposits and calcifications, respectively [44,45,46,47]. Interpretation based solely upon phase images, however, does not permit reliable classification of arbitrarily shaped susceptibility variations. This is due to the non-local relation between phase and the underlying magnetic susceptibility distribution as well as due to the strong dependence of phase on geometry and orientation of the object to the static magnetic field [35,48]. As known from the observed tumor-related SBS, glioblastoma exhibit arbitrarily shaped susceptibility variations. Thus, only the conversion of properly pre-processed phase information into quantitative magnetic susceptibility maps can provide reliable differentiation between brain lesions of blood products or calcium [30].

In conclusion, quantitative susceptibility mapping (QSM) uses the conventional 3D GRE data that is routinely acquired in the course of the established susceptibility weighted imaging protocol and, thus, requires no additional scan time. Clinically, QSM provides a novel quantitative MRI contrast that enables reliable differentiation between tumor-related calcification and blood products. As calcifications appear promising as a biomarker for evaluating patient response and outcome in the treatment of glioblastoma, it is anticipated that QSM will influence differential diagnosis of enhancing brain lesions, progression-assessment, understanding of pathophysiology, and ultimately daily clinical decision making.

Acknowledgments

This research was funded by the German Research Foundation (DFG, RE 1123/9-2) and by a Carl Zeiss Foundation dissertation fellowship for Ferdinand Schweser. We are grateful to Ryan Topfer for proofreading the manuscript.

Author Contributions

Conceived and designed the experiments: AD F. Schweser AR. Performed the experiments: AD F. Schweser AR. Analyzed the data: AD F. Schweser AR. Contributed reagents/materials/analysis tools: AD F. Schweser BW MA MR F. Sahm WW AMN SH HPS MB JRR AR. Wrote the paper: AD F. Schweser MA MR F. Sahm WW AMN SH HPS MB JRR AR.

References

1. Wen PY, Kesari S (2008) Malignant gliomas in adults. N Engl J Med 359: 492–507.
2. Wong ET, Hess KR, Gleason MJ, Jaeckle KA, Kyritsis AP, et al. (1999) Outcomes and prognostic factors in recurrent glioma patients enrolled onto phase II clinical trials. J Clin Oncol 17: 2572–2578.
3. Kim HS, Jahng GH, Ryu CW, Kim SY (2009) Added value and diagnostic performance of intratumoral susceptibility signals in the differential diagnosis of solitary enhancing brain lesions: preliminary study. AJNR Am J Neuroradiol 30: 1574–1579.
4. Toh CH, Wei KC, Chang CN, Hsu PW, Wong HF, et al. (2012) Differentiation of Pyogenic Brain Abscesses from Necrotic Glioblastomas with Use of Susceptibility-Weighted Imaging. AJNR Am J Neuroradiol 33(8): 1534–8.
5. Sehgal V, Delproposto Z, Haddar D, Haacke EM, Sloan AE, et al. (2006) Susceptibility-weighted imaging to visualize blood products and improve tumor contrast in the study of brain masses. J Magn Reson Imaging 24: 41–51.
6. Peters S, Knoss N, Wodarg F, Cnyrim C, Jansen O (2012) Glioblastomas vs. Lymphomas: More Diagnostic Certainty by Using Susceptibility-Weighted Imaging (SWI). Rofo 184(8):713–8.
7. Park SM, Kim HS, Jahng GH, Ryu CW, Kim SY (2010) Combination of high-resolution susceptibility-weighted imaging and the apparent diffusion coefficient: added value to brain tumour imaging and clinical feasibility of non-contrast MRI at 3 T. Br J Radiol 83: 466–475.
8. Reichenbach JR, Venkatesan R, Schillinger DJ, Kido DK, Haacke EM (1997) Small vessels in the human brain: MR venography with deoxyhemoglobin as an intrinsic contrast agent. Radiology 204: 272–277.
9. Haacke EM, Xu Y, Cheng YC, Reichenbach JR (2004) Susceptibility weighted imaging (SWI). Magn Reson Med 52: 612–618.
10. Reichenbach JR, Haacke EM (2001) High-resolution BOLD venographic imaging: a window into brain function. NMR Biomed 14: 453–467.
11. Li C, Ai B, Li Y, Qi H, Wu L (2010) Susceptibility-weighted imaging in grading brain astrocytomas. Eur J Radiol 75: e81–85.
12. Sedlacik J, Kutschbach C, Rauscher A, Deistung A, Reichenbach JR (2008) Investigation of the influence of carbon dioxide concentrations on cerebral physiology by susceptibility-weighted magnetic resonance imaging (SWI). Neuroimage 43: 36–43.
13. Pinker K, Noebauer-Huhmann IM, Stavrou I, Hoeftberger R, Szomolanyi P, et al. (2008) High-field, high-resolution, susceptibility-weighted magnetic resonance imaging: improved image quality by addition of contrast agent and higher field strength in patients with brain tumors. Neuroradiology 50: 9–16.
14. Rauscher A, Sedlacik J, Barth M, Haacke EM, Reichenbach JR (2005) Nonnvasive assessment of vascular architecture and function during modulated blood oxygenation using susceptibility weighted magnetic resonance imaging. Magn Reson Med 54: 87–95.
15. Rauscher A, Sedlacik J, Fitzek C, Walter B, Hochstetter A, et al. (2005) High resolution susceptibility weighted MR-imaging of brain tumors during the application of a gaseous agent. Rofo 177: 1065–1069.
16. Park MJ, Kim HS, Jahng GH, Ryu CW, Park SM, et al. (2009) Semiquantitative assessment of intratumoral susceptibility signals using non-contrast-enhanced high-field high-resolution susceptibility-weighted imaging in patients with gliomas: comparison with MR perfusion imaging. AJNR Am J Neuroradiol 30: 1402–1408.
17. Radbruch A, Wiestler B, Kramp L, Lutz K, Baumer P, et al. (2012) Differentiation of glioblastoma and primary CNS lymphomas using susceptibility weighted imaging. Eur J Radiol 2012 Dec 10 [Epub ahead of print].
18. Kraus JA, Lamszus K, Glesmann N, Beck M, Wolter M, et al. (2001) Molecular genetic alterations in glioblastomas with oligodendroglial component. Acta Neuropathol 101: 311–320.

19. He J, Mokhtari K, Sanson M, Marie Y, Kujas M, et al. (2001) Glioblastomas with an oligodendroglial component: a pathological and molecular study. J Neuropathol Exp Neurol 60: 863–871.
20. Nakamura H, Makino K, Kuratsu J (2011) Molecular and clinical analysis of glioblastoma with an oligodendroglial component (GBMO). Brain Tumor Pathol 28: 185–190.
21. Louis DW, Ohgaki H; Wiestler · OD, Cavenee WK (Eds.) (2007) WHO Classification of Tumours of the Central Nervous System. IARC: Lyon.
22. Hilton DA, Penney M, Pobereskin L, Sanders H, Love S (2004) Histological indicators of prognosis in glioblastomas: retinoblastoma protein expression and oligodendroglial differentiation indicate improved survival. Histopathology 44: 555–560.
23. Salvati M, Formichella AI, D'Elia A, Brogna C, Frati A, et al. (2009) Cerebral glioblastoma with oligodendrogliomal component: analysis of 36 cases. J Neurooncol 94: 129–134.
24. Bahr O, Hattingen E, Rieger J, Steinbach JP (2011) Bevacizumab-induced tumor calcifications as a surrogate marker of outcome in patients with glioblastoma. Neuro Oncol 13: 1020–1029.
25. Oot RF, New PF, Pile-Spellman J, Rosen BR, Shoukimas GM, et al. (1986) The detection of intracranial calcifications by MR. AJNR Am J Neuroradiol 7: 801–809.
26. Tsuchiya K, Makita K, Furui S, Nitta K (1993) MRI appearances of calcified regions within intracranial tumours. Neuroradiology 35: 341–344.
27. Anderson HC (1980) Calcification processes. Pathol Annu 15: 45–75.
28. Spees WM, Yablonskiy DA, Oswood MC, Ackerman JJ (2001) Water proton MR properties of human blood at 1.5 Tesla: magnetic susceptibility, T(1), T(2), T*(2), and non-Lorentzian signal behavior. Magn Reson Med 45: 533–542.
29. Plyavin YA, Blum EY (1984) Magnetic parameters of blood cells and high gradient paramagnetic and diamagnetic phoresis. Magnetohydrodynamics 19: 349–359.
30. Schweser F, Deistung A, Lehr BW, Reichenbach JR (2010) Differentiation between diamagnetic and paramagnetic cerebral lesions based on magnetic susceptibility mapping. Med Phys 37: 5165–5178.
31. Griswold MA, Jakob PM, Heidemann RM, Nittka M, Jellus V, et al. (2002) Generalized autocalibrating partially parallel acquisitions (GRAPPA). Magn Reson Med 47: 1202–1210.
32. Roemer PB, Edelstein WA, Hayes CE, Souza SP, Mueller OM (1990) The NMR phased array. Magn Reson Med 16: 192–225.
33. Hammond KE, Lupo JM, Xu D, Metcalf M, Kelley DA, et al. (2008) Development of a robust method for generating 7.0 T multichannel phase images of the brain with application to normal volunteers and patients with neurological diseases. Neuroimage 39: 1682–1692.
34. Schofield MA, Zhu Y (2003) Fast phase unwrapping algorithm for interferometric applications. Opt Lett 28: 1194–1196.
35. Schweser F, Deistung A, Lehr BW, Reichenbach JR (2011) Quantitative imaging of intrinsic magnetic tissue properties using MRI signal phase: an approach to in vivo brain iron metabolism? Neuroimage 54: 2789–2807.
36. Schweser F, Sommer K, Atterbury M, Deistung A, Lehr BW, et al. (2011) On the impact of regularization and kernel type on SHARP-corrected GRE phase images.; 2011 7–13 May; Montreal, QC, Canada. 2267.
37. Schweser F, Sommer K, Deistung A, Reichenbach JR (2012) Quantitative susceptibility mapping for investigating subtle susceptibility variations in the human brain. Neuroimage 2012 Sep; 62(3): 2083–100.
38. Lehr BW SF, Deistung A, Güllmar D, Reichenbach J R (2011) McCS - Integrating prototype processing programs into clinical routine. Proc Intl Soc Mag Reson Med 19 p. 2553.
39. Wang Y, Li S, Chen L, You G, Bao Z, et al. (2012) Glioblastoma with an oligodendroglioma component: distinct clinical behavior, genetic alterations, and outcome. Neuro Oncol 14: 518–525.
40. Abayomi O, Chun MS, Kelly K (1990) Cerebral calcification and learning disabilities following cranial irradiation for medulloblastoma. J Natl Med Assoc 82: 833–836.
41. Haacke EM, Tang J, Neelavalli J, Cheng YC (2010) Susceptibility mapping as a means to visualize veins and quantify oxygen saturation. J Magn Reson Imaging 32: 663–676.
42. Ziener CH, Bauer WR, Jakob PM (2005) Transverse relaxation of cells labeled with magnetic nanoparticles. Magn Reson Med 54: 702–706.
43. Ziener CH KT, Melkus G, Herold V, Weber T, Reents G, et al. (2007) Local frequency density of states around field inhomogeneities in magnetic resonance imaging: effects of diffusion. Phys Rev (2007) E 76, 031915.
44. Deistung A, Mentzel HJ, Rauscher A, Witoszynskyj S, Kaiser WA, et al. (2006) Demonstration of paramagnetic and diamagnetic cerebral lesions by using susceptibility weighted phase imaging (SWI). Z Med Phys 16: 261–267.
45. Deistung A, Rauscher A, Sedlacik J, Witoszynskyj S, Reichenbach JR (2008) Informatics in Radiology: GUIBOLD: a graphical user interface for image reconstruction and data analysis in susceptibility-weighted MR imaging. Radiographics 28: 639–651.
46. Yamada N, Imakita S, Sakuma T, Takamiya M (1996) Intracranial calcification on gradient-echo phase image: depiction of diamagnetic susceptibility. Radiology 198: 171–178.
47. Gronemeyer SA, Langston JW, Hanna SL, Langston JW Jr (1992) MR imaging detection of calcified intracranial lesions and differentiation from iron-laden lesions. J Magn Reson Imaging 2: 271–276.
48. Schafer A, Wharton S, Gowland P, Bowtell R (2009) Using magnetic field simulation to study susceptibility-related phase contrast in gradient echo MRI. Neuroimage 48: 126–137.

5

ErbB2 and NFκB Overexpression as Predictors of Chemoradiation Resistance and Putative Targets to Overcome Resistance in Muscle-Invasive Bladder Cancer

Fumitaka Koga[1*¶], Soichiro Yoshida[1¶], Manabu Tatokoro[1], Satoru Kawakami[1], Yasuhisa Fujii[1], Jiro Kumagai[2], Len Neckers[3], Kazunori Kihara[1]

1 Department of Urology, Tokyo Medical and Dental University Graduate School, Tokyo, Japan, **2** Department of Surgical Pathology, Tokyo Medical and Dental University Graduate School, Tokyo, Japan, **3** Urologic Oncology Branch, National Cancer Institute, Bethesda, Maryland, United States of America

Abstract

Radical cystectomy for muscle-invasive bladder cancer (MIBC) patients frequently impairs their quality of life (QOL) due to urinary diversion. To improve their QOL, a bladder-sparing alternative strategy using chemoradiation has been developed. In bladder-sparing protocols, complete response (CR) to induction chemoradiation is a prerequisite for bladder preservation and favorable survival. Thus predicting chemoradiation resistance and overcoming it would increase individual MIBC patients' chances of bladder preservation. The aim of this study is to investigate putative molecular targets for treatment aimed at improving chemoradiation response. Expression levels of erbB2, NFκB, p53, and survivin were evaluated immunohistochemically in pretreatment biopsy samples from 35 MIBC patients in whom chemoradiation sensitivity had been pathologically evaluated in cystectomy specimens, and associations of these expression levels with chemoradiation sensitivity and cancer-specific survival (CSS) were investigated. Of the 35 patients, 11 (31%) achieved pathological CR, while tumors in the remaining 24 patients (69%) were chemoradiation-resistant. Multivariate analysis identified erbB2 and NFκB overexpression and hydronephrosis as significant and independent risk factors for chemoradiation resistance with respective relative risks of 11.8 ($P = 0.014$), 15.4 ($P = 0.024$) and 14.3 ($P = 0.038$). The chemoradiation resistance rate was 88.5% for tumors overexpressing erbB2 and/or NFκB, but only 11.1% for those negative for both ($P < 0.0001$). The 5-year CSS rate was 74% overall. Through multivariate analysis, overexpression of erbB2 and/or NFκB was identified as an independent risk factor for bladder cancer death with marginal significance (hazard ratio 21.5, $P = 0.056$) along with chemoradiation resistance ($P = 0.003$) and hydronephrosis ($P = 0.018$). The 5-year CSS rate for the 11 patients achieving pathological CR was 100%, while that for the 24 with chemoradiation-resistant disease was 61% ($P = 0.018$). Thus, erbB2 and NFκB overexpression are relevant to chemoradiation resistance and are putative targets aimed at overcoming chemoradiation resistance in MIBC.

Editor: Eliana Saul Furquim Werneck Abdelhay, Instituto Nacional de Câncer, Brazil

Funding: This work was supported, in part, by grants-in-aids for scientific research (19791102, 19791103), from the Ministry of Education, Culture, Sports, Science and Technology of Japan. The funders had no role in study design, data collection and analysis, decision to publish, or preparation of the manuscript. No additional external funding received for this study.

Competing Interests: The authors have declared that no competing interests exist.

* E-mail: f-koga.uro@tmd.ac.jp

¶ These authors contributed equally to this work.

Introduction

Bladder cancer is the 5th most common cancer in the US, with 70,530 new patients and 14,680 deaths recorded in 2010 [1]. Muscle-invasive bladder cancer (MIBC) accounts for one-third of all bladder cancer cases [2]. Radical cystectomy is the reference standard of care for patients with MIBC, but urinary diversion, which must be performed concurrently with radical cystectomy, and postsurgical morbidity potentially compromise patients' quality of life. To overcome these issues, bladder-sparing approaches with various modalities have been investigated. Among them, trimodality protocols consisting of transurethral resection (TUR), chemotherapy, and radiotherapy have yielded the most favorable oncological outcomes, with 5-year overall survival rates of 50 to 60%, which are comparable to contemporary survival rates of immediate radical cystectomy series [3,4]. In most chemoradiotherapy (CRT)-based bladder-sparing protocols, patients who achieve complete response (CR) after induction CRT are selectively subjected to consolidative therapies for bladder preservation, whereas those who do not achieve CR are recommended to undergo radical cystectomy [5]. In addition, the response to induction CRT has a strong impact on the survival of MIBC patients regardless of subsequent radical cystectomy with curative intent [6,7]. Thus, the ability to predict non-CR patients and the development of a novel strategy to improve their response to CRT would increase the chances of bladder preservation and potentially improve survival outcomes in MIBC patients.

A number of translational studies have been conducted to identify molecular markers that predict therapeutic response to chemotherapy and/or radiotherapy in patients with MIBC or more advanced forms of the disease. Several molecules and genetic modifications have been identified as predictors of CRT response in MIBC [8,9,10,11,12]. Yet most studies have focused on predicting CRT response without also specifically attempting to improve CRT response by targeting the molecules responsible for CRT resistance.

The aim of the current study is to identify putative molecular targets to improve CRT sensitivity and thereby to improve patient prognosis. Of several molecular markers reportedly predicting unfavorable tumor response to CRT or radiotherapy [8,13,14,15,16,17,18,19,20], those that can be targeted by small molecules or monoclonal antibodies include erythroblastic leukemia viral oncogene homolog 2 (erbB2, also known as HER2/neu) [8], nuclear factor-κB (NFκB) [13,14], mutant p53 [17,18], and survivin [19]. We investigated associations of the expression profiles of these oncoproteins with both CRT sensitivity and cancer-specific survival (CSS) in a cohort of MIBC patients in whom CRT sensitivity of tumors had been pathologically evaluated in cystectomy specimens.

Methods

Ethical statement

The ethical committee of Tokyo Medical and Dental University reviewed and approved the current study protocol (approval number 602). Written informed consent was obtained from all patients whose tumor tissues were examined for expression of CRT resistance-associated proteins.

Patients

Between 1997 and 2008, 162 MIBC patients without clinical metastasis were treated in accordance with our institutional therapeutic protocol, which is described elsewhere [7,21,22]. Briefly, patients underwent transurethral resection (TUR) of bladder tumor and induction CRT consisting of external beam radiotherapy to the small pelvis (40 Gy) and two cycles of concurrent intravenous cisplatin (20 mg/day for 5 days) separated by a three-week interval. When bladder cancer was intravesically localized and did not involve the bladder neck and trigone, and residual disease was clinically absent or present only in a small quantity after induction CRT, the patient could selectively undergo consolidative partial cystectomy with pelvic lymph node dissection for bladder preservation; otherwise radical cystectomy was recommended. Of the 162 patients, 88 who underwent visibly complete TUR before CRT and another 39 who did not undergo cystectomy were excluded. In the remaining 35 patients in whom tumor sensitivity to CRT was assessed pathologically in cystectomy specimens, we investigated clinical and molecular variables relevant to CRT resistance, which was defined as the presence of pathological residual disease (non-CR) in cystectomy specimens.

TNM stage

Clinical stage was determined according to the 2002 TNM system [23] based on findings obtained through TUR, bimanual examination and CT of the chest, abdomen and pelvis. MRI of the pelvis was also included starting in 2007.

Follow-up

Patients were followed essentially at 3-month intervals for the first 2 years, at 6-month intervals for the following 3 years, and yearly thereafter. Evaluations consisted of medical history, physical examination, complete blood counts and blood chemistry, and CT of the chest, abdomen and pelvis. Urine cytology, cystoscopy and pelvic MRI were added for bladder-spared patients. Survival intervals were calculated from the first day of CRT to the date of death.

Immunohistochemistry

Immunostaining was performed as previously described [24] using formalin-fixed paraffin-embedded tumor tissues obtained at TUR before induction CRT. Primary antibodies used were prediluted rabbit polyclonal anti-erbB2 antibody (Dako Cytomation, Glostrup, Denmark; at 1:300), rabbit monoclonal antibody against survivin (Cell Signaling Technology, Danvers, MA, USA; at 1:200), mouse monoclonal antibody against p53 (Pab1801; at 1:40) and NFκB p65 (F-6; Santa Cruz Biotechnology, Santa Cruz, CA, USA; at 1:100). Percentages of tumor cells positive for immunostaining were scored. Since NFκB p65 exerts its oncogenic properties as a nuclear transcription factor, nuclear immunoreactivity was evaluated as positive. The slides were reviewed at a magnification of ×200 by two independent observers (Y.S. and J.K.) who were blinded to clinicopathological data. In cases of observer disagreement, a final decision was made by consensus between the two observers.

Statistical Analysis

Differences between groups were assessed using the Chi-square test for categorical data. Cut-off values of continuous variables best predicting CRT resistance were determined by partition analysis. Risk factors for CRT resistance and bladder cancer death were evaluated using logistic regression analysis and the Cox proportional hazard model, respectively. In multivariate analysis, variables were selected using the backward stepwise method. Survival curves were plotted using the Kaplan-Meier method and their differences were assessed by log-rank test. These statistical analyses were performed using JMP 8.0 statistical software (SAS Institute, Cary, NC, USA). Differences were considered significant at $P < 0.05$.

Results

Baseline statistics of the 35 eligible patients are listed in Table 1. All MIBCs comprised high-grade urothelial carcinomas. Four (11%) underwent partial cystectomy as consolidative therapy for bladder preservation while 31 (89%) underwent radical cystectomy. Of the 35 patients, 11 (31%) achieved pathological CR; of the remaining 24 patients with CRT-resistant MIBC, pathological T stages were Tis in 2 (6%), T1 in 8 (23%), T2 in 4 (11%), T3 in 9 (26%), and T4a in 1 (3%). Pathological lymph node metastasis was found in 3 patients (9%).

Immunoreactivity for erbB2, NFκB, p53, and survivin was observed in 20 (57%), 16 (46%), 25 (71%), and 28 patients (80%), respectively (Figure 1). The cut-off value of immunoreactivity that best predicted clinical CRT resistance was 20% for erbB2, NFκB, and survivin. For p53, a previously reported cut-off value of 10% was used [25].

Among the clinical and molecular variables listed in Table 1, univariate analysis revealed that erbB2 overexpression was significantly associated with CRT resistance ($P = 0.003$, Table 2); NFκB overexpression, the presence of hydronephrosis, and tumor size ≥5 cm were also associated with CRT resistance despite not reaching statistical significance ($P = 0.055$, 0.056, and 0.075, respectively). Multivariate analysis identified erbB2 and NFκB overexpression and the presence of hydronephrosis as significant and independent risk factors for CRT resistance, with respective relative risks of 11.8 ($P = 0.014$), 15.4 ($P = 0.024$) and 14.3 ($P = 0.038$, Table 2). Neither p53 nor survivin was significantly associated with CRT resistance. Ability to predict CRT resistance was strengthened when data on the expression of both erbB2 and NFκB were used; the CRT resistance rate was 88.5% among tumors overexpressing erbB2 and/or NFκB but only 11.1%

Table 1. Baseline statistics of the 35 MIBC patients who underwent induction CRT followed by cystectomy.

Variables	**No. of patients (%)**
Gender	
Female	15 (43)
Male	20 (57)
Median (range) age, years	71 (45-83)
Clinical T stage	
T2	14 (40)
T3	18 (51)
T4a	3 (9)
Tumor size	
<5 cm	17 (49)
≥5 cm	18 (51)
Multifocality	
No	12 (34)
Yes	23 (66)
Presence of CIS	
No	28 (80)
Yes	7 (20)
Presence of hydronephrosis	
No	23 (66)
Yes	12 (34)
Pathological T stage of cystectomy specimens	
T0	11 (31)
Tis/1/2	2 (6)/8 (23)/4 (11)
T3/4a	9 (26)/1 (3)
Pathological N stage	
N0	32 (91)
N1/2	2 (6)/1 (3)
ErbB2	
Negative (<20%)	15 (43)
Positive (≥20%)	20 (57)
NFκB	
Negative (<20%)	23 (66)
Positive (≥20%)	12 (34)
p53	
Negative (<10%)	10 (29)
Positive (≥10%)	25 (71)
Survivin	
Negative (<20%)	7 (20)
Positive (≥20%)	28 (80)

among those negative for both (P <0.0001). Thus, erbB2 and NFκB overexpression are relevant to CRT resistance in MIBC.

During the follow-up period (median 60 months, range 19-104), 10 patients died of bladder cancer. The 5-year CSS rate was 74%. Clinicopathological and molecular variables associated with bladder cancer death are listed in Table 3. Univariate analysis revealed that CRT resistance and the presence of hydronephrosis were significantly associated with bladder cancer death (P=0.003 and 0.008, respectively). Multivariate analysis revealed that CRT resistance was the strongest and most independent risk factor

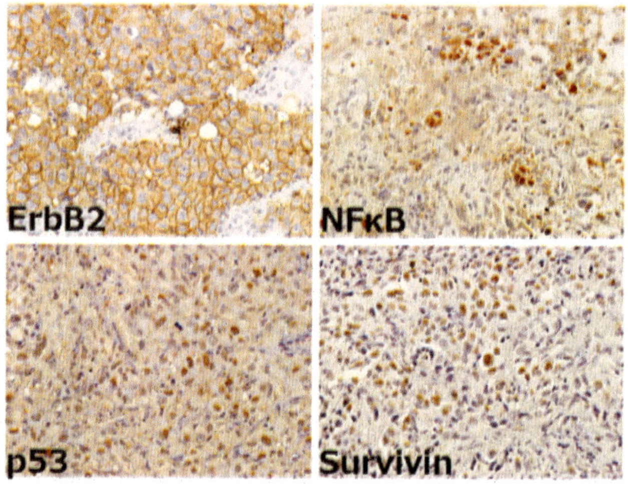

Figure 1. Representative microphotographs of MIBC positive for erbB2 (upper left), NFκB (upper right), p53 (lower left), and survivin (lower right). Reduced from ×400.

(P=0.003) followed by the presence of hydronephrosis (P=0.018). Overexpression of ErbB2 and/or NFκB was also identified as an independent risk factor for bladder cancer death with marginal statistical significance (P=0.056). The 5-year CSS rate among the 11 patients with pathological CR was 100%, while that for the remaining 24 with CRT-resistant MIBC was 61% (P=0.018). Thus high sensitivity to CRT is associated with excellent survival outcomes among MIBC patients.

Discussion

The current study showed that erbB2 and NFκB overexpression play a potential role in CRT resistance and are independently associated with unfavorable CSS with marginal significance in MIBC patients treated with induction CRT plus cystectomy. This indicates that erbB2 and NFκB are putative therapeutic targets for treatments aimed at improving CRT sensitivity in MIBC. This is the first study to demonstrate the relationship between NFκB overexpression and CRT resistance in MIBC and the potential prognostic impact of a combined expression profile of erbB2 and NFκB in patients treated with induction CRT and cystectomy. As we and others have demonstrated, a better response to CRT is associated with more favorable survival outcomes [4,7,26]. Thus, enhancing CRT sensitivity by targeting erbB2 and NFκB may improve survival times among patients treated with CRT.

ErbB2 is a member of the epidermal growth factor receptor (EGFR) family of receptor tyrosine kinases, which generate a complex program of signal transduction events that modulates cell proliferation, differentiation, invasion, and survival [27]. Unlike EGFR, erbB2 does not have its own ligand; instead, it heterodimerizes with other activated EGFR members to enhance and prolong their signaling. In cancer cells overexpressing erbB2 due to gene amplification, high basal autophosphorylation of erbB2 promotes oncogenic activities including metastasis and therapeutic resistance [27]. According to previous reports on MIBC, erbB2 overexpression is an independent risk factor for cancer death in patients undergoing radical cystectomy [28] and an independent predictor of non-CR after CRT but not a risk factor for cancer death in patients treated with CRT [8]. The results of our study are consistent with those of the latter study, theoretically supporting the adjunctive use of erbB2 inhibitors to improve CRT sensitivity.

Table 2. Risk factors predicting CRT resistance.

Variables	Univariate		Multivariate	
	CRT resistance rate (%)	***P* value**	**RR**	***P* value**
Gender		0.28		0.062
Female	80.0		7.79	
Male	60.0		1	
Age		0.17		
<71	81.3			
≥71	57.9			
Clinical T stage		0.28		
T2	57.1			
T3-4a	76.2			
Tumor size		0.075		
<5 cm	52.9			
≥5 cm	83.3			
Multifocality		0.71		
No	75.0			
Yes	65.2			
Presence of CIS		1.00		
No	67.9			
Yes	71.4			
Presence of hydronephrosis		0.056		0.038
No	56.5		1	
Yes	91.7		14.3	
ErbB2		0.003		0.014
Negative (<20%)	46.7		1	
Positive (≥20%)	85.0		11.8	
NFκB		0.055		0.024
Negative (<20%)	56.5		1	
Positive (≥20%)	91.7		15.4	
p53		0.45		
Negative (<10%)	80.0			
Positive (≥10%)	64.0			
Survivin		1.00		
Negative (<20%)	71.4			
Positive (≥20%)	67.9			
Combination of erbB2 and NFκB		<0.0001		-
Dual negative	11.1			
Single or dual positive	88.5			

RR, relative risk.

Table 3. Risk factors predicting bladder cancer death.

	Univariate		Multivariate	
Variables	**HR**	***P* value**	**HR**	***P* value**
Gender		0.94		
Female vs Male	1.05			
Age		0.80		
<71 vs ≥71	1.18			
Clinical T stage		0.057		
T3-4a vs 2	3.91			
Tumor size		0.37		
≥5 cm vs <5 cm	1.78			
Multifocality		0.20		
Yes vs No	2.54			
Presence of CIS		0.32		
Yes vs No	0.40			
Presence of hydronephrosis		0.008		0.018
Yes vs No	5.71		5.56	
ErbB2		0.97		
Positive vs Negative	1.03			
NFκB		0.24		
Positive vs Negative	2.13			
Combination of erbB2 and NFκB		0.19		0.056
Single or dual positive vs dual negative	3.26		21.5	
p53		0.53		
Positive vs Negative	0.64			
Survivin		0.30		
Positive vs Negative	0.46			
CRT resistance		0.003		0.003
Yes vs No	6.9×10^7		5.2×10^6	

HR, hazard ratio.

NFκB is a transcription factor involved in cellular response to various extracellular stimuli such as stress and cytokines [29]. In cancer cells, NFκB is often activated aberrantly, promoting the invasion, metastasis, and survival of these cells. Indeed, NFκB overexpression is associated with poor prognosis in various malignancies including MIBC [30] and with CRT resistance in esophageal cancer [13,14]. The current study showed that NFκB overexpression is closely related to CRT resistance in MIBC and that, in cooperation with erbB2 overexpression, it potentially affects the prognoses of MIBC patients treated with induction CRT and cystectomy. These results strengthen the case for a putative role of NFκB inhibitors, of which many types are under clinical investigation [29], in overcoming CRT resistance in MIBC overexpressing NFκB.

The current study indicates that both erbB2 and NFκB are putative targets for treatments to overcome CRT resistance in MIBC. Among the small molecules currently being investigated in clinical studies, heat shock protein 90 (Hsp90) inhibitors can simultaneously block the activity of both of these oncoproteins [31]. Hsp90 is a ubiquitous molecular chaperone required for the stability and function of numerous client proteins, including a number of oncoproteins essential for the acquisition and maintenance of cancer hallmarks [31,32,33]. Hsp90 inhibitors destabilize Hsp90 clients by dissociating Hsp90-Hsp90 client complexes and thereby exerting antitumor activity [34]. Since both erbB2 and inhibitor of κB kinase β (IKKβ), which mediates NFκB activation, are Hsp90 client proteins [31], adjunctive use of Hsp90 inhibitors is expected to efficiently sensitize MIBCs overexpressing erbB2 and/or NFκB to CRT. Indeed, we have confirmed that low-dose Hsp90 inhibitors effectually potentiate the effects of CRT on bladder cancer cells overexpressing erbB2 and NFκB in preclinical models [35].

In most bladder-sparing protocols for MIBC, CR after induction CRT is a prerequisite for bladder preservation; patients with residual disease are at higher risk for bladder cancer death despite undergoing salvage radical cystectomy [4,7,26]. This is the reason why CRT resistance was stringently defined as pathological non-CR in the current study. When CRT resistance was instead defined as the presence of disease at pathological stage T2 or greater remaining in a cystectomy specimen, overexpression of survivin (with a cut-off value of 40%) was also identified as an independent predictor of CRT resistance. Survivin, a member of the inhibitor of apoptosis protein family, is reportedly associated with local failure in high-grade T1 bladder cancer patients treated with CRT [19]. Recently, a small molecule inhibiting survivin has been identified and is now in clinical trials [36]. This compound is also expected to sensitize MIBC to CRT in clinical settings.

The current study has some limitations including a small cohort size, selection bias, and its retrospective nature. To precisely assess CRT sensitivity in cystectomy specimens from patients who had visible tumors before CRT, only 35 out of 162 patients were eligible for analysis. The fact that statistically significant results were obtained despite such a small number of subjects might be attributed to the stringent selection of subjects for analysis. A prospective study in a larger cohort is needed to validate the findings obtained in the current retrospective study.

In conclusion, erbB2 and NFκB overexpression are relevant to CRT resistance of MIBC, and overexpression of at least one of these oncoproteins potentially increases the risk for cancer death in MIBC patients treated with induction CRT and cystectomy. ErbB2 and NFκB are potential targets for treatment to overcome CRT resistance of MIBC.

Author Contributions

Conceived and designed the experiments: FK KK. Performed the experiments: SY MT JK. Analyzed the data: FK SY SK YF LN. Wrote the paper: FK SY.

References

1. Jemal A, Siegel R, Xu J, Ward E (2010) Cancer statistics, 2010. CA Cancer J Clin 60: 277–300.
2. Lee R, Droller MJ (2000) The natural history of bladder cancer. Implications for therapy. Urol Clin North Am 27: 1–13, vii.
3. Krause FS, Walter B, Ott OJ, Haberle L, Weiss C, et al. (2011) 15-year survival rates after transurethral resection and radiochemotherapy or radiation in bladder cancer treatment. Anticancer Res 31: 985–990.
4. Rodel C, Weiss C, Sauer R (2006) Trimodality treatment and selective organ preservation for bladder cancer. J Clin Oncol 24: 5536–5544.
5. Shipley WU, Kaufman DS, Tester WJ, Pilepich MV, Sandler HM (2003) Overview of bladder cancer trials in the Radiation Therapy Oncology Group. Cancer 97: 2115–2119.
6. Sandler HM, Mirhadi AJ (2010) Current status of radiation therapy for bladder cancer. Expert Rev Anticancer Ther 10: 895–901.
7. Koga F, Yoshida S, Kawakami S, Kageyama Y, Yokoyama M, et al. (2008) Low-dose chemoradiotherapy followed by partial or radical cystectomy against muscle-invasive bladder cancer: an intent-to-treat survival analysis. Urology 72: 384–388.
8. Chakravarti A, Winter K, Wu CL, Kaufman D, Hammond E, et al. (2005) Expression of the epidermal growth factor receptor and Her-2 are predictors of favorable outcome and reduced complete response rates, respectively, in patients with muscle-invading bladder cancers treated by concurrent radiation and cisplatin-based chemotherapy: a report from the Radiation Therapy Oncology Group. Int J Radiat Oncol Biol Phys 62: 309–317.
9. Kawashima A, Nakayama M, Kakuta Y, Abe T, Hatano K, et al. (2011) Excision repair cross-complementing group 1 may predict the efficacy of chemoradiation therapy for muscle-invasive bladder cancer. Clin Cancer Res 17: 2561–2569.
10. Matsumoto H, Matsuyama H, Fukunaga K, Yoshihiro S, Wada T, et al. (2004) Allelic imbalance at 1p36 may predict prognosis of chemoradiation therapy for bladder preservation in patients with invasive bladder cancer. Br J Cancer 91: 1025–1031.
11. Matsumoto H, Wada T, Fukunaga K, Yoshihiro S, Matsuyama H, et al. (2004) Bax to Bcl-2 ratio and Ki-67 index are useful predictors of neoadjuvant chemoradiation therapy in bladder cancer. Jpn J Clin Oncol 34: 124–130.
12. Rodel C, Grabenbauer GG, Rodel F, Birkenhake S, Kuhn R, et al. (2000) Apoptosis, p53, bcl-2, and Ki-67 in invasive bladder carcinoma: possible predictors for response to radiochemotherapy and successful bladder preservation. Int J Radiat Oncol Biol Phys 46: 1213–1221.
13. Izzo JG, Correa AM, Wu TT, Malhotra U, Chao CK, et al. (2006) Pretherapy nuclear factor-kappaB status, chemoradiation resistance, and metastatic progression in esophageal carcinoma. Mol Cancer Ther 5: 2844–2850.
14. Izzo JG, Malhotra U, Wu TT, Ensor J, Luthra R, et al. (2006) Association of activated transcription factor nuclear factor kappa B with chemoradiation resistance and poor outcome in esophageal carcinoma. J Clin Oncol 24: 748–754.
15. Lara PC, Perez S, Rey A, Santana C (1999) Apoptosis in carcinoma of the bladder: relation with radiation treatment results. Int J Radiat Oncol Biol Phys 43: 1015–1019.
16. Lara PC, Rey A, Santana C, Afonso JL, Diaz JM, et al. (1998) The role of Ki67 proliferation assessment in predicting local control in bladder cancer patients treated by radical radiation therapy. Radiother Oncol 49: 163–167.
17. Moonen L, Ong F, Gallee M, Verheij M, Horenblas S, et al. (2001) Apoptosis, proliferation and p53, cyclin D1, and retinoblastoma gene expression in relation to radiation response in transitional cell carcinoma of the bladder. Int J Radiat Oncol Biol Phys 49: 1305–1310.
18. Ong F, Moonen LM, Gallee MP, ten Bosch C, Zerp SF, et al. (2001) Prognostic factors in transitional cell cancer of the bladder: an emerging role for Bcl-2 and p53. Radiother Oncol 61: 169–175.
19. Weiss C, von Romer F, Capalbo G, Ott OJ, Wittlinger M, et al. (2009) Survivin expression as a predictive marker for local control in patients with high-risk T1 bladder cancer treated with transurethral resection and radiochemotherapy. Int J Radiat Oncol Biol Phys 74: 1455–1460.
20. Wijkstrom H, Tribukait B (1990) Deoxyribonucleic acid flow cytometry in predicting response to radical radiotherapy of bladder cancer. J Urol 144: 646–650; discussion 650-651.
21. Koga F, Kihara K, Fujii Y, Yoshida S, Saito K, et al. (2009) Favourable outcomes of patients with clinical stage T3N0M0 bladder cancer treated with induction low-dose chemo-radiotherapy plus partial or radical cystectomy vs immediate radical cystectomy: a single-institutional retrospective comparative study. BJU Int 104: 189–194.
22. Koga F, Kihara K, Yoshida S, Yokoyama M, Saito K, et al. (2011) Selective bladder-sparing protocol consisting of induction low-dose chemoradiotherapy plus partial cystectomy with pelvic lymph node dissection against muscle-invasive bladder cancer: oncological outcomes of the initial 46 patients. BJU Int. [Epub ahead of print].
23. Sobin LH, Wittekind C, eds (2002) Classification of Malignant Tumours. 6th ed. New York: Wiley-Liss.
24. Koga F, Kawakami S, Fujii Y, Saito K, Ohtsuka Y, et al. (2003) Impaired p63 expression associates with poor prognosis and uroplakin III expression in invasive urothelial carcinoma of the bladder. Clin Cancer Res 9: 5501–5507.
25. Esrig D, Spruck CH, 3rd, Nichols PW, Chaiwun B, Steven K, et al. (1993) p53 nuclear protein accumulation correlates with mutations in the p53 gene, tumor grade, and stage in bladder cancer. Am J Pathol 143: 1389–1397.
26. Rodel C, Grabenbauer GG, Kuhn R, Papadopoulos T, Dunst J, et al. (2002) Combined-modality treatment and selective organ preservation in invasive bladder cancer: long-term results. J Clin Oncol 20: 3061–3071.
27. Marmor MD, Skaria KB, Yarden Y (2004) Signal transduction and oncogenesis by ErbB/HER receptors. Int J Radiat Oncol Biol Phys 58: 903–913.
28. Kruger S, Weitsch G, Buttner H, Matthiensen A, Bohmer T, et al. (2002) HER2 overexpression in muscle-invasive urothelial carcinoma of the bladder: prognostic implications. Int J Cancer 102: 514–518.
29. Lin Y, Bai L, Chen W, Xu S (2010) The NF-kappaB activation pathways, emerging molecular targets for cancer prevention and therapy. Expert Opin Ther Targets 14: 45–55.
30. Levidou G, Saetta AA, Korkolopoulou P, Papanastasiou P, Gioti K, et al. (2008) Clinical significance of nuclear factor (NF)-kappaB levels in urothelial carcinoma of the urinary bladder. Virchows Arch 452: 295–304.
31. Trepel J, Mollapour M, Giaccone G, Neckers L (2010) Targeting the dynamic HSP90 complex in cancer. Nat Rev Cancer 10: 537–549.
32. Hanahan D, Weinberg RA (2000) The hallmarks of cancer. Cell 100: 57–70.
33. Koga F, Kihara K, Neckers L (2009) Inhibition of cancer invasion and metastasis by targeting the molecular chaperone heat-shock protein 90. Anticancer Res 29: 797–807.
34. Whitesell L, Mimnaugh EG, De Costa B, Myers CE, Neckers LM (1994) Inhibition of heat shock protein HSP90-pp60v-src heteroprotein complex formation by benzoquinone ansamycins: essential role for stress proteins in oncogenic transformation. Proc Natl Acad Sci U S A 91: 8324–8328.
35. Koga F, Yoshida S, Tatokoro M, Kawakami S, Fujii Y, et al. (2011) Potential Role of Heat Shock Protein 90 Inhibitors to Overcome Chemoradiotherapy Resistance Associated with Her-2 and Nf-Kappa B Overexpression in Muscle-Invasive Bladder Cancer. Eur Urol Suppl 10: 167–167.
36. Tolcher AW, Quinn DI, Ferrari A, Ahmann F, Giaccone G, et al. (2011) A phase II study of YM155, a novel small-molecule suppressor of survivin, in castration-resistant taxane-pretreated prostate cancer. Ann Oncol. [Epub ahead of print].

Quantitative CT Variables Enabling Response Prediction in Neoadjuvant Therapy with EGFR-TKIs: Are They Different from Those in Neoadjuvant Concurrent Chemoradiotherapy?

Yousun Chong[1]❡, Jae-Hun Kim[1]❡, Ho Yun Lee[1]*, Yong Chan Ahn[2], Kyung Soo Lee[1], Myung-Ju Ahn[3], Jhingook Kim[4], Young Mog Shim[4], Joungho Han[5], Yoon-La Choi[5]

1 Department of Radiology and Center for Imaging Science, Sungkyunkwan University School of Medicine, Seoul, Korea, **2** Department of Radiation Oncology, Sungkyunkwan University School of Medicine, Seoul, Korea, **3** Division of Hemato-Oncology, Department of Internal Medicine, Sungkyunkwan University School of Medicine, Seoul, Korea, **4** Department of Thoracic Surgery, Sungkyunkwan University School of Medicine, Seoul, Korea, **5** Department of Pathology, Samsung Medical Center, Sungkyunkwan University School of Medicine, Seoul, Korea

Abstract

Background and Purpose: To correlate changes of various CT parameters after the neoadjuvant treatment in patients with lung adenocarcinoma with pathologic responses, focused on their relationship with different therapeutic options, particularly of EGFR-TKI and concurrent chemoradiation therapy (CCRT) settings.

Materials and Methods: We reviewed pre-operative CT images of primary tumors and surgical specimens obtained after neoadjuvant therapy (TKI, n = 23; CCRT, n = 28) from 51 patients with lung adenocarcinoma. Serial changes in tumor volume, density, mass, skewness/kurtosis, and size-zone variability/intensity variability) were assessed from CT datasets. The changes in CT parameters were correlated with histopathologic responses, and the relationship between CT variables and histopathologic responses was compared between TKI and CCRT groups.

Results: Tumor volume, mass, kurtosis, and skewness were significant predictors of pathologic response in CCRT group in univariate analysis. Using multivariate analysis, kurtosis was found to be independent predictor. In TKI group, intensity variability and size-zone variability were significantly decreased in pathologic responder group. Intensity variability was found to be an independent predictor for pathologic response on multivariate analysis.

Conclusions: Quantitative CT variables including histogram or texture analysis have potential as a predictive tool for response evaluation, and it may better reflect treatment response than standard response criteria based on size changes.

Editor: Prasad S. Adusumilli, Memorial Sloan-Kettering Cancer Center, United States of America

Funding: The authors have no support or funding to report.

Competing Interests: The authors have declared that no competing interests exist.

* E-mail: hoyunlee96@gmail.com

❡ These authors contributed equally to this work.

Introduction

Locally advanced non-small cell lung cancer (NSCLC) has a dismal prognosis with a median overall survival (OS) of 25–35 months despite multimodal treatment including radiation therapy (RT), chemotherapy and surgery [1,2]. Induction concurrent chemoradiation therapy (CCRT) is known to result in short-term gross tumor volume reduction, with aggressive locoregional control. Previous studies demonstrated variable responses with volume reduction averaging 38% to 73% [3], with improved survival compared with the treatment of surgery alone [4]. This may be explained by the potent local control effect of irradiation. Therefore, there is a need for studies directed toward predicting treatment benefit versus risk of treatment failure. Clinically, such predictors would allow further individualization of treatment during radiotherapy [5].

On the other hand, during the last decade, several molecular-targeted agents—for example, epidermal growth factor receptor tyrosine kinase inhibitors (EGFR-TKIs) such as erlotinib and gefitinib—have emerged for treatment of NSCLC [6], as well as in the neoadjuvant setting, which has also shown to be effective in a subset of patients with NSCLC [7–10]. Furthermore, although TKI agents are most active in patients with an EGFR mutation, patients without documented mutation still showed survival benefit compared with placebo [9].

With the advancement in imaging techniques and their increasing application to oncology practice, imaging-based tumor volume regression rate evaluated at mid-RT has been shown to predict local control rate and disease-free survival (DFS) after RT or CCRT [11,12]. In addition, quantitative measurement of tumor regression rate becomes more realistic with the use of imaging — particularly during therapy when the morphologic changes remain subtle and difficult to assess by clinical examination [12,13]. Evaluation of treatment response to TKI agents is also challenging. It is well established that the conventional RECIST underestimates response rates than the proportion of patients who actually experience clinically effective disease control [7,10,14–20]. Since TKI agents aim for inhibition of tumor cell growth, but not necessarily tumor cell death, tumor response may not emerge as early decrease in tumor size [19]. Very recently, histogram analysis or texture analysis is receiving attention as a method for quantifying tumor heterogeneity and evaluating treatment response [14,21,22].

Here, the question remains which is more effective to predict treatment response in the various imaging-based quantitative assessment methods, and whether or not each method acts differently depending on therapeutic regimen.

Given the need for clinical validation of any updated analysis tool, our main objectives were to identify differences in serial changes of various CT-based parameters in patients with lung adenocarcinoma scheduled to undergo surgical resection after neoadjuvant therapy, and to correlate those changes with pathologic responses, focused on their relationship with different neoadjuvant therapeutic options, particularly of EGFR-TKI and concurrent chemoradiation therapy (CCRT) settings.

Materials and Methods

The institutional review board of Samsung Medical Center (SMC IRB) approved this retrospective study with a waiver of informed consent.

Patients

From September 2005 through December 2011, 398 patients with stage IIIA NSCLC underwent curative surgical resection of lung cancer at our institution, after neoadjuvant treatment (chemotherapy, radiation therapy, or both). Among these patients, patients with pathologically proven adenocarcinoma were only included, while other histologic subtypes (such as squamous cell carcinoma, large cell carcinoma, small cell lung cancer, neuroendocrine cancer, etc.) were excluded. We subdivided the patients into three groups, depending on different neoadjuvant treatment options: chemotherapy with TKI agents, chemotherapy with conventional agents, and CCRT. Since our interest lay in comparing the imaging parameter changes for treatment response prediction between novel TKI and CCRT as a neoadjuvant option, patients who underwent neoadjuvant chemotherapy with conventional agents were excluded. As a result, two groups of patients were enrolled in our study: patients who underwent neoadjuvant chemotherapy with TKI agents, and those who underwent CCRT. Patients for neoadjuvant TKI agent were assembled from a selected population fulfilling ≥ two of the following features: female, adenocarcinoma, nonsmoker, and Asian. Regimen of TKI group comprised 1 tablet of 150 mg of erlotinib daily for 3 weeks. Neoadjuvant CCRT included chemotherapy and concurrent thoracic radiotherapy (TRT). The chemotherapy regimen was weekly paclitaxel (50 mg/m^2 per week IV) plus cisplatin (25 mg/m^2 per week IV) or weekly paclitaxel (50 mg/m^2 per week IV) plus carboplatin (AUC 1.5/week IV) for 5 weeks. The concurrent TRT dose was 45 Gy over 5 weeks (1.8 Gy/fraction per day, 5 fractions/week). Surgical resection was planned around 6 weeks after the completion of neoadjuvant therapy for CCRT group, and was scheduled in the fourth week after start of treatment for TKI group. Surgical resection involved a radical resection of the tumor, preferably by lobectomy, and regional lymph node dissection.

Ultimately, 51 patients (25 men and 26 women) satisfied our inclusion criteria. Twenty-three patients received neoadjuvant chemotherapy with TKI, while 28 patients underwent concurrent chemoradiation therapy.

Imaging protocol

In all patients, baseline contrast-enhanced CT before treatment commencement, and follow up contrast-enhanced CT after 4–6 weeks of neoadjuvant treatment were performed.

Image data analysis

A thoracic radiologist (Y.C., with 4 years of experience in thoracic CT interpretation) who was unaware of other patient data evaluated the acquired images semiquantitatively. Only the primary tumors were analyzed. Tumors were segmented by drawing a region of interest (ROI) covering as large an area as possible of the whole tumor. Next, voxel-based CT numbers were collected from lesion segmentations. Since the lesions were segmented to cover the entire tumor, larger lesions had more number of segments than smaller lesions.

For tumor density and volume, the computer automatically calculated the density (g/cm^3) from mean attenuation of total voxels and volume (cm^3) by multiplying the number of voxels by the unit volume of a voxel [23]. Tumor mass (in grams) was calculated by multiplying tumor volume (in cubic centimeters) by mean tumor density [24]. Next, a spreadsheet of all of the values was created, which was used to compute histogram distribution parameters of kurtosis and skewness [25]. The skewness and kurtosis were computed from the segmented tumor region. On histograms, skewness represented the distribution pattern of CT attenuation values; negative and positive skewness indicated that the data were more spread to the left and right of the mean, respectively. Kurtosis represented the position of peak height that indicates CT attenuation value of the maximum number of voxels, with leptokurtic indicated by a sharper peak and platykurtic indicated by a flatter peak (Figure 1).

Texture analysis was performed by a radiology physicist (J.H.K.) with four years of experience in radiology physics. Voxel values within the segmented tumors were resampled to yield 16 of discrete values in order to reduce the noise in image and to normalize the intensity across subjects by clustering voxels with similar intensities [26]. From the discrete tumor images (16 gray levels), the gray level size zone matrix was computed. The value of the matrix's (m, n) is defined by the number of homogenous regions given the homogeneous tumor size (n) to their intensity (m). For example, 'Matrix's (3, 5) is 6.' means that there are 6 homogenous regions, in which the grey level of each cluster is 3, and the size of each cluster is 5 voxels. This gray level size zone matrix was used to compute the variability in the size and the intensity of homogeneous tumor regions [26,27].

Pathologic evaluation of treatment response

Pathologic response was used as the reference standard of therapeutic response. An experienced lung pathologist (J.H. with 20 years of experience in lung pathology) retrospectively interpreted entire tissue sections sliced at 5- to 10-mm intervals and measured the proportion (%) of viable tumor cells in the primary tumor of the resected surgical specimens [28]. Tumor regression was scored as 'pathologic response' if more than 50% necrosis was present with morphologic signs of therapy-induced regression or 'no response' when either 0%–50% necrosis or

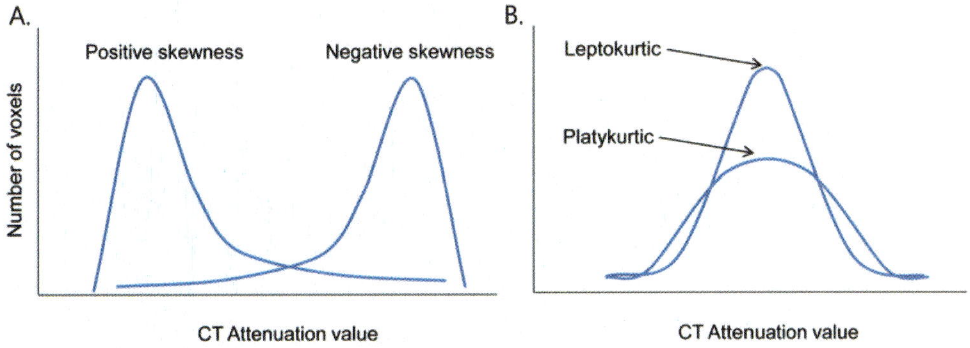

Figure 1. Histogram distributions of CT attenuation value. (a) Skewness. A negative skewness indicates an elongated tail on the left side of the mean, with most values lying to the right of the mean. A positive skewness indicates an elongated tail on the right side of the mean, with most values lying to the left of the mean. (b) Kurtosis. Leptokurtosis indicates a sharper peak, and platykurtosis indicates a flatter peak.

necrosis that could not be attributed to the therapy effect was seen [6]. If more than 90% necrosis was present in the resected specimen, tumor regression was defined as 'near- complete pathologic response' [6].

In addition, comprehensive histologic subtyping was made for the primary tumor in a semi-quantitative manner. Tumors were stratified into the following three grades based on histologically predominant subtypes as: low grade; intermediate grade; and high grade [29,30].

EGFR/KRAS mutational status had been determined by a pathologist (Y.L.C.) by using polymerase chain reaction (PCR) and a direct DNA sequencing method, as previously described [31].

Statistical analysis

Statistical differences between TKI group and CCRT group were analyzed by using either the Mann Whitney test or the Fisher exact test. To identify variables that could be used in differentiating pathologic responders from nonresponders, logistic regression analysis was conducted. Characteristics with a p value of less than 0.50 at univariate analysis were used as the input variables for multiple logistic regression analysis. In multiple logistic regression analysis, a backward stepwise selection mode was used, with iterative entry of variables on the basis of test results ($p < 0.05$). The removal of variables was based on likelihood ratio statistics with a probability of 0.10. ROC analysis was also performed to evaluate the differentiating performance of multiple logistic regression models in discriminating pathologic responders from nonresponders. All analysis was performed using SPSS for Windows, version 12.0 (SPSS, Inc., Chicago, IL).

Results

Baseline characteristics

The TKI group consisted of 23 patients, and the CCRT group included 28 patients. There was a discrepancy in gender distribution and smoking habit, with female predominance(17 out of 23) in the TKI group and male predominance(19 out of 28) in the CCRT group ($p = 0.004$). This was because never smoker females were selected and included in the neoadjuvant TKI treatment planning. Otherwise, all baseline CT and PET features did not show significant difference between the two groups (Table 1). Also, all pathologic and genetic features did not differ significantly in each group.

CT parameters and pathologic response

Percent changes of CT parameters in pathologic responders and pathologic nonresponders were tabulated and compared in both CCRT group and TKI group (Table 2, Figure 2). In case of CCRT group, percent decreases of tumor volume and mass were significantly greater in pathologic responders, as compared with pathologic nonresponders (ps = 0.028 and 0.018, respectively).

As for histogram analysis, in pathologic responders, the lesion showed negative changes in skewness and kurtosis, indicating platykurtosis and negative skewness (Figure 3). Percent changes of kurtosis and skewness were significantly different between pathologic responders and nonresponders in CCRT group (ps = 0.001 and 0.005, respectively), while those were not in TKI group.

On the other hand, in TKI group, intense variability and size-zone variability was significantly decreased in pathologic responders group (ps = 0.005 and 0.003, respectively), as compared with nonresponders (Figure 3). These significant differences were not found in CCRT group. Decrease in intense variability and size-zone variability reflects homogeneous change of vascularity [14,26].

Logistic Regression Analysis and ROC Analysis

In TKI group, intense variability and size-zone variability were used as input variables for multivariate logistic regression analysis. Multivariate analysis disclosed that intense variability was the sole significant predictor of pathologic response ($p = 0.028$; 95% confidence interval: 1.009, 1.184; adjusted odds ratio, 1.093) (Table 3). ROC analysis showed that the area under the ROC curve (AUC) for intense variability was 0.931 and that the optimal cut-off value of percent change of intense variability for predicting pathologic response was less than −6.9 (sensitivity, 92.3%; specificity, 80%).

In CCRT group, tumor volume, mass, kurtosis, and skewness were used as input variables for multivariate logistic regression analysis. Multivariate analysis displayed that kurtosis was the sole significant predictor of pathologic response ($p = 0.009$; 95% confidence interval: 1.026, 1.195; adjusted odds ratio, 1.107) (Table 3). ROC analysis showed that the AUC for kurtosis was 0.943 and that the optimal cut-off value of percent change of kurtosis for predicting pathologic response was less than −23 (sensitivity, 87.5%; specificity, 84.3%).

Discussion

Our study showed various imaging-based quantitative assessment methods worked differently with different therapeutic

Table 1. Clinicopathologic and baseline radiologic characteristics according to the neoadjuvant regimen.

	TKI group (n = 23)	CCRT group (n = 28)	*P* values
Age (y)**	55.6±9.1	56.5±10.5	.732
Gender			**.004***
Male	6 (26)	19 (68)	
Female	17 (74)	9 (32)	
Smoking habit			<.001*
Never	22 (96)	14 (50)	
Ever	1 (4)	14 (50)	
Histology type			
Adenocarcinoma	23 (100)	28 (100)	1.00
Stage			
IIIA	23 (100)	28 (100)	1.00
Baseline CT features			
Volume (cm^3)	22.7±23.8	31.9±47.8	.405
Density	1.13±0.51	1.14±0.34	.458
Mass (g)	25.9±28.1	36.6±55.2	.403
Histogram Analysis			
Kurtosis	35.5±87.5	17.2±11.9	.280
Skewness	−1.91±4.58	−2.42±1.99	.600
Texture Analysis			
Intensity variability	8.00±3.83	6.87± 4.42	.338
Size-zone variability	23.5±10.8	22.7±18.6	.857
Baseline PET features			
SUVmax**	10.3±3.8	12.7±6.5	.180
Pathologic features			
Response			.924
Responder+	10 (43)	12 (43)	
Near complete responder++	4 (17)	7 (25)	
Nonresponder	13 (57)	16 (57)	
Differentiation			.066
Well-	1 (4)	0 (0)	
Moderately-	21 (92)	21 (75)	
Poorly-	1 (4)	7 (25)	
***EGFR* mutation**			.721
Positive	11 (48)	5 (18)	
Negative	10 (43)	6 (21)	
Unknown	2 (9)	17 (61)	
***KRAS* mutation**			.467
Positive	0 (0)	2 (7)	
Negative	7 (30)	6 (21)	
Unknown	16 (70)	20 (72)	

TKI, tyrosine kinase inhibitors; CCRT, concurrent chemoradiation therapy.
Note.—Unless otherwise indicated, data in parentheses are percentages.
* $P < .05$.
** Data are the range.
+Less than 50% of viable tumor cells in the resected specimen.
++Less than 10% of viable tumor cells in the resected specimen.

regimens, particularly of EGFR-TKI setting and CCRT setting. We found tumor volume, mass, kurtosis, and skewness were all significant predictors of pathologic response in CCRT group in univariate analysis. Using multivariate analysis, kurtosis was found to be independent predictor. On the other hand, in TKI group, heterogeneity from texture analysis was an independent predictor for pathologic response. Our results suggest the possible value of adapting various combination of imaging parameters for response evaluation beyond size-based measurement according to the different treatment modality used. Since there is raising request for personalized and optimized therapy, an advanced diagnostic tool to predict treatment response more accurately is required.

Prognostic factors are an essential requirement in the management of NSCLC and this is reflected in recent changes in the TNM staging [32], where each sub-group is indicative of outcome. However, despite such refinements, there remains uncertainty and more predictive data are required. This is particularly true in Stage 3A disease where outcome remains variable [33]. Moreover, the selection and benefit of surgical patients for neo-adjuvant/adjuvant treatment is also unclear [34,35]. It is important that the possible survival benefits of chemoradiation should be balanced by the adverse effects of toxicity to the patient [36]. Through the early identification of patients who will not get a clinical benefit from treatment, patients could be saved from drug toxicity and they could be switched to an alternative treatment earlier. Moreover, there are potential cost savings if drugs are used in only those patients who will benefit from them [14]. Recent additional option of targeted agents makes the situation more complicated. Imaging-defined response assessment (RECIST) is a cornerstone of modern oncologic practice; however, it is limited in a number of targeted therapies, including treatment with TKIs. In a recent study evaluating tumor response to neoadjuvant erlotinib in 60 patients with NSCLC, radiologic response by RECIST was observed in only 5% of the patients, while pathologic response was shown in 23% of the patients [10]. Furthermore, as our figure 2A, the ground-glass opacity component of the tumor may remain at the exact area of pretreatment solid component of the tumor, where volume reduction of the lesion is not significant [19], Therefore, even near complete pathologic response was not predicted by CT-driven RECIST, suggesting that RECIST was suboptimal for short-term radiologic response evaluation. This is because apoptosis, transition of necrosis to fibrosis, or lymphocytic and granulomatous reactions may not result in early decrease in tumor size [10]. These results support the need for development of an optimal imaging parameter for early response evaluation and accurate prediction. In that regard, quantitative CT analysis may be emerging as a potential tool for doing this task.

In the CCRT group, volume decrease was significantly greater in the pathologic responder group, with mean volume reduction of 56.4%. Early volume decrease is achieved by potent locoregional control with cytotoxic effect of irradiation. Volume reduction rate in our study correlates with the results of previous studies [3].

Moreover, skewness and kurtosis could predict pathologic response in the CCRT group. Two values all decreased greater in the pathologic responders, as compared in the nonresponders. Decreased skewness or positive skewness reflects decreased enhancement, which may result from decreased neovascularization.

Meanwhile, CT variables reflecting tumoral heterogeneity were significant prognostic factors for pathologic response in TKI group. A previous study assessing tumor heterogeneity using CT texture in NSCLC patients reported poorer survival in patients who had heterogeneous tumors with low uniformity values [21]. In addition, Tixier et al. analyzed textural features on FDG-PET

Table 2. Percent changes of CT parameters in relation to pathologic response.

	TKI group (n = 23)			CCRT group (n = 28)		
	Pathologic responder	Pathologic nonresponder		Pathologic responder	Pathologic nonresponder	
CT parameters	(n = 10)	(n = 13)	*P* values	(n = 12)	(n = 16)	*P* values
%Volume (cm^3)	-51.5±28.1	-42.5±21.7	.266	-56.4±42.2	-14.3±42.5	**.028***
%Density	-9.5±12.5	-5.1±9.7	.349	-8.5±11.8	-5.1±12.1	.209
%Mass (g)	-56.9±23.7	-40.0±31.9	.095	-61.8±36.2	-17.9±43.7	**.018***
Histogram Analysis						
%Kurtosis	-27.7±47.8	-18.4±36.9	.605	-48.0±23.1	1.7±38.6	**.001***
%Skewness	-26.8±39.8	-22.4±29.1	.760	-34.2±28.9	-1.7±26.9	**.005***
Texture Analysis						
%Intensity variability	-35.3±31.3	21.6±50.7	**.005***	92.1±33.3	60.4±81.5	.689
%Size-zone variability	-50.2±23.7	-1.3±40.9	**.003***	-32.9±21.5	-28.0±32.6	.652

TKI, tyrosine kinase inhibitors; CCRT, concurrent chemoradiation therapy.
Note.—Data are mean ± standard deviation of the percent change n the given parameter.
* $P < .05$.

images in patients with esophageal cancer who underwent concomitant chemoradiation therapy, and found textural features can predict responders (complete and partial) better than can SUV [26]. In their study regional tumor heterogeneity represented by intensity and size-zone variability was a significant predictor of response, rather than global measurement including SUV. Similar results were found in our study, in which intensity variability was a significant independent predictor for pathologic response in patients treated with neoadjuvant TKI agents. Significantly decreased intensity variability and size-zone variability in the pathologic responder group reflects increased tumoral homogeneity, including homogeneous change of vascularity. However, these texture parameters were not helpful in predicting response in the CCRT group. Such reasoning may be explained in part by the difference in pharmagophysiologic reactions according different treatment regimens.

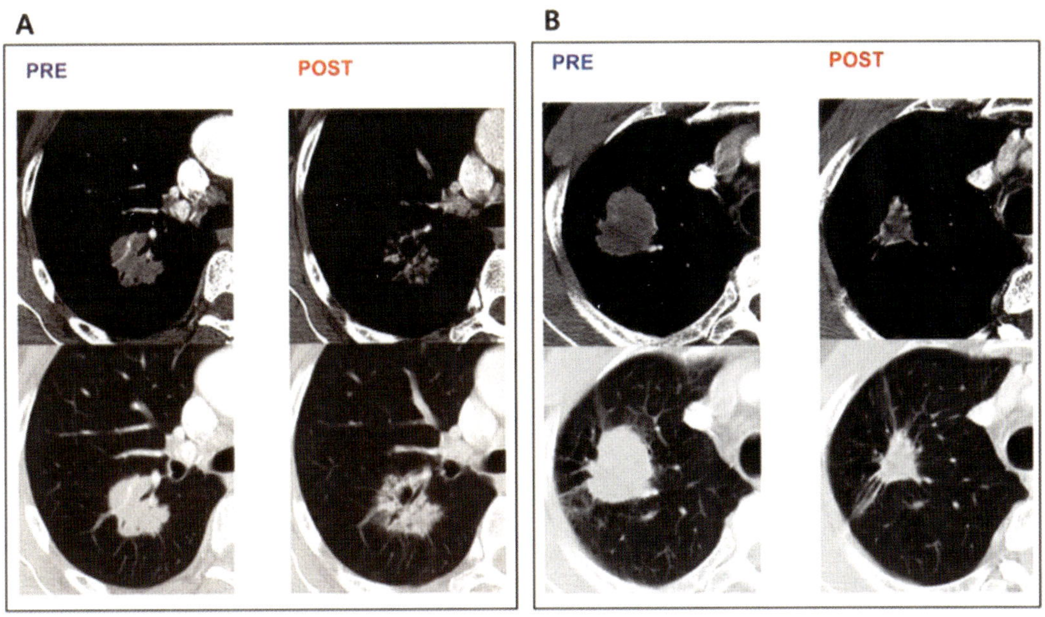

Figure 2. Quantitative CT parameters of pathologic responder. (a) Combined histogram distributions of the treatment before (blue) and after (red). As for histogram distribution, the vertical axis in each histogram shows the number of pixels in the segmented tumor. The horizontal axis shows the CT attenuation values. Attenuation value is shifted to the left from the blue to the red graph. (b) Intensity size-zone matrix of the treatment before (blue) and after (red). The horizontal axis shows size of homogenous area. Divergent distribution on the horizontal axis indicates increased size-zone variability. The vertical axis shows intensity. Divergent distribution on the vertical axis indicates increased intensity variability. Distributions of the points on the matrix become more convergent and clustered both in the horizontal axis and the vertical axis from the pre-treatment matrix to the post-treatment matrix.

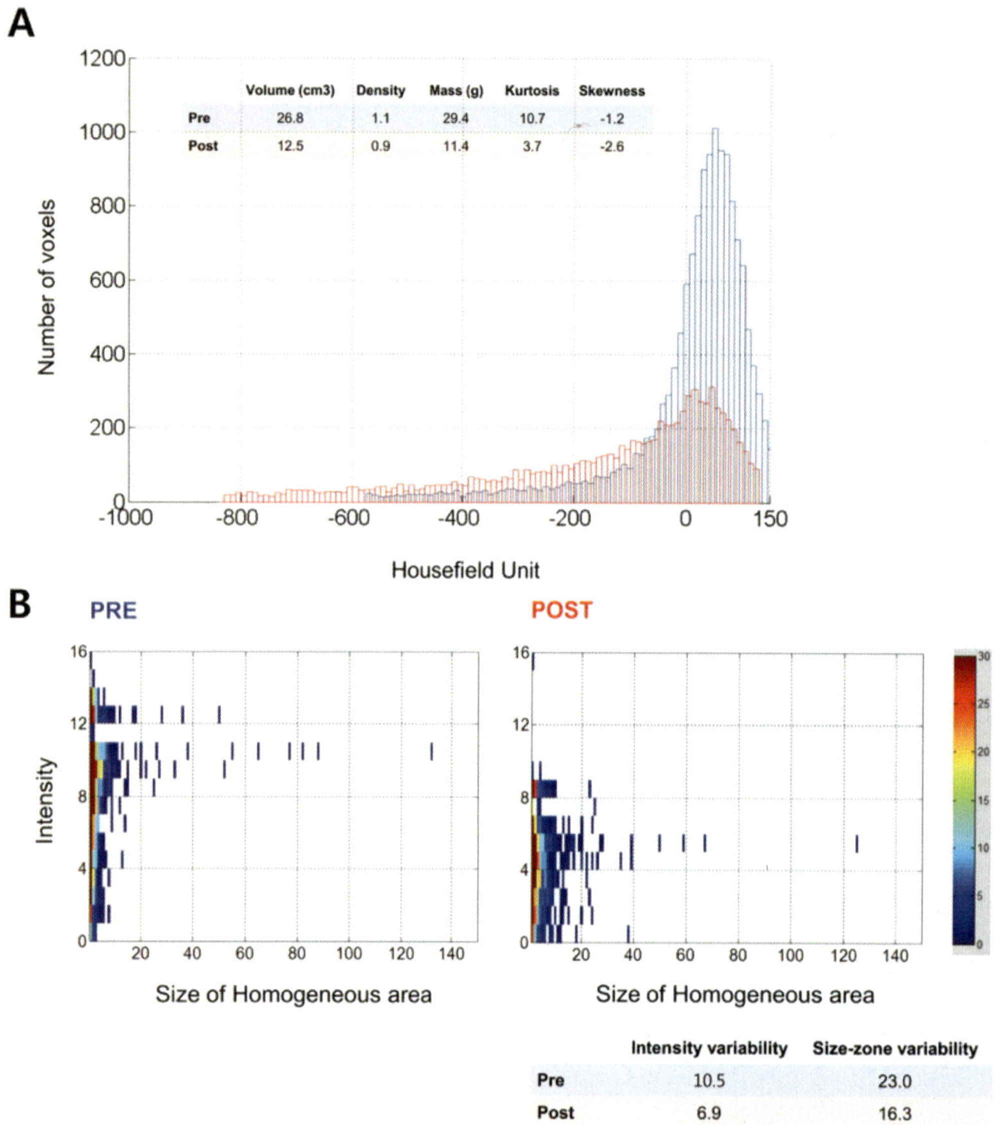

Figure 3. CT images of TKI group and CCRT group. (a) A 56-year-old woman with lung adenocarcinoma who underwent neoadjuvant treatment with EGFR-TKI. Pretreatment CT scans on mediastinal and lung window images show a lobulating sold mass. CT scans obtained after treatment show that the ground-glass opacity component of lesion is remaining on lung window image at the exact area of pretreatment solid component, and reduction of the lesion extent is not significant, (b) A 68-year-old man with lung adenocarcinoma who underwent neoadjuvant treatment with CCRT. Pretreatment CT scans on mediastinal and lung window images show a lobulating sold mass. CT scans obtained after treatment show significant volume reduction of the tumor.

Some authors explain potential significance of tumoral heterogeneity by correlation with genomic heterogeneity [36]. It has recently been shown that a genomic heterogeneity exists within tumors, and this observation has significant implications for Darwinist theories of tumor resistance [37]. Whether textural heterogeneity on imaging relates to underlying genomics would be important to investigate. Given the challenges and expense of measuring tumor genomic signatures, then imaging may be more viable option. Another possible meaning is the possible relationship between tumor heterogeneity and hypoxia. It has been recently shown that tumor textural analysis was associated with tumor hypoxia on histological examinations from NSCLC patients who were administered intravenous pimonidazole prior to surgery [38]. Hypoxia is a recognized marker of poor outcome, and as such, a positive relationship between tumor hypoxia and tumor heterogeneity would be biologically consistent. Additional potential merit of texture analysis is that texture methods can quantify the spatial variations in parametric maps, not the absolute values of the maps. Therefore, texture analysis can provide additional and independent information compared to histogram-based measures of parametric maps [39].

A potential limitation of our study is its retrospective design. However, the majority of baseline characteristics did not differ between the two study populations. Even though there was considerable difference in gender distribution and smoking habit, this occurred because never smoker females were enrolled in the neoadjuvant TKI agent treatment arm, in the clinical setting. A relatively small number of patients were included in our study. Further studies with a larger sample size are necessary for validation of our results. Since tumor regions of interest (ROI)

Table 3. Logistic regression analysis of CT variables for predicting pathologic response.

	Variables	Odds ratio	95% CI	P value
TKI group	Intensity variability	**1.093**	**1.009, 1.184**	**0.028**
	Size-zone variability	1.026	0.980, 1.075	0.270
CCRT group	Tumor volume (cm^3)	1.188	0.441, 3.202	0.733
	Tumor mass (g)	0.855	0.320, 2.286	0.756
	Kurtosis	**1.092**	**1.028, 1.160**	**0.004**
	Skewness	1.001	0.919, 1.090	0.982

TKI, tyrosine kinase inhibitors; CCRT, concurrent chemoradiation therapy; AUC, area under the curve; CI, confidence interval.

were drawn manually by a single operator, inter- and intra-observer variation may be present. Assistance of an automated software tool could improve this limitation, and furthermore help decrease the time consumed in the tedious work. Despite limitations in our study, it presented novel methodologies that went beyond the traditional size-based analytical method, to evaluate treatment outcomes in NSCLC patients. Our study provides a proof-of-concept that a multiparametric image-feature-based approach holds promise in planning individualized treatment, and that prospective clinical trials may be warranted to better understand the extent of this approach [5].

In conclusion, quantitative CT variables including histogram analysis or texture analysis has potential as a predictive biomarker, and it may better reflect treatment response than standard response criteria based on size change. Also, different combinations of imaging parameters may be correlated to physiologic processes occurring after various different treatment modalities.

Author Contributions

Conceived and designed the experiments: YC JHK HYL. Performed the experiments: JHK KSL YCA MJA JK YMS JH YLC. Analyzed the data: YC JHK. Contributed reagents/materials/analysis tools: JHK YLC. Wrote the paper: YC JHK HYL KSL YCA MJA JK YMS JH YLC.

References

1. Ahn HK, Choi YL, Han JH, Ahn YC, Kim K, et al. (2013) Epidermal growth factor receptor mutation and treatment outcome of mediastinoscopic N2 positive non-small cell lung cancer patients treated with neoadjuvant chemoradiotherapy followed by surgery. Lung Cancer 79: 300–306.
2. Park BB, Park JO, Kim H, Ahn YC, Choi YS, et al. (2006) Is trimodality approach better then bimodality in stage IIIA, N2 positive non-small cell lung cancer? Lung Cancer 53: 323–330.
3. Kozak MM, Murphy JD, Schipper ML, Donington JS, Zhou L, et al. (2011) Tumor volume as a potential imaging-based risk-stratification factor in trimodality therapy for locally advanced non-small cell lung cancer. J Thorac Oncol 6: 920–926.
4. Katakami N, Tada H, Mitsudomi T, Kudoh S, Senba H, et al. (2012) A phase 3 study of induction treatment with concurrent chemoradiotherapy versus chemotherapy before surgery in patients with pathologically confirmed N2 stage IIIA nonsmall cell lung cancer (WJTOG9903). Cancer 118: 6126–6135.
5. Vaidya M, Creach KM, Frye J, Dehdashti F, Bradley JD, et al. (2012) Combined PET/CT image characteristics for radiotherapy tumor response in lung cancer. Radiother Oncol 102: 239–245.
6. Aukema TS, Kappers I, Olmos RA, Codrington HE, van Tinteren H, et al. (2010) Is 18F-FDG PET/CT useful for the early prediction of histopathologic response to neoadjuvant erlotinib in patients with non-small cell lung cancer? J Nucl Med 51: 1344–1348.
7. Dingemans AM, de Langen AJ, van den Boogaart V, Marcus JT, Backes WH, et al. (2011) First-line erlotinib and bevacizumab in patients with locally advanced and/or metastatic non-small-cell lung cancer: a phase II study including molecular imaging. Ann Oncol 22: 559–566.
8. Sunaga N, Tomizawa Y, Yanagitani N, Iijima H, Kaira K, et al. (2007) Phase II prospective study of the efficacy of gefitinib for the treatment of stage III/IV non-small cell lung cancer with EGFR mutations, irrespective of previous chemotherapy. Lung Cancer 56: 383–389.
9. O'Brien ME, Myerson JS, Coward JI, Puglisi M, Trani L, et al. (2012) A phase II study of (1)(8)F-fluorodeoxyglucose PET-CT in non-small cell lung cancer patients receiving erlotinib (Tarceva); objective and symptomatic responses at 6 and 12 weeks. Eur J Cancer 48: 68–74.
10. Schaake EE, Kappers I, Codrington HE, Valdes Olmos RA, Teertstra HJ, et al. (2012) Tumor response and toxicity of neoadjuvant erlotinib in patients with early-stage non-small-cell lung cancer. J Clin Oncol 30: 2731–2738.
11. Johnson CR, Thames HD, Huang DT, Schmidt-Ullrich RK (1995) The tumor volume and clonogen number relationship: tumor control predictions based upon tumor volume estimates derived from computed tomography. Int J Radiat Oncol Biol Phys 33: 281–287.
12. Mayr NA, Taoka T, Yuh WT, Denning LM, Zhen WK, et al. (2002) Method and timing of tumor volume measurement for outcome prediction in cervical cancer using magnetic resonance imaging. Int J Radiat Oncol Biol Phys 52: 14–22.
13. Hong JH, Chen MS, Lin FJ, Tang SG (1992) Prognostic assessment of tumor regression after external irradiation for cervical cancer. Int J Radiat Oncol Biol Phys 22: 913–917.
14. Goh V, Ganeshan B, Nathan P, Juttla JK, Vinayan A, et al. (2011) Assessment of response to tyrosine kinase inhibitors in metastatic renal cell cancer: CT texture as a predictive biomarker. Radiology 261: 165–171.
15. Shim JH, Lee HC, Kim SO, Shin YM, Kim KM, et al. (2012) Which response criteria best help predict survival of patients with hepatocellular carcinoma following chemoembolization? A validation study of old and new models. Radiology 262: 708–718.
16. William WN, Jr., Pataer A, Kalhor N, Correa AM, Rice DC, et al. (2013) Computed tomography RECIST assessment of histopathologic response and prediction of survival in patients with resectable non-small-cell lung cancer after neoadjuvant chemotherapy. J Thorac Oncol 8: 222–228.
17. Zhao B, Oxnard GR, Moskowitz CS, Kris MG, Pao W, et al. (2010) A pilot study of volume measurement as a method of tumor response evaluation to aid biomarker development. Clin Cancer Res 16: 4647–4653.
18. Kang H, Lee HY, Lee KS, Kim JH (2012) Imaging-based tumor treatment response evaluation: review of conventional, new, and emerging concepts. Korean J Radiol 13: 371–390.
19. Lee HY, Lee KS, Ahn MJ, Hwang HS, Lee JW, et al. (2011) New CT response criteria in non-small cell lung cancer: proposal and application in EGFR tyrosine kinase inhibitor therapy. Lung Cancer 73: 63–69.
20. Lee HY, Lee KS, Hwang HS, Lee JW, Ahn MJ, et al. (2010) Molecularly targeted therapy using bevacizumab for non-small cell lung cancer: a pilot study for the new CT response criteria. Korean J Radiol 11: 618–626.
21. Ganeshan B, Panayiotou E, Burnand K, Dizdarevic S, Miles K (2012) Tumour heterogeneity in non-small cell lung carcinoma assessed by CT texture analysis: a potential marker of survival. Eur Radiol 22: 796–802.
22. Baek HJ, Kim HS, Kim N, Choi YJ, Kim YJ (2012) Percent change of perfusion skewness and kurtosis: a potential imaging biomarker for early treatment response in patients with newly diagnosed glioblastomas. Radiology 264: 834–843.
23. de Hoop B, Gietema H, van de Vorst S, Murphy K, van Klaveren RJ, et al. (2010) Pulmonary ground-glass nodules: increase in mass as an early indicator of growth. Radiology 255: 199–206.
24. Lee HY, Jeong JY, Lee KS, Kim HJ, Han J, et al. (2012) Solitary pulmonary nodular lung adenocarcinoma: correlation of histopathologic scoring and patient survival with imaging biomarkers. Radiology 264: 884–893.
25. Chandarana H, Rosenkrantz AB, Mussi TC, Kim S, Ahmad AA, et al. (2012) Histogram analysis of whole-lesion enhancement in differentiating clear cell from papillary subtype of renal cell cancer. Radiology 265: 790–798.
26. Tixier F, Le Rest CC, Hatt M, Albarghach N, Pradier O, et al. (2011) Intratumor heterogeneity characterized by textural features on baseline 18F-FDG PET images predicts response to concomitant radiochemotherapy in esophageal cancer. J Nucl Med 52: 369–378.
27. Thibault G, Fertil B, Navarro C, Pereira S, Cau P, et al. (2009) Texture indexes and gray level size zone matrix: application to cell nuclei classification. Pattern Recognition Inf Process: 140–145.
28. Lee HY, Lee HJ, Kim YT, Kang CH, Jang BG, et al. (2010) Value of combined interpretation of computed tomography response and positron emission

tomography response for prediction of prognosis after neoadjuvant chemotherapy in non-small cell lung cancer. J Thorac Oncol 5: 497–503.
29. Kadota K, Colovos C, Suzuki K, Rizk NP, Dunphy MP, et al. (2012) FDG-PET SUVmax combined with IASLC/ATS/ERS histologic classification improves the prognostic stratification of patients with stage I lung adenocarcinoma. Ann Surg Oncol 19: 3598–3605.
30. Lee HY, Jeong JY, Lee KS, Yi CA, Kim BT, et al. (2013) Histopathology of Lung Adenocarcinoma Based on New IASLC/ATS/ERS Classification: Prognostic Stratification With Functional and Metabolic Imaging Biomarkers. J Magn Reson Imaging.
31. Yoon HJ, Lee HY, Lee KS, Choi YL, Ahn MJ, et al. (2012) Repeat biopsy for mutational analysis of non-small cell lung cancers resistant to previous chemotherapy: adequacy and complications. Radiology 265: 939–948.
32. Edge SB, Byrd DR, Compton CC, Fritz AG, Greene FL, et al. (2010) AJCC Cancer Staging Manual New York, NY: Springer.
33. Brunelli A, Charloux A, Bolliger CT, Rocco G, Sculier JP, et al. (2009) ERS/ESTS clinical guidelines on fitness for radical therapy in lung cancer patients (surgery and chemo-radiotherapy). Eur Respir J 34: 17–41.
34. Kamal NS, Soria JC, Mendiboure J, Planchard D, Olaussen KA, et al. (2010) MutS homologue 2 and the long-term benefit of adjuvant chemotherapy in lung cancer. Clin Cancer Res 16: 1206–1215.
35. Waller D, Peake MD, Stephens RJ, Gower NH, Milroy R, et al. (2004) Chemotherapy for patients with non-small cell lung cancer: the surgical setting of the Big Lung Trial. Eur J Cardiothorac Surg 26: 173–182.
36. Win T, Miles K, Janes SM, Ganeshan B, Shastry M, et al. (2013) Tumor Heterogeneity as measured on the CT component of PET/CT Predicts Survival in Patients with Potentially Curable Non-Small Cell Lung Cancer. Clin Cancer Res.
37. Gerlinger M, Rowan AJ, Horswell S, Larkin J, Endesfelder D, et al. (2012) Intratumor heterogeneity and branched evolution revealed by multiregion sequencing. N Engl J Med 366: 883–892.
38. Ganeshan B, Goh V, Mandeville HC, Ng QS, Hoskin PJ, et al. (2013) Non-small cell lung cancer: histopathologic correlates for texture parameters at CT. Radiology 266: 326–336.
39. Alic L, van Vliet M, van Dijke CF, Eggermont AM, Veenland JF, et al. (2011) Heterogeneity in DCE-MRI parametric maps: a biomarker for treatment response? Phys Med Biol 56: 1601–1616.

Regional Variation in Brain White Matter Diffusion Index Changes following Chemoradiotherapy: A Prospective Study Using Tract-Based Spatial Statistics

Christopher H. Chapman[1]*, Mohammad Nazem-Zadeh[1], Oliver E. Lee[2], Matthew J. Schipper[1], Christina I. Tsien[1], Theodore S. Lawrence[1], Yue Cao[1,3,4]

1 Department of Radiation Oncology, University of Michigan, Ann Arbor, Michigan, United States of America, **2** Department of Biostatistics, University of Michigan, Ann Arbor, Michigan, United States of America, **3** Department of Radiology, University of Michigan, Ann Arbor, Michigan, United States of America, **4** Department of Biomedical Engineering, University of Michigan, Ann Arbor, Michigan, United States of America

Abstract

Purpose: There is little known about how brain white matter structures differ in their response to radiation, which may have implications for radiation-induced neurocognitive impairment. We used diffusion tensor imaging (DTI) to examine regional variation in white matter changes following chemoradiotherapy.

Methods: Fourteen patients receiving two or three weeks of whole-brain radiation therapy (RT) ± chemotherapy underwent DTI pre-RT, at end-RT, and one month post-RT. Three diffusion indices were measured: fractional anisotropy (FA), radial diffusivity (RD), and axial diffusivity (AD). We determined significant individual voxel changes of diffusion indices using tract-based spatial statistics, and mean changes of the indices within fourteen white matter structures of interest.

Results: Voxels of significant FA decreases and RD increases were seen in all structures ($p<0.05$), with the largest changes (20–50%) in the fornix, cingula, and corpus callosum. There were highly significant between-structure differences in pre-RT to end-RT mean FA changes ($p<0.001$). The inferior cingula had a mean FA decrease from pre-RT to end-RT significantly greater than 11 of the 13 other structures ($p<0.00385$).

Conclusions: Brain white matter structures varied greatly in their response to chemoradiotherapy as measured by DTI changes. Changes in FA and RD related to white matter demyelination were prominent in the cingula and fornix, structures relevant to radiation-induced neurocognitive impairment. Future research should evaluate DTI as a predictive biomarker of brain chemoradiotherapy adverse effects.

Editor: Wang Zhan, University of Maryland, College Park, United States of America

Funding: This study was supported by National Institutes of Health grants RO1 NS064973 and R21 CA113699. The funders had no role in study design, data collection and analysis, decision to publish, or preparation of the manuscript.

Competing Interests: The authors have declared that no competing interests exist.

* E-mail: chchap@med.umich.edu

Introduction

Radiation therapy for brain neoplasms–with or without chemotherapy–is limited by toxicity to healthy brain tissue, which is not easily predicted by dose alone [1]. One major symptom is neurocognitive impairment, a delayed and irreversible effect characterized by selective declines in short-term memory and attention [2–6]. While this toxicity is thought to be a result of many interacting processes, it is known that brain white matter, composed of axonal fibers and their myelin sheaths, is particularly sensitive to radiation [7]. Radiation therapy-induced white matter degradation has been associated with neurocognitive impairment in animals and humans [2], [8]. However, non-invasive anatomical studies in humans have been difficult in the past, because white matter degradation may not be visible on conventional magnetic resonance imaging (MRI) [2], [9].

Diffusion tensor imaging (DTI) is a non-invasive MRI-based technique that is more sensitive to white matter structure than conventional MRI [10]. DTI measures water molecule diffusion in the brain, which varies with the direction, density, and myelination of white matter fibers. Two derived indices of this measurement are radial diffusivity (RD) and axial diffusivity (AD), which are associated with the magnitudes of diffusion perpendicular and parallel to white matter fibers respectively. Increased RD has been correlated to decreased myelination in several models of brain injury, including radiation-induced demyelination [11–15]. Decreased AD has been correlated to axonal degeneration and radiation-induced reactive astrogliosis [11], [14–16]. Another commonly used diffusion index is fractional anisotropy (FA), a normalized index which ranges from zero (equal diffusion in all directions) to one (diffusion along a single axis only). FA reflects overall white matter density and integrity, and decreased FA has been seen in many brain pathologies [10]. The first uses of DTI to

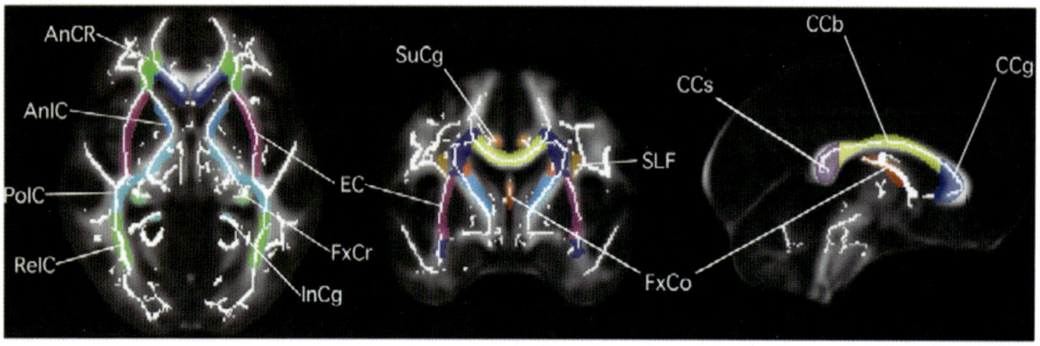

Figure 1. White matter regions of interest. ICBM DTI-81 white matter atlas [33] depicted on FMRIB58 standard-space FA map [35]. Data-derived white matter skeleton mask in white. AnCr, anterior corona radiata; AnIC, anterior internal capsules; PoIC, posterior internal capsules; ReIC, retrolenticular internal capsules; EC, external capsules; FxCr, fornix crura; InCg, inferior cingula; SuCg, superior cingula; SLF, superior longitudinal fasciculi; FxCo, fornix columns; CCs, corpus callosum splenium; CCb, corpus callosum body; CCg, corpus callosum genu. Posterior corona radiata not depicted.

assess chemoradiotherapy effects were in pediatric patients, where a reduction in FA was found without white matter lesions on conventional MRI [17], [18]. Along with preclinical data, this demonstrates that DTI is sensitive to treatment-induced white matter degradation.

DTI's sensitivity to white matter degradation can be used to determine whether there is regional variation in the toxic effects of radiation therapy within the brain. This is important because the brain is currently considered a homogeneous structure for radiation dose-volume calculations and toxicity prediction, but it is not known whether this is accurate [19]. Identifying structures of particular sensitivity to radiation could support proposals of targeted dose-sparing in order to prevent neurocognitive impairment [20], [21]. The majority of current dose-sparing proposals have focused on protecting the hippocampus, including an ongoing phase II clinical trial [22]. Evidence that radiation impairs hippocampal neural stem cell differentiation has advanced the hypothesis that this is the primary mechanism behind late-delayed cognitive decline [23]. Support for neural stem cell-sparing radiation techniques makes the presumption that preserving neurogenesis alone will prevent neurocognitive impairment. However, if the associated white matter is damaged, then the networks that produce neurocognitive functions are not intact. Our approach is to determine whether preferential damage to any white matter structures may also contribute to neurocognitive impairment. Previous studies have compared diffusion indices in pediatric brain radiation patients to controls, and found lower FA in frontal lobe, temporal lobe, and periventricular white matter, demonstrating localized white matter damage [18], [24], [25]. Longitudinal studies have looked at diffusion index changes in a few selected regions [26–30], but there has not yet been a study which has systematically analyzed longitudinal diffusion index changes in whole brain white matter. This information could impartially identify sensitive white matter structures, which would be valuable for developing radiation dose-sparing techniques and imaging biomarkers.

The current study aimed to (i) examine regional variation in white matter chemoradiotherapy sensitivity throughout the whole brain, and (ii) investigate changes in diffusion indices which are influenced by distinct pathological processes. To accomplish this, we obtained diffusion tensor images from brain metastasis patients before and after whole-brain radiation and chemotherapy. Maps of the diffusion indices FA, RD, and AD were calculated for each patient at each time point. Using tract-based spatial statistics (TBSS), we evaluated individual voxel changes in these indices with automated white matter tract finding [31]. We then partitioned these results into volumes representing the major white matter structures in the brain, in order to analyze diffusion index changes within these structures over time. Our final analysis evaluated differences between structures in the magnitude of diffusion index changes, in order to identify regional variation in white matter chemoradiotherapy sensitivity. Completion of these aims is important for better understanding the pathogenesis of treatment-induced toxicity, and designing techniques for predicting and preventing this outcome.

Table 1. Fourteen white matter structures.

White Matter Structure	Paired
Corpus Callosum Body	No
Corpus Callosum Genu	No
Corpus Callosum Splenium	No
Cingula, Inferior	Yes
Cingula, Superior	Yes
Corona Radiata, Anterior	Yes
Corona Radiata, Posterior	Yes
External Capsules	Yes
Fornix Columns	No
Fornix Crura	Yes
Internal Capsules, Anterior	Yes
Internal Capsules, Posterior	Yes
Internal Capsules, Retrolenticular	Yes
Superior Longitudinal Fasiculi	Yes

Materials and Methods

Ethics Statement

A prospective imaging study with human subjects was approved by the Institutional Review Boards of the University of Michigan Medical School (Federal Wide Assurance #00004969). Written informed consent was obtained for all participants.

Table 2. Patient characteristics.

No.	Sex	Age (y)	Dose (Gy)	Chemotherapy	Primary Cancer	Metastases (>5 mm)	Location (lobe)	Scans
1	Male	40	37.5	Bortezomib	Melanoma	2	Left Frontal, Left Occipital	2/3
2	Female	60	37.5	None	Non-small cell lung	0	–	2/3
3	Male	41	37.5	Bortezomib	Melanoma	1	Left Thalamus	3/3
4	Female	52	37.5	Bortezomib	Melanoma	1	Left Parietal	3/3
5	Male	49	30	Bortezomib	Melanoma	2	Left Temporal, Left Temporal	3/3
6	Female	45	30	Bortezomib	Melanoma	1	Right Frontal	3/3
7	Male	52	30	Paclitaxel & Carboplatin	Non-small cell lung	0	-	3/3
8	Female	55	30	Bortezomib	Melanoma	1	Right Frontal	3/3
9	Male	76	30	Bortezomib	Melanoma	1	Left Frontal	3/3
10	Female	64	37.5	Gemcitabine	Non-small cell lung	0	–	3/3
11	Female	57	30	Bortezomib	Melanoma	2	Right Thalamus, Right Occipital	3/3
12	Male	60	30	Bortezomib	Melanoma	2	Left Cerebellum, Right Temporal	3/3
13	Male	43	30	Cetuximab	Squamous cell, tonsil	0	–	3/3
14	Female	66	37.5	None	Non-small cell lung	1	Left Frontal	3/3

Study Design and MRI

Patients with cancer metastatic to the brain received fractionated whole-brain radiation. Radiation was delivered in opposed lateral fields to 30 Gy in 3 Gy daily fractions or 37.5 Gy in 2.5 Gy daily fractions. Treatment dose was calculated at the point of maximum field separation. Patients underwent MRI scans at three time points: within two weeks before starting RT (pre-RT), within one week after finishing RT (end-RT), and one month after finishing RT (one month post-RT). All images were obtained on a 3T Achieva scanner (Phillips, The Netherlands). MRI sequences included diffusion tensor imaging (DTI), T1- and T2-weighted images. DTI was acquired using a spin-echo echo-planar imaging sequence with a repetition time of 7032 ms, echo time of 62 ms, $224\times224\times120$ mm^3 field of view, 128×128 matrix, and $1.75\times1.75\times2.0$ mm^3 voxels with no gap between slices. For each axial slice, diffusion sensitizing gradient encoding with a diffusion weighting factor of $b=1000$ s/mm^2 was applied in 15 non-collinear directions, plus one null image with $b=0$ s/mm^2.

Image Pre-processing and Diffusion Tensor Calculation

All image pre-processing before TBSS analysis was done with FIAT (Functional Imaging Analysis Tool), an in house software package [32]. All diffusion weighted images were registered to the null image of the same series using mutual information and rigid body transformation. Diffusion tensors were then computed at each voxel and eigenvalues were determined, from which three diffusion index maps were generated: axial diffusivity (AD), radial diffusivity (RD), and fractional anisotropy (FA).

Image Selection Criteria

Before analysis, fourteen white matter structures representing the major supratentorial white matter tracts of the brain were selected from the International Consortium of Brain Mapping (ICBM) DTI-81 white matter atlas, which is registered to the ICBM-152 standard-space anatomical template (Table 1; Figure 1) [33]. To choose patients with major white matter tracts free from metastasis influence, FIAT was used to compare the non-diffusion weighted images to the white matter atlas structures by the following steps. All T1- and T2-weighted images were interpolated to 1 mm^3 voxels. T1-weighted images were registered to the ICBM-152 anatomical template by affine transformation [34]. The same transformation matrix was then used to deform the T2-weighted images. Masks of the fourteen white matter structure volumes were overlaid on the template-registered T1- and T2-weighted images, and any patients with non-punctate metastases (defined as >5 mm diameter), edema, or mass effect in the structures at any time point were excluded from further analysis. Punctate metastases (≤5 mm diameter) were permitted in white matter structures if there was no surrounding edema or interval change on T1- and T2-weighted images. The original non-deformed images were used to visually confirm that the structures were free from tumor influence.

Computation of Image Skeletons

The FMRIB Software Library (FSL) was used for the following image processing steps previously explained in detail [31], [35]. Briefly, FA maps from all patients and time points were interpolated to 1 mm^3 voxels and registered to the FMRIB58 standard-space FA image by nonlinear transformation. This target was chosen instead of the "most typical" subject method [31] to minimize potential registration error due to metastases. These co-registered FA maps were averaged to produce a mean FA map. On this mean FA map, the local direction of greatest FA slope was found around each voxel, defining the direction perpendicular to the local white matter tract at each voxel. The voxels representing the local FA maximum along these directions were labeled, producing a one-voxel thick "skeleton" near the center of white matter tracts. The volume of this mean FA skeleton above threshold $FA=0.2$ was then used to create a skeleton mask, in order to exclude minor tracts, non-white matter voxels, and areas of possible misalignment. The skeleton mask was projected using the same voxel assignments back to the original individual FA maps to confirm correct registration of white matter tracts. FA maps for each patient and all time points were then projected onto the skeleton mask by assigning the maximum FA value along the direction perpendicular to the skeleton mask (defined above) to the

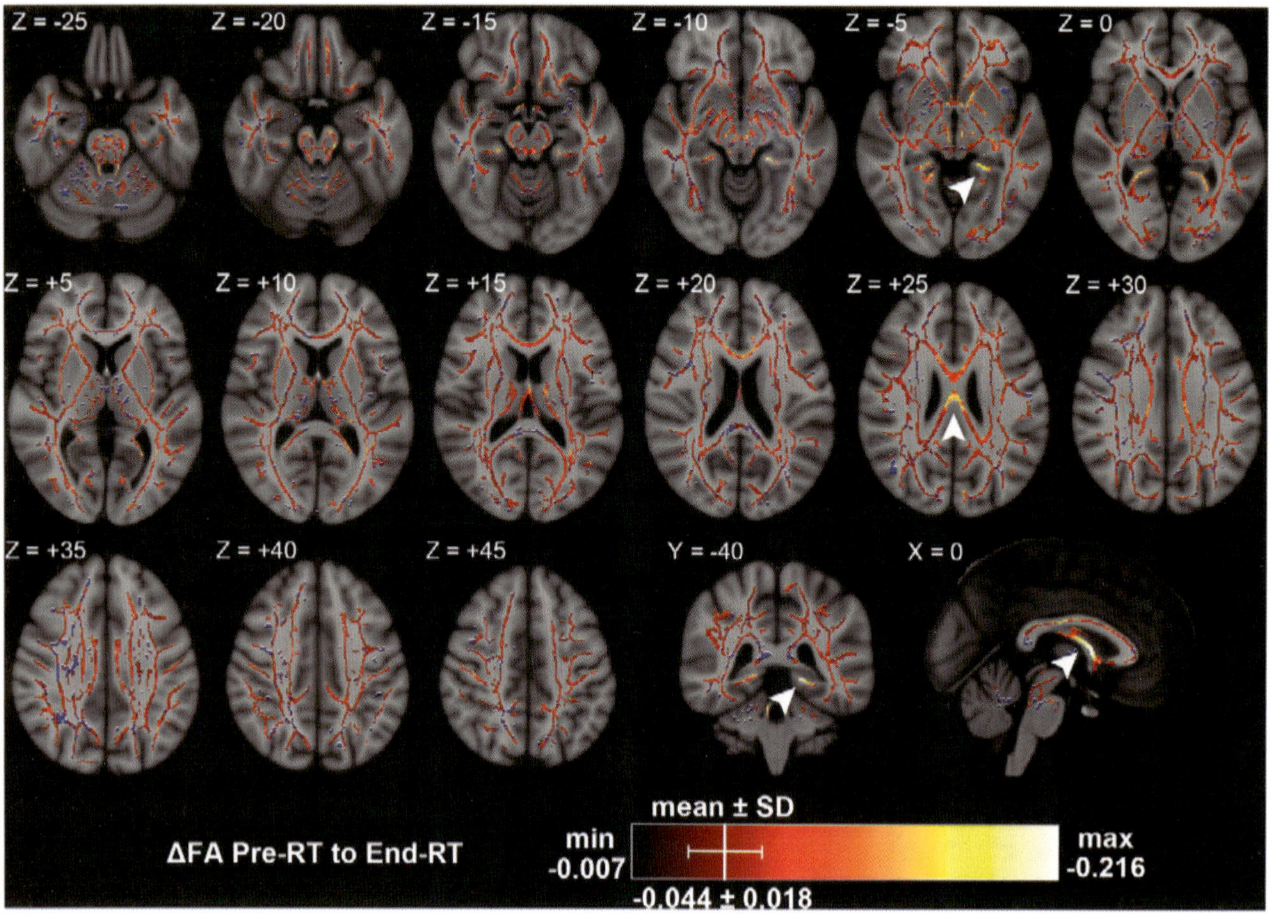

Figure 2. Significant changes in FA from pre-RT to end-RT. Arrowheads: Z = −5, left inferior cingulum; Z = +25, corpus callosum body; Y = −40, left inferior cingulum; X = 0, fornix columns. Significant results per color chart, blue is TBSS skeleton without significant results. Depicted on Montreal Neurological Institute (MNI) ICBM152 standard brain T1-weighted image [34].

nearest skeleton mask voxel. This created a one-to-one voxel correlation between all subjects' FA maps, allowing for individual voxel statistics. The same nonlinear transformation matrices and perpendicular projections were also applied to all AD and RD maps to generate skeletonized forms of these maps as well.

Tract-based Spatial Statistics

Tract-based spatial statistics were performed using FSL. Significant differences in FA, AD, and RD values between all time points (pre-RT to end-RT, pre-RT to one month post-RT, end-RT to one month post-RT) were determined by subject-paired two-sided *t*-tests. Maps of *t* values were augmented with threshold-free cluster enhancement to reduce noise [36], and correction for multiple comparisons was achieved using a non-parametric permutation test with 5000 permutations [37]. Significance level was set at $\alpha = 0.05$. At this point in analysis, all white matter skeleton voxels were used, including those outside the fourteen white matter structures defined above.

Within-Structure Analysis

We identified fourteen volumes of the skeleton mask representing the white matter structures of interest. These were labeled as the spatial intersection between the corresponding ICBM DTI-81 white matter atlas structure and the skeleton mask, with visual confirmation of appropriate fit. Mean values for FA, AD, and RD within each skeletonized structure of interest for all patients and time points were calculated from the voxel values. The longitudinal changes of mean diffusion index values within each structure of interest were calculated for all patients and time intervals (pre-RT to end-RT, pre-RT to one month post-RT, end-RT to one month post-RT). Statistical analysis consisted of two steps. First, significant left-right asymmetries of diffusion index longitudinal changes were determined by subject-paired two-sided *t*-tests. Paired structures were combined where significant asymmetry of diffusion index longitudinal changes did not exist. Second, the significance of the longitudinal changes themselves was determined by subject-paired two-sided *t*-tests. At both steps, corrections for multiple comparisons were performed by a Bonferroni-type sequential procedure to control false discovery rate. A comparison was considered statistically significant when $p_i < \alpha_i$ where p_i is the ith smallest *p*-value from *m* comparisons and $\alpha_i = 0.05i/m$ [38].

Between-Structure Group Analysis

Change in FA from pre-RT to end-RT was chosen as a representative diffusion index and time interval. Mean FA changes were compared between structures using repeated-measures ANOVA in two steps. First, repeated-measures ANOVA was performed with different structures representing the within-subject factor and different patients representing the between-

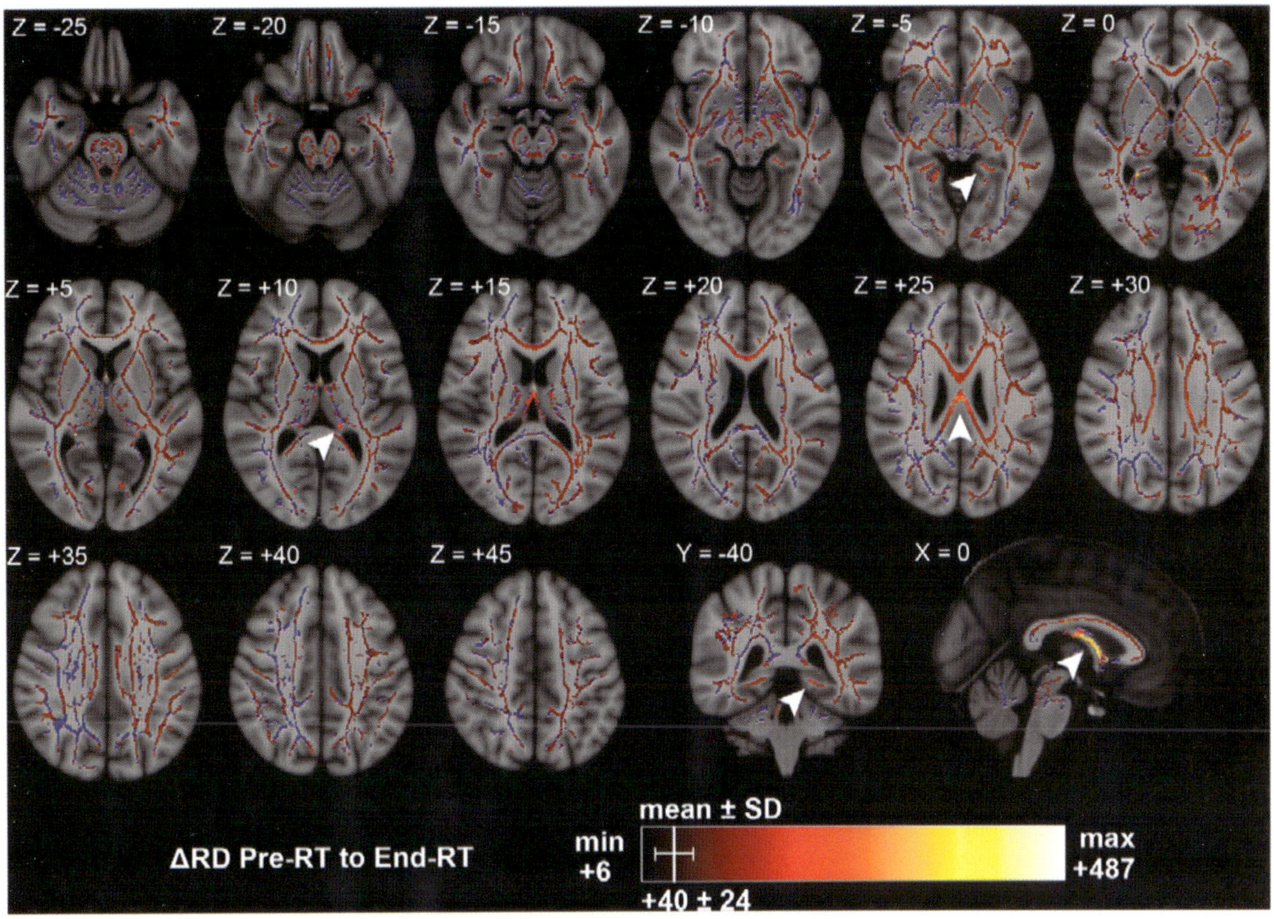

Figure 3. Significant changes in RD from pre-RT to end-RT. Arrowheads: Z = −5, left inferior cingulum; Z = +10, left fornix crus; Z = +25, corpus callosum body; Y = −40, left inferior cingulum; X = 0, fornix columns. Significant results per color chart, blue is TBSS skeleton without significant results. Depicted on MNI ICBM152 standard brain T1-weighted image [34]. Units are $\mu m^2/s$.

subject factor. Additional between-subject dichotomous factors were evaluated: patient age (above and below median age), radiation dose (30 Gy and 37.5 Gy), and sex (male and female). Levene's test and Mauchly's test were used to assess homoscedasticity and sphericity, assumptions of repeated-measures ANOVA. Violation of sphericity was corrected using the Greenhouse-Geisser method to reduce type I error. Significance level was set at $\alpha = 0.05$. Second, post hoc comparisons were performed using subject-paired two-sided *t*-tests to compare mean FA change in the structure with the greatest change to changes in all other structures (thirteen comparisons). For these post hoc comparisons, Bonferroni correction was used with $\alpha = 0.05/13 \approx 0.00385$.

Results

Study Completion and Image Selection

Of thirty-one enrolled patients who underwent imaging at pre-RT, fourteen underwent imaging at end-RT and were free from metastasis influence in the white matter regions of interest, permitting inclusion for analysis (Table 2). Ten of the fourteen included patients had one or fewer non-punctate metastases. These were fairly evenly distributed throughout the brain across patients, minimizing the average effect of tumor influence in any single brain area. Nine patients received bortezomib concurrent with RT on a separate clinical trial, 1.7 mg/m^2 every 72 hours for four doses. Three other patients (7, 10, and 13) received one cycle of chemotherapy between end-RT and one month post-RT. Two patients did not complete imaging at one month post-RT and were excluded from analysis at that time point.

TBSS Voxel Analysis

The white matter skeleton used for individual voxel statistics consisted of 112,388 voxels of 1 mm^3. From pre-RT to end-RT, statistically significant FA decreases were seen in 87.8% of white matter skeleton voxels, representing widespread treatment-induced changes. Of voxels with significant FA decreases, the minimum was −0.007 (−3.1%), the maximum was −0.216 (−34.4%), and the mean was −0.044 with a standard deviation of 0.018 (−9.7±4.2%), a skewed distribution towards larger FA decreases. These larger FA decreases were clustered in the columns of the fornix at approximately −0.200 (−30%), in the left inferior cingulum at approximately −0.180 (−30%), and in the posterior corpus callosum body at approximately −0.130 (−20%) (Figure 2).

There were significant RD increases from pre-RT to end-RT in 64.6% of white matter skeleton voxels, also representing treatment-induced changes. Of voxels with significant RD increases, the minimum was +6 $\mu m^2/s$ (+1.5%), the maximum was +487 $\mu m^2/s$ (+86.6%), and the mean was +40 $\mu m^2/s$ with a standard deviation of 24 $\mu m^2/s$ (+10.0±6.7%), also a skewed

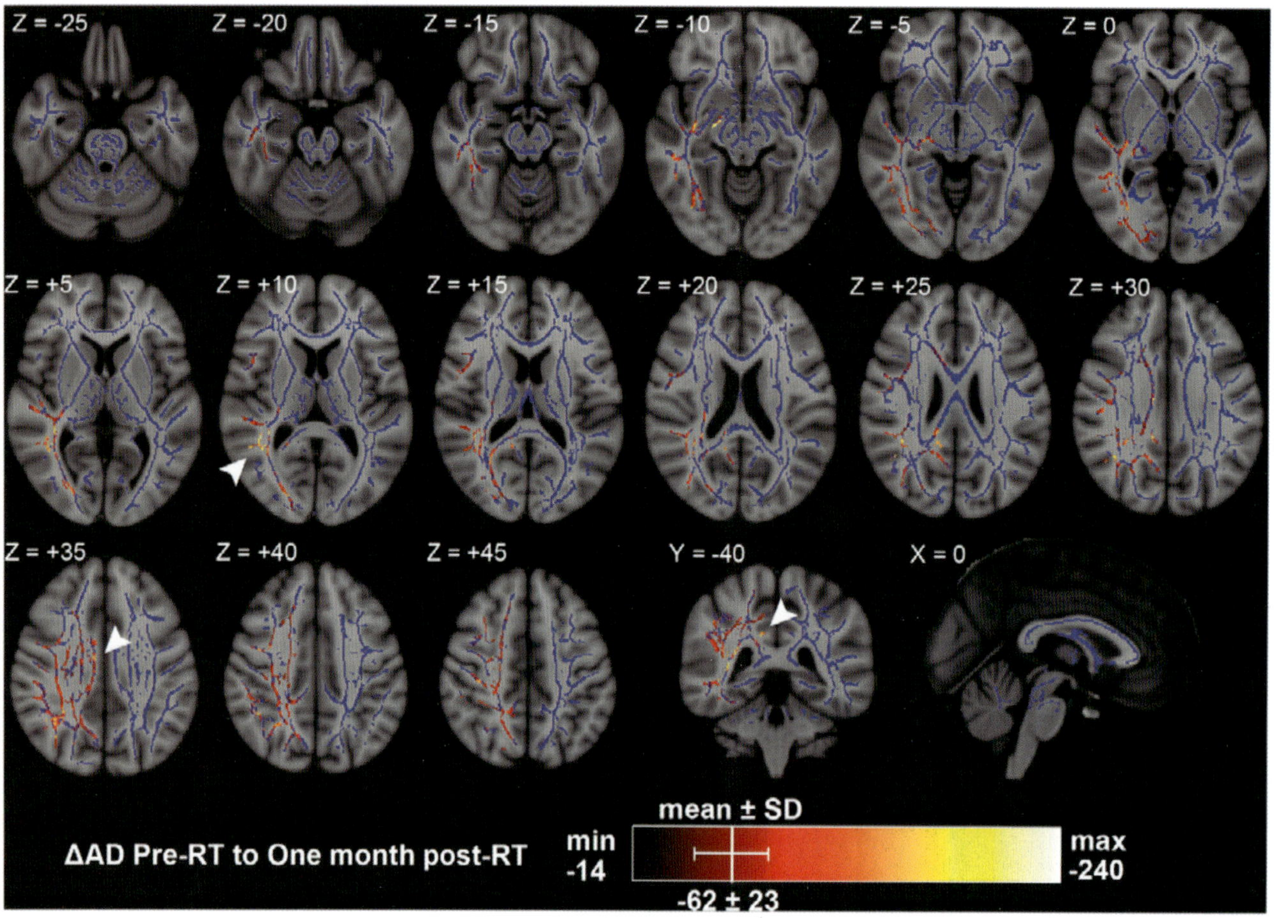

Figure 4. Significant changes in AD from pre-RT to one month post-RT. Arrowheads: Z = +10, right superior longitudinal fasciculus; Z = +35, right superior cingulum; Y = −40, right superior cingulum. Significant results per color chart, blue is TBSS skeleton without significant results. Depicted on MNI ICBM152 standard brain T1-weighted image [34]. Units are $\mu m^2/s$.

distribution towards larger RD increases. These larger RD increases were clustered in the columns and crura of the fornix at approximately +300 $\mu m^2/s$ (+50%), in the left and right inferior cingulum at approximately +250 $\mu m^2/s$ (+40%), and the posterior corpus callosum body at approximately +175 $\mu m^2/s$ (+45%) (Figure 3). These clusters of large RD increases were very similar in distribution to the large FA decreases. Of all white matter skeleton voxels, 63.1% of white matter skeleton voxels showed significant changes in both FA and RD. Nearly all areas showing significant RD increases also showed significant FA increases.

There were no significant changes in AD between pre-RT and end-RT. However, between pre-RT and one month post-RT there were significant AD decreases in 12.9% of white matter skeleton voxels. Of voxels with significant AD decreases, the minimum was −14 $\mu m^2/s$ (−1.7%), the maximum was −240 $\mu m^2/s$ (−18.7%), and the mean was −62 $\mu m^2/s$ with a standard deviation of −23 $\mu m^2/s$ (−6.4±2.3%), a skewed distribution towards larger AD decreases. These larger AD decreases were clustered in the right superior longitudinal fasciculus at approximately −200 $\mu m^2/s$ (−18%), and in the right superior cingulum at approximately −120 $\mu m^2/s$ (−12%) (Figure 4). Significant AD changes were seen at different locations and time intervals than significant RD changes.

From pre-RT to one month post-RT, there continued to be significant FA decreases in 82.9% of white matter skeleton voxels, with clusters of relatively large FA decreases in the same regions as seen from pre-RT to end-RT (Figure S1). From pre-RT to one month post-RT, there continued to be relatively large RD increases in the same regions as before, however only 37.4% of white matter skeleton voxels showed significant increases in RD, a large reduction from the fraction showing significant RD increases from pre-RT to end-RT (64.6%). There were fewer voxels showing significant RD increases in the peripheral white matter (Figure S2), suggesting partial resolution of an RD specific process by one month after radiation. Between pre-RT and one month post-RT, 33.5% of white matter skeleton voxels showed significant changes in both FA and RD, and 10.4% of the skeleton voxels showed significant changes in both FA and AD, indicating large spatial overlap between FA and the other two diffusion indices. Only 0.1% of the skeleton voxels showed significant changes in both AD and RD between pre-RT and one month post-RT, indicating virtually no spatial overlap between AD and RD changes (Figure 5). From end-RT to one month post-RT there were no significant voxel changes in RD, AD, or FA.

Within-Structure Analysis

Of the total white matter skeleton, 91,222 voxels (81.2%) were labeled as one of fourteen structures representing the major supratentorial white matter tracts. The ten laterally paired structures (Table 1) did not show any statistically significant left-right asymmetry in mean FA, AD, or RD changes between any

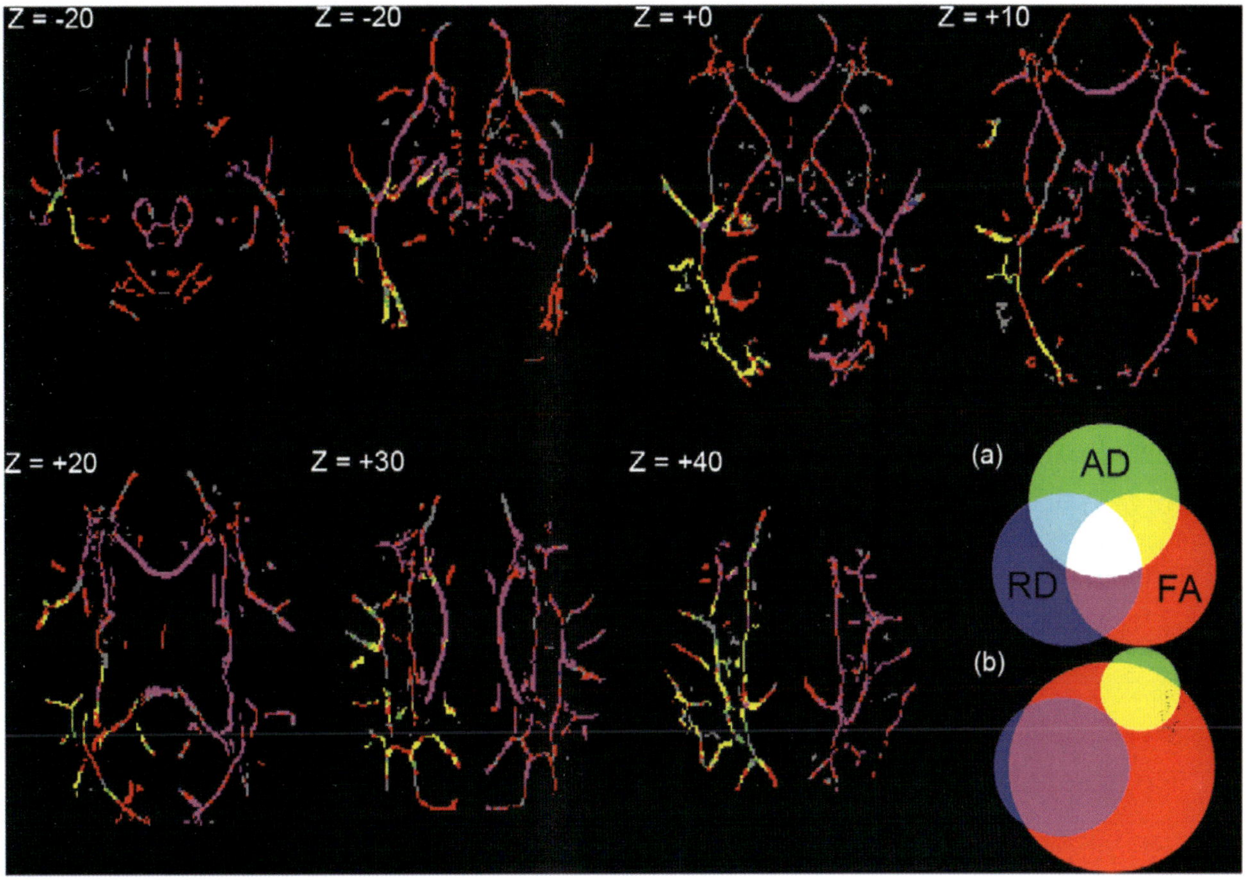

Figure 5. Pre-RT to one month post-RT significant voxel overlap. (a) Color key to significant voxel changes from pre-RT to one month post-RT in AD, RD, and FA with overlapping voxels. Underlying white matter skeleton with no significant changes is gray. (b) Venn diagram depicting proportion of white matter skeleton with significant changes. FA = 82.9%; RD = 37.4%; AD = 12.9%; FA ∩ RD = 33.5%; FA ∩ AD = 10.4%; RD ∩ AD = 0.1%. Labels are MNI coordinates.

Table 3. Fractional anisotropy (FA) longitudinal changes by structure.

		Pre-RT to End-RT			Pre-RT to One Month Post-RT			End-RT to One Month Post-RT	
White Matter Structure	**Pre-RT FA**	**Mean ΔFA**	**95% CI**	**Rank**	**Mean ΔFA**	**95% CI**	**Rank**	**Mean ΔFA**	**95% CI**
Corpus Callosum Body	0.701	**−0.066**	**±0.014**	**2**	**−0.070**	**±0.016**	**2**	*−0.007*	*±0.012*
Corpus Callosum Genu	0.711	**−0.051**	**±0.016**	**6**	**−0.057**	**±0.018**	**3**	*−0.008*	*±0.014*
Corpus Callosum Splenium	0.781	**−0.034**	**±0.014**	**13**	**−0.038**	**±0.015**	**10**	*−0.007*	*±0.009*
Cingula, Inferior	0.559	**−0.085**	**±0.017**	**1**	**−0.078**	**±0.022**	**1**	*+0.003*	*±0.020*
Cingula, Superior	0.597	**−0.052**	**±0.015**	**5**	**−0.050**	**±0.009**	**6**	*−0.002*	*±0.011*
Corona Radiata, Anterior	0.457	**−0.036**	**±0.008**	**11**	**−0.035**	**±0.008**	**12**	*+0.000*	*±0.006*
Corona Radiata, Posterior	0.495	**−0.036**	**±0.008**	**12**	**−0.037**	**±0.010**	**11**	*−0.001*	*±0.006*
External Capsules	0.453	**−0.045**	**±0.012**	**8**	**−0.045**	**±0.010**	**7**	*−0.004*	*±0.008*
Fornix Columns	0.333	**−0.054**	**±0.021**	**4**	**−0.051**	**±0.018**	**5**	*−0.002*	*±0.012*
Fornix Crura	0.531	**−0.054**	**±0.010**	**3**	**−0.052**	**±0.021**	**4**	*+0.000*	*±0.018*
Internal Capsules, Anterior	0.585	**−0.043**	**±0.013**	**9**	**−0.039**	**±0.015**	**9**	*−0.001*	*±0.009*
Internal Capsules, Posterior	0.685	**−0.034**	**±0.016**	**14**	**−0.030**	**±0.014**	**14**	*+0.003*	*±0.022*
Internal Capsules, Retrolenticular	0.601	**−0.046**	**±0.012**	**7**	**−0.043**	**±0.017**	**8**	*+0.001*	*±0.015*
Superior Longitudinal Fasiculi	0.505	**−0.037**	**±0.012**	**10**	**−0.033**	**±0.010**	**13**	*+0.002*	*±0.012*

Statistically significant changes after correction for false discovery rate bolded; non-significant italicized.

Table 4. Radial diffusivity (RD) longitudinal changes by structure.

White Matter Structure	Pre-RT RD	Pre-RT to End-RT			Pre-RT to One Month Post-RT			End-RT to One Month Post-RT	
		Mean ΔRD	95% CI	Rank	Mean ΔRD	95% CI	Rank	Mean ΔRD	95% CI
Corpus Callosum Body	323	**+71**	**±17**	**2**	**+71**	**±18**	**1**	*+1*	*±13*
Corpus Callosum Genu	314	**+55**	**±20**	**4**	**+55**	**±23**	**3**	*+2*	*±15*
Corpus Callosum Splenium	252	**+32**	**±20**	**8**	**+33**	**±25**	**6**	*+4*	*±11*
Cingula, Inferior	357	**+67**	**±24**	**3**	**+52**	**±23**	**4**	*−8*	*±17*
Cingula, Superior	370	**+34**	**±13**	**7**	**+27**	**±11**	**8**	*−4*	*±9*
Corona Radiata, Anterior	458	**+28**	**±11**	**10**	**+21**	**±11**	**13**	*−7*	*±8*
Corona Radiata, Posterior	438	**+26**	**±18**	**12**	**+23**	**±18**	**10**	*−3*	*±12*
External Capsules	446	**+28**	**±14**	**11**	**+26**	**±14**	**9**	*+0*	*±9*
Fornix Columns	211	**+112**	**±38**	**1**	*+60*	*±73*	*2*	*−48*	*±58*
Fornix Crura	437	**+51**	**±11**	**5**	**+45**	**±19**	**5**	*−3*	*±18*
Internal Capsules, Anterior	359	**+29**	**±18**	**9**	**+22**	**±18**	**11**	*−5*	*±14*
Internal Capsules, Posterior	308	**+25**	**±14**	**13**	**+22**	**±15**	**12**	*−2*	*±20*
Internal Capsules, Retrolenticular	396	**+36**	**±14**	**6**	**+30**	**±23**	**7**	*−4*	*±18*
Superior Longitudinal Fasiculi	432	**+24**	**±12**	**14**	*+13*	*±14*	*14*	*−11*	*±12*

Statistically significant changes after correction for false discovery rate bolded; non-significant italicized.
Units are $\mu m^2/s$.

time points. Therefore, longitudinal analysis was performed using the mean values from combined paired structures.

From pre-RT to end-RT, all fourteen structures showed statistically significant mean FA decreases and mean RD increases (Table 3, Table 4). Similar to the individual voxel results, the largest mean FA decreases ($< -0.05\ \mu m^2/s$) from pre-RT to end-RT were seen in the inferior and superior cingula, corpus callosum body and genu, and fornix columns and crura. The largest mean RD increases ($> +50\ \mu m^2/s$) from pre-RT to end-RT were in the fornix columns and crura, inferior cingula, and corpus callosum body and genu. Also similar to the voxel results, the superior cingula and superior longitudinal fasciculi showed significant decreases in mean AD from pre-RT to one month post-RT. However, these structures also showed significant mean AD decreases from pre-RT to end-RT, unlike the voxel results and

Table 5. Axial diffusivity (AD) longitudinal changes by structure.

Structure	Pre-RT AD	Pre-RT to End-RT		Pre-RT to One Month Post-RT		End-RT to One Month Post-RT	
		Mean ΔAD	95% CI	Mean ΔAD	95% CI	Mean ΔAD	95% CI
Corpus Callosum Body	1287	*+8*	*±23*	*−12*	*±19*	**−23**	**±19**
Corpus Callosum Genu	1275	*+13*	*±30*	*−9*	*±27*	*−24*	*±22*
Corpus Callosum Splenium	1317	*−5*	*±30*	*−21*	*±35*	*−17*	*±16*
Cingula, Inferior	908	*+8*	*±35*	*−4*	*±41*	*−3*	*±18*
Cingula, Superior	1048	**−40**	**±20**	**−54**	**±30**	*−15*	*±17*
Corona Radiata, Anterior	954	*−3*	*±15*	*−15*	*±14*	*−12*	*±14*
Corona Radiata, Posterior	985	*−9*	*±15*	*−15*	*±25*	*−7*	*±16*
External Capsules	927	*−16*	*±15*	*−22*	*±2*	*−7*	*±18*
Fornix Columns	1996	*+32*	*±61*	*−35*	*±91*	**−89**	**±70**
Fornix Crura	1028	*+3*	*±18*	*−10*	*±28*	*−6*	*±18*
Internal Capsules, Anterior	1006	*−11*	*±24*	*−18*	*±24*	*−5*	*±19*
Internal Capsules, Posterior	1108	*−13*	*±16*	*−19*	*±24*	*−8*	*±23*
Internal Capsules, Retrolenticular	1135	*−20*	*±21*	*−30*	*±26*	*−12*	*±19*
Superior Longitudinal Fasiculi	977	**−22**	**±16**	**−37**	**±27**	*−17*	*±18*

Statistically significant changes after correction for false discovery rate bolded; non-significant italicized.
Units are $\mu m^2/s$.

Table 6. Repeated-measures ANOVA of FA changes from pre-RT to end-RT.

Within-Subject Effects				
Source	**Type III Sum of Squares**	**Degrees of Freedom**	**F-value**	***P*-value**
Structure	0.036	4.127	8.831	<0.001
Structure * Dose	0.004	4.127	1.102	0.369
Structure * Age	0.002	4.127	0.512	0.732
Structure * Sex	0.001	4.127	0.344	0.852
Error	0.041	41.271	–	–
Between-Subject Effects				
Source	**Type III Sum of Squares**	**Degrees of Freedom**	**F-value**	***P*-value**
Intercept	0.452	1	108.798	<0.001
Dose	0.002	1	0.542	0.478
Age	0.007	1	1.799	0.210
Sex	<0.001	1	0.006	0.942
Error	0.042	10	–	–

Degrees of freedom for within-subject effects corrected for lack of sphericity by Greenhouse-Geisser method, $\varepsilon = 0.311$.

possibly due to averaging of individual voxel changes within these structures (Table 5).

From pre-RT to one month post-RT, there were again significant mean FA decreases in all structures, greatest in the inferior cingula, corpus callosum body and genu, and fornix columns and crura (Table 3). Again similar to the voxel results, there were fewer structures showing significant mean RD increases from pre-RT to one month post-RT as compared to pre-RT to end-RT. Notably, the fornix columns no longer showed a significant change despite having the second highest mean RD increase from pre-RT to one month post-RT, due to a wide variation in this change across patients and large confidence interval. Of the structures showing a significant mean RD increase between pre-RT and one month post-RT, the greatest changes were in the corpus callosum body and genu, inferior cingula, and fornix crura (Table 4).

Between end-RT to one month post-RT, there were no significant changes seen in FA and RD, again similar to the voxel results. However, there were significant AD decreases seen in the corpus callosum body and in the fornix columns between end-RT and one month post-RT, despite no significant AD changes in these structures from pre-RT to end-RT or to one month post-RT (Table 5). This was unlike the voxel results, and may again be due to the averaging of individual voxel changes within these structures.

Between-Structure Analysis

Repeated-measures ANOVA revealed a highly significant ($p<0.001$) difference between structures in pre-RT to end-RT FA changes following chemoradiotherapy (Table 6). Levene's test of equality revealed no significant differences in error variance between patients for all structures (all $p>0.05$), indicating applicability of ANOVA. Mauchly's test of sphericity revealed a significant departure from sphericity across structures ($p<0.001$), therefore degrees of freedom for estimating within-subject effects were adjusted using the Greenhouse-Geisser method with $\varepsilon = 0.311$. For within-subject and between-subject variance, there were no statistically significant contributions by age, sex, or radiation dose.

Post hoc comparisons were performed between the structure with the greatest pre-RT to end-RT FA change (inferior cingula) and all other structures using subject-paired two-sided *t*-tests. All 13 comparisons had $p<0.05$, and 11 remained statistically significant after Bonferroni correction ($p<0.00385$). This indicates that the inferior cingula show greater FA decrease from pre-RT to end-RT than almost all other structures (Figure 6).

Discussion

This study found (i) large regional variation in white matter diffusion index changes following radiation, representing varying susceptibility to treatment toxicity; and (ii) differences in the time course and spatial extent of changes in diffusion indices, implying specificity to distinct processes. Regional variation in diffusion index changes was greatest in fractional anisotropy (FA) and radial diffusivity (RD), and more extreme FA and RD changes were seen in inferior and superior cingula, the fornix columns and crura, and in sections of the corpus callosum. This likely represents greater vulnerability to the toxic effects of chemoradiotherapy in these structures, and may be related to the specific neurocognitive deficits seen following treatment. Temporal and spatial differences were seen between changes in RD and axial diffusivity (AD), demonstrating that that these diffusion indices may be specific for distinct pathologies and can be used to better examine white matter toxicity following chemoradiotherapy.

The inferior cingula and fornix showed large diffusion index changes, representing greater white matter degradation. These two structures are components of the limbic system, a functional circuit which also includes the hippocampus [39]. The limbic system as a whole functions to assist memory and learning and regulate emotional states and attention [40], processes commonly reported to be specifically impaired following brain radiation therapy [2–6]. This raises the hypothesis that selective sensitivity of the limbic circuit may be responsible for the specific pattern of functional impairments seen after chemoradiotherapy. This has previously been proposed, and could be tested by limbic circuit

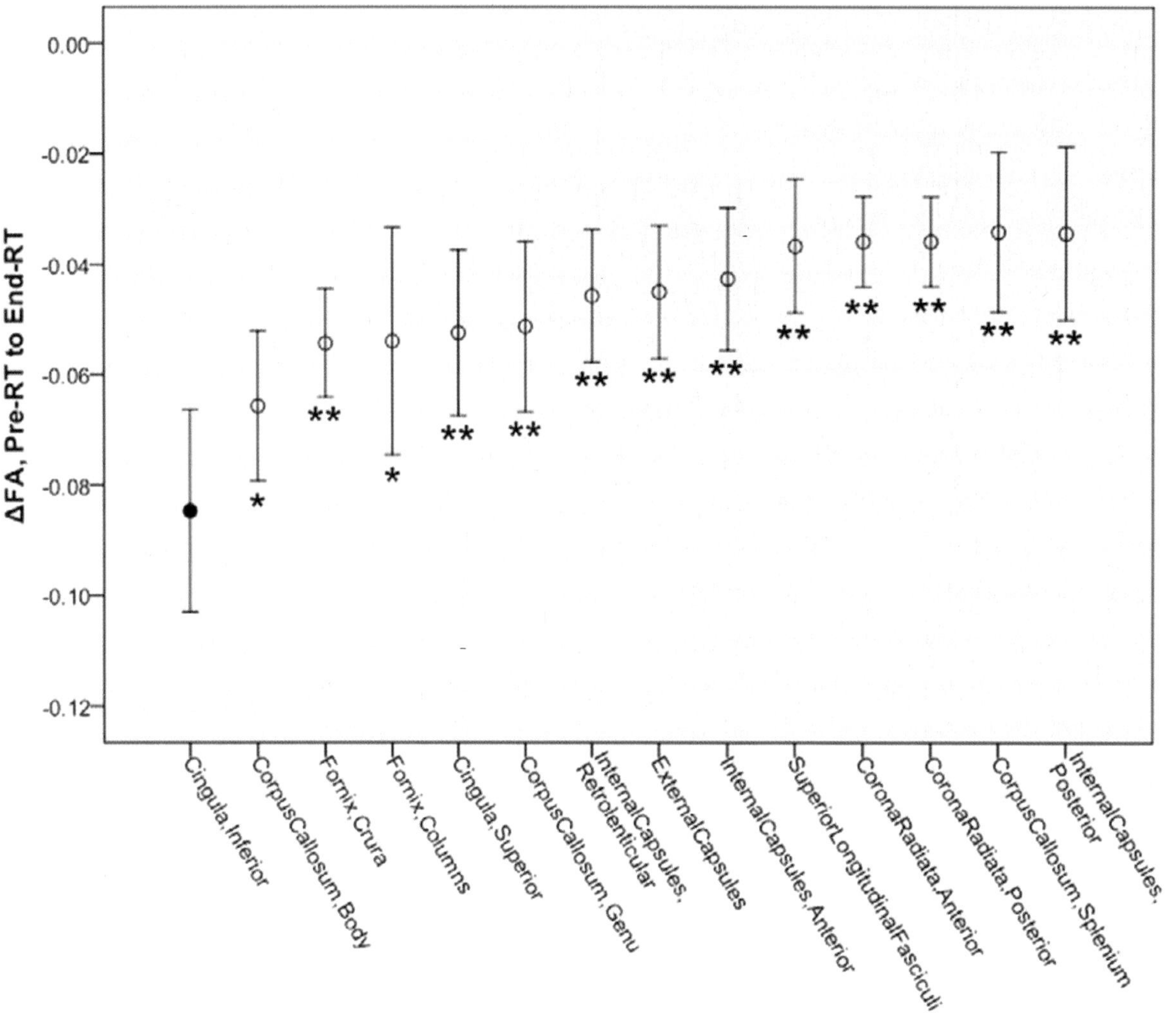

Figure 6. Mean FA changes from pre-RT to end-RT in fourteen structures. Comparisons by subject-paired two-sided *t*-test to Inferior Cingula (filled marker). *$p<0.05$; **$p<0.00385$ (Bonferroni correction). Error bars are 95% confidence interval.

sparing during radiation therapy [21]. The present study also supports investigating diffusion tensor imaging of limbic circuit structures as a biomarker of radiation-induced neurocognitive impairment, just as reduced FA in the fornix and inferior cingula have been associated with other forms of neurocognitive impairment [41–43]. In a prior study, we found that neurocognitive tests after radiation were significantly correlated with diffusion index changes in the inferior cingula, but not in other temporal lobe white matter [26].

Changes in RD and AD occurred at different time intervals and locations. RD increases appeared to peak at the end of radiation, consistent with demyelination as the predominant early effect of radiation [12], [13], [28]. Fewer structures showed significant RD increases at one month after radiation, which may represent partial remyelination at this time point. Early demyelination and remyelination following brain irradiation has been observed in animal models [44]. By TBSS analysis, AD decreases appeared at one month after radiation, and there was virtually no spatial intersection between significant AD and RD changes. One possible explanation is that these reflect distinct pathologic processes, as has been seen in animal models [11–16]. Decreased AD could represent reactive astrogliosis and/or axonal degradation [11], [14–16]. Alternatively, decreased AD emerging in areas of previously increased RD could be due to resolving extracellular edema, which can affect both diffusion indices [10], [11]. However, this alternative is less plausible, as there was no edema detected by T2-weighted imaging. There was apparent left-right asymmetry in the occurrence of significant individual voxel changes, especially in AD (Figure 4). However, with direct comparison there was no significant asymmetry in mean diffusion index changes between paired structures. This could be due to within-structure variation, because we did not examine asymmetry in a voxel-wise manner. A previous study [18] also saw apparent asymmetry in diffusion index differences, but did not perform a direct comparison. At least one other study with direct comparison found no significant asymmetry in diffusion index changes after radiation [30].

The mechanism behind regional variation in white matter changes is still unclear. In addition to limbic circuit structures, large diffusion index changes were also seen in the corpus callosum and posterior superior longitudinal fasciculus, structures which like the limbic circuit are periventricular. These locations may be more susceptible to compressive damage from increased intracranial pressure, and a similar pattern has been seen with hydrocephalus

[45]. However, increased intracranial pressure is not known to be a major effect of chemoradiotherapy in the absence of tumor progression or radiation necrosis. Alternatively, the deep location from the cortex means that these structures have lower capillary density and less blood flow [46], which has been associated with more severe white matter degradation after radiation [47–49]. A combination of mechanisms may be present, as animal models show early periventricular and vascular damage simultaneously [49], [50]. The addition of functional imaging techniques sensitive to vascular changes such as dynamic contrast enhanced MRI may help clarify this question [51].

One limitation of any imaging study is the potential for partial volume effect, i.e. values in the voxels of interest representing multiple tissue types. An advantage of tract based spatial statistics is that by identifying the tract center, voxels likely to contain partial volume effect at the periphery of the tract are excluded [31]. This remains a concern for small-caliber tracts, especially when the tract diameter approaches voxel size. For example, mean diameter of the fornix columns has been reported to be 2.3 mm [39], compared with our 1.75 mm original voxel size. This is reflected by the greater uncertainty in our estimates of diffusion index changes in the fornix columns, especially in AD and RD, due to partial volume effect from neighboring cerebrospinal fluid. Repeat imaging minimizes the impact of partial volume effect on our conclusions, as diffusion properties of cerebrospinal fluid are not expected to be systematically influenced by chemoradiotherapy. Additionally, tumor burden may still have affected our results despite no apparent tumor influence on the structures of interest by T1- and T2-weighted imaging. This was likely also minimized by repeat imaging allowing for within-patient compensation of tumor effects, and the fact that tumors were fairly evenly distributed throughout the brain across patients.

No interaction effect was found by age, sex or radiation dose on diffusion index changes, strengthening the validity of our results but also possibly reflecting our small sample size. A previous study has observed greater radiation-induced diffusion index changes in adults over sixty-five [30], however only two of our subjects were older than sixty-five years. A variation with radiation dose may have been expected, as previous studies have shown a dose-response relationship in diffusion index changes [26], [28]. However, this relationship was seen over larger ranges of 5 to 60 Gy. In this study, dose distribution between structures within a single patient was assumed to be uniform. Although this cannot be precisely true, opposed lateral field technique typically results in 97% of the brain receiving between 98% and 110% of the prescription dose [52]. We would not expect to see major differences in response within this range. The distribution of chemotherapy and primary cancer types in our study did not allow for statistically powerful comparisons between these groups. Bortezomib has been associated with peripheral neuropathy [53] and platinum-based agents such as carboplatin are associated with ototoxicity and peripheral neuropathy [54], however the short term effects of these agents on the central nervous system and possible interactions with radiation therapy are not known. A larger number of subjects, as well as longer follow up and neurocognitive testing could help determine the relationship between these factors and neurocognitive impairment.

Conclusion

Our study demonstrates regional variation in white matter diffusion index changes following chemoradiotherapy, with larger changes implying greater white matter degradation. Large changes in the inferior cingula and fornix have implications for predicting and preventing treatment-induced neurocognitive impairment. We also address the specificity of diffusion indices and their potential utility for clarifying the mechanisms of white matter radiation injury.

Supporting Information

Figure S1 Significant changes in FA from pre-RT to one month post-RT. Arrowheads: Z = −15, left inferior cingulum; Z = +25, corpus callosum body; Y = −40, left inferior cingulum; X = 0, fornix columns. Significant results per color chart, blue is TBSS skeleton without significant results. Depicted on MNI ICBM152 standard brain T1-weighted image [34].

Figure S2 Significant changes in RD from pre-RT to one month post-RT. Arrowheads: Z = +10, left fornix crus; Z = +25, corpus callosum body; Y = −40, left inferior cingulum; X = 0, fornix columns. Significant results per color chart, blue is TBSS skeleton without significant results. Depicted on MNI ICBM152 standard brain T1-weighted image [34]. Units are $\mu m^2/s$.

Acknowledgments

We would like to acknowledge our patients and their families for their gracious participation in this study.

Author Contributions

Enrolled participants: CIT TSL. Designed software used in part of analysis: YC. Conceived and designed the experiments: CHC CIT TSL YC. Performed the experiments: CHC CIT TSL YC. Analyzed the data: CHC MN OEL MJS. Contributed reagents/materials/analysis tools: CIT TSL YC. Wrote the paper: CHC MN OEL CIT TSL YC.

References

1. Taphoorn MJB, Klein M (2004) Cognitive deficits in adult patients with brain tumours. Lancet Neurol 3: 159–168. doi:10.1016/S1474-4422(04)00680-5.
2. Crossen JR, Garwood D, Glatstein E, Neuwelt EA (1994) Neurobehavioral sequelae of cranial irradiation in adults: a review of radiation-induced encephalopathy. J Clin Oncol 12: 627–642.
3. Douw L, Klein M, Fagel SS, van den Heuvel J, Taphoorn MJ, et al. (2009) Cognitive and radiological effects of radiotherapy in patients with low-grade glioma: long-term follow-up. Lancet Neurol 8: 810–818. doi:10.1016/S1474-4422(09)70204-2.
4. Hsiao K-Y, Yeh S-A, Chang C-C, Tsai P-C, Wu J-M, et al. (2010) Cognitive function before and after intensity-modulated radiation therapy in patients with nasopharyngeal carcinoma: a prospective study. Int J Radiat Oncol Biol Phys 77: 722–726. doi:10.1016/j.ijrobp.2009.06.080.
5. Roman DD, Sperduto PW (1995) Neuropsychological effects of cranial radiation: current knowledge and future directions. Int J Radiat Oncol Biol Phys 31: 983–998.
6. Surma-aho O, Niemela M, Vilkki J, Kouri M, Brander A, et al. (2001) Adverse long-term effects of brain radiotherapy in adult low-grade glioma patients. Neurology 56: 1285–1290. doi:10.1212/WNL.56.10.1285.
7. Okada S, Okeda R (2001) Pathology of radiation myelopathy. Neuropathology 21: 247–265.
8. Akiyama K, Tanaka R, Sato M, Takeda N (2001) Cognitive dysfunction and histological findings in adult rats one year after whole brain irradiation. Neurol Med Chir (Tokyo) 41: 590–598.
9. Constine LS, Konski A, Ekholm S, McDonald S, Rubin P (1988) Adverse effects of brain irradiation correlated with MR and CT imaging. Int J Radiat Oncol Biol Phys 15: 319–330.
10. Assaf Y, Pasternak O (2008) Diffusion tensor imaging (DTI)-based white matter mapping in brain research: a review. J Mol Neurosci 34: 51–61. doi:10.1007/s12031-007-0029-0.
11. Mac Donald CL, Dikranian K, Bayly P, Holtzman D, Brody D (2007) Diffusion Tensor Imaging Reliably Detects Experimental Traumatic Axonal Injury and Indicates Approximate Time of Injury. Journal of Neuroscience 27: 11869–11876. doi:10.1523/jneurosci.3647-07.2007.

12. Song S-K, Sun S-W, Ramsbottom MJ, Chang C, Russell J, et al. (2002) Dysmyelination revealed through MRI as increased radial (but unchanged axial) diffusion of water. Neuroimage 17: 1429–1436.
13. Song S-K, Yoshino J, Le TQ, Lin S-J, Sun S-W, et al. (2005) Demyelination increases radial diffusivity in corpus callosum of mouse brain. Neurology 26: 132–140. doi:10.1016/j.neuroimage.2005.01.028.
14. Sun S-W, Liang H-F, Cross AH, Song S-K (2008) Evolving Wallerian degeneration after transient retinal ischemia in mice characterized by diffusion tensor imaging. Neuroimage 40: 1–10. doi:10.1016/j.neuroimage.2007.11.049.
15. Wang S, Wu EX, Qiu D, Leung LHT, Lau H-F, et al. (2009) Longitudinal diffusion tensor magnetic resonance imaging study of radiation-induced white matter damage in a rat model. Cancer Res 69: 1190–1198. doi:10.1158/0008-5472.CAN-08-2661.
16. Song S-K, Sun S-W, Ju W-K, Lin S-J, Cross AH, et al. (2003) Diffusion tensor imaging detects and differentiates axon and myelin degeneration in mouse optic nerve after retinal ischemia. Neuroimage 20: 1714–1722.
17. Khong P-L, Kwong DLW, Chan GCF, Sham JST, Chan F-L, et al. (2003) Diffusion-tensor imaging for the detection and quantification of treatment-induced white matter injury in children with medulloblastoma: a pilot study. AJNR Am J Neuroradiol 24: 734–740.
18. Leung LHT, Ooi GC, Kwong DLW, Chan GCF, Cao G, et al. (2004) White-matter diffusion anisotropy after chemo-irradiation: a statistical parametric mapping study and histogram analysis. Neuroimage 21: 261–268.
19. Lawrence YR, Li XA, Naqa el I, Hahn CA, Marks LB, et al. (2010) Radiation dose-volume effects in the brain (QUANTEC). Int J Radiat Oncol Biol Phys 76: S20–S27. doi:10.1016/j.ijrobp.2009.02.091.
20. Ghia A, Tomé W, Thomas S, Cannon G, Khuntia D, et al. (2007) Distribution of brain metastases in relation to the hippocampus: implications for neurocognitive functional preservation. Int J Radiat Oncol Biol Phys 68: 971.
21. Marsh JC, Godbole R, Diaz AZ, Gielda BT, Turian JV (2011) Sparing of the hippocampus, limbic circuit and neural stem cell compartment during partial brain radiotherapy for glioma: A dosimetric feasibility study. J Med Imaging Radiat Oncol 55: 442–449. doi:10.1111/j.1754-9485.2011.02282.x.
22. Radiation Therapy Oncology Group; National Cancer Institute (2010) Avoiding the Hippocampus During Whole-Brain Radiation Therapy in Treating Patients With Brain Metastases. Available: http://clinicaltrials.gov/show/NCT01227954. Accessed 2012 Oct 29.
23. Monje ML, Mizumatsu S, Fike JR, Palmer TD (2002) Irradiation induces neural precursor-cell dysfunction. Nat Med 8: 955–962. doi:10.1038/nm749.
24. Dellani PR, Eder S, Gawehn J, Vucurevic G, Fellgiebel A, et al. (2008) Late structural alterations of cerebral white matter in long-term survivors of childhood leukemia. Journal of magnetic resonance imaging : JMRI 27: 1250–1255. doi:10.1002/jmri.21364.
25. Qiu D, Kwong DLW, Chan GCF, Leung LHT, Khong P-L (2007) Diffusion tensor magnetic resonance imaging finding of discrepant fractional anisotropy between the frontal and parietal lobes after whole-brain irradiation in childhood medulloblastoma survivors: reflection of regional white matter radiosensitivity? Int J Radiat Oncol Biol Phys 69: 846–851. doi:10.1016/j.ijrobp.2007.04.041.
26. Chapman CH, Nagesh V, Sundgren PC, Buchtel H, Chenevert TL, et al. (2012) Diffusion tensor imaging of normal-appearing white matter as biomarker for radiation-induced late delayed cognitive decline. Int J Radiat Oncol Biol Phys 82: 2033–2040. doi:10.1016/j.ijrobp.2011.01.068.
27. Hua C, Merchant TE, Gajjar A, Broniscer A, Zhang Y, et al. (2012) Brain tumor therapy-induced changes in normal-appearing brainstem measured with longitudinal diffusion tensor imaging. Int J Radiat Oncol Biol Phys 82: 2047–2054. doi:10.1016/j.ijrobp.2011.03.057.
28. Nagesh V, Tsien CI, Chenevert TL, Ross BD, Lawrence TS, et al. (2008) Radiation-induced changes in normal-appearing white matter in patients with cerebral tumors: a diffusion tensor imaging study. Int J Radiat Oncol Biol Phys 70: 1002–1010. doi:10.1016/j.ijrobp.2007.08.020.
29. Nazem-Zadeh M-R, Chapman CH, Lawrence TL, Tsien CI, Cao Y (2012) Radiation therapy effects on white matter fiber tracts of the limbic circuit. Med Phys 39: 5603. doi:10.1118/1.4745560.
30. Welzel T, Niethammer A, Mende U, Heiland S, Wenz F, et al. (2008) Diffusion tensor imaging screening of radiation-induced changes in the white matter after prophylactic cranial irradiation of patients with small cell lung cancer: first results of a prospective study. AJNR Am J Neuroradiol 29: 379–383. doi:10.3174/ajnr.A0797.
31. Smith SM, Jenkinson M, Johansen-Berg H, Rueckert D, Nichols TE, et al. (2006) Tract-based spatial statistics: voxelwise analysis of multi-subject diffusion data. Neuroimage 31: 1487–1505. doi:10.1016/j.neuroimage.2006.02.024.
32. Cao Y (2005) Development of Image Software Tools for Radiation Therapy Assessment. Med Phys 32: 2136.
33. Mori S, Oishi K, Jiang H, Jiang L, Li X, et al. (2008) Stereotaxic white matter atlas based on diffusion tensor imaging in an ICBM template. Neuroimage 40: 570–582. doi:10.1016/j.neuroimage.2007.12.035.
34. Mazziotta J, Toga A, Evans A, Fox P, Lancaster J, et al. (2001) A probabilistic atlas and reference system for the human brain: International Consortium for Brain Mapping (ICBM). Philosophical Transactions of the Royal Society of London Series B 356: 1293. doi:10.1098/rstb.2001.0915.
35. Smith SM, Jenkinson M, Woolrich MW, Beckmann CF, Behrens TEJ, et al. (2004) Advances in functional and structural MR image analysis and implementation as FSL. Neuroimage 23 Suppl 1: S208–S219. doi:10.1016/j.neuroimage.2004.07.051.
36. Smith SM, Nichols TE (2009) Threshold-free cluster enhancement: Addressing problems of smoothing, threshold dependence and localisation in cluster inference. Neuroimage 44: 83–98. doi:10.1016/j.neuroimage.2008.03.061.
37. Nichols TE, Holmes AP (2002) Nonparametric permutation tests for functional neuroimaging: a primer with examples. Hum Brain Mapp 15: 1–25.
38. Benjamini Y, Hochberg Y (1995) Controlling the false discovery rate: a practical and powerful approach to multiple testing. Journal of the Royal Statistical Society Series B (Methodological): 289–300.
39. Shah A, Jhawar SS, Goel A (2012) Analysis of the anatomy of the Papez circuit and adjoining limbic system by fiber dissection techniques. Journal of Clinical Neuroscience 19: 289–298. doi:10.1016/j.jocn.2011.04.039.
40. Lautin A (2002) The Limbic Brain. New York, NY: Kluwer Academic Publishers.
41. Chua TC, Wen W, Chen X, Kochan N, Slavin MJ, et al. (2009) Diffusion tensor imaging of the posterior cingulate is a useful biomarker of mild cognitive impairment. Am J Geriatr Psychiatry 17: 602–613. doi:10.1097/JGP.0b013e3181a76e0b.
42. Wu TC, Wilde EA, Bigler ED, Yallampalli R, McCauley SR, et al. (2010) Evaluating the relationship between memory functioning and cingulum bundles in acute mild traumatic brain injury using diffusion tensor imaging. J Neurotrauma 27: 303–307. doi:10.1089/neu.2009.1110.
43. Zhuang L, Wen W, Zhu W, Trollor J, Kochan N, et al. (2010) White matter integrity in mild cognitive impairment: a tract-based spatial statistics study. Neuroimage 53: 16–25. doi:10.1016/j.neuroimage.2010.05.068.
44. van der Kogel AJ (1986) Radiation-induced damage in the central nervous system: an interpretation of target cell responses. Br J Cancer Suppl 7: 207–217.
45. Hattori T, Ito K, Aoki S, Yuasa T, Sato R, et al. (2012) White matter alteration in idiopathic normal pressure hydrocephalus: tract-based spatial statistics study. AJNR Am J Neuroradiol 33: 97–103.
46. Nonaka H, Akima M, Hatori T, Nagayama T, Zhang Z, et al. (2003) Microvasculature of the human cerebral white matter: arteries of the deep white matter. Neuropathology 23: 111–118.
47. Calvo W, Hopewell JW, Reinhold HS, Yeung TK (1988) Time- and dose-related changes in the white matter of the rat brain after single doses of X rays. Br J Radiol 61: 1043–1052.
48. Hodges H, Katzung N, Sowinski P, Hopewell JW, Wilkinson JH, et al. (1998) Late behavioural and neuropathological effects of local brain irradiation in the rat. Behav Brain Res 91: 99–114.
49. Reinhold HS, Calvo W, Hopewell JW, van der Berg AP (1990) Development of blood vessel-related radiation damage in the fimbria of the central nervous system. Int J Radiat Oncol Biol Phys 18: 37–42.
50. Miot-Noirault E, Akoka S, Hoffschir D, Pontvert D, Gaboriaud G, et al. (1996) Potential of T2 relaxation time measurements for early detection of radiation injury to the brain: experimental study in pigs. AJNR Am J Neuroradiol 17: 907–912.
51. Cao Y (2011) The promise of dynamic contrast-enhanced imaging in radiation therapy. Semin Radiat Oncol 21: 147–156. doi:10.1016/j.semradonc.2010.11.001.
52. Yu JB, Shiao SL, Knisely JPS (2007) A dosimetric evaluation of conventional helmet field irradiation versus two-field intensity-modulated radiotherapy technique. Int J Radiat Oncol Biol Phys 68: 621–631.
53. Richardson PG, Briemberg H, Jagannath S, Wen PY, Barlogie B, et al. (2006) Frequency, characteristics, and reversibility of peripheral neuropathy during treatment of advanced multiple myeloma with bortezomib. J Clin Oncol 24: 3113–3120.
54. Bokemeyer C, Berger CC, Kuczyk MA, Schmoll H (1996) Evaluation of long-term toxicity after chemotherapy for testicular cancer. J Clin Oncol 14: 2923–2932.

8

Polymorphisms in Radio-Responsive Genes and Its Association with Acute Toxicity among Head and Neck Cancer Patients

Goutham Hassan Venkatesh[1], Vadhiraja Bejadi Manjunath[3], Kamalesh Dattaram Mumbrekar[1], Hitendra Negi[2], Donald Jerard Fernandes[5], Krishna Sharan[5], Sourjya Banerjee[4], Satish Rao Bola Sadashiva[1]*

1 Division of Radiobiology & Toxicology, School of Life Sciences, Manipal University, Manipal, Karnataka, India, **2** Division of Biotechnology, School of Life Sciences, Manipal University, Manipal, Karnataka, India, **3** Manipal Hospital, Bangalore, Karnataka, India, **4** Department of Radiotherapy & Oncology, Kasturba Medical College and Hospital, Mangalore, Karnataka, India, **5** Department of Radiotherapy & Oncology, Shiridi SaiBaba Cancer Hospital and Research Centre, Kasturba Hospital, Manipal, Karnataka, India

Abstract

Cellular and molecular approaches are being explored to find a biomarker which can predict the development of radiation induced acute toxicity prior to radiation therapy. SNPs in radiation responsive genes may be considered as an approach to develop tools for finding the inherited basis of clinical radiosensitivity. The current study attempts to screen single nucleotide polymorphisms/deletions in DNA damage response, DNA repair, profibrotic cytokine as well as antioxidant response genes and its predictive potential with the normal tissue adverse reactions from 183 head and neck cancer patients undergoing platinum based chemoradiotherapy or radiotherapy alone. We analysed 22 polymorphisms in 17 genes having functional relevance to radiation response. Radiation therapy induced oral mucositis and skin erythema was considered as end point for clinical radiosensitivity. Direct correlation of heterozygous and mutant alleles with acute reactions as well as haplotype correlation revealed NBN variants to be of predictive significance in analysing oral mucositis prior to radiotherapy. In addition, genetic linkage disequilibrium existed in XRCC1 polymorphisms for >grade 2 oral mucositis and skin reaction indicating the complex inheritance pattern. The current study indicates an association for polymorphism in NBN with normal tissue radiosensitivity and further warrants the replication of such studies in a large set of samples.

Editor: Jian Jian Li, University of California Davis, United States of America

Funding: Funded by Department of Biotechnology, Government of India, grant number BT/01/COE/06/02/07 (http://dbtindia.nic.in/index.asp). The funders had no role in study design, data collection and analysis, decision to publish, or preparation of the manuscript.

Competing Interests: The authors have declared that no competing interests exist.

* E-mail: satishraomlsc@gmail.com

Introduction

Precise radiation delivery methodologies have significantly improved tumor cure and survival rate owing to recent developments, however it has been at the expense of significant increase in normal tissue toxicity. Heterogeneity in normal tissue radioresponse is observed among patients treated with identical doses of radiation, which further leads to a dynamic and cumulative process of normal tissue toxicity. In head and neck cancer (HNC) patients, oral mucositis and skin erythema are the major complications during the course of chemoradiotherapy. It affects pain control and adequate treatment delivery, thereby leading to unanticipated radiotherapy (RT) breaks, compromising treatment efficacy [1]. Earlier clinical experiences have indicated that only 20% of the variability was because of stochastic or random events, whereas the rest 80% were because of patient related genetic factors [2]. The association between severe radiosensitivity and genetic syndromes like Ataxia-telangiectasia, Fanconi's anemia, and Bloom syndrome, etc., provides us a proof of the principle about the involvement of genetic component behind normal tissue acute reactions [3]. Also, previous findings demonstrate genotype-dependent cause for acute and late effects of RT seen in normal tissues [4] [5]. Apart from molecular aspects, our earlier studies suggest that there exist a cellular basis for normal tissue radiation sensitivity [6]. Two-third of the studies conducted till date report the association of genetic variation in candidate genes with radiation induced toxicity, but most of these studies are with small patient numbers and lacks independent validation [7]. Although studies have been conducted to associate the polymorphism in selected candidate genes with clinically observed normal tissue adverse effects, its clinical applicability as biomarker/s is still questionable [8] [9]. Therefore, well designed clinical studies with hundreds of samples are needed to seek a biomarker for developing individual treatment protocols [10] [11].

In the present study, single nucleotide polymorphisms/deletions in selected candidate genes related to DNA damage and repair, antioxidant response and detoxification enzymes and profibrotic cytokine were analysed. SNPs in candidate radiation responsive genes like ATM, XRCC1, XRCC3, XRCC4, Ku70, Ku80, LIG4, OGG1, NBN, RAD51, TGFβ1, SOD2, CAT and GST were selected. The severity of oral mucositis and skin reaction was recorded according to Radiation Therapy Oncology Group

(RTOG) criteria [12] and the association between genetic polymorphism and oral mucositis and skin reaction was evaluated for the increased risk of developing these normal tissue adverse reactions.

Materials and Methods

Patients and clinical data

The study was conducted from 183 HNC patients undergoing chemoradiotherapy at Kasturba Hospital, with a prior approval by the University Ethical Committee (UEC/15/2007) and a written informed consent from the patients before collecting blood prior to RT. All patients were treated using 3-Dimensional Conformal Radiotherapy. Gross tumor volume (GTV), Clinical Target Volume (CTV) and Planning target volume (PTV) were defined by using these planning CT scan. Gross tumor volume encompassed all known gross disease as defined by clinical physical examination and imaging findings. Patients with gross disease were treated using Linac 6-MV X-ray linear accelerator (Elekta Precise digital, Stockholm, Sweden) with the total tumor dose of 70 Gy (2 Gy per day for 5 days week). Patients after surgical resection having positive margins were given a dose of 66 Gy in 33 fractions. Patients with no positive margins were given 60 Gy in 30 fractions. Dose to parotid gland, submandibular salivary glands, constrictor muscles and other structures were not restricted in view of 3-Dimensional treatment planning in all the patients. Cisplatin chemotherapy (100 mg/m^2 for once in 3 weeks) was given to majority of the patients when serum creatinine was normal. Elderly patients received a weekly dose of 40 mg/m^2 for 6 weeks and patients having borderline elevation of serum creatinine received carboplatin (area under curve (AUC) @ 1.5) on a weekly basis for 6 weeks. A total of 148 patients received concurrent chemoradiotherapy and the remaining patients were received radiotherapy alone. Patients with recurrent tumour and distant metastasis were excluded. Acute adverse events (oral mucositis and skin reaction) were recorded during and after completion of therapy according to RTOG criteria [10]. The details of HNC patient characteristics are described in table 1.

Table 1. Demographic and clinical details of head and neck cancer patients.

Patient clinical details		
Number of patients		183
Mean age		55 (26–80)
Males		157
Females		26
Smoking/Tobacco chewing		122
Alcohol consumption		66
Region	Hypopharynx	32
	Oropharynx	85
	Nasopharynx	5
	Larynx	27
	Oral cavity	15
	Para nasal region	11
	Parotid	4
	Thyroid	3
	Unknown origin of region	1
Tumor staging	T1	9
	T2	32
	T3	48
	T4	65
	Tx	12
Treatment	Chemoradiotherapy	148
	RT alone	35
Skin reaction (RTOG Grading)	Grade 0	3
	Grade I	27
	Grade II	97
	Grade III	36
	Grade IV	3
Mucositis (RTOG Grading)	Grade 0	1
	Grade I	8
	Grade II	57
	Grade III	48
	Grade IV	6

Genotyping, haplotype and linkage disequilibrium analysis

Genomic DNA isolation was performed by employing the conventional phenol chloroform extraction and ethanol precipitation procedure. Genotyping was performed by Polymerase Chain Reaction based Restriction Fragment Length Polymorphism. The details are available in table 2. Five percent of the samples were randomly selected and re-genotyped to assess the consistency in results.

Statistical analysis

Each polymorphism was tested for deviation from Hardy-Weinberg equilibrium. Statistical significance was analysed by Fisher exact test. Odds ratio was estimated to test whether any association exist between the grade of acute toxicity and selected SNP/haplotypes. Haplotype analysis and linkage disequilibrium estimates were done using SHEsis software [13]. All statistical tests were performed using Prism v.5.0 (GraphPad Software, San Diego, California, USA) and Statistical Package for Social Science (Version 16.0, Chicago, USA).

Results

The distribution of patients based on histopathological grading, tumor stage and acute toxicity grades is provided in table 1. The mean age group of the patients considered in the study was 54.74 years. Radiation doses ranging from 60 to 70 Gy (median = 66 Gy) in 30 to 35 fractions were given to the patients. A total of 148 patients underwent platinum-based chemoradiotherapy, while the remaining was given radiotherapy alone. Out of 183 patients, 71 (38.79%) patients experienced severe mucositis (grade 3 and 4) and 44 (24.04%) experienced severe skin reactions. We analysed the presence of confounding factors like diabetes, hypertension, smoking, alcohol, surgery and chemotherapy and found that patients with alcoholism was associated with grade ≤2 mucositis ($p = 0.02$) (Table 3).

According to radiation oncologists, toxicity upto grade 2 is usually tolerated by patients without any therapeutic intervention but grade 3 and 4 requires intervention with therapeutic agents. Based on this, and considering reports from earlier studies [14] [15], we grouped the patient normal tissue toxicity data as grade ≤ 2 or >2. Since the dose exposed to oral cavity/pharyngeal region varies from 0–40% in hypopharynx, larynx, thyroid and region of

Table 2. The list of candidate genes selected in the present study.

Gene	rs number	Amino acid/nucleotide change	Chromosome	PCR product size (bp)	Enzyme	Dominant (wild type)	Heterozygous	Recessive (mutant)
DNA damage and repair genes								
XRCC1	rs25487	Gln399Arg (A>G)	Chr 19	615	*Msp I*	615	615, 377, 238	377, 238
XRCC1	rs1799782	Arg194Trp (C>T)	Chr 19	491	*Msp I*	292,178,21	313, 292, 178, 21	313, 178
XRCC1	rs25489	Arg280His (G>A)	Chr 19	280	*Rsa I*	280	280, 140	140
XRCC1	rs3213245	−77 (C>T)	Chr 19	219	*BsrB I*	173, 46	173,116, 57, 46	116, 57, 46
XRCC3	rs861539	Thr241Met (C>T)	Chr 14	336	*Nla III*	336	336, 231, 105	231, 105
XRCC4	rs1805377	894–7 (A>G)	Chr 5	170	*Tsp509 I*	170	170, 88, 82	88, 82
XRCC5 (Ku80)	rs3835	2110–2408 (G>A)	Chr 2	151	*Alu I*	78, 73	151,78,73	151
XRCC6 (Ku70)	rs2267437	88+57 (C>G)	Chr 22	178	*Nar I*	178	178,147, 31	147,31
LIG4	rs1805388	Thr9Ile, 26C>T	Chr 13	121	*HpyCH4 III*	65, 56	121, 65, 56	121
NBN	rs1805794	Glu185Gln, 553G>C	Chr 8	174	*Hinf I*	125, 49	174, 125, 49	174
NBN	rs1805787	1125–520 G>C	Chr 8	197	*Ear I*	172, 25	197, 172, 25	197
RAD51	rs1801320	−98G>C	Chr 19	131	*BstN I*	71, 60	131, 71, 60	131
RAD51	rs1801321	−61G>T	Chr 19	131	*NgoM IV*	110, 21	131, 110, 21	131
ATM	rs3218698	3285-10delT	Chr 11	200	*Fnu4H I*	200	200, 176, 24	176,24
OGG1	rs1052133	Ser326Cys (C>G)	Chr 3	156	*Fnu4HI*	156	156, 100, 56	100, 56
Profibrotic and inflammatory cytokine								
TGF-β1	rs1800469	509C>T	Chr 19	418	*Bsu36I*	229,189	418,229,189	418
Antioxidant genes								
CAT	rs7943316	−21A>T	Chr 11	250	*Hinf I*	177, 73	250, 177, 73	250
SOD2	rs4880	Val16Ala (C>T)	Chr 6	207	*BsaWI*	207	207, 167, 40	167, 40
NQO1	rs1131341	C>T	Chr 16	194	*Msp I*	102,92	194,102,94	194
Detoxification genes								
GSTP1	rs1695	Ile105Val (G>A)	Chr 11	433	*BsmAI*	222,106,105	328,222,106,105	328, 106, 105
GSTT1	-	Present/Null	Chr 22	480				
GSTM1	-	Present/Null	Chr 1	240				

unknown origin, data from cancers in these regions were excluded for analysing oral mucositis. Of all the polymorphisms tested, RAD51 (rs1801321) Ku70 (rs2267437) and XRCC4 (rs1805377) were found to deviate from Hardy-Weinberg equilibrium. Univariate analysis showed that none of the polymorphisms presented any significant association to skin reaction (Table 4). However, it indicated that odds of patients experiencing severe oral mucositis (grade >2) with recessive allele of NBN (rs1805794) was 3.75 times higher having a confidence interval of 1.201–11.70 and $p = 0.023$. Also, heterozygous variants in CAT (rs7943316) displayed 0.452 (odds value) times lesser prone to experience severe oral mucositis (grade >2) with a confidence interval of 0.206–0.993 and $p = 0.048$. In continuation, multivariate analysis indicated that odds of patients experiencing severe oral mucositis

Table 3. Effect of confounding factors on the set of samples analysed.

Confounding factors	Grade ≤2 Skin reaction (n = 139)	Grade >2 Skin reaction (n = 44)	p-value	Grade ≤2 Mucositis (n = 66)	Grade >2 Mucositis (n = 54)	p-value
Age	54.55±11.041	54.41±13.191	0.948	51.98±11.48	54.15±12.49	0.326
Gender	120m, 19f	37m, 7f	0.805	57m, 9f	45m, 9f	0.798
Diabetes	19	4	0.305	7	7	0.778
Hypertension	14	9	0.114	7	8	0.583
Alcohol	53	13	0.369	29	12	**0.020***
Smoking	93	29	1.000	47	35	0.555
Surgery	51	15	0.858	27	18	0.451
Chemotherapy	111	37	0.148	52	47	0.429

Table 4. Univariate analysis of candidate single nucleotide polymorphisms and radiation-induced oral mucositis and skin reactions in head and neck cancer patients.

Gene name	Genotype	Skin reaction ≤2 (n = 139)	Skin reaction >2 (n = 44)	Odds ratio	95% CI	p-value	Oral Mucositis ≤2 (N = 66)	Oral Mucositis >2 (N = 54)	Odds ratio	95% CI	p-value
XRCC1 (rs25487)	AA	50	17	Reference			29	23	Reference		
	GA	62	14	0.411	0.154–1.096	0.076	28	25	1.339	0.418–4.295	0.623
	GG	15	8	0.545	0.204–1.458	0.227	9	6	1.190	0.370–3.829	0.771
XRCC1 (rs1799782)	CC	95	31	Reference			48	40	Reference		
	CT	30	6	0.624	0.253–1.537	0.305	15	12	.960	.403–2.285	0.927
	TT	2	2	1.962	0.315–12.228	0.470	3	2	.800	.127–5.026	0.812
XRCC1 (rs25489)	AA	97	30	Reference			52	41	Reference		
	GA	30	8	0.727	0.307–1.722	0.469	14	13	1.087	.454–2.603	0.851
	GG	0	1	3.000	0.183–49.239	0.442	0	0	2.049	000	1.000
XRCC1 (rs3213245)	TT	58	21	Reference			28	27	Reference		
	TC	53	16	0.955	0.469–1.943	0.898	27	23	0.883	0.410–1.903	0.751
	CC	16	2	0.452	0.122–1.677	0.235	11	4	0.377	0.107–1.330	0.129
RAD51 (rs1801321)*	GG	81	20	Reference			45	30	Reference		
	GT	21	11	1.891	0.842–4.247	0.123	12	14	1.750	0.712–4.299	0.222
	TT	25	8	1.164	0.466–2.909	0.745	9	10	1.667	0.606–4.586	0.323
RAD51 (rs1801320)	GG	90	29	Reference			48	35	Reference		
	CG	34	9	.842	0.377–1.880	0.674	17	17	1.371	0.616–3.055	0.440
	CC	3	1	1.010	0.102–10.04	0.993	1	2	2.743	0.239–31.45	0.418
NBN (rs1805794)	GG	44	13	Reference			24	16	Reference		
	CG	62	13	0.906	0.409–2.010	0.808	36	23	0.958	0.422–2.178	0.919
	CC	21	13	2.110	0.853–5.223	0.106	6	15	3.750	1.201–11.70	**0.023**
NBN (rs1805787)	GG	87	30	Reference			44	40	Reference		
	GC	36	8	0.599	0.254–1.411	0.241	22	12	0.550	0.237–1.275	0.164
	CC	4	1	0.554	0.063–4.911	0.596	0	2	1.777E9	.000	0.999
OGG1 (rs1052133)	CC	57	13	Reference			31	26	Reference		
	CG	53	19	1.235	0.586–2.605	0.579	25	23	1.097	0.508–2.368	0.814
	GG	17	7	1.560	0.583–4.176	0.376	10	5	0.596	0.181–1.955	0.396
GSTP1 (rs1695)	AA	63	21	Reference			37	30	Reference		
	AG	52	14	0.737	0.355–1.528	0.412	25	18	0.888	0.410–1.925	0.764
	GG	12	4	0.933	0.275–3.162	0.912	4	6	1.850	0.478–7.163	0.373
GSTM1	1	88	28	Reference			47	33	Reference		
	0	39	11	0.866	0.422–1.778	0.695	19	21	0.635	0.296–1.363	0.244
GSTT1	1	100	32	Reference			48	46	Reference		
	0	27	7	1.394	0.563–3.446	0.473	18	8	2.156	0.854–5.442	0.104

Table 4. Cont.

Gene name	Genotype	Skin reaction ≤2 (n = 139)	Skin reaction >2 (n = 44)	Odds ratio	95% CI	p-value	Oral Mucositis ≤2 (N = 66)	Oral Mucositis >2 (N = 54)	Odds ratio	95% CI	p-value
CAT (rs7943316)	TT	55	14	Reference			21	25	Reference		
	TA	62	17	0.532	0.532–2.356	0.766	39	21	0.452	0.206–0.993	**0.048**
	AA	10	8	0.874	0.874–7.151	0.087	6	8	1.120	0.335–3.745	0.854
ATM (rs3218698)	T/T	113	36	Reference			56	49	Reference		
	T/−T	14	3	0.718	0.228–2.258	0.571	10	5	0.571	0.183–1.787	.336
Ku80 (rs3835)	AA	96	27	Reference			53	39	Reference		
	GA	25	12	1.543	0.701–3.400	0.282	11	14	1.730	0.709–4.218	0.228
	GG	6	0	0.000	0.000 -	0.999	2	1	0.679	0.059–7.763	0.756
KU70 (rs2267437)*	CC	82	27	Reference			41	37	Reference		
	CG	33	10	0.812	0.370–1.784	0.605	19	13	0.758	0.329–1.745	0.515
	GG	12	2	0.401	0.086–1.865	0.244	6	4	0.739	0.193–2.824	0.658
XRCC4 (rs1805377)*	GG	94	28	Reference			44	40	Reference		
	GA	28	9	1.028	0.455–2.325	0.947	20	11	0.605	0.258–1.417	0.247
	AA	5	2	1.062	0.204–5.526	0.943	2	3	1.650	0.262–10.386	0.594
XRCC3 (rs861539)	CC	87	29	Reference			42	32	Reference		
	CT	46	15	0.978	0.477–2.007	0.952	22	22	1.313	0.621–2.775	0.477
	TT	6	0	0.000	0.000	0.999	2	0	0.000	0.000	0.999
LIG4 (rs1805388)	CC	100	32	Reference			52	48	Reference		
	CT	26	6	0.724	0.292–1.794	0.486	13	4	0.333	0.102–1.093	0.070
	TT	1	1	1.500	0.132–17.03	0.744	1	2	2.167	0.190–24.66	0.533
SOD2 (rs4880)	CC	29	11	Reference			15	18	Reference		
	CT	71	17	0.688	0.307–1.542	0.364	35	24	0.571	0.242–1.350	0.202
	TT	27	11	0.992	0.386–2.548	0.987	16	12	0.625	0.227–1.724	0.364
TGF β1(rs1800469)	CC	62	16	Reference			30	23	Reference		
	CT	50	16	1.361	0.646–2.869	0.417	29	23	1.034	0.478–2.237	0.931
	TT	15	7	1.855	0.686–5.015	0.224	7	8	1.491	0.472–4.711	0.496
NQO1 (rs1131341)	CC	103	33	Reference			55	45	Reference		
	CT	21	6	0.818	0.309–2.168	0.687	9	8	1.086	0.388–3.045	0.875
	TT	3	0	0.000	0.000	0.999	2	1	0.611	0.054–6.959	0.692

* Not in HWE.

Table 5. Multivariate analysis for CAT and NBN polymorphisms with radiation-induced oral mucositis in presence of alcohol among head and neck cancer patients.

Gene name	Genotype	Oral mucositis ≤2 (n = 66)	Oral mucositis >2 (n = 54)	Adjusted Odds ratio	95% CI	p- value
CAT (rs7943316)	TT	21	25	Reference		
	TA	39	21	0.463	0.199–1.076	0.074
	AA	6	8	1.675	0.427–6.575	0.460
NBN (rs1805794)	GG	24	16	Reference		
	CG	36	23	1.275	0.531–3.062	0.587
	CC	6	15	4.728	1.384–16.151	**0.013**

(grade >2) with recessive allele of NBN (rs1805794) was 4.72 times higher having a confidence interval of 1.384–16.151 and p = 0.013 (Table 5). However, when we categorized the data as chemoradiotherapy and radiotherapy as separate groups, we did not observe any such significant association with normal tissue toxicity in chemoradiotherapy group (Table S1 and Table S2). Further, as the sample number is less in radiation therapy alone (n = 35) it is difficult to effectively conclude the findings.

Haplotyping and combination of risk alleles

Haplotype analysis was done for 4 SNPs in XRCC1, 2 polymorphisms in RAD51 as well as 2 polymorphisms in NBN to explore association of the combinatorial effect of these variants with increased normal tissue radiosensitivity. Haplotype analysis of NBN (rs1805787, rs1805794) gene demonstrated G-C haplotype to be associated with development of oral mucositis (odds ratio of 1.687 and 95% CI of 1.005–2.831 with p = 0.047) (Table 6). Further, to determine if any multiple SNP has an additive effect on the oral mucositis as well as skin reaction, the average number of variant alleles per patient in each RTOG group was analysed (Figure 1). Based on the allele frequency reported in the dbSNP database, we have reported the wild type, heterozygous and recessive genotypes. We considered the minor allele in this group as the risk allele and counted the number of risk alleles in each patient. The results suggest that the number of variant alleles has no effect on severity of normal tissue toxicity.

Furthermore, we analysed the linkage disequilibrium pattern for SNPs in XRCC1 and found that rs3213245, rs1799782, rs25489 and rs25487 were linked with severe oral mucositis while, rs1799782 and rs25489 were linked with severe skin reaction. Also, to validate this linked SNPs were analysed for linkage disequilibrium pattern separately in normal tissue overreactor and non-overreactor phenotypes. The d′ values were strikingly higher in normal tissue radiosensitive phenotypes (Figure 2).

Discussion

Although, the growing volume of SNP data suggests the genetic basis for susceptibility to radiotherapy induced acute effects, it is

Table 6. Haplotype analysis for XRCC1 (rs3213245, rs1799782, rs25489 and rs25487), *RAD51* (rs1801320, rs1801321) and *NBN* (rs1805787, rs1805794) and radiation-induced oral mucositis and skin reactions in head and neck cancer patients.

Gene		Haplotype	Skin reactions			Oral mucositis			
		OR frequency	NOR frequency	Fisher's p-value	Odds ratio (95% CI)	OR frequency	NOR frequency	Fisher's p-value	Odds ratio (95% CI)
XRCC1	C-C-A-A	20.00 (0.256)	72.86 (0.287)	0.406	0.782 (0.438–1.397)				
	C-C-A-G	-	-	-	-	28.05 (0.260)	43.53 (0.330)	0.195	0.687 (0.389–1.215)
	T-C-A-A	9.07 (0.116)	33.72 (0.133)	0.573	0.799 (0.365–1.747)	32.20 (0.298)	39.81 (0.302)	0.873	0.955 (0.544–1.676)
	T-C-A-G	28.93 (0.371)	76.49 (0.301)	0.414	1.250 (0.731–2.136)	16.05(0.149)	12.94 (0.098)	0.252	1.576 (0.719–3.453)
	T-C-G-A	10.0 (0.128)	25.78 (0.101)	0.627	1.213 (0.556–2.648)	-	-	-	-
	T-C-G-G	-	-	-	-	12.75 (0.118)	9.71 (0.074)	0.258	1.654 (0.687–3.986)
	T-T-A-A	8.93 (0.114)	26.28 (0.103)	0.918	1.043 (0.465–2.338)				
	T-T-A-G	-	-	-	-	13.90 (0.129)	17.38 (0.132)	0.897	0.951 (0.445–2.033)
RAD	G-C	7.97 (0.102)	32.60 (0.128)	0.537	0.773 (0.340–1.754)	16.65 (0.154)	16.70 (0.127)	0.538	1.258 (0.605~2.616)
	G-G	43.03 (0.552)	150.40 (0.592)	0.526	0.848 (0.508–1.414)	57.35 (0.531)	85.30 (0.646)	0.070	0.620 (0.369~1.043)
	T-C	3.03 (0.039)	7.40 (0.029)	0.667	1.347 (0.345–5.258)	4.35 (0.040)	2.30 (0.017)	0.282	2.371 (0.470~11.968)
	T-G	23.97 (0.307)	63.60 (0.250)	0.319	1.328 (0.760–2.322)	29.65 0.275)	27.70 (0.210)	0.242	1.425 (0.786~2.583)
NBN	C-G	39.0 (0.500)	103.99 (0.409)	0.158	1.442 (0.867–2.401)	16.00 (0.148)	21.99 (0.167)	0.696	0.870 (0.431~1.753)
	G-C	10.0 (0.128)	43.99 (0.173)	0.346	0.702 (0.335–1.470)	53.00 (0.491)	47.99 (0.364)	**0.047**	1.687 (1.005~2.831)
	G-G	29.0(0.372)	106.01 (0.417)	0.473	0.826 (0.490–1.393)	39.00 (0.361)	62.01 (0.470)	0.089	0.638 (0.379~1.074)

All those haplotypes with frequency <0.03 were ignored during the analysis.

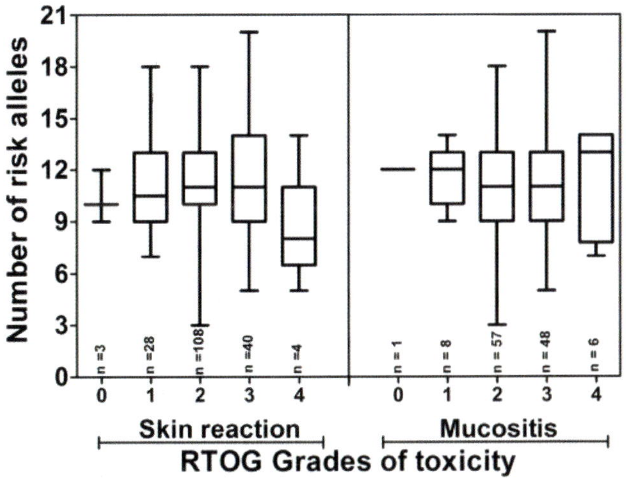

Figure 1. Association of average number of risk allele with the increasing RTOG grades of normal tissue toxicity. The results of Kruskal-Wallis test demonstrate that the comparison between the groups are non-significant (p>0.05). The error bars represent the minimum to maximum values of risk allele represented in each group.

less clear whether the SNPs can serve as a biomarker for predicting the normal tissue toxicity. Identifying the genetic profiles associated with an enhanced or reduced risk for radiotherapy complications seems to be a most promising factor to improve the efficacy of radiotherapy [9] [16]. The amount of human genetic diversity is immense, and we are just now beginning to understand how such changes influence the specific phenotypic expression. Remarkable genetic variations exist among populations and understanding this variation will help us to tailor the therapy with a personalised approach for safer and effective outcome.

Based on the functional significance of genes in radiation response, we analysed the association of some of the important gene variants belonging to DNA damage response, DNA repair, profibrotic cytokine, antioxidant genes with normal tissue over-reactor phenotype (grade >2 toxicity). We did not find any significant association for either the selected SNPs or for the haplotypes with the risk of developing oral mucositis and skin reaction in HNC patients. However, we observed an association for NBN (rs1805794) polymorphism in univariate as well as multivariate model of analysis. In addition, one of the NBN haplotype was associated with severe oral mucositis. NBN is a component of MRE complex (MRE11-RAD50-NBN) which is

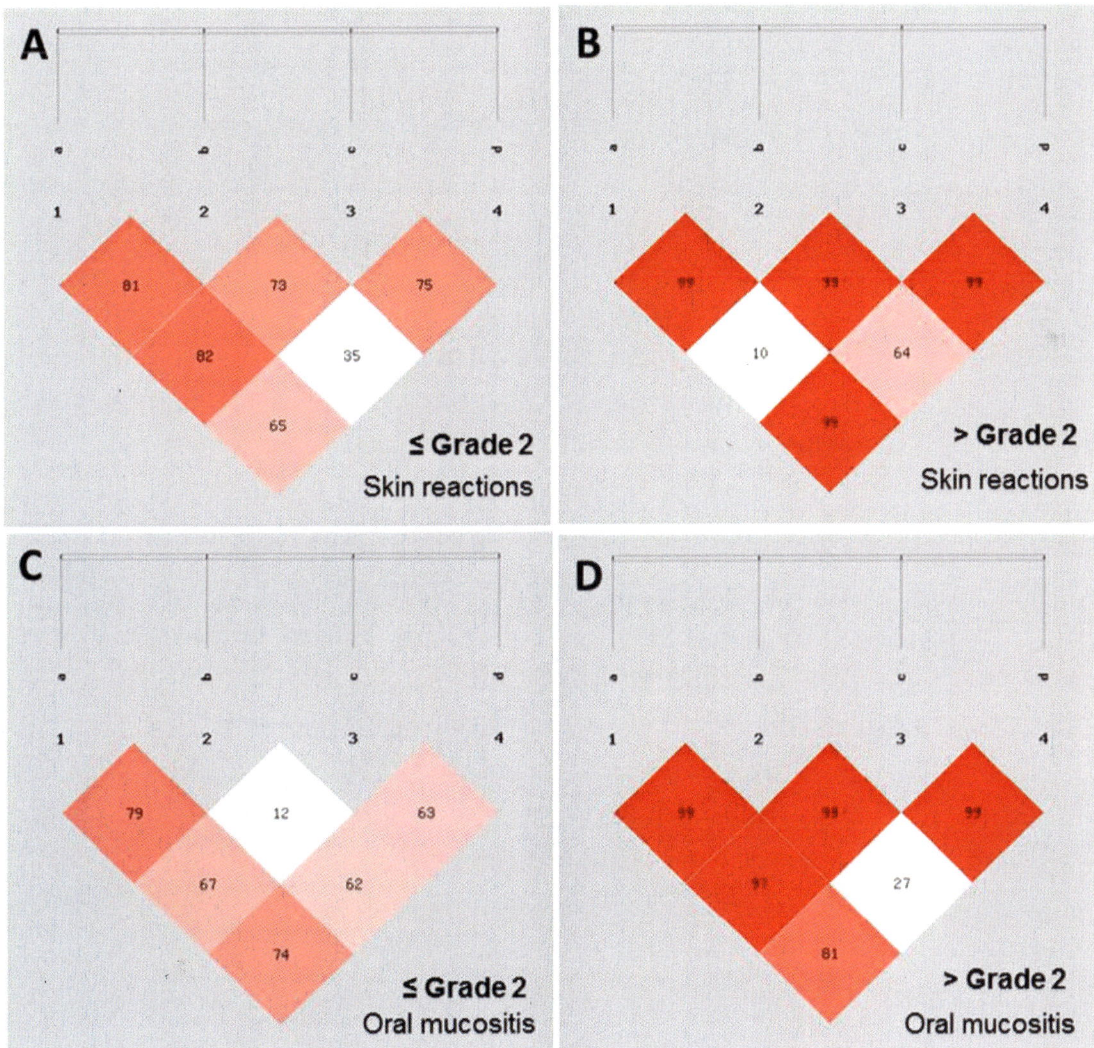

Figure 2. Linkage disequilibrium analysis for XRCC1 polymorphisms (a = rs3213245, b = rs1799782, c = rs25487, d = rs25489) for skin reaction (A and B) and oral mucositis (C and D). The numbers inside every box represent r2 values (%) of the linkage disequilibrium.

involved in damage sensing, signaling and responding to DSBs [17]. This polymorphism brings about the change in Nibrin protein at 185th codon position from glutamic acid to glutamine and the functional significance of this change still remains unclear [18]. It was reported that rs1805794 was not associated with acute side effects of radiotherapy in breast cancer patients [18] [19]. Also, there are studies which report no association for rs1805794 and late radiation toxicities [20] [21].

Currently there are only few studies related to normal tissue toxicity and genotype analysis in HNC patients, and it is less clear whether the SNPs can serve as a biomarker for predicitng the normal tissue toxicity. Werbrouck and co-workers [22] report that SNPs in DNA repair genes XRCC3 (rs861539) and Ku70 (rs2267437) may help in determining the risk for acute dysphagia. Study conducted by Pratesi et al. [23] has suggested that patients with XRCC1 (rs25487) and RAD51 (rs1801320) have higher likelihood of developing oral mucositis and dysphagia in HNC patients. Unlike previous reports, null variants of GSTM1 and GSTT1 also showed no association with the development of acute reactions [24]. Also, a large-scale analysis for screening 3,144 SNPs from 156 breast cancer patients has revealed that ABCA1 and IL12RB2 polymorphism are highly susceptible to radiation-induced dermatitis [25]. Conversely, several studies aimed at validating the effect of TGFβ1 [26], [27], ATM, GSTP1, SOD2, TGFβ1, XPD and XRCC1 [28] have indicated no such association for the risk of developing normal tissue toxicity. Earlier reports with the approach of haplotype analysis have revealed several haplotypes with significant evidence for predicting acute reactions of radiotherapy [4] [29] [30]. Our analysis for XRCC1 haplotype did not associate with the risk of increased acute reactions, but NBN haplotype had an association for oral mucositis.. Studies suggest that SNPs or haplotypes in functionally important candidate genes alone may not contribute to radiation induced acute reactions. In addition, extensive literature review [8], [31] has indicated a contradictory association for susceptibility to radiation induced toxicity, which supports the need for further studies.

In conclusion, we report that gene variants and haplotypes of NBN are associated with the risk of developing oral mucositis in head and neck cancer patients undergoing chemoradiotherapy/radiotherapy. In addition to the screening for rare variants having large effects and common variants with small effects, we need to identify other types of variation and explore gene environment interactions for developing predictive models. Further replication of our results in large data sets with pathway-based approach and large genome wide association studies with methodological approach can be of great use to develop predictive biomarkers for this complex trait and the findings must be independently confirmed in different populations.

Acknowledgments

We are grateful to all the participating patients for their co-operation. We are indebted to Dr. K. Satyamoorthy, Director, School of Life Sciences for his encouragement and Manipal University for providing the facilities while undertaking this study. We thank Prof. P. Gopalakrishna Bhat, Prof. Padmalatha Rai S. and Dr. Saadi Abdul Vahab for helpful comments on the manuscript.

Author Contributions

Conceived and designed the experiments: VBM DJF SRBS. Performed the experiments: GHV KDM HN. Analyzed the data: GHV KDM HN SRBS. Contributed reagents/materials/analysis tools: VBM SB DJF KS SB. Wrote the manuscript: GHV KDM SRBS.

References

1. Trotti A (2000) Toxicity in head and neck cancer: a review of trends and issues. Int J Radiat Oncol Biol Phys 47:1–12.
2. Safwat A, Bentzen SM, Turesson I, Hendry JH (2002) Deterministic rather than stochastic factors explain most of the variation in the expression of skin telangiectasia after radiotherapy. Int J Radiat Oncol Biol Phys 52:198–204.
3. Barnett GC, West CM, Dunning AM, Elliott RM, Coles CE, et al. (2009) Normal tissue reactions to radiotherapy: towards tailoring treatment dose by genotype. Nat Rev Cancer 9:134–142.
4. Ishikawa A, Suga T, Shoji Y, Kato S, Ohno T, et al. (2011) Genetic variants of NPAT-ATM and AURKA are associated with an early adverse reaction in the gastrointestinal tract of patients with cervical cancer treated with pelvic radiation therapy. Int J Radiat Oncol Biol Phys 81:1144–52.
5. Giotopoulos G, Symonds RP, Foweraker K, Griffin M, Peat I, et al. (2007) The late radiotherapy normal tissue injury phenotypes of telangiectasia, fibrosis and atrophy in breast cancer patients have distinct genotype-dependent causes. Br J Cancer 96:1001–1007.
6. Goutham HV, Mumbrekar KD, Vadhiraja BM, Fernandes DJ, Sharan K, et al. (2012) DNA Double-strand break analysis by γ-H2AX Foci: a useful method for determining the overreactors to radiation-induced acute reactions among head-and-neck cancer patients. Int J Radiat Oncol Biol Phys 84:e607–12.
7. Andreassen CA, Dikomey E, Parliament M, West CML (2012) Will SNPs be useful predictors of normal tissue radiosensitivity in the future? Radiother Oncol 105:283–288
8. Popanda O, Marquardt JU, Chang-Claude J, Schmezer P (2009) Genetic variation in normal tissue toxicity induced by ionizing radiation. Mut Res 667:58–69.
9. Barnett GC, Coles CE, Elliott RM, Baynes C, Luccarini C, et al. (2012) Independent validation of genes and polymorphisms reported to be associated with radiation toxicity: a prospective analysis study. Lancet Oncol 13: 65–77.
10. Zackrisson B, Mercke C, Strander H, Wennerberg J, Cavallin-Ståhl E (2003) A systematic overview of radiation therapy effects in head and neck cancer. Acta Oncol 42:443–61.
11. Parliament MB, Murray D (2010) Single nucleotide polymorphisms of DNA repair genes as predictors of radioresponse. Semin Radiat Oncol 20:232–40.
12. Cox JD, Stetz J, Pajak TF (1995) Toxicity criteria of the Radiation Therapy Oncology Group (RTOG) and the European Organization for Research and Treatment of Cancer (EORTC). Int J Radiat Oncol Biol Phys 31:1341–1346.
13. Li Z, Zhang Z, He Z, Tang W, Li T, et al. (2009) A partition-ligation combinationsubdivision EM algorithm for haplotype inference with multiallelic markers: update of the SHEsis. Available: http://analysis.bio-x.cn. Cell Res 19:519–23.
14. Guerra JL, Gomez D, Wei Q, Liu Z, Wang LE, et al. (2012) Association between single nucleotide polymorphisms of the transforming growth factor β1 gene and the risk of severe radiation esophagitis in patients with lung cancer. Radiother Oncol 105:299–304.
15. Bentzen SM (2006) Preventing or reducing late side effects of radiation therapy: radiobiology meets molecular pathology. Nat Rev Cancer 6:702–13.
16. West CM, Barnett GC (2012) Genetics and genomics of radiotherapy toxicity: towards prediction. Genome Med 3:e52.
17. Silva J, Teixeira AL, Lobo F, Maurício J, Medeiros R (2012) DNA repair system and prostate cancer progression: the role of NBS1 polymorphism (rs1805794). DNA Cell Biol 3: 1182–6.
18. Popanda O, Tan XL, Ambrosone CB, Kropp S, Helmbold I, et al. (2006) Genetic polymorphisms in the DNA double-strand break repair genes XRCC3, XRCC2, and NBS1 are not associated with acute side effects of radiotherapy in breast cancer patients. Cancer Epidemiol Biomarkers Prev 15: 1048–50.
19. Millikan RC, Player JS, Decotret AR, Tse CK, Keku T (2012) Polymorphisms in DNA repair genes, medical exposure to ionizing radiation, and breast cancer risk. Cancer Epidemiol Biomarkers Prev 14: 2326–34.
20. Damaraju S, Murray D, Dufour J, Carandang D, Myrehaug S et al. (2006) Association of DNA repair and steroid metabolism gene polymorphisms with clinical late toxicity in patients treated with conformal radiotherapy for prostate cancer. Clin Cancer Res 12: 2545–54.
21. Chang-Claude J, Ambrosone CB, Lilla C, Kropp S, Helmbold I, et al. (2009) Genetic polymorphisms in DNA repair and damage response genes and late normal tissue complications of radiotherapy for breast cancer. Br J Cancer 100: 1680–6.
22. Werbrouck J, De Ruyck K, Duprez F, Veldeman L, Claes K, et al. (2009) Acute normal tissue reactions in head-and-neck cancer patients treated with IMRT: influence of dose and association with genetic polymorphisms in DNA DSB repair genes. Int J Radiat Oncol Biol Phys 73:1187–1195.

23. Pratesi N, Mangoni M, Mancini I, Paiar F, Simi L, et al. (2011) Association between single nucleotide polymorphisms in the XRCC1 and RAD51 genes and clinical radiosensitivity in head and neck cancer. Radiother Oncol 99:356–361.
24. Ambrosone CB, Tian C, Ahn J, Kropp S, Helmbold I, et al. (2006) Genetic predictors of acute toxicities related to radiation therapy following lumpectomy for breast cancer: a case-series study. Breast Can Res 8:R40.
25. Isomura M, Oya N, Tachiiri S, Kaneyasu Y, Nishimura Y, et al. (2008) IL12RB2 and ABCA1 genes are associated with susceptibility to radiation dermatitis. Clin Cancer Res 14:6683–9.
26. Voets AM, Oberije C, Struijk RB, Reymen B, De Ruyck K, et al. (2012) No association between TGFβ1 polymorphisms and radiation-induced lung toxicity in a European cohort of lung cancer patients. Radiother Oncol 105:296–8.
27. Reuther S, Metzke E, Bonin M, Petersen C, Dikomey E, et al. (2013) No effect of the transforming growth factor b1 promoter polymorphism c-509t on TGFβ1 gene expression, protein secretion, or cellular radiosensitivity. Int J Radiat Oncol Biol Phys 85: 460–65.
28. Zschenker O, Raabe A, Boeckelmann IK, Borstelmann S, Szymczak S, et al. (2010) Association of single nucleotide polymorphisms in ATM, GSTP1, SOD2, TGFβ1, XPD and XRCC1 with clinical and cellular radiosensitivity, Radiother Oncol 97:26–32.
29. Suga T, Ishikawa A, Kohda M, Otsuka Y, Yamada S, et al. (2007) Haplotype-based analysis of genes associated with risk of adverse skin reactions after radiotherapy in breast cancer patients. Int J Radiat Oncol Biol Phys 69:685–93.
30. Schirmer MA, Brockmöller J, Rave-Fränk M, Virsik P, Wilken B, et al. (2011) A putatively functional haplotype in the gene encoding transforming growth factor beta- 1 as a potential biomarker for radiosensitivity. Int J Radiat Oncol Biol Phys 79:866–74.
31. Andreassen CN, Alsner J (2009) Genetic variants and normal tissue toxicity after radiotherapy: a systematic review. Radiother Oncol 92:299–309.

9

Outcomes of Anterolateral Thigh Flap Reconstruction for Salvage Laryngopharyngectomy for Hypopharyngeal Cancer after Concurrent Chemoradiotherapy

Wei F. Chen[1], Kai-Ping Chang[2], Chih-Hao Chen[3], Victor Bong-Hang Shyu[3], Huang-Kai Kao[3]*

1 Division of Plastic and Reconstructive Surgery, Department of Surgery, University of Iowa Hospitals and Clinics, Iowa City, Iowa, United States of America, **2** Department of Otolaryngology – Head and Neck Surgery, Chang Gung Memorial Hospital & Chang Gung University College of Medicine, Taoyuan, Taiwan, **3** Department of Plastic and Reconstructive Surgery, Chang Gung Memorial Hospital & Chang Gung University College of Medicine, Taoyuan, Taiwan

Abstract

Objective: To evaluate the functional and oncological outcomes of anterolateral thigh flap reconstruction for salvage laryngopharyngectomy after concurrent chemoradiotherapy for patients with hypopharyngeal carcinoma.

Materials/Methods: A retrospective review was conducted on patients who underwent pharyngoesophageal reconstruction using anterolateral thigh flap after salvage laryngopharyngectomy for recurrent hypopharyngeal carcinoma between June 2003 and May 2010 at Chang Gung Memorial Hospital. The perioperative morbidity, mortality, functional outcomes, and oncological outcomes were evaluated.

Results: 33 patients were entered into the study. The mean follow-up time was 19.5±12.3 months. Recurrent pathological TNM stages included 3 (9.1%), 2 (6.1%), and 28 (84.8%) patients with stage II, III, and IV disease, respectively. Mean ICU stay was 10.3 days and the mean hospital stay was 39.9 days. Peri-operative mortality occurred in one patient (3%). 16 patients (48.5%) developed recipient site complications. Among them, 14 patients (42.4%) developed fistulas and 9 patients (27.3%) developed strictures. Except for 4 patients (12.1%), all achieved varying degree of oral intake with 29 patients (60.6%) being completely independent from tube feeding. The mean interval to start oral intake was 15.1 days. The 5-year overall survival and disease-free survival rates were 51.8% and 53.7%, respectively. The pN status is an independent predictor of overall survival and disease-free survival ($P = 0.027$ and 0.038, respectively).

Conclusion: Pharyngoesophageal reconstruction after salvage laryngopharyngectomy remains challenging even in the experienced hands. Reconstructive microsurgeons who are prepared to take on these cases should be equally well prepared to manage the potential postoperative complications.

Editor: Samuel J. Lin, Harvard Medical School, United States of America

Funding: The authors have no support or funding to report.

Competing Interests: The authors have declared that no competing interests exist.

* E-mail: kai3488@gmail.com

Introduction

Hypopharyngeal cancer has one of the worst prognoses of head and neck cancers because patients are often diagnosed at advanced stages. Chemoradiotherapy (CRT) has emerged as the mainstay of initial treatments of hypopharyngeal squamous cell carcinoma. In comparison to primary laryngopharyngectomy, it promises organ preservation and provides comparable survival benefits. Local recurrence after CCRT, however, remains a challenging problem. Salvage laryngopharyngectomy is considered to be the most effective treatment, especially in long-term disease control and restoration of oral intake. However, the technical difficulty of both tumor ablation and reconstruction, the expectedly high perioperative morbidity and mortality rates, the diminished quality of life due to functional sacrifice, and the overall poor prognoses of the patients with disease recurrence make the choice of salvage surgery for treatment of locally recurrent hypopharygeal cancer controversial.

Accepted reconstructive modalities include anterolateral thigh (ALT) flap, radial forearm flaps, jejunal flap, gastro-omental flap, and pectoralis flap. The choice of flap depends on individual surgeon's expertise and preference. A consensus on the flap selection has not been reached [1–4].

Our favorable and rather extensive experience of ALT flap in head and neck reconstruction had led us to use this versatile flap as the flap of choice in pharyngoesophageal reconstruction after salvage laryngopharyngectomy [5]. The advantages of ALT flap include consistent and reliable anatomy, long vascular pedicle, being far from the ablative site and allowing a two-team approach, the feasibility to create multiple skin paddles by recruiting additional perforators, the flexibility to reconstruct composite defects by recruiting different tissue types (adipose, muscle, and fascial components) all based on a single pedicle, and low donor site morbidity [6].

The aim of this study was to review our experience of using ALT flap for pharyngoesophageal reconstruction in patients undergoing salvage laryngopharyngectomy for disease recurrence after CCRT. We analyzed the oncological outcomes, complication rates, and the postoperative functional status of these patients.

Materials and Methods

Patients

This study was approved by the ethics committee of Chang Gung Memorial Hospital – Linkou Medical Center. Informed consent was not needed since the data were analyzed anonymously. The ethics committee specifically waived the need for consent. A retrospective review was conducted on all patients who underwent pharyngoesophageal reconstruction after salvage laryngopharyngectomy for recurrent hypopharyngeal carcinoma between June 2003 and May 2010 at Chang Gung Memorial Hospital (CCMH), Taiwan. Only patients who had resectable tumors and received ALT flap reconstruction when local recurrence was detected after CCRT were included in the study. All patients were regularly followed every two months until either October 2011 or death.

Reconstruction

The pharyngoesophageal reconstruction was circumferential in 30 patients (90.9%) and near-circumferential in 3 patients (9.1%). All were reconstructed with ALT flaps. The design and harvest of the ALT flaps were performed as previously described [5,6]. When additional bulk was needed, vastus lateralis (VL) muscle was recruited in a chimeric fashion to provide the needed volume (Fig. 1). 16 patients (48.5%) received ALT fasciocutaneous flap and 17 patients (51.5%) received ALT-VL chimeric flap. The ALT flap was tubularized either by itself or in combination with residual pharyngeal mucosa to form a neoesophagus. The average length of the flap was 16.2±5.8 cm (range, 8–25 cm) and the average width of the flap was 8.6±1.6 cm (range, 6–12 cm). When anterior neck resurfacing was needed and given permissible anatomy, a separate skin island based on independent perforator was harvested for this purpose. Contralateral superior thyroid artery (STA) was preferentially used as recipient artery as it tended to be minimally affected by CCRT. Contralateral transverse cervical artery was used as an alternative when STA was not available.

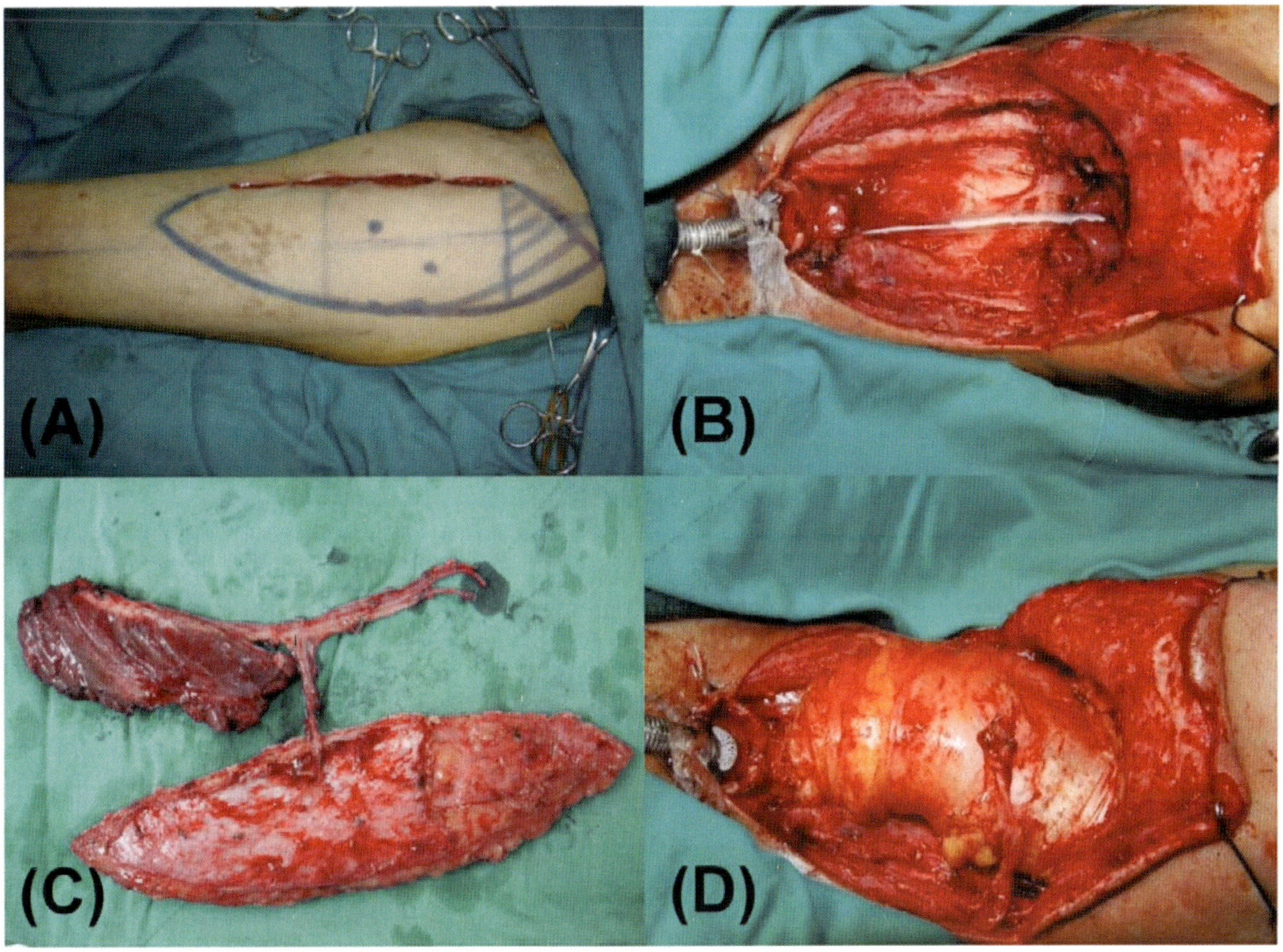

Figure 1. Pharyngoesophageal reconstruction with the anterolateral thigh flap after total laryngopharyngectomy. (A) Preoperative marking. (B) After salvage pharyngolaryngectomy with neck dissection, an "empty" neck was noted. (C) A chimeric flap was composed of a skin paddle and a piece of vastus lateralis (VL) muscle. The skin paddle was tubularized to form a neoesophagus and the VL muscle was used to increase tissue bulk and to obliterate the dead space. (D) Immediate photograph after reconstruction.

Table 1. Patients' details.

	No. of patients (%)
Age (yrs)	
Range	39–79
Mean (SD)	57.4 (9.4)
Gender	
M	33 (100)
BMI[a]	
Range	28.6–16.5
Mean (SD)	21.8 (3.3)
≦20	13 (39.4)
20–25	13 (39.4)
≧25	7 (21.2)
Location	
Piriform sinus	29 (87.8)
Postcricoid	2 (6.1)
Post-pharyngeal wall	2 (6.1)
T stage	
T2	4 (12.1)
T3	1 (3.0)
T4	27 (81.8)
N stage	
N0	20 (60.6)
N1	5 (15.2)
N2	8 (24.2)
Overall Stage	
II	3 (9.1)
III	2 (6.1)
IV	28 (84.8)

[a]body mass index.

Postoperative Care

All patients were admitted to a specialized microsurgery intensive care unit (ICU) postoperatively for flap monitoring. Tube feeding was started on the first postoperative day. The patients were routinely transferred to regular wards on postoperative day 8. Liquid diet was started as soon as a contrast esophagogram on postoperative day 10 demonstrated intact anastomoses. The diet was advanced as tolerated. Fistulae identified on the contrast esophagram were managed conservatively. Surgical treatments were performed when the conservative management failed.

Statistical Analysis

All data is described as mean ± SD. Statistical analyses was performed using SAS software (version 9.1, SAS institute Inc., Cary, NC). Survival analysis was plotted using the Kaplan-Meyer method and differences were evaluated using the log-rank test. Univariate and multivariate regression analyses were used to define specific risk factors for overall survival and disease-free survival. All *P* values were 2-sided and statistical significance was accepted when $P<0.05$.

Table 2. Operative data.

	No. of patients (%)
Operative time (min)	
Range	436–790
Mean (SD)	730.7 (123.5)
Blood loss (mL)	
Range	50–1100
Mean (SD)	312.1 (207.7)
ICU[f] stay (day)	
Range	6–41
Mean (SD)	10.3 (8.3)
Hospital stay (day)	
Range	13–92
Mean (SD)	39.9 (22.1)
In-hospital death	1 (3.0)
Flap related	
Defect	
Circumferential	30 (90.9)
Near-Circumferential	3 (9.1)
Type	
ALT[a] skin tube	16 (48.5)
ALT+chimeric VL[b] muscle	17 (51.5)
Flap width (cm)	
Range	6–12
Mean (SD)	8.6 (1.6)
Flap length (cm)	
Range	8–25
Mean (SD)	16.2 (5.8)
Recipient artery	
STA[c]	29 (87.9)
TCA[d]	4 (12.1)
Donor site closure	
Primary	28 (84.8)
STSG[e]	5 (15.2)

[a]anterolateral thigh;
[b]vastus lateralis;
[c]superior thyroid artery;
[d]transverse cervical artery;
[e]split thickness skin graft;
[f]intensive care unit.

Results

Patient Characteristics

During the study period, 47 patients underwent pharyngoesophageal reconstruction for salvage ablation for local recurrence. After excluding those reconstructed with non-ALT flaps, a cohort of 33 patients remained. The mean follow-up period was 2.6 years (range, 0.6–6.9 years). All patients were male, with a mean age of 57.4 years (Table 1). Mean body mass index (BMI) was 21.8 (range, 16.5 to 28.6).

Operative Details

Intraoperative data are summarized in Table 2. The operative time was 730.7±123.5 min (range, 436–790 min). This represent-

Table 3. Postoperative complications.

	No. of patients (%)
Recipient site	
Partial necrosis	4 (12.1)
Flap failure	1 (3.0)
Venous insufficiency	2 (6.1)
Neck infection	15 (45.5)
Hematoma	2 (6.1)
Carotid artery blow out	2 (6.1)
Re-operation within 1 week	5 (15.2)
Fistula	14 (42.4)
Stricture	9 (27.3)
Donor site	
Seroma	1 (3.0)
Hematoma	1 (3.0)
Infection	1 (3.0)
Wound dehiscence	1 (3.0)
Medical complications	
Cardiac	1 (3.0)
Pulmonary	2 (6.1)
Renal	1 (3.0)
Hepatic	1 (3.0)

ed the combined operative time of the ablative and reconstructive procedures, as a two-team approach was consistently used. The intraoperative blood loss was 312.1±207.7 mL (range, 50–1100 mL). Primary closure of the donor site was achieved in 28 patients (84.8%) of the patients.

Postoperative Course and Morbidities

Mean ICU stay was 10.3 days (range, 6–41 days) and the mean hospital stay was 39.9 days (range, 13–92 days) (Table 2). There was 1 (3.0%) in-hospital mortality. Recipient site complications developed in 16 patients (48.5%) and 11 patients (33%) experienced more than one complication (Table 3). Reoperation within 7 days from the initial surgery was necessary in 5 patients (15.2%). Among patients who underwent reoperative surgery, one had unsalvageable flap failure and was replaced with pectoralis major flap, two had venous insufficiency that were successfully salvaged, and the remaining two developed carotid blowout manifested as acute neck hematoma. Both cases of carotid blowout were successfully treated with vessel ligation without neurologic sequelae.

Esophagocutaneous fistulae were identified in 14 patients (42.4%) upon barium contrast study. Among them, 5 fistulae responded favorably to conservative management and went on to complete healing without surgical intervention. In the remaining 9 cases that failed conservative management, 5 underwent successful surgical revision; the remaining 4 patients could not undergo revision due to disease recurrence.

During follow-up, 9 patients (27.3%) developed anastomotic strictures, 7.2±5.1 months (range, 3–12 months) after surgery. 2 patients developed strictures at upper anastomosis (pharyngeal junction) and 7 patients developed strictures at the lower anastomosis (thoracic esophageal junction). All were successfully

Table 4. Postoperative diet.

Interval to start oral intake, d, mean±SD (range)[a]	15.1±6.2 (9–30)
Diet, no. (%)	
Soft	20 (60.6)
Liquid	3 (9.1)
Partial TF[b]	6 (18.2)
Total TF	4 (12.1)

[a]29 patients achieve oral intake.
[b]tube feeding.

treated by mechanical dilatation and the average duration of treatment was 3.3 months.

Swallowing Function

The time interval from the time of operation to the time of oral intake was 15.1±6.2 days (range, 9–30 days) (Table 4). Swallowing function was determined by the highest level of diet achieved after surgery. Among them, 29 patients (87.9%) achieved oral intake. 23 patients (69.7%) achieved soft or liquid diet. 20 patients (60.6%) were completely independent from tube feeding. 6 patients remained partially dependent on tube feedings due to strictures. Four patients remained completely dependent on tube-feeding due to persistent fistulas.

Pathology

All recurrent disease was local, regional, or both. None of the patients had distant metastasis after preoperative systemic workups. Recurrent pathological T stage included 4 (9.1%), 1 (6.1%), and 28 (84.8%) patients with T2, T3, and T4, respectively. 13 patients (39.4%) had lymph node metastasis, in which 5 patients (15.2%) had N1 and 8 patients (24.2%) had N2 (Table 1). The overall stages included 3 (9.1%), 2 (6.1%), and 28 (84.8%) patients with stage II, III, and IV disease, respectively. After ablative resection, the pathological examination demonstrated the nearest resection margin to be 4±2.9 mm (range, 0–20 mm).

Disease Control and Survival

The 5-year overall survival and disease-free survival for this specific group of patients were 51.8% and 53.7%, respectively (Figure 2).

Correlation of BMI, Surgical Margins and Nodal Status (pN) to Patient Overall Survival (OS)

Using data from these 33 patients undergoing salvage resection and free ALT flap reconstruction, we further evaluated whether BMI, surgical margins, and pN status had any impact upon OS. BMI and surgical margins were stratified into two groups by median, and pN status was stratified by pN0 and pN+. We found that the 3-year survival of pN0 and pN+ was 65.1% and 32.9%, respectively. This difference in OS was significant when compared using a log-rank test ($P=0.034$) (Figure 3). Conversely, 3-year OS shown by Kaplan-Meier plots of patients stratified by lower and higher BMI values was not significantly different (50.0% and 50.1%, respectively; $P=0.749$) (Figure 3). Likewise 3-year OS of the patients stratified by lower and higher surgical margins were not significantly different either (38.5% and 62.7%, respectively; $P=0.182$). To determine whether pN status is an independent predictor of OS, a multivariate analysis was carried out using age,

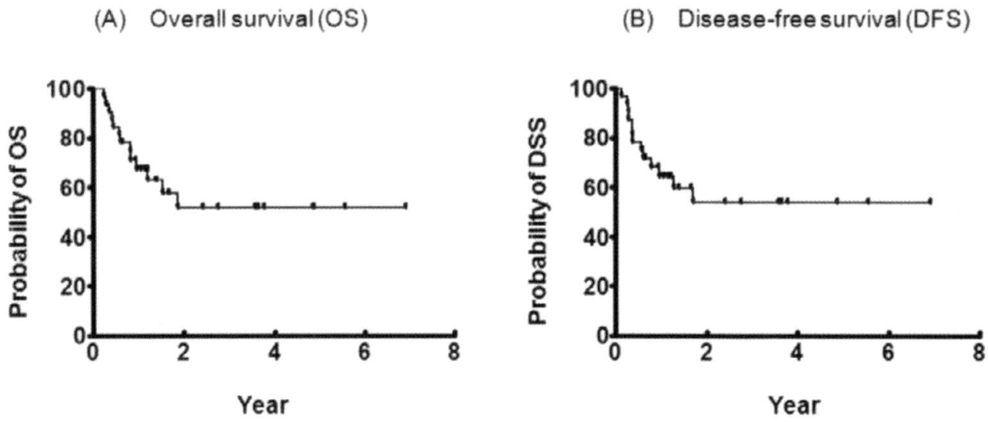

Figure 2. Kaplan-Meier survival analysis in patients with recurrent hypopharyngeal cancers after concurrent chemoradiotherapy receiving ablating salvage surgery and anterolateral thigh flap reconstruction. (A) & (B), Kaplan-Meier plots indicated that 5-year overall survival (OS) and disease-free survival (DFS) were 51.8% and 53.7%, respectively.

gender, pT status, pN status, BMI values and surgical margins as parameters. We found pN status was the only independent predictors of OS ($P = 0.027$).

Correlation of BMI, Surgical Margins and pN Status to Patient Disease-free Survival (DFS)

We also evaluated whether BMI, surgical margins, and pN status have any impact on DFS and found that the 3-year survival of pN0 and pN+ were 65.1% and 32.9%, respectively. This difference in DFS was significant when compared using a log-rank test ($P = 0.034$) (Figure 3). Conversely, 3-year DFS shown by Kaplan-Meier plots of patients stratified by lower and higher BMI values was not significantly different (51.4% and 51.7%, respectively; $P = 0.711$) (Figure 3). Likewise 3-year DFS of the patients stratified by lower and higher surgical margins were not significantly different either (38.8% and 66.0%, respectively; $P = 0.149$). To determine whether pN status is an independent predictor of DFS, a multivariate analysis was carried out using age, gender, pT status, pN status, BMI values and surgical margins as parameters. The results indicate that only pN status is an independent predictor of DFS ($P = 0.038$), and the remaining factors are not. Overall, these results indicate that only pN status has a vital impact on OS in these patients through survival analyses.

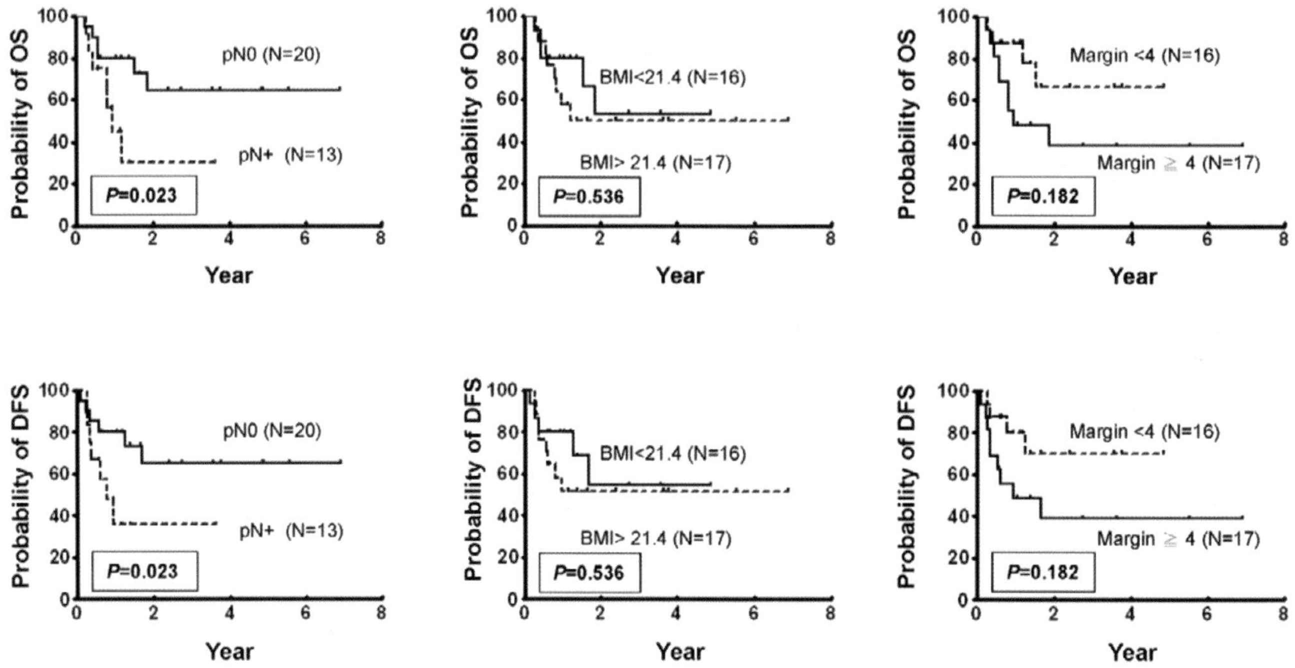

Figure 3. Kaplan-Meier plot analyses of the overall survival (OS) and disease-free survival (DFS) of patient subgroups stratified by pathological nodal status (pN), BMI values, and surgical margins (mm). The inlets indicate statistically significant differences measured by log-rank test.

Discussion

CCRT as initial treatment for hypopharyngeal carcinoma has recently gained popularity due to its comparable disease control and the potential for organ preservation when compared with primary surgery [7–12]. In accordance with the literature, our experience at CGMH demonstrated no survival difference between patients receiving primary CCRT and those receiving primary radical surgery [7,8]. However, when those who received primary CCRT develop recurrent disease and now require salvage ablation, the reconstruction becomes more challenging than ever. More so than reconstruction after primary laryngopharyngectomy, these patients are compromised by poor nutrition, cachexia, depression, and other morbidities related to chemotherapy and radiation.

Over the past 10 years, we have consolidated our approach for pharyngoesophageal reconstruction. We have increasingly relied on ALT for parital and circumferential reconstructions and jejunum flaps for circumferential reconstructions [5,13]. For the patients in this study, all of whom had severely compromised physiologic reserves, we favored the ALT flap over the jejunum flap to avoid the morbidities associated with open abdominal surgery, such as postoperative ileus, risks of bowel adhesion and obstruction, incisional hernia, and pulmonary embarrassment. ALT flap also excels over jejunum in producing superior tracheoesophageal speech while providing similar fistula and stricture rates, as demonstrated by Yu et al [14]. The thickness of an ALT flap could be problematic in obese patients. However, this had not been an issue in our study population. None of the patients, even those who were previously obese, had thick thigh tissue when presented for salvage ablation and reconstruction. This was not surprising considering their disease courses and the treatment histories. Before salvage surgery, almost all of the patients could not tolerate oral intake and experienced malnutrition. The skin laxity secondary to soft tissue wasting ironically facilitated ALT donor site closure. Primary closure was achieved in 84.8% of patients despite the harvests of relatively large flaps.

The postoperative complication rate was an important parameter for surgical success because it had significant impact on the hospitalization length, permanent sequelae, functional status, and quality of life. Pharyngocutaneous fistula is the most common early complication after major laryngopharyngeal surgery, reported from 5% to 65% [15]. Our rate of fistula of 42.4% was high when compared with other studies of pharyngoesophageal reconstruction using ALT flap, which reported fistula rates ranging from 0 to 25 percent [2–4,16]. This was likely secondary to our selection criteria of including only the patients with disease recurrence after CCRT. With preoperative CCRT, cancer recurrence, aggressive salvage surgery, and significant co-morbidities, the tissue's capacity to heal was likely compromised. Tsou et al. found preoperative CCRT to be an independent risk factor that significantly raised the risk of fistula formation, from 21.4% in 112 patients receiving primary total laryngopharyngectomy and reconstruction to 58.3% in 48 patients undergoing post-irradiated salvage laryngopharyngectomy and reconstruction [17].

Compared to previously published literature, in which 5 to 25 percent of transferred flaps require re-exploration within the first week postoperatively due to circulatory compromise or neck hematoma, the re-operative rate of 15.2% in the present study is concerning, especially considering that 2 patients (6.1%) developed life-threatening vascular blowouts [18,19]. This relatively high re-operative rate, again, reflects the highly morbid nature of the patient population. At the same time, it emphasizes the importance of ICU monitoring. We routinely monitor these patients for a week in a specialized microsurgical ICU. The successful treatment of vascular blowouts and flap salvage was attributed to timely diagnosis and prompt return to the operating room.

To reduce these complications, the ALT flap can be adjusted with the inclusion of partial VL muscle to meet the requirements of the reconstruction, such as increasing tissue bulk, obliteration of dead space, or coverage of the great vessels in the neck. Moreover, the underlying fascia of the ALT flap could provide a vascularized second layer to reinforce the suture lines and mucosal anastomoses.

We found donor wound healing to be reflective of patients' tissue healing capacity, and useful as an easily monitored tool in assessing patients' overall metabolic status. Delayed donor wound healing indicates an underlying cause that tipped the balance toward catabolic metabolism. The cause was most frequently poor nutrition in the study's patient population.

Variable results of postoperative locoregional control and survival have been reported. Kadota et al. reported the results of an analysis on 14 patients who underwent salvage surgery after definitive chemoradiotherapy in a single-institution study. The 5-year disease-free survival and local control rates were 57.1% and 92.9%, respectively [20]. However, less favorable results have also been reported. In a series reported by Relic et al., only 2 out of 20 patients undergoing surgery for histologically proven recurrence after radiochemotherapy (10%) were actually tumor-free and alive after a mean follow-up period of 43.9 months [21]. In our study, the 5-year overall survival and disease-free survival rate for this specific group of patients were 51.8% and 53.7%, respectively. Our results also indicate that only pN status has a vital impact on the overall survival rates. It should be noted that all of the patients in our study had favorable response to CCRT initially and only those with feasibility of complete surgical resection were included. This may introduce selection bias and mask the negative oncological outcomes in the study.

Conclusion

Despite advances in microsurgical techniques, pharyngoesophageal reconstruction after salvage laryngopharyngectomy remains challenging. Meaningful oncologic and functional outcomes can be obtained by meticulous attention to surgical techniques and postoperative care. Among the techniques available, we continue to favor the ALT flap as it proves to be reliable and versatile. Reconstructive microsurgeons who are prepared to take on these cases should be equally well prepared to manage the potential postoperative complications.

Author Contributions

Conceived and designed the experiments: HKK WFC KPC. Performed the experiments: WFC CHC VBHS. Analyzed the data: WFC HKK KPC. Contributed reagents/materials/analysis tools: KPC. Wrote the paper: WFC HKK.

References

1. Chan YW, Ng RW, Liu LH, Chung HP, Wei WI (2011) Reconstruction of circumferential pharyngeal defects after tumour resection: Reference or preference. J Plast Reconstr Aesthet Surg 64: 1022–1028.
2. Sagar B, Marres HAM, Hartman EHM (2010) Hypopharyngeal reconstruction with an anterolateral thigh flap after laryngopharyngeal resection: Results of a retrospective study on 20 patients. J Plast Reconstr Aesthet Surg 63: 970–975.

3. Yu P, Hanasono MM, Skoracki RJ, Baumann DP, Lewin JS, et al. (2010) Pharyngoesophageal reconstruction with the anterolateral thigh flap after total laryngopharyngectomy. Cancer 116: 1718–1724.
4. Murray DJ, Gilbert RW, Vesely MJ, Novak CB, Zaitlin-Gencher S, et al. (2007) Functional outcomes and donor site morbidity following circumferential pharyngoesophageal reconstruction using an anterolateral thigh flap and salivary bypass tube. Head Neck 29: 147–154.
5. Wong CH, Wei FC (2009) Microsurgical free flap in head and neck reconstruction. Head Neck 32: 1236–1245.
6. Ali RS, Bluebond-Langner R, Rodriguez ED, Cheng MH (2009) The Versatility of the Anterolateral Thigh Flap. Plast Reconstr Surg 124: e395–e407.
7. Chang MF, Wang HM, Kang CJ, Huang SF, Lin CY, et al. (2010) Treatment results for hypopharyngeal cancer by different treatment strategies and its secondary primary- an experience in Taiwan. Radiat Oncol 5: 91.
8. Wang HM, Wang CS, Chen JS, Chen IH, Liao CT, et al. (2002) Cisplatin, tegafur, and leucovorin: a moderately effective and minimally toxic outpatient neoadjuvant chemotherapy for locally advanced squamous cell carcinoma of the head and neck. Cancer 94: 2989–2995.
9. Guibert M, Lepage B, Woisard V, Rives M, Serrano E, et al. (2011) Quality of life in patients treated for advanced hypopharyngeal or laryngeal cancer. Eur Ann Otorhinolaryngol Head Neck Dis 128: 218–223.
10. Shellenberger TD, Madero-Visbal R, Weber RS (2011) Quality indicators in head and neck operations: a comparison with published benchmarks. Arch Otolaryngol Head Neck Surg 137: 1086–1093.
11. Paximadis P, Yoo G, Lin HS, Jacobs J, Sukari A, et al. (2012) Concurrent Chemoradiotherapy Improves Survival in Patients with Hypopharyngeal Cancer. Int J Radiat Oncol Biol Phys 82: 1515–1521.
12. Takes RP, Strojan P, Silver CE, Brandley PJ, Haigentz M, et al. (2012) Current trends in initial management of hypopharyngeal cancer: The declining use of open surgery. Head Neck 34: 270–281.
13. Lutz BS, Wei FC (2005) Microsurgical Workhorse Flaps in Head and Neck Reconstruction. Clin Plast Surg 32: 421–430.
14. Yu P, Lewin JS, Reece GP, Robb GL (2006) Comparison of Clinical and Functional Outcomes and Hospital Costs following Pharyngoesophageal Reconstruction with the Anterolateral Thigh Free Flap versus the Jejunal Flap. Plast Reconstr Surg 117: 968–974.
15. Chu PY, Chang SY (2005) Reconstruction after resection of hypopharyngeal carcinoma: comparison of the postoperative complications and oncologic result of different methods. Head Neck 27: 901–908.
16. Lewin JS, Barringer DA, May AH, Gillenwate AM, Arnold KA, et al. (2005) Functional Outcomes after Circumferential Pharyngoesophageal Reconstruction. Laryngoscope 115: 1266–1271.
17. Tsou YA, Hua CH, Lin MH, Tseng HC, Tsai MH, et al. (2010) Comparison of pharyngocutaneous fistula between patients followed by primary laryngopharyngectomy and salvage laryngopharyngectomy for advanced hypopharyngeal cancer. Head Neck 32: 1494–1500.
18. Chen KT, Mardini S, Chung DCC, Lin CH, Cheng MH, et al. (2007) Timing of presentation of the first signs of vascular compromise dictates the salvage outcome of free flap transfers. Plast Reconstr Surg 120: 187–195.
19. Kao HK, Chang KP, Ching WC, Tsao CK, Cheng MH, et al. (2009) Tha impacts of liver cirrhosis on head and neck cancer patients undergoing microsurgical free tissue transfer: An evaluation of flap outcome and flap-related complications. Oral Oncol 45: 1058–1062.
20. Kadota H, Fukushima J, Nakashima T, Kumamoto Y, Yoshida S, et al. (2010) Comparison of salvage and planned pharyngolaryngectomy with jejunal transfer for hypopharyngeal carcinoma after chemoradiotherapy. Laryngoscope 120: 1103–1108.
21. Relic A, Scheich M, Stapf J, Voelter C, Hoppe F, et al. (2009) Salvage surgery after induction chemotherapy with paclitaxel/cisplatin and primary radiotherapy for advanced laryngeal and hypopharyngeal carcinomas. Eur Arch Otorhinolaryngol 266: 1799–1805.

10

Lymphangiogenesis in Regional Lymph Nodes Is an Independent Prognostic Marker in Rectal Cancer Patients after Neoadjuvant Treatment

Christiane Jakob[1], Daniela E. Aust[1], Birgit Liebscher[1], Gustavo B. Baretton[1], Kaustubh Datta[1,2]*, Michael H. Muders[1]*

1 Institute of Pathology, University Hospital Carl Gustav Carus, University of Technology, Dresden, Germany, **2** Department of Biochemistry, University of Nebraska Medical Center, Omaha, Nebraska, United States of America

Abstract

One of the major prognostic factors in rectal cancer is lymph node metastasis. The formation of lymph node metastases is dependent on the existence of a premetastatic niche. An important factor preceding metastasis are lymph vessels which are located in the lymph node. Accordingly, the occurrence of intranodal lymphangiogenesis is thought to indicate distant metastasis and worse prognosis. To evaluate the significance of lymph node lymphangiogenesis, we studied formalin fixed, paraffin embedded adenocarcinomas and regional lymph nodes of 203 rectal cancer patients who were treated with neoadjuvant radiochemotherapy and consecutive curative surgery with cancer free surgical margins (R0). Regional lymph node lymph vessels were detected by immunohistochemistry for podoplanin (D2-40). Our results show that the presence of lymphatic vessels in regional lymph nodes significantly affects the disease-free survival in univariate and multivariate analyses. In contrast, there was no correlation between peritumoral or intratumoral lymph vessel density and prognosis. Indeed, our study demonstrates the importance of lymphangiogenesis in regional lymph nodes after neoadjuvant radiochemotherapy and consecutive surgery as an independent prognostic marker. Staining for intranodal lymphangiogenesis and methods of intravital imaging of lymphangiogenesis and lymphatic flow may be a useful strategy to predict long-term outcome in rectal cancer patients. Furthermore, addition of VEGF-blocking agents to standardized neoadjuvant treatment schemes might be indicated in advanced rectal cancer.

Editor: Soumitro Pal, Children's Hospital Boston & Harvard Medical School, United States of America

Funding: No current external sources fund this specific study. Generally, the work of the researchers was supported by grants to MHM (Wilhelm Sander Stiftung fur Krebsforschung) and KD (R01-NIH, CA140432).

Competing Interests: The authors have declared that no competing interests exist.

* E-mail: michael.muders@uniklinikum-dresden.de (MHM); kaustubh.datta@unmc.edu (KD)

Introduction

Preoperative (neoadjuvant) radiochemotherapy followed by curative surgery has become standard treatment in locally advanced rectal cancer [1]. The histopathological tumor regression as a correlate for local treatment efficacy varies from no to minimal regressive changes to complete response [2,3]. The lymph node status after neoadjuvant radiochemotherapy, however, remains the most important independent prognostic factor for disease-free survival, as patients with post-therapeutic positive lymph nodes (ypN+) have an unfavourable prognosis irrespective of regression of the primary tumor [2,3,4,5,6]. Thus, inhibition of regional lymph node metastases might be an effective future avenue in treating rectal cancer patients. Therefore, efforts have been made to uncover the mechanisms of lymph node metastasis. It has been suggested that the induction of lymphangiogenesis in the primary tumor and in lymph nodes significantly contributes to tumor metastases [7,8]. In this study we have validated lymphangiogenesis in regional lymph nodes as a predictor for poor prognosis and facilitator for distant metastasis in a cohort of neoadjuvant treated advanced rectal cancer patients. It is a better predictor than peri- and intratumoral lymph vessel densities or standardized tumor regression grading systems for this group of rectal cancer patients.

Results

Clinicopathological characterization of the evaluated cohort

All patients underwent rectum resection with total mesorectal excision after neoadjuvant radiochemotherapy. In all patients a locally curative resection was achieved (R0-situation). Pathological staging is reported in Table 1. Complete tumor regression [9] was observed in 10 cases (5%). 57 patients experienced tumor regression grade 3 (28%). 85 patients showed tumor regression grade 2 (42%) and 48 patients had tumor regression grade 1 (23%). No tumor regression was observed in 3 patients (1.5%). At median follow-up of 223 weeks (95% confidence interval 216.9 to 247.3 weeks) 38 patients had disease recurrence, 32 developed distant metastasis and 6 local recurrences. Distant metastases were detected in the following organs: hepatic 15 (HEP), pulmonary 6 (PUL), distant non-regional lymph nodes 3 (LYM), pleura 1 (PLE), skin 1 (SKIN), peritoneum 1 (PER), bone 2 (OSS), hepatic and pulmonary 2 (HEP and PUL) and others 1 (OTH). In these cases

Table 1. Characterization of the evaluated cohort and the correlation of the presence of lymph node lymph vessels (nLV+) with clinicopathological parameters.

Variable	Numbers	Detectable LVD in lymph nodes (nLV+)	p-value
Sex			0.4052 (Pearson)
Male	148 (73%)	71 (47%)	
Female	55 (27%)	30 (55%)	
Age, years			0.7188 (Pearson)
≤70	112 (55%)	57 (51%)	
>70	91 (45%)	44 (48%)	
yUICC stage			***0.0026 (Pearson)***
0	10 (5%)	3 (30%)	
I	66 (33%)	22 (33%)	
IIA	58 (29%)	31 (53%)	
IIB	3 (1%)	1 (33%)	
IIC	1	1 (100%)	
IIIA	9 (4%)	8 (89%)	
IIIB	32 (16%)	17 (53%)	
IIIC	5 (2%)	5 (100%)	
IVA	19 (9%)	13 (68%)	
Relapse			***0.0171 (Pearson)***
yes	46 (23%)	30 (65%)	
No	157 (77%)	71 (45%)	

disease recurrence and distant metastases were confirmed by pathologic evaluation and examination. In eight cases clinical information (accessed by a documentation assistant) was used to detect disease recurrence.

To detect metastatic tumor cells in lymph nodes we used standard HE staining as well as Pan-Cytokeratin staining using a commercially available monoclonal antibody (Dako Inc) in at least three serial sections of the lymph node. A median of 14 regional lymph nodes per case was studied. The presence of Pancytokeratin positive tumor cells indicated lymph node metastasis (Fig. 1A).

Association of regression of primary tumor and lymph node metastasis with clinicopathological parameters and prognostic parameters

A significant correlation was found between the grades of tumor regression (Fig. 2) and progression free survival when dichotomized for high and low tumor regression ($p = 0.0033$ Log-Rank) (Fig. 3A) in Kaplan Meier analysis. Multivariate analysis revealed a statistically significant difference when comparing TRG 1 and TRG 3 (Table 2). As in previously published reports [2,3,4,5,6], we also demonstrated that lymph node metastasis is an important independent prognostic factor in our cohort ($p = 0.0017$ Log-Rank) (Fig. 3B).

Association of peritumoral and intratumoral lymph vessel density with lymph node metastasis, UICC stage, and prognostic parameters

In a next step we evaluated the peritumoral and intratumoral lymphangiogenesis (pLVD and iLVD) and its relationship to metastasis in our cohort. Lymphangiogenesis was assessed using a commercially available antibody that detects podoplanin (D2-40, Dako) (Fig. 1B and 1C). The staining is specific for lymphatic endothelium and does not stain any blood vessels with detectable intraluminal erythrocytes. pLVD was not significantly correlated with lymph node metastases ($p = 0.08$ χ^2). There was no significant correlation of pLVD and ypUICC stage or disease free survival. Additionally, iLVD did not correlate with prognosis, lymph node metastasis, or ypUICC stage.

Association of intranodal lymphangiogensis in regional lymph nodes with UICC stage, progression free survival, and type of relapse

table-1-captionIn parallel, we assessed intranodal lymphangiogenesis by staining regional mesorectal lymph nodes with D2-40 as previously described. A lymph node is classified as positive for intranodal lymphangiogenesis when at least one lymph vessel can be detected in the follicular or/and interfollicular region of at least one mesorectal lymph node (designated as nLV+). In essence, in 102 patients all lymph nodes were negative for lymph node lymphangiogenesis, whereas in 43 patients in only one lymph node detectable lymphangiogenesis could be seen. In 58 patients more than one regional lymph node has detectable lymphangiogenesis.

We found a statistically significant correlation between nLV+ (lymphangiogenesis in at least one mesorectal/regional lymph node) and tumor relapse as well as ypUICC stage (Table 1). Kaplan Meier Analysis revealed a significant correlation of nLV+ with progression free survival time ($p = 0.0071$ LogRank) in the whole cohort (Fig. 4A). Furthermore, nLV+ was an independent prognostic factor as studied by the Cox proportional hazards regression model with the covariates ypUICC-stage, age, gender, tumor regression, intratumoral lymph vessel density, peritumoral lymph vessel density, and lymph node lymph vessel density (Table 2). Accordingly, subgroup analysis of node-negative patients presented a significant correlation between nLV+ and disease-free survival (Fig. 4B) using Kaplan-Meier analysis. When comparing the frequency of hepatic metastasis in patients with and without mesorectal intranodal lymphangiogenesis (nLV+), we found more hepatic metastasis in patients with nodal lymphangiogenesis (13 hepatic metastasis in patients with intranodal lymphangiogenesis versus 2 hepatic metastasis in patients without intranodal lymphangiogenesis). We also evaluated the number of lymph vessels (lymph vessel density, nLVD) detected in the regional lymph nodes. Here, the maximal number of lymph vessels detected in a lymph node with lymphangiogenesis correlates significantly with the node status (ypN0 or ypN+; $p = 0.01$ χ^2) (Fig. 5B). In contrast, there was no correlation of the maximal number of lymph vessels with distant metastasis. When dichotomizing according to the median of the maximum lymph node lymph vessel density, we could not detect any significant correlation with time to progression. Also, the number of lymph nodes with lymphangiogenesis did not correlate with ypUICC stage or tumor relapse in the subgroup of patients with nLV+. In summary, the presence of regional lymph node lymph vessels represents an independent prognostic parameter, while the nodal lymph vessel density as well as the number of lymph nodes with detectable nodal lymphangiogenesis might be of minor importance for overall prognosis.

Association of lymph node metastasis regression grading and prognosis

In our cohort, there was no statistically significant correlation between lymph node metastasis regression grading and tumor recurrence / disease free survival in the Kaplan Meier model in all

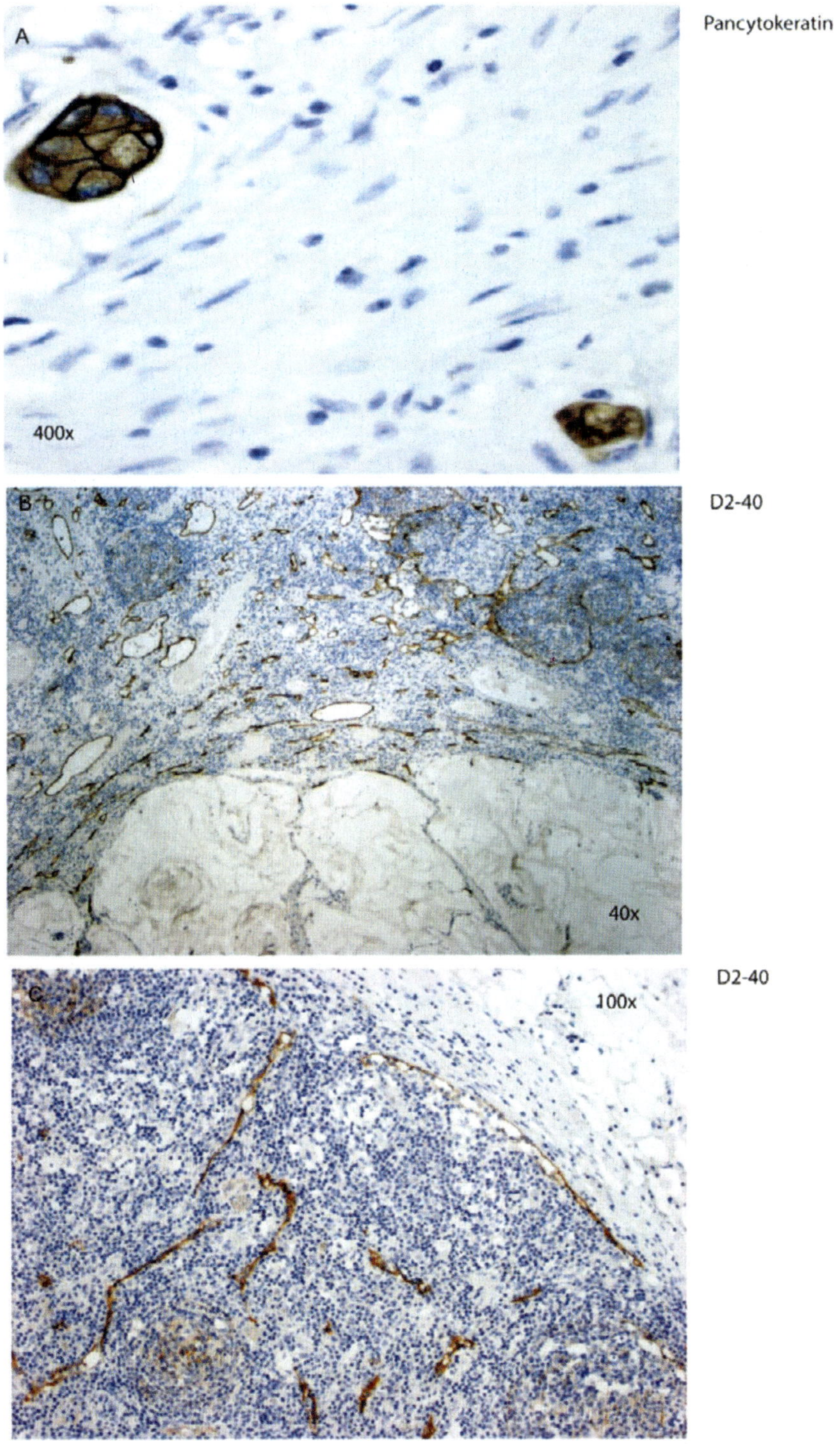

Figure 1. Immunohistochemistry of regional lymph nodes. A. Immunohistochemistry for Pancytokeratin to detect lymph node micrometastases. B. Podoplanin staining with D2-40 in a lymph node with metastasis. The red to brown staining marks lymph vessels. C. Podoplanin staining with D2-40 in a lymph node without metastasis.

patients and in subgroup analyses. In multivariate analyses no statistically relevant correlation could be found.

Discussion

Regardless of tumor size and extent of invasion, regional lymph node metastasis (ypN+) is an important prognostic factor in patients treated with neoadjuvant radiochemotherapy [2,3,4,5,6]. Therefore, it is important to elucidate the mechanisms of lymph node metastasis as well as how lymph node metastasis might influence overall patient survival. Although controversial, peritumoral lymphatics are reported by some to play a role in promoting lymph node metastasis in colorectal carcinoma [10,11,12,13] [12,14,15]. We used D2-40 antibody (Podoplanin, cell surface sialylated

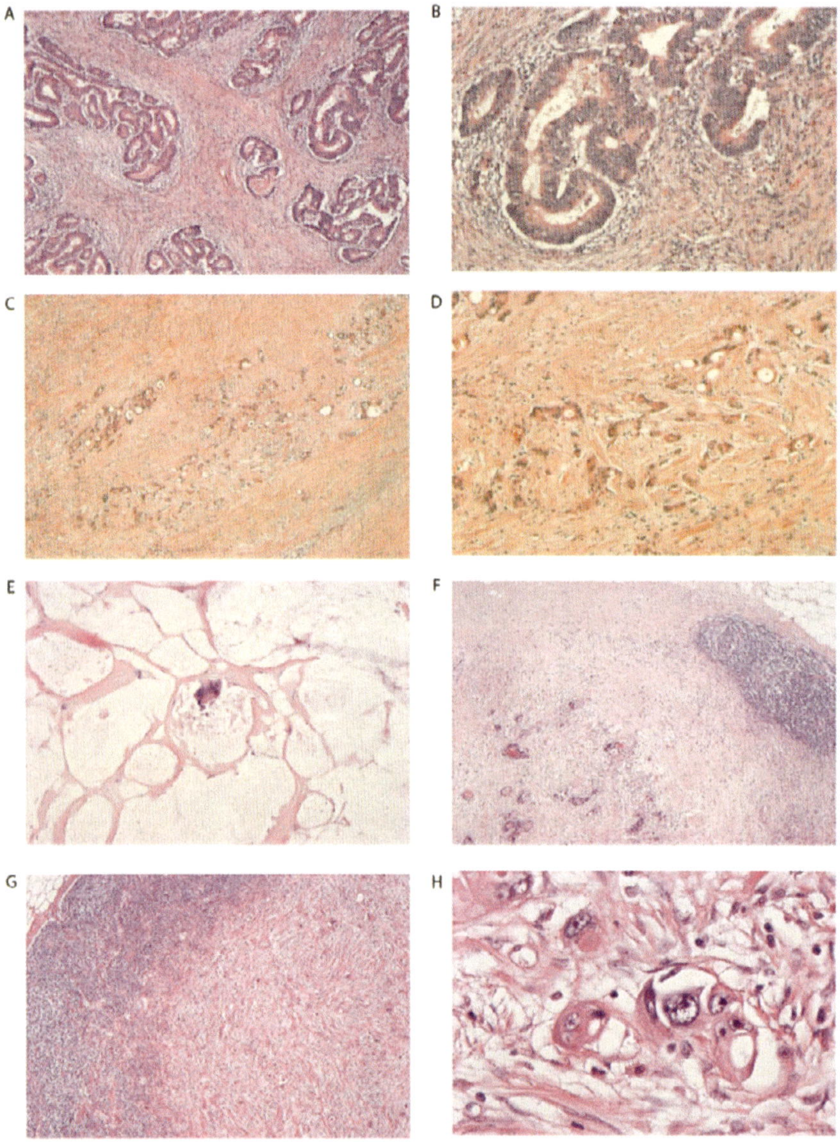

Figure 2. Stages of primary tumor regression and regional lymph node metastasis regression after neoadjuvant radiochemotherapy. A. HE stained rectal adenocarcinoma with tumor regression grade 1 (40x). B. HE stained rectal cancer tissue with tumor regression grade 1 (100x) C. Rectal carcinoma with tumor regression grade 2 (40x) D. Rectal adenocarcinoma with tumor regression grade 2 (100x). E. Tumor regression grade 3 (100x) in rectal cancer with extracellular mucin accumulation. F. Lymph node metastasis regression grade 2 (40x). G. Lymph node metastasis regression grade 3 (40x). H. Regional lymph node metastasis (400x) in standard HE staining.

glycoprotein)[16,17] to stain lymphatic vessels in primary adenocarcinomas and mesorectal lymph nodes of 203 rectal cancer patients. These patients were treated with preoperative radiochemotherapy followed by complete surgical removal of the tumor (R0). Our results indicate no significant correlation between peritumoral and intratumoral lymphangiogenesis and patient prognosis. Interestingly, we observed lymph node lymphangiogenesis was an important prognostic parameter in this patient cohort. As previously reported, lymphangiogenic growth factors such as VEGF-C and VEGF-A can migrate to the regional lymph nodes from primary tumors and promote lymphangiogenesis [7,18]. We can predict a similar phenomenon in colorectal cancer as the level of VEGF-C was shown to be elevated in the blood serum of patients with colorectal cancer [19]. It has been hypothesized that lymph node lymph vessels can act as a metastatic niche for cancer cells [7,8,20,21] and facilitate further metastatic transformation of the tumor cells. This might lead to therapy-resistant metastatic cancer and is therefore responsible for poor patient prognosis. Studies in other cancers also indicate a similar prognostic significance of lymph node lymphangiogenesis. In a B16 melanoma mouse model it was demonstrated that lymph node lymphangiogenesis is an early response to tumor growth and precedes tumor metastasis [22]. The significance of sentinel lymph node lymphangiogenesis in metastatic spread of breast cancer to non-sentinel lymph nodes has been shown in human patients. [23]. Similar results indicating the importance of lymph node lymphangiogenesis were reported in pancreatic cancer [8], squamous head and neck cancer [21], and extramammary Paget's disease [20].

Multimodal pretreatment of locally advanced rectal cancer has shown therapeutic benefits to the patients [24]. Previously, it has

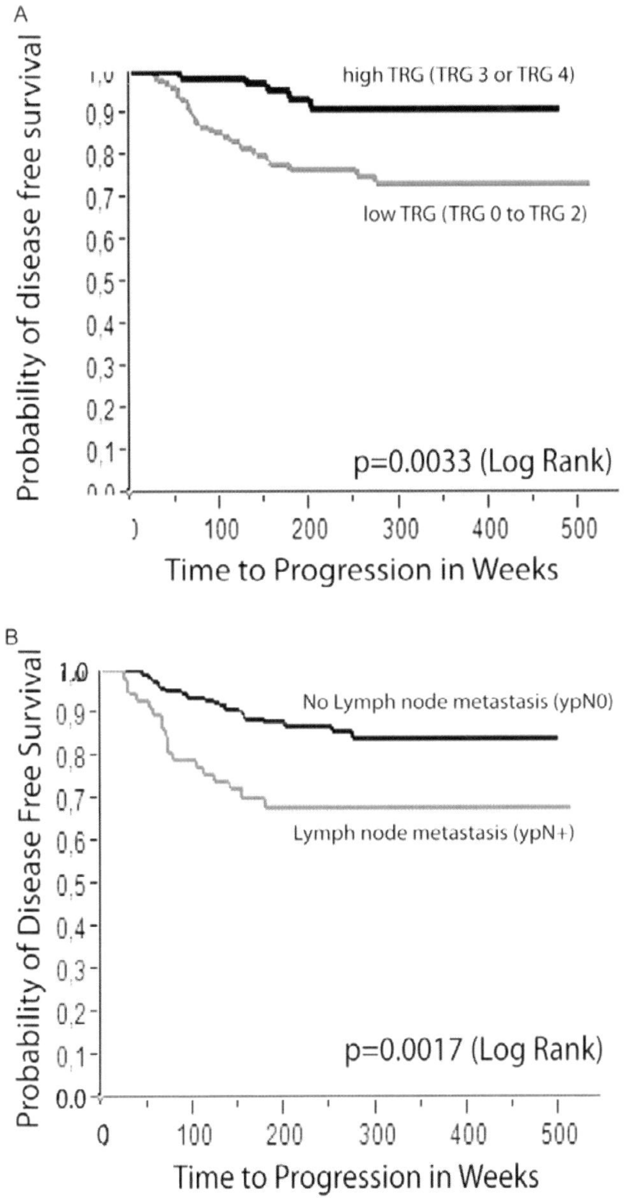

Figure 3. Kaplan Meier diagrams for the time to progression. A. Time to progression in weeks in relation to the probability of progression free survival stratified for a dichotomized tumor regression grading (TRG 0/1/2 = no regression or dominant tumor mass with obvious fibrosis or mucin or dominantly fibrotic or mucinous changes, with tumor cells or groups; TRG 3/4 = very few tumor cells in fibrotic or mucinous tissue or no tumor cells, only fibrotic or mucinous mass / total regression; according to Dworak et al. 1997). B. Time to progression in weeks in relation to the probability of progression free survival stratified for lymph node metastasis (ypN0 and ypN+).

been shown that lymphangiogenic growth factors e.g. VEGF-C were upregulated by tumor cells during stress and promoted their stress-resistance ability [25][26]. Therefore, it is possible that therapeutic stress during neoadjuvant treatment of rectal cancer enhances the level of synthesis of lymphangiogenic growth factors and increases the formation of lymph vessels in regional lymph nodes. This eventually leads to tumor recurrence and metastasis. Blocking the lymphangiogenic axis during neoadjuvant therapy should therefore improve the outcome of current treatment modalities for advanced stage rectal cancer. The association of lymph node lymphangiogenesis and worse prognosis further suggests the routine detection of lymph node lymphangiogenesis as an important parameter for the prediction of cancer relapse and as an indicator for a more aggressive adjuvant treatment.

In conclusion, our study demonstrates that the presence of intranodal lymphangiogenesis represents an independent prognostic marker associated with shorter progression free survival in patients with locally advanced rectal cancer, who are treated with neoadjuvant radiochemotherapy. Therefore, strategies to detect lymph node lymphangiogenesis in the clinical setting might help to identify patients who would benefit from more aggressive treatment options. Also, inclusion of a therapeutic approach to block lymphangiogenesis would be beneficial to neoadjuvantly treated advanced rectal cancer patients.

Materials and Methods

Patient material

Material used in this study is covered by the approval of ethic's committee of the University Hospital "Carl Gustav Carus", TUD-Medical Faculty, for the use in research (EK59032007; "Feingewebliche und molekularpathologische Untersuchung in langzeitarchiviertem Gewebsmaterial des Instituts fuer Pathologie des Universitaetsklinikum Dresden/Medizinische Fakultaet Carl Gustav Carus, TU Dresden"; Chairman of the Committee: W. Kirch, MD). The decision of the ethic's committee specifically approved the use of tissue material for this minimally invasive and retrospective study that uses patient material that has been stored for more than three years. All patients consented to the use of tissue material for research (as noted in the files of the patients). According to the Ethic's committee oral consent is sufficient in this case (this consent procedure is approved by the Ethic's committee) because the material used here is not associated with the name of the patient and is coded. Two hundred and three patients (male: n = 152, female: n = 51, median age = 70 years) with locally advanced rectal adenocarcinoma (UICC stage II/III) between 2001 and 2008 were included in this study (Figure 1). All patients underwent preoperative (neoadjuvant) 5-fluorouracil (5-FU) based radiochemotherapy and curative R0 surgery in analogy to the randomized phase III German Rectal Cancer Trials CAO/ARO/AIO-94 [1]. The data for disease relapses (distant metastasis or local recurrences) as well as other relevant data were retrieved from the database of the Institute of Pathology, University

Table 2. Significant relationships as depicted in the multivariate Cox proportional hazard regression model.

Prognostic factors	Hazard Ratio	95% confidence interval	P-value
ypUICC stage I,II/III,IV	0.11	0.1828–0.7194	*0.0037*
Tumor regression TRG 1/TRG 3	3.31	1.2373–10.3846	*0.0163*
nodular LVD (nLV) absent (-)/present (+)	0.41	0.1896–0.8562	*0.0168*

A

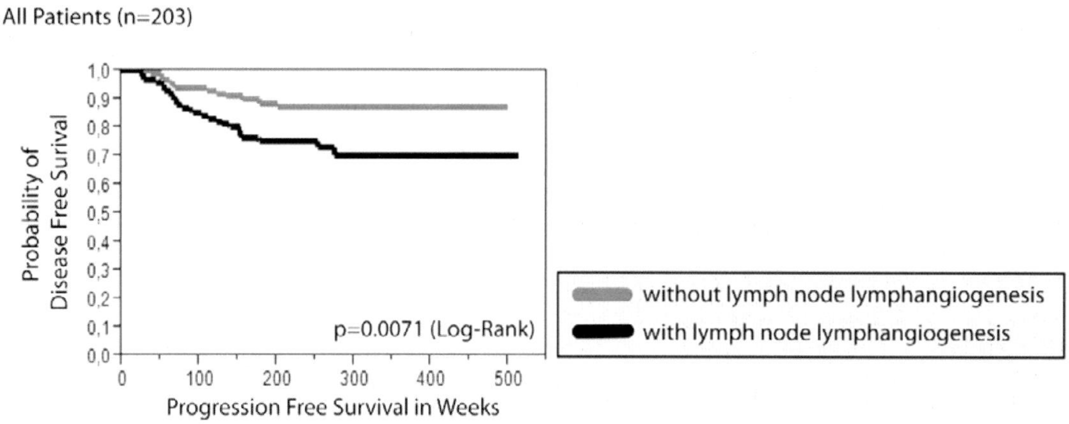

B

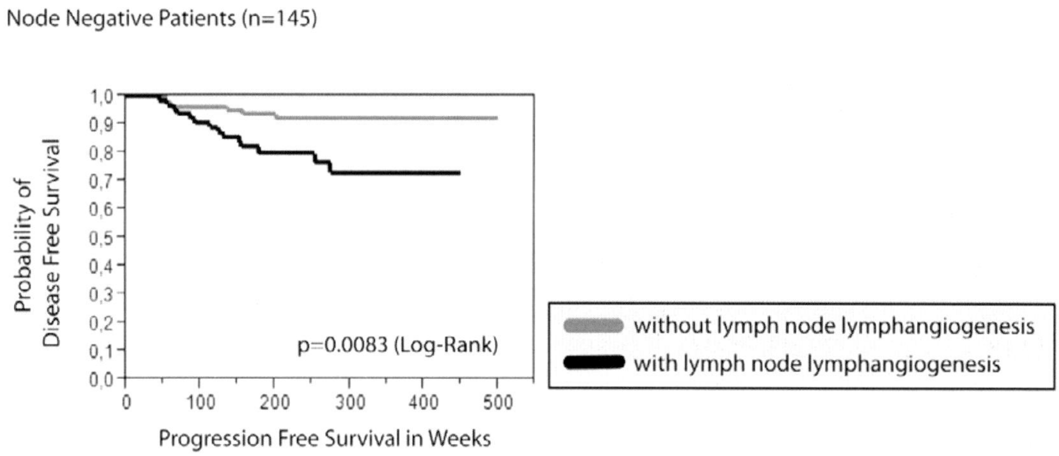

Figure 4. Lymph node lymphangiogenesis (nLV+) and its correlation with clinicopathological parameters and time to progression. "With lymph node lymphangiogenesis" is defined as at least one regional/mesorectal lymph node with detectable lymphangiogenesis in the follicular or interfollicular area. A. Time to progression in weeks in relation to the probability of disease free survival stratified for the presence of lymph node lymphangiogenesis in all patients. B. Time to progression in weeks in relation to the probability of disease free survival stratified for the presence of lymph node lymphangiogenesis in node negative patients.

Hospital "Carl Gustav Carus", Medical Faculty of the University of Dresden, Germany.

Pathological examination of cancer specimen after neoadjuvant therapy

At least four samples were taken and evaluated from the primary rectal cancer. In the case of occult residual cancer during gross examination, the complete former cancer area was embedded and studied by histology. In case of the absence of residual cancer cells in the HE staining vital epithelial cancer cells were detected by cytokeratin staining. This procedure ensures that therapy induced tissue fibrosis as well as extracellular mucin accumulations were not considered as residual cancer tissue and incuded in the tumor regression grading. Mesorectal regional lymph nodes were dissected according to the "Union internationale contre cancer" (UICC). In case of examination of less than twelve regional mesorectal lymph nodes perirectal fatty tissue (minimum ten paraffin blocks) were embedded and evaluated for the presence of further lymph nodes that were not detectable by gross examination. To detect residual cancer cells Pancytokeratin staining was performed as described.

Tumor and lymph node metastasis regression grading

Histopathological tumor regression (TRG) within the primary tumor was graded according to the semiquantitative system established by Dworak et al. [9]: TRG 0 = no regression; TRG 1 = dominant tumor mass with obvious fibrosis or mucin; TRG 2 = dominantly fibrotic or mucinous changes, with few tumor cells or groups; TRG 3 = very few tumor cells in fibrotic or mucinous tissue; TRG 4 = no tumor cells, only fibrotic or mucinous mass / total regression [2] (Fig. 2).

Evidence of tumor response to preoperative radiochemotherapy within the perirectal lymph nodes was defined as the presence of nodal fibrosis or mucin pools (with or without residual tumor cells), as described previously [27,28]. Lymph node metastasis regression (LRG) was evaluated with the same parameters like the primary tumor regression considering each metastatic lymph node: LRG 0 = no regression; LRG 1 = dominant tumor mass with obvious fibrosis or mucin; LRG 2 = dominantly fibrotic or mucinous changes, with few tumor cells or groups; LRG 3 = very few tumor cells in fibrotic or mucinous tissue; LRG 4 = no tumor cells, only fibrotic or mucinous mass / total regression. Non-metastatic lymph nodes were distinguished from those with total metastatic regression (LRG 4) by absence of fibrosis or mucin (Fig. 2). When

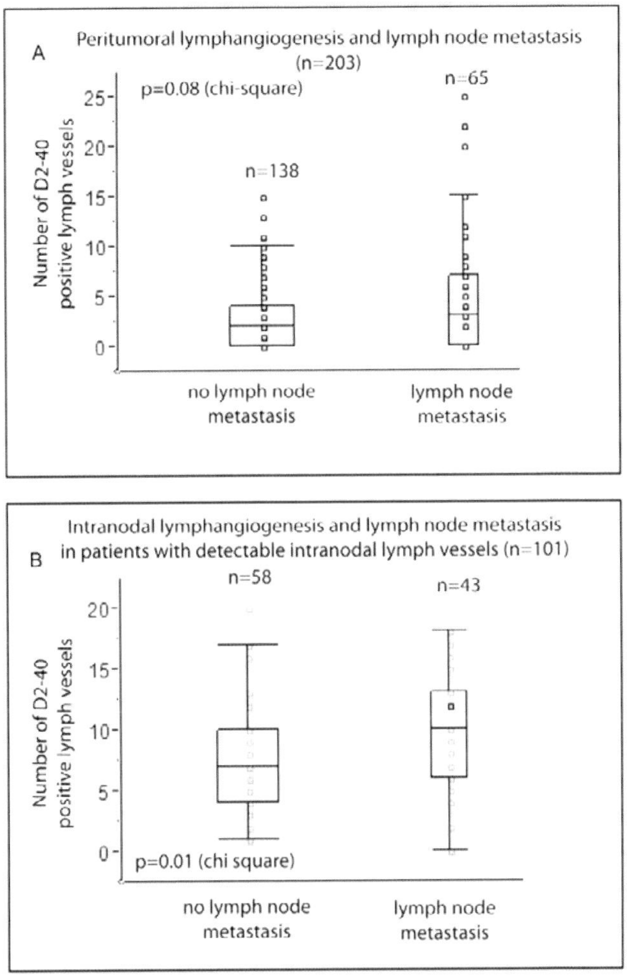

Figure 5. Lymphangiogenesis and metastasis. A. Box plots comparing the number of lymph vessels in the peritumoral region with the presence or absence of lymph node metastasis. B. Box plots comparing the number of regional lymph node lymph vessels in relation with the presence or absence of lymph node metastasis in patients with detectable lymph vessels in the regional lymph nodes.

different LRGs were found in one patient, only the lymph node with the worst regression was considered.

Immunohistochemistry

Immunohistochemistry was performed on 2 µm sections of paraffin-embedded blocks from the primary tumor and regional lymph nodes. Deparaffination, rehydration, and antigen retrieval were performed by steam cooking (98°C, 45 min) in PT Module buffer (pH 8.0) (Thermo scientific, Medac, Hamburg, Germany). The tissues were washed in Tris-buffered saline (TBS) (Thermo scientific, Medac, Hamburg, Germany) and incubated with monoclonal mouse anti human podoplanin detecting D2-40-antibody (DAKO, Hamburg, Germany, 1:400 dilution) for 30 min at room temperature. Then, endogenous peroxidase activity was inhibited by incubating the slides in 3% H_2O_2 for 10 minutes. After washing in TBS, Ultravision LP large volume detection system HRP Polymer (Thermo scientific, Medac, Hamburg, Germany) was used according to the manufacturer's recommendation. The sections were stained with 0.5 mg/ml diaminobenzidin tetrahydrochlorid (DAB) and counter-stained with hematoxylin. In all experiments, positive and negative controls were included.

Evaluation of immunohistochemistry

Lymph vessel density was assessed by the "hot-spot" method as described previously and was also referred to as the Chalkley point graticule method [29]. Briefly, all slides were scanned at low magnification (x40) and the areas with the highest density of D2-40 positive vessels were identified. Then, the number of D2-40 positive vessels was counted in those areas in five high-power fields (HPF, x400) by two independent pathologists (C.J. and M.H.M.) without knowledge of the clinicopathological findings, and the mean value of vessel counts were calculated. Intratumoral (lymph vessels within the tumor mass) and peritumoral (lymph vessels outside of the tumor, but within 2 mm from the tumor invasion front) LVD was determined separately. Vessels close to ulcerated areas were not counted. LVD was assessed on all dissected mesorectal lymph nodes including nodal metastases, residual lymphoid tissue of metastatic lymph nodes (if existing), and all non-metastatic lymph nodes. Preexisting intranodal vessels (intermediate as well as marginal sinus) were not counted. During evaluation high interobserver agreement was confirmed by using Cohen's Kappa coefficient ($\kappa = 0.8$; $p<0.001$). In case of interobserver differences, the case was reevaluated by simultaneous reassessment of the specimen.

Statistical analysis

All tests are performed using SAS JMP Version 9. Associations between different categorical variables were assessed using the χ^2 test. Continuous variables were compared using Mann-Whitney's U-test or ANOVA. Time to progression rates were compared using the univariate analysis of Kaplan-Meier, multivariate analysis was performed using the Cox proportional hazards regression model with the covariates ypUICC-stage, age, gender, tumor regression, intratumoral lymph vessel density, peritumoral lymph vessel density, lymph node lymph vessel density. P-values smaller than 0.05 were considered statistically significantly.

Acknowledgments

The authors thank Marissa J Stanton, University of Nebraska Medical Center, for the critical review of the manuscript.

Author Contributions

Conceived and designed the experiments: MHM KD CJ. Performed the experiments: CJ MHM BL. Analyzed the data: MHM CJ. Wrote the paper: MHM KD. Designed and built up the patient cohort used in this study: CJ DEA GBB.

References

1. Sauer R, Fietkau R, Wittekind C, Rodel C, Martus P, et al. (2003) Adjuvant vs. neoadjuvant radiochemotherapy for locally advanced rectal cancer: the German trial CAO/ARO/AIO-94. Colorectal Dis 5: 406–415.
2. Jakob C, Liersch T, Meyer W, Baretton GB, Schwabe W, et al. (2006) Prognostic value of histologic tumor regression, thymidylate synthase, thymidine phosphorylase, and dihydropyrimidine dehydrogenase in rectal cancer UICC Stage II/III after neoadjuvant chemoradiotherapy. Am J Surg Pathol 30: 1169–1174.
3. Rodel C, Martus P, Papadoupolos T, Fuzesi L, Klimpfinger M, et al. (2005) Prognostic significance of tumor regression after preoperative chemoradiotherapy for rectal cancer. J Clin Oncol 23: 8688–8696.

4. Chang GJ, Rodriguez-Bigas MA, Eng C, Skibber JM (2009) Lymph node status after neoadjuvant radiotherapy for rectal cancer is a biologic predictor of outcome. Cancer 115: 5432–5440.
5. Klos CL, Shellito PC, Rattner DW, Hodin RA, Cusack JC, et al. (2010) The effect of neoadjuvant chemoradiation therapy on the prognostic value of lymph nodes after rectal cancer surgery. Am J Surg 200: 440–445.
6. Yeo SG, Kim DY, Kim TH, Chang HJ, Oh JH, et al. (2010) Pathologic complete response of primary tumor following preoperative chemoradiotherapy for locally advanced rectal cancer: long-term outcomes and prognostic significance of pathologic nodal status (KROG 09-01). Ann Surg 252: 998–1004.
7. Sleeman JP, Thiele W (2009) Tumor metastasis and the lymphatic vasculature. Int J Cancer 125: 2747–2756.
8. Kurahara H, Takao S, Shinchi H, Maemura K, Mataki Y, et al. (2010) Significance of lymphangiogenesis in primary tumor and draining lymph nodes during lymphatic metastasis of pancreatic head cancer. J Surg Oncol 102: 809–815.
9. Dworak O, Keilholz L, Hoffmann A (1997) Pathological features of rectal cancer after preoperative radiochemotherapy. Int J Colorectal Dis 12: 19–23.
10. Kaneko I, Tanaka S, Oka S, Kawamura T, Hiyama T, et al. (2007) Lymphatic vessel density at the site of deepest penetration as a predictor of lymph node metastasis in submucosal colorectal cancer. Dis Colon Rectum 50: 13–21.
11. Matsumoto K, Nakayama Y, Inoue Y, Minagawa N, Katsuki T, et al. (2007) Lymphatic microvessel density is an independent prognostic factor in colorectal cancer. Dis Colon Rectum 50: 308–314.
12. Omachi T, Kawai Y, Mizuno R, Nomiyama T, Miyagawa S, et al. (2007) Immunohistochemical demonstration of proliferating lymphatic vessels in colorectal carcinoma and its clinicopathological significance. Cancer Lett 246: 167–172.
13. Longatto-Filho A, Pinheiro C, Ferreira L, Scapulatempo C, Alves VA, et al. (2008) Peritumoural, but not intratumoural, lymphatic vessel density and invasion correlate with colorectal carcinoma poor-outcome markers. Virchows Arch 452: 133–138.
14. Gao J, Knutsen A, Arbman G, Carstensen J, Franlund B, et al. (2009) Clinical and biological significance of angiogenesis and lymphangiogenesis in colorectal cancer. Dig Liver Dis 41: 116–122.
15. Duff SE, Jeziorska M, Kumar S, Haboubi N, Sherlock D, et al. (2007) Lymphatic vessel density, microvessel density and lymphangiogenic growth factor expression in colorectal cancer. Colorectal Dis 9: 793–800.
16. Van der Auwera I, Van den Eynden GG, Colpaert CG, Van Laere SJ, van Dam P, et al. (2005) Tumor lymphangiogenesis in inflammatory breast carcinoma: a histomorphometric study. Clin Cancer Res 11: 7637–7642.
17. Royston D, Jackson DG (2009) Mechanisms of lymphatic metastasis in human colorectal adenocarcinoma. The Journal of Pathology 217: 608–619.
18. Halin C, Tobler NE, Vigl B, Brown LF, Detmar M (2007) VEGF-A produced by chronically inflamed tissue induces lymphangiogenesis in draining lymph nodes. Blood 110: 3158–3167.
19. Alabi AA, Suppiah A, Madden LA, Monson JR, Greenman J (2009) Preoperative serum levels of serum VEGF-C is associated with distant metastasis in colorectal cancer patients. Int J Colorectal Dis 24: 269–274.
20. Hirakawa S, Detmar M, Kerjaschki D, Nagamatsu S, Matsuo K, et al. (2009) Nodal lymphangiogenesis and metastasis: Role of tumor-induced lymphatic vessel activation in extramammary Paget's disease. Am J Pathol 175: 2235–2248.
21. Ishii H, Chikamatsu K, Sakakura K, Miyata M, Furuya N, et al. (2010) Primary tumor induces sentinel lymph node lymphangiogenesis in oral squamous cell carcinoma. Oral Oncol 46: 373–378.
22. Harrell MI, Iritani BM, Ruddell A (2007) Tumor-induced sentinel lymph node lymphangiogenesis and increased lymph flow precede melanoma metastasis. Am J Pathol 170: 774–786.
23. Van den Eynden GG, Vandenberghe MK, van Dam PJ, Colpaert CG, van Dam P, et al. (2007) Increased sentinel lymph node lymphangiogenesis is associated with nonsentinel axillary lymph node involvement in breast cancer patients with a positive sentinel node. Clin Cancer Res 13: 5391–5397.
24. Roh MS, Colangelo LH, O'Connell MJ, Yothers G, Deutsch M, et al. (2009) Preoperative multimodality therapy improves disease-free survival in patients with carcinoma of the rectum: NSABP R-03. J Clin Oncol 27: 5124–5130.
25. Rinaldo F, Li J, Wang E, Muders M, Datta K (2007) RalA regulates vascular endothelial growth factor-C (VEGF-C) synthesis in prostate cancer cells during androgen ablation. Oncogene 26: 1731–1738.
26. Muders MH, Zhang H, Wang E, Tindall DJ, Datta K (2009) Vascular endothelial growth factor-C protects prostate cancer cells from oxidative stress by the activation of mammalian target of rapamycin complex-2 and AKT-1. Cancer Res 69: 6042–6048.
27. Perez RO, Habr-Gama A, Nishida Arazawa ST, Rawet V, Coelho Siqueira SA, et al. (2005) Lymph node micrometastasis in stage II distal rectal cancer following neoadjuvant chemoradiation therapy. Int J Colorectal Dis 20: 434–439.
28. Caricato M, Ausania F, De Dominicis E, Vincenzi B, Rabitti C, et al. (2007) Tumor regression in mesorectal lymphnodes after neoadjuvant chemoradiation for rectal cancer. Eur J Surg Oncol 33: 724–728.
29. Weidner N, Semple JP, Welch WR, Folkman J (1991) Tumor angiogenesis and metastasis–correlation in invasive breast carcinoma. N Engl J Med 324: 1–8.

Nanostring-Based Multigene Assay to Predict Recurrence for Gastric Cancer Patients after Surgery

Jeeyun Lee[1]❡, Insuk Sohn[2]❡, In-Gu Do[2,3]❡, Kyoung-Mee Kim[3]❡, Se Hoon Park[1], Joon Oh Park[1], Young Suk Park[1], Ho Yeong Lim[1], Tae Sung Sohn[4], Jae Moon Bae[4], Min Gew Choi[4], Do Hoon Lim[5], Byung Hoon Min[6], Joon Haeng Lee[6], Poong Lyul Rhee[6], Jae J. Kim[6], Dong Il Choi[7], Iain Beehuat Tan[8], Kakoli Das[9], Patrick Tan[8,9,10], Sin Ho Jung[2], Won Ki Kang[1]*, Sung Kim[4]*

1 Division of Hematology-Oncology, Department of Medicine, Samsung Medical Center Sungkyunkwan University School of Medicine, Seoul, Korea, **2** Samsung Cancer Research Institute, Samsung Medical Center, Seoul, Korea, **3** Department of Pathology, Samsung Medical Center Sungkyunkwan University School of Medicine, Seoul, Korea, **4** Department of Surgery, Samsung Medical Center, Sungkyunkwan University School of Medicine, Seoul, Korea, **5** Department of Radiation Oncology, Samsung Medical Center, Sungkyunkwan University School of Medicine, Seoul, Korea, **6** Department of Gastroenterology, Samsung Medical Center, Sungkyunkwan University School of Medicine, Seoul, Korea, **7** Department of Radiology, Samsung Medical Center, Sungkyunkwan University School of Medicine, Seoul, Korea, **8** Cancer and Stem Cell Biology, Duke-NUS Graduate Medical School Singapore, Singapore, **9** Genome Institute of Singapore, Singapore, Singapore, **10** Cancer Science Institute of Singapore, Singapore, Singapore

Abstract

Despite the benefits from adjuvant chemotherapy or chemoradiotherapy, approximately one-third of stage II gastric cancer (GC) patients developed recurrences. The aim of this study was to develop and validate a prognostic algorithm for gastric cancer (GCPS) that can robustly identify high-risk group for recurrence among stage II patients. A multi-step gene expression profiling study was conducted. First, a microarray gene expression profiling of archived paraffin-embedded tumor blocks was used to identify candidate prognostic genes (N = 432). Second, a focused gene expression assay including prognostic genes was used to develop a robust clinical assay (GCPS) in stage II patients from the same cohort (N = 186). Third, a predefined cut off for the GCPS was validated using an independent stage II cohort (N = 216). The GCPS was validated in another set with stage II GC who underwent surgery without adjuvant treatment (N = 300). GCPS was developed by summing the product of Cox regression coefficients and normalized expression levels of 8 genes (LAMP5, CDC25B, CDK1, CLIP4, LTB4R2, MATN3, NOX4, TFDP1). A prospectively defined cut-point for GCPS classified 22.7% of validation cohort treated with chemoradiotherapy (N = 216) as high-risk group with 5-year recurrence rate of 58.6% compared to 85.4% in the low risk group (hazard ratio for recurrence = 3.16, p = 0.00004). GCPS also identified high-risk group among stage II patients treated with surgery only (hazard ratio = 1.77, p = 0.0053).

Editor: Ju-Seog Lee, University of Texas MD Anderson Cancer Center, United States of America

Funding: This study was supported by an Intramural grant from the Samsung Medical Center. The funders had no role in study design, data collection and analysis, decision to publish, or preparation of the manuscript.

* E-mail: wkkang@skku.edu (WK); sungkimm@skku.edu (SK)

❡ These authors contributed equally to this work.

Introduction

Gastric cancers are highly lethal malignancies with five-year survival rates being one of the worst reported for any solid tumors. According to data from the National Cancer Institute Surveillance, Epidemiology and End Results (SEER) Program, the five-year survival for patients with gastric cancer (GC) improved only modestly over the last 50 years, from 12 to 22 percent [1]. The propensity of GC for early metastatic dissemination has been well documented in previous studies [2,3]. Based on the recent adjuvant phase III trials, survival benefit from adjuvant chemotherapy or chemoradiation therapy has been documented in GC [4–7]. However, 25 to 40% of all surgically resected GC patients still develop recurrences that are not amenable to re-resection [4,7–9]. For pathologic stage III and IV GC, 5-year disease-free survival rates are very poor (stage IIIA, 57.6%, stage IIIB, 39.6%; and stage IV 26.3%) [8] implicating that these tumors have inherently aggressive behaviour. In contrast, pathologic stage II GC patients have more favorable clinical outcome with 5-year disease free survival rates of 76% −90% following surgery and adjuvant treatment [8,9]. Nevertheless, there is a wide spectrum of clinical aggressiveness even within the same stage with some patients being cured with surgery alone while some patients recur shortly after surgery and adjuvant chemoradiation therapy. Hence, based on the hypothesis that there is a significant molecular heterogeneity, we designed a large-scaled gene expression profiling study to develop a molecular test which may efficiently discriminate low-risk from high-risk GC groups for recurrence after surgery.

A molecular test that identifies high-risk patients for recurrence may lead to optimized perioperative treatment strategies in GC. The discovery phase included GC patients from all clinical stages treated with chemoradiotherapy (N = 520). Tumor blocks from these patients were subjected to prognostic gene discovery using Whole Genome DASL assay (WG-DASL) (Illumina, San Diego, CA), a microarray gene expression profiling method for formalin-fixed paraffin-embedded tissue (FFPE). The purpose was to develop hypothesis for clinical utility and discover candidate prognostic or internal reference genes that will help design focused gene expression assay. Results from this phase suggested that clinical utility of a gene expression based prognostic algorithm may potentially distinguish a high-risk group among stage II patients.

The objective of the project was to develop a hypothesis with clinical utility and discover candidate prognostic or internal reference genes in order to design focused gene expression assays. The results from the discovery phase suggest that clinical utility of a gene expression-based prognostic algorithm may potentially distinguish a high-risk group among stage II patients. With the use of a robust multistep prognostic algorithm, Gastric Cancer Prognostic Score (GCPS) for stage II GC patients was developed to identify high-risk patients for recurrence after surgery.

Methods

From September 1994 to December 2005, 1,557 GC patients underwent curative gastrectomy at Samsung Medical Center. Among those, 1,107 patients were selected based on following criteria: histologically confirmed adenocarcinoma of the stomach; surgical resection of tumour without macroscopic or microscopic residual disease; age ≥18; pathology stage IB (T2bN0, T1N1 but not T2aN0) to IV, according to the American Joint Committee on Cancer (AJCC) staging system (6th Ed); complete surgical record and treatment record, and patients receiving the INT-0116 regimen as adjuvant treatment [7]. The study was approved by the institutional review board of the Samsung Medical Center, Seoul, South Korea (IRB approval number: SMC 2010-10-025). All study participants provided written informed consent form recommended by the IRB. In the patients who have deceased at the time of study entry, written informed consent forms were waived by the IRB. Study design and patient cohorts are provided according to REMARK guideline (**Figure 1A, 1B**, **File S1, Section 1**). Of the cohort of 1,107 patients, a discovery set of 520 patients and a validation set of 587 patients were randomly assigned and allocated to 6 batches stratified by tumor size and year of surgery for WG-DASL assay.

To avoid false-positive conclusions due to over-fitting, prognostic algorithms and their predefined cut-points were tested in independent cohorts that were not used for prognostic gene discovery and algorithm building. A 4-phase study was designed, with 4 pre-defined independent cohorts recruited from the Samsung Medical Center. The first 3 cohorts include patients with similar clinical and pathological features from chemoradiotherapy-treated study cohorts (**File S1, Section 2**). The **first phase (discovery phase)** of the study included GC patients from all clinical stages who were treated with chemo-radiotherapy (N = 520) [8]. Tumor blocks from these patients were subjected to prognostic gene discovery using the WG-DASL (Illumina, San Diego, CA), a microarray gene expression profiling method for FFPE [7]. An ad-hoc external validation of the gene set was performed to minimize any bias from single institutional cohort. The **second phase (algorithm development)** was to translate findings from the first phase into a clinically applicable test format. We chose the nCounter platform (Nanostring Technologies, Seattle, WA), because of its ability to interrogate the expression levels of up to 800 genes using total RNA extracted from FFPE in a single-tube reaction [8]. We screened stage II patients from the first phase (N = 186) for *de novo* discovery of prognostic genes, selected ideal combinations of genes using the gradient least absolute shrinkage and selection operator (LASSO) algorithm [10], and then built a first-generation GCPS (GCPS-g1) by adding the products of normalized gene expression and coefficients from the Cox model for DFS. In the **third** cohort of stage II patients (N = 216). In the **fourth phase (testing of clinical utility in a surgery-only setting)**, we tested the potential clinical utility of GCPS in stage II patients treated with surgery only. A time stamp protocol (**Figure S12**) was developed before processing of this final cohort. We subsequently developed a refined second-generation GCPS (GCPS-g2) (the final gene set) by analyzing the combined stage II cohorts from the second and third phases of the study.

Gene expression profiling using whole genome-DASL assay

Before each gene profiling experiment, tissue samples were randomly allocated to different batches stratified by surgery time (before 2000 vs. after 2000) and tumor size (≤5 cm vs >5 cm) to minimize any variations from the DNA quality. Total RNA was extracted from 2–4 sections of 4-μm thick FFPE sections from representative primary tumor blocks using the High Pure RNA

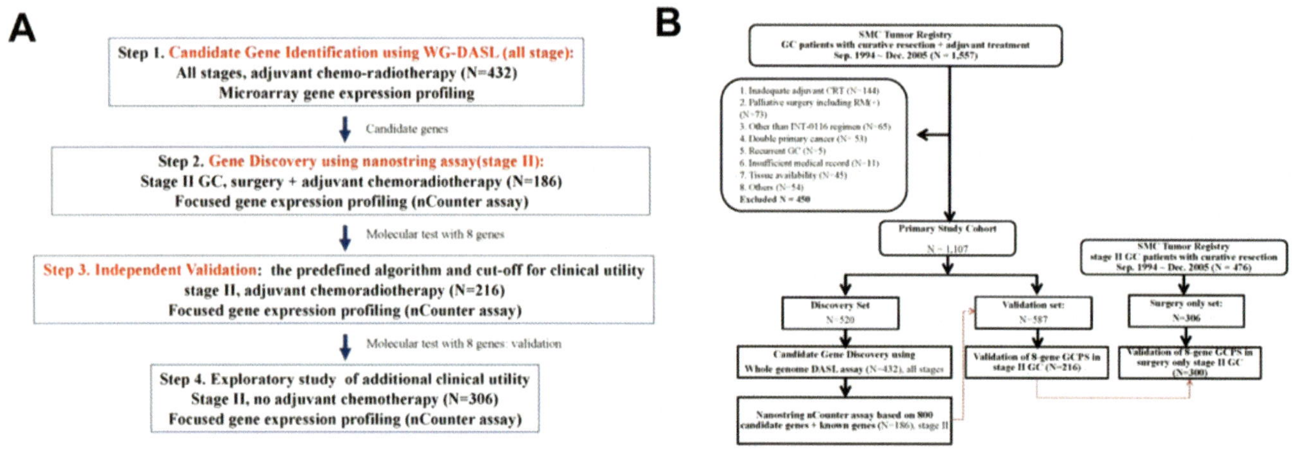

Figure 1. The Consort Diagram. (A) A multi-step approach gene expression profiling design, (B) Consort Diagram.

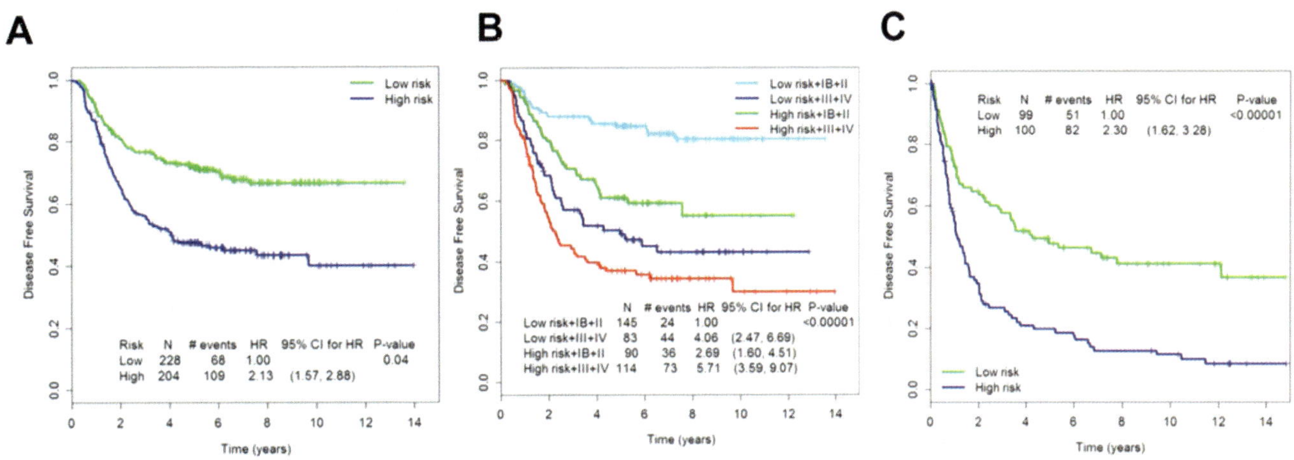

Figure 2. Kaplan-Meier curves for high risk and low risk groups classified by leave one out cross validation procedure. HR denotes hazard ratio and p-value is calculated from 100 permutations. (A) all stage patients, high vs low risk; (B) according to stage and risk groups; (C) External validation of the initial gene expression profiling.

Paraffin kit (Roche Diagnostic, Mannheim, Germany) after removing non-tumor elements by manual macrodissection guided by hematoxylin and eosin stained slides. WG-DASL assay was performed using 200 ng of RNA following the manufacturer's instruction [11]. For nCounter assay, 200 ng of total RNA was hybridized with the custom designed code set of 800 genes for 18 hours at 65°C and processed according to manufacturer's instruction [12]. The data were normalized to average expression levels of 48 internal reference genes selected from microarray experiment. The detailed description of the discovery phase using WG-DASL assay is provided in **File S1, Section 3**. The comparability in DNA quality of FFPE tissue and fresh frozen tissues using DASL assay was published previously [13,14].

Prognostic model building and validation

The algorithm for n-Counter-based assay development for clinical utility based on WG-DASL is provided in **File S1, Sections 4–6**. We used the gradient lasso algorithm to fit a prediction model based on Cox's proportional hazards model for DFS using the probes with marginal p value<0.01 (**Figure S2 in File S1**) [10]. We used leave one out cross validation with de novo discovery at each leave one out step to assess the performance of the prognostic model within the discovery cohort. Optimal cut-point was determined by creating a plot for p-values for each cut-point for the prognostic score. For validation study, a priori defined algorithm and cut-point values were used. The validation method for GCPS is outlined in **File S1, Section 7**.

Results

Microarray gene expression profiling of GC patients treated with adjuvant chemoradiotherapy (phase 1)

We performed gene expression profiling of FFPE from the discovery cohort of 520 cases of stage IB–IV GC treated with standard chemoradiotherapy after curative resection using the WG-DASL assay (**Figure 1**). Among them, 432 samples passed RNA quality control (GEO database GSE 26253) (**File S1, Section 3**). The primary end point was DFS. Univariate analysis identified 369 probes that were significantly associated with disease-free survival at p<0.01 without adjustment for other clinical variables (**File S1, Section 3d**). Next, gradient Lasso was used to develop a prognostic algorithm to predict recurrence (**File S1, Section 3e**). The leave-one-out cross-validation (LOOCV) procedure with *de novo* discovery of prognostic genes and the building of a prognostic algorithm at each step was used to examine the robustness of the prognostic algorithm. According to prognostic gene signatures (26 genes, **File S1, Section 3f**) and pathologic stages (localized vs. advanced), 432 patients were categorized into the following groups: low-risk and stage IB/II (N = 145; 5-year DFS, 84.8%), high-risk and stage IB/II (N = 90; 5-year DFS, 61.1%), low-risk and stage III/IV (N = 83; 5-year DFS, 48.9%), and high-risk and stage III/IV (N = 114; 5-year DFS, 36.9%) (**Figure 2**). As an ad-hoc analysis, we tested this gene signature using gene expression profiling data from the Singapore patient cohort (N = 199) to minimize any inherent bias from a single institution cohort [15]. In the external patient cohort, the gene signature was able to separate the high-risk group (N = 100) from the low-risk group (N = 99) for recurrence with statistical significance (p<0.00001; hazard ratio (HR), 2.3; 95% CI, 1.62–3.28) (**Figure 2**). These data suggest the main clinical utility of gene expression profiling of GC in the identification of high-risk patients among stage II patients (low vs. high risk stage IB/II, 84.8% vs. 61.1%; low vs. high risk stage III/IV, 48.9% vs. 36.9%). Therefore, for the development of clinical assay and validation, we focused on developing a gene-set which can robustly predict recurrence in stage II patients.

Development of Gastric Cancer Prognostic Score (GCPS) for stage II GC using the nCounter assay (phase 2)

We custom designed an nCounter probe set comprised of candidate prognostic genes from WG-DASL microarray data (phase 1), as well as known cancer genes, kinase genes, and G protein-coupled receptor genes. To address the variability problem in the integrity of RNA molecules in archived FFPE due to pre-analytical variables, such as fixation time and age of the blocks, we applied within-sample normalization using a set of 48 internal reference genes selected from microarray data based on minimum variation across cases and lack of association with prognosis (**File S1, Section 4**). Correlation between hazard ratios of prognostic genes based on nanostring and WG-DASL are provided in **File S1, Section 4b**, and **Figure S3 in File S1**.

We profiled 186 stage II patients from the discovery set. After assessing the robustness of prognostic algorithms built by gradient LASSO through LOOCV, we applied gradient LASSO to all 186 patients and identified 8 genes (LAMP5, CDC25B, CDK1, CLIP4, LTB4R2, MATN3, NOX4, and TFDP1) that in combination provided robust prognostic information (**Table 1**). The GCPS was then developed as a linear combination of the Cox regression estimates and normalized expression levels of these 8 genes. The cut-point analysis demonstrates that the GCPS was most robust in identifying 25% of patients with worst outcomes (**File S1, Section 4**). We chose a cut-point of 0.2205 for prospective validation in the independent validation cohort.

Validation of GCPS and its predefined cut-point in stage II GC patients treated with chemoradiotherapy (phase 3)

To avoid the potential over-fitting issue associated with cross-validation [16], we validated GCPS with the fixed algorithm and cut-points in an independent patient cohort that was not used in gene discovery. The clinical and pathological features of 216 stage II patients from the validation set were similar to those from the discovery cohort (**File S1, Section 6**, and **Figures S4–6 in File S1**). When we applied GCPS-g1 to the validation set, the risk score distribution was very similar, suggesting the robust analytical performance of the assay (**File S1, Section 7a**, and **Figure S7 is File S1**). The predefined cut-point (0.2205) for GCPS-g1 classified 22.7% of tumors from the validation set as the high-risk group. The Kaplan Meier estimate of 5-year DFS for the high-risk patients was 58.6%, compared to 85.4% for the low-risk patients (HR for recurrence, 3.16; $p = 0.00004$) (**Figure 3**). GCPS was significant in both intestinal- and diffuse- type GCs, as shown in Figure S8 in File S1 (**File S1, Section 7b**). The multivariate analysis further shows that GCPS-g1 provided additional prognostic information, besides other known factors such as Lauren classification, differentiation grade, age, and surgery type (HR, 3.027; $p = 0.00016$; **Table 2**). Therefore, GCPS may be used to identify stage II patients who remain at high risk even after standard adjuvant chemoradiotherapy and who have similar risk of recurrence as stage III patients.

GCPS as a prognostic factor for stage II GC patients treated with surgery only based on a prospectively designed protocol (phase 4)

The review of the clinical database identified 306 patients who did not receive postoperative treatment based on shared decision between physicians and patients (**File S1, Section 1, Table S1 in File S1**). These patients were subjected to exploratory analyses for assessing the prognostic role of GCPS in patients treated with surgery only and testing the hypothesis that the benefit from chemoradiotherapy is limited in high-risk patients defined by GCPS. For this step, we developed GCPS-g2 (**Table S8 in File S1**), the second-generation GCPS, by analyzing all stage II cases from phases 2 and 3 to maximize the sample size. We prospectively tested the predefined GCPS-g2 algorithm and cut-point as described in the time stamp protocol (**Figure S12 in File S1**). The GCPS-g2 predicted recurrence in 300 stage II tumors with a hazard ratio of 2.131 (95% CI, 1.428–3.180; $p = 0.00021$) (HR, 3.16) (**Figure S9 in File S1**). To minimize the possibility of over-fitting of the algorithm to chemoradiotherapy-treated patients, we also tested the GCPS-g1, which was previously validated in the chemoradiotherapy-treated cohort, in surgery alone cohort (**Figure S10 in File S1**). The hazard ratio for GCPS-g1 (HR, 1.77; 95% CI, 1.18–2.67; $p = 0.0053$) is similar to that for GCPS-g2 (**Figure 3**). Therefore, the GCPS robustly predicted recurrence in stage II GC with or without postoperative treatment. Based on this data, it can be speculated that high-risk stage II patients defined by GCPS did not gain a tremendous benefit from chemoradiotherapy.

Expression of adverse prognostic genes in tumor microenvironments

In all 3 stage II cohorts included in this study, increased expression levels of 4 genes from GCPS (NOX4, LAMP5, MATN3, and CLIP4) were associated with poor prognosis. Since the known functions of these genes suggest their expression in microenvironments rather than actual tumor cells, we performed the nCounter assay for microdissected tumors versus stromal components from 4 representative high-risk tumors (**Figure S11 in File S1**). The expression of these genes was significantly higher in stromal components, compared to epithelial cancer cells, with NOX4 showing the most pronounced differences ($p = 0.04$).

Discussion

In an initial discovery phase, we performed WG-DASL in all stage GC patients. Then, based on the WG-DASL data, we observed that the segregation of high risk group from low risk group was most significant in early stage Ib/II patients (low vs. high risk stage IB/II, 84.8% vs. 61.1%; low vs. high risk stage III/IV, 48.9% vs. 36.9%). Therefore, for the development of clinical assay and validation, we focused on developing a gene-set which can robustly predict recurrence in stage II patients. We developed

Table 1. List of genes that constitute Gastric Cancer Prognostic Score and their Cox regression estimates used to calculate the score.

Gene Symbol	Chromosomal location	Gene Name	Cox regression estimate
LAMP5(BAD-LAMP, C20orf103)	20p12	Lysosomal-associated membrane protein family, member 5	0.0636
CDC25B	20p13	Cell division cycle 25 homolog B (S. pombe)	−0.0175
CDK1	10q21.1	Cyclin-dependent kinase 1	−0.1005
CLIP4 (UBASH3A, TULA, STS-2, TULA-1)	2p23.2	CAP-GLY domain containing linker family, member 4; Suppressor of T cell receptor signaling-2	0.4822
LTB4R2	14q11.2-q12	Leukotriene B4 receptor	−0.3950
MATN3	2p24-p23	Matrillin 3	0.2982
NOX4	11q14.2-q21	NADPH oxidase 4	0.0288
TFDP1	13q34	Transcription factor Dp-1	−0.2886

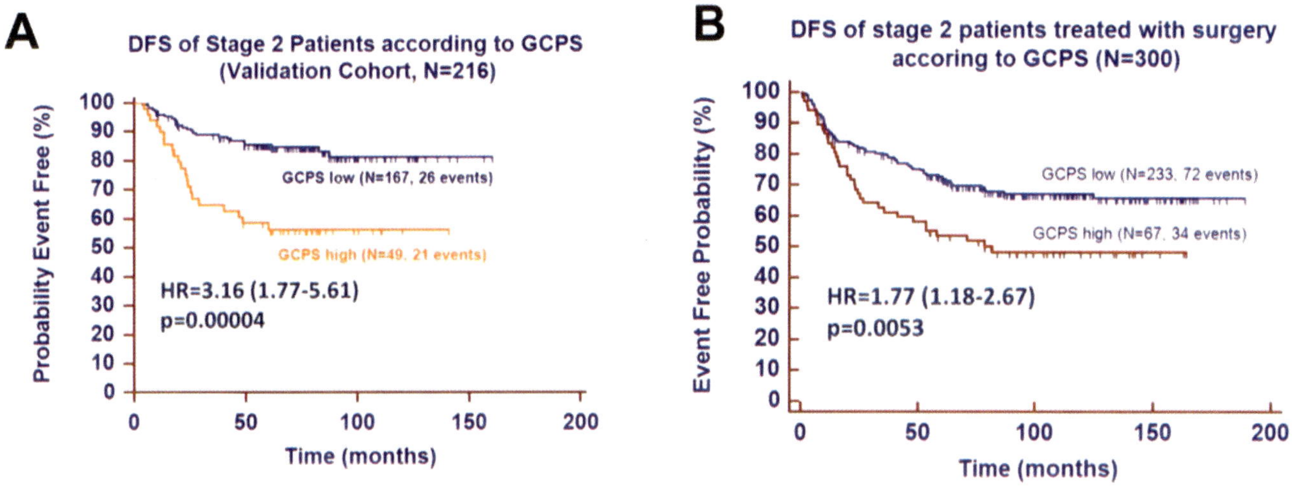

Figure 3. (A) DFS of stage 2 patients according to GCPS. (B) DFS of stage 2 patients treated with surgery according to GCPS.

and validated a prognostic algorithm for gastric cancer, GCPS, which can robustly identify high-risk groups for recurrence among stage II patients. GCPS, developed using the nCounter platform, showed the robust performance in FFPE samples. In addition, the inclusion of internal reference genes allowed the application of GCPS to individual patients. Therefore, we suggest that GCPS can be readily applied to routine clinical use. The GCPS of 8 genes (LAMP5, CDC25B, CDK1, CLIP4, LTB4R2, MATN3, NOX4, and TFDP1) were discovered and validated in over 700 stage II GC patients. We found that the GCPS identified high-risk GC patients for recurrence regardless adjuvant treatment and that high-risk stage II GC patients showed similar DFS to stage III patients. Notably, the GCPS predicted recurrence of both Lauren types (diffuse or intestinal) (**Figure S8 in File S1**).

Our data clearly demonstrate the presence of molecular heterogeneity in GC, which was associated with clinical outcomes but independent of clinicopathologic staging information. Our data indicate that stage IB/II patients had very poor prognosis when their tumors expressed poor-risk gene signatures. There was a difference of 23.7% in 5-year DFS between high-risk and low-risk gene signatures in stage IB/II patients, and 5-year DFS of high-risk stage IB/II patients was below 60%, despite the use of adjuvant chemoradiotherapy (**Figure 1**). Therefore, it may be necessary to prospectively design a trial to question whether chemoradiotherapy is required for stage IB/II patients with low-risk gene expression profiles. In order to minimize any potential bias from variations in clinical practice or surgery at a single center, we performed an ad hoc external validation of the signature to validate the signature. As shown in the Results, the signature consistently predicted recurrence in Singapore cohort.

Among the 8 final GCPS genes (LAMP5, CDC25B, CDK1, CLIP4, LTB4R2, MATN3, NOX4, and TFDP1), CDC25B and CDK1, which are known to be associated with cell proliferation, were found to correlate with favorable prognosis (negative Cox regression estimates in Table 2). Notably, a similar trend has been observed for colon cancer by a gene expression assay [17,18]. These findings may reflect the differentiation status of these tumor cells, since normal gastric and colon mucosal epithelial cells have high turnover rates. TFDP1 encodes the transcriptional factor DP-1, which acts as a positive regulator of the G1/S transition during the cell cycle [19,20]. Particularly in hepatocellular carcinoma, TFDP1 overexpression was substantially associated with disease progression [19]. Since the scope of this current study does not include the functional study of these genes, their biological significance should be investigated in future studies. Recently, Cho *et al.* has performed the largest gene expression profiling in 213 GC patients using fresh frozen tissues [21]. They identified 6 prognostic genes (CTNBB1, EXOCS3, TOP2A, LBA1, CCL5, and LZTR1) for patient survival after curative resection. However, to the best of our knowledge, GCPS is the only gene set which has now been validated in more than 700 stage II GC patients, regardless Lauren classification (diffuse or intestinal), a known prognostic factor, or adjuvant treatment.

In conclusion, with the use of a multistep approach, we developed 8-gene GCPS, which was able to robustly identify high-risk stage II GC patients for recurrence after surgery regardless of adjuvant treatment. Currently, with the ongoing ARTIST-II trial (NCT#01761461), we plan to validate our GCPS in a prospectively designed phase III trial.

Table 2. Multivariate Cox regression analysis results on the validation set (N = 216).

	Hazard ratio	P-value
GCPS (low vs high-risk)	3.027	0.00016
LAUREN (intestinal vs diffuse)	0.541	0.18000
WHO (W/D~M/D vs P/D*)	2.491	0.07600
AGE (65< = vs 65>)	1.496	0.19000
Surgery types (subtotal vs total gastrectomy)	1.121	0.71000

*W/D, well differentiated; M/D, moderately differentiated; P/D, poorly differentiated.

Supporting Information

File S1 1. Patient characteristics of study cohorts at each step (**Table S1**). a. Table S1. Patients characteristics. **2.** Clinical and pathological characteristics of cases examined at each phase. **3.** Detailed description of the discovery step using WG-DASL assay (step 1). a. **Figure S1**. QA of WG-DASL data. b. **Table S2**. Comparison of FISH and IHC results for HER2 status in gastric cancer in Step 1. c. **Table S3**. List of probes that are differentially

expressed between HER2-positive and HER2- negative patient groups in Step 1. d. **Table S4**. List of all probes with univariate p-values<0.01 in Step 1. e. **Figure S2**. Gradient Lasso algorithm. f. **Table S5**. List of 26 probes included in the prediction model fitted by the whole data set (n = 432). g. **Table S6**. Multivariate Cox regression analysis results in gene discovery set (n = 432). **4.** Design of focused gene expression assay using nCounter platform. a. **Table S7**. List of reference genes for nCounter assay. b. **Figure S3**. Correlation between hazard ratios of prognostic genes based on quantile normalization and self-normalization using WG-DASL assay. **5.** nCounter assay and quality control. **6.** Selection of cut-off for Gastric Cancer Prognostic Score (GCPS(**Figure S4, S5, & S6**). a. **Figure S4**. DFS according to each quartiles of GCPS-g1. b. Figure S5. Cut-point analysis for GCPS-g1. c. **Figure S6**. DFS according to optimized cut-point of GCPS-g1. **6.** Distribution of GCPS between discovery set and validation set. a. **Figure S7**. Distribution of GCPS-g1 within the discovery and validation set. b. **Figure S8**. GCPS: intestinal vs diffuse type. **7.** Testing of clinical utility of GCPS-g2 in patients treated with surgery only. a. **Figure S9**. DFS of stage II patients treated with chemoradiotherapy based on quartile of GCPS-g2. b. **Figure S10**. DFS of stage II patients treated with surgery alone based on quartile of GCPS-g2. c. **Figure S11**. Expression of adverse prognostic genes included in Gastric Cancer Prognostic Score according to tissue compartments (tumor versus stroma). Normalized expression levels are shown. d. **Table S8**. List of nCounter probes included in GCPS-g2. **8.** Gastric cancer validation study protocol. a. **Figure S12**. Gastric cancer validation study protocol.
(DOCX)

Author Contributions

Conceived and designed the experiments: JL WK SK. Performed the experiments: IGD KMK. Contributed reagents/materials/analysis tools: SHP JOP YSP HYL TSS JMB MGC DHL BHM JHL PLR JJK DIC IBT KD PT. Wrote the paper: JL IS IGD WK SK. Performed statistics: IS SHJ.

References

1. Levi F, Lucchini F, Gonzalez JR, Fernandez E, Negri E, et al. (2004) Monitoring falls in gastric cancer mortality in Europe. Ann Oncol 15: 338–345.
2. Folli S, Morgagni P, Roviello F, De Manzoni G, Marrelli D, et al. (2001) Risk factors for lymph node metastases and their prognostic significance in early gastric cancer (EGC) for the Italian Research Group for Gastric Cancer (IRGGC). Jpn J Clin Oncol 31: 495–499.
3. Nigro JJ, Hagen JA, DeMeester TR, DeMeester SR, Theisen J, et al. (1999) Occult esophageal adenocarcinoma: extent of disease and implications for effective therapy. Ann Surg 230: 433–438; discussion 438–440.
4. Bang YJ, Kim YW, Yang H, Chung HC, Park YK, et al. (2011) Adjuvant capecitabine and oxaliplatin for gastric cancer: results of the Phase III CLASSIC trial. J of Clin Oncol 29 (Abstr LBA 4002).
5. Bang YJ, Kim YW, Yang HK, Chung HC, Park YK, et al. (2012) Adjuvant capecitabine and oxaliplatin for gastric cancer after D2 gastrectomy (CLASSIC): a phase 3 open-label, randomised controlled trial. Lancet 379: 315–321.
6. Lee J, Lim do H, Kim S, Park SH, Park JO, et al. (2012) Phase III trial comparing capecitabine plus cisplatin versus capecitabine plus cisplatin with concurrent capecitabine radiotherapy in completely resected gastric cancer with D2 lymph node dissection: the ARTIST trial. J Clin Oncol 30: 268–273.
7. Macdonald JS, Smalley SR, Benedetti J, Hundahl SA, Estes NC, et al. (2001) Chemoradiotherapy after surgery compared with surgery alone for adenocarcinoma of the stomach or gastroesophageal junction. N Engl J Med 345: 725–730.
8. Kim S, Lim DH, Lee J, Kang WK, MacDonald JS, et al. (2005) An observational study suggesting clinical benefit for adjuvant postoperative chemoradiation in a population of over 500 cases after gastric resection with D2 nodal dissection for adenocarcinoma of the stomach. Int J Radiat Oncol Biol Phys 63: 1279–1285.
9. Lee K, Kye M, Jang JS, Lee OJ, Kim T, et al. (2004) Proteomic analysis revealed a strong association of a high level of alpha1-antitrypsin in gastric juice with gastric cancer. Proteomics 4: 3343–3352.
10. Sohn I, Kim J, Jung SH, Park C (2009) Gradient lasso for Cox proportional hazards model. Bioinformatics 25: 1775–1781.
11. Bibikova M, Talantov D, Chudin E, Yeakley JM, Chen J, et al. (2004) Quantitative gene expression profiling in formalin-fixed, paraffin-embedded tissues using universal bead arrays. Am J Pathol 165: 1799–1807.
12. Geiss GK, Bumgarner RE, Birditt B, Dahl T, Dowidar N, et al. (2008) Direct multiplexed measurement of gene expression with color-coded probe pairs. Nat Biotechnol 26: 317–325.
13. Hoshida Y, Villanueva A, Kobayashi M, Peix J, Chiang DY, et al. (2008) Gene expression in fixed tissues and outcome in hepatocellular carcinoma. N Engl J Med 359: 1995–2004.
14. Fan JB, Yeakley JM, Bibikova M, Chudin E, Wickham E, et al. (2004) A versatile assay for high-throughput gene expression profiling on universal array matrices. Genome Res 14: 878–885.
15. Tan IB, Ivanova T, Lim KH, Ong CW, Deng N, et al. (2011) Intrinsic subtypes of gastric cancer, based on gene expression pattern, predict survival and respond differently to chemotherapy. Gastroenterology 141: 476–485, 485 e471–411.
16. Simon R, Radmacher MD, Dobbin K, McShane LM (2003) Pitfalls in the use of DNA microarray data for diagnostic and prognostic classification. J Natl Cancer Inst 95: 14–18.
17. Allegra CJ, Paik S, Colangelo LH, Parr AL, Kirsch I, et al. (2003) Prognostic value of thymidylate synthase, Ki-67, and p53 in patients with Dukes' B and C colon cancer: a National Cancer Institute-National Surgical Adjuvant Breast and Bowel Project collaborative study. J Clin Oncol 21: 241–250.
18. Clark-Langone KM, Wu JY, Sangli C, Chen A, Snable JL, et al. (2007) Biomarker discovery for colon cancer using a 761 gene RT-PCR assay. BMC Genomics 8: 279.
19. Yasui K, Okamoto H, Arii S, Inazawa J (2003) Association of over-expressed TFDP1 with progression of hepatocellular carcinomas. J Hum Genet 48: 609–613.
20. Yasui K, Arii S, Zhao C, Imoto I, Ueda M, et al. (2002) TFDP1, CUL4A, and CDC16 identified as targets for amplification at 13q34 in hepatocellular carcinomas. Hepatology 35: 1476–1484.
21. Cho JY, Lim JY, Cheong JH, Park YY, Yoon SL, et al. (2011) Gene expression signature-based prognostic risk score in gastric cancer. Clin Cancer Res 17: 1850–1857.

Survival Benefit of Adding Chemotherapy to Intensity Modulated Radiation in Patients with Locoregionally Advanced Nasopharyngeal Carcinoma

Xuemei Ji[1,2]*, Conghua Xie[2]*, Desheng Hu[3], Xia Fan[2], Yajuan Zhou[3], Yingjie Zheng[1]

1 Department of Radiation Oncology, Beijing Chaoyang Hospital, Capital Medical University, Beijing, China, **2** Department of Radiation and Medical Oncology, Zhongnan Hospital, Wuhan University, Wuhan, China, **3** Department of Radiation Oncology, Tumor Hosptal of Hubei Province, Wuhan, China

Abstract

Background: To evaluate the contribution of chemotherapy for patients with locoregionally advanced nasopharyngeal carcinoma (NPC) treated by intensity modulated radiotherapy (IMRT) and to identify the optimal combination treatment strategy.

Patients and Methods: Between 2006 and 2010, 276 patients with stage II-IVb NPC were treated by IMRT alone or IMRT plus chemotherapy. Cisplatin-based chemotherapy included neoadjuvant or concurrent, or neoadjuvant plus concurrent protocols. The IMRT alone and chemoradiotherapy groups were well-matched for prognostic factors, except N stage, with more advanced NPC in the chemoradiotherapy arm.

Results: With a mean follow-up of 33.8 months, the 3-year actuarial rates of overall survival (OS), metastasis-free survival (MFS), relapse-free survival (RFS), and disease-free survival (DFS) were 90.3%, 84.2%, 80.3%, and 69.2% for all of the patients, respectively. Compared with the IMRT alone arm, patients treated by concurrent chemoradiotherapy had a significantly better DFS (HR = 2.64; 95% CI, 1.12−6.22; P = 0.03), patients with neoadjuvant-concurrent chemoradiotherapy had a significant improvement in RFS and DFS (HR = 4.03; 95% CI, 1.35−12.05; P = 0.01 and HR = 2.43; 95% CI, 1.09−5.44; P = 0.03), neoadjuvant chemoradiotherapy provided no significant benefit in OS, MFS, RFS, and DFS. Stage group and alcohol consumption were prognostic factors for OS and N stage was a significant predictor for DFS.

Conclusions: Addition of concurrent or neoadjuvant-concurrent chemotherapy to IMRT is available to prolong RFS or DFS for locoregionally advanced NPC. Such work could be helpful to guide effective individualized therapy.

Editor: Jingwu Xie, Indiana University School of Medicine, United States of America

Funding: This work was supported by National Natural Science Foundation of China (81101561); a UICC American Cancer Society Beginning Investigators Fellowship funded by the American Cancer Society; the Scientific Research Foundation for the Returned Overseas Chinese Scholars from State Education Ministry, China to Xuemei Ji. URL of National Natural Science Foundation of China: http://www.nsfc.gov.cn/Portal0/default152.htm, URL of the American Cancer Society:http://www.cancer.org/, and URL of State Education Ministry, China:http://www.moe.edu.cn/. There are no grant numbers for a UICC American Cancer Society Beginning Investigators Fellowship funded by the American Cancer Society, whose certification is available if needed or can be found in URL: http://www.uicc.org/fellowships/beginning-investigators. There are also no grant numbers for the Scientific Research Foundation for the Returned Overseas Chinese Scholars from State Education Ministry to Xuemei Ji, which is available if needed. The funders had no role in study design, data collection and analysis, decision to publish, or preparation of the manuscript.

Competing Interests: The authors have declared that no competing interests exist.

* E-mail: xuemei.ji@yahoo.com (XJ); chxie65@hotmail.com (CX)

Introduction

Nasopharyngeal carcinoma (NPC), a relatively rare cancer in most contraries and regions worldwide, is endemic in China, being the eighth most common cause of cancer mortality in China and accounting for 1.45 deaths per 100,000 Chinese people annually [1]. The incidence-to-mortality rate ratios of NPC vary according to different countries, with China having a higher incidence relative to mortality than other populations [2], which might be attributed to distinct treatment regimens, various carcinogenetic factors, and the histologic distribution of NPC in diverse regions.

Radiotherapy (RT) to the nasopharynx, with elective radiation to the neck, used to be the standard treatment for all stages of NPC. Intensity modulated radiotherapy (IMRT), which delivers a high dose of radiation to the tumor while keeping a reduced dose to normal tissues surrounding the NPC region and excellent tumor coverage, has become widely accepted for the treatment of NPC, and has been shown to be more advanced than the conventional two-dimensional technique and three-dimensional conformal radiation in local or regional control. [3] IMRT is target specific (sparingcritical non-target organs) and yields superior treatment outcomes in patients with NPC compared to the conventional treatments mentioned above [4,5,6,7]. Locoregional control has been improved with IMRT, but distant metastasis is the main cause of treatment failure and death [8]. Chemotherapy is important to control distant metastasis of chemoradiosensitive NPC, and thus should play an important role in the treatment of NPC. Alternatively, considering that patients with advanced stage tumors have been shown to have a relatively poor prognosis when treated with IMRT alone [6] and cisplatin-based concurrent chemotherapy has been shown to provide significant survival benefit for patients with locoregionally advanced NPC treated with conventional radiotherapy [9], the addition of chemotherapy to IMRT has been suggested in an attempt to reduce failures and prolong survival. However, the most effective combination of chemotherapy and IMRT has not been well-established. Three retrospective studies have evaluated the contribution of chemotherapy for patients with NPC treated by IMRT and revealed no significant improvement in metastasis-free survival (MFS), disease-free survival (DFS), and overall survival (OS) [10,11,12], which were distinct from the efficacy of adding chemotherapy to conventional radiation [9]. The conflicting results might be attributable to basic differences in the radiation technique and confounding factors of NPC treatment in the various patient populations.

We followed a cohort of NPC patients to compare OS, DFS, MFS, and relapse-free survival (RFS) between IMRT alone and IMRT combined with concurrent or neoadjuvant chemotherapy or both to determine the efficacy of chemotherapy and the most effective combined strategy of chemotherapy and IMRT for patients with locoregionally advanced NPC. We also identified the prognostic factors which might affect the prognosis and predict the outcome of patient with locoregionally advanced NPC. Such work could be helpful to achieve an improvement in survival for patients with locoregionally advanced NPC.

Patients and Methods

Clinical Data

The current retrospective cohort is composed of 276 newly diagnosed and previously untreated patients with histopathologically-confirmed NPC treated with IMRT at a Hubei Cancer Center in Wuhan, China between January 2006 and December 2010. All patients were Chinese Han. Patients with stage I NPC, had known distant metastases at the time of diagnosis of NPC or were treated with adjuvant chemotherapy, and were excluded from the current study. Patients, alive with <1 year of follow-up were also excluded from this study. Human participant approval was obtained from the ethical committee of Zhongnan Hospital of Wuhan University.

We reviewed the medical records regarding demographic data (age, gender, cigarette smoking, alcohol use, and family history), and clinical characteristics (histologic type, clinical presentation, cancer stage, medical history, physical examination findings, and treatment). According to the World Health Organization (WHO) criteria, NPC was classified into three categories based on the histologic type: type I, squamous cell carcinoma; type II, non-keratinizing carcinoma; and type III, undifferentiated carcinoma [13]. Patients were followed until the date of death or the last contact date, which was 31 May 2012. Response to treatment, survival, pattern of relapse, and distant metastasis were obtained through telephone interviews and follow-up examinations, which included a chest X-ray, abdominal sonography, a whole-body bone scan, and computed tomography or magnetic resonance imaging of the head and neck.

Treatment

All patients underwent IMRT, with a total radiation dose of 70–74 Gy delivered to gross disease in the nasopharynx, a dose of 60–66 Gy delivered to positive lymph node areas, and a dose of 50–56 Gy to the low-risk local area, in 30–33 fractions, in approximately 7–8 weeks. Clinical target volumes were designed and planning target volumes expanded as per the RTOG 0225 protocol. Doses were modified according to the cancer stage and the size of the positive regional lymph nodes. Irradiation was performed primarily using 6 MV photons and electrons from linear accelerators.

Cisplatin-based chemotherapy, with various sequences and regimens, was added to IMRT in the chemotadiotherapy group. Concurrent chemotherapy was given to 47 patients, mainly with 75–100 mg/m^2 on day 1 every 3 weeks. A total of 93 patients received neoadjuvant chemotherapy, primarily consisted of 2–3 cycles of DF (cisplatin [25 mg/m^2 on day 1–3] and 5-fluorouracil [1000 mg/m^2 on days 1–5]/Tegafur 1000 mg on days 1–5 every 3 weeks) or TP regimen (cisplatin [25 mg/m^2 on day 1, 2, 3] and docetaxel [75 mg/m^2 on day 1 every 3 weeks]). Ninety-six patients received neoadjuvant plus concurrent chemotherapy. Among the patients who received neoadjuvant chemotherapy or neoadjuvant plus concurrent chemotherapy, 149 patients were treated with DF regimen, 28 with TP regimen, and 12 with mixed regimens including DF and/or TP regimens and/or other regimen.

Statistical Analysis

Descriptive statistical analyses were performed to characterize the patients in the IMRT alone and IMRT plus chemotherapy groups. The differences in the distribution of selected demographic variables (age, gender, smoking status, alcohol status, family history of cancer) and clinical characteristics (histologic types, cancer stage group, T stage, N stage, and treatment) were evaluated using a χ^2 test.

Actuarial rates of OS, DFS, MFS, and RFS were calculated by the Kaplan-Meier method. The primary endpoint for OS, DFS, MFS, and RFS was death, occurrence of relapse or distant metastasis, distant metastasis occurrence, and relapse occurrence of local or nodal tumors, respectively. The time-to-event was calculated from the date of therapy for newly diagnosed NPC to the date-of-event occurrence. Patients who were not known to have an event at the date of last contact or who were lost to follow-up were censored for OS, DFS, MFS, and RFS. Moreover, patients who died during follow-up without an occurrence of the event were censored for DFS, MFS, and RFS. To balance the distribution bias, a multivariate Cox model was built using the demographic variables and clinical characteristics. Associations were quantified using hazard ratios and the 95% confidence intervals. Statistical significance was set at a $P<0.05$. SAS version 9.1 was used to perform all statistical analyses.

Results

Patient Characteristics

The mean duration of follow-up was 33.8 months for all patients (33.8±14.6) and 35.1 months for survivors (35.1±13.8). In our cohort study, the median interval was 20 months for occurrence of distant metastasis, 22 months for occurrence of relapse, and 23 months for death before the end of the study. The characteristics of the 276 patients, including 236 patients treated by IMRT combined with neoadjuvant or concurrent chemotherapy or both and 40 patients treated by IMRT alone, are summarized in **Table 1**. The mean age at the time of diagnosis of NPC was 47.1±11.4 years in our cohort study. The distribution of patients was well-balanced among the two groups by major potential prognostic factors, such as the age at the time of diagnosis, gender, cigarette smoking, alcohol use, family history, histologic type, stage group, and T stage (P = 0.092 for age, 0.293 for gender, 0.503 for cigarette smoking, 0.693 for alcohol use, 0.268 for family history, 0.180 for histologic type, 0.470 for stage group, and 0.169 for T stage). Patients treated by combined treatment were more

Table 1. Characteristics of patients treated with IMRT alone versus combination of IMRT and chemotherapy.

	IMRT (n = 40)	IMRT plus chemotherapy (n = 236)	
	Number (%)	Number (%)	P*
Ages (Years)			
≤50 y	20 (50.0)	151 (64.0)	
>50y	20 (50.0)	85 (36.0)	0.092
Gender			
Female	8 (20.0)	66 (28.0)	
Male	32 (80.0)	170 (72.0)	0.293
Cigarette smoking			
Never	25 (62.5)	136 (57.6)	
Ever	15 (37.5)	100 (42.4)	0.563
Alcohol use			
Never	29 (72.5)	178 (75.4)	
Ever	11 (27.5)	58 (24.6)	0.693
Family history			
Yes	5 (12.5)	47 (19.9)	
No	35 (87.5)	189 (80.1)	0.268
WHO Histology			
I	4 (10.0)	13 (5.5)	
II	23 (57.5)	112 (47.5)	
III	13 (32.5)	111 (47.0)	0.180
Stage group			
II	8 (20.0)	35 (14.8)	
III	22 (55.0)	121 (51.3)	
IV	10 (25.0)	80 (33.9)	0.470
T stage			
T1	4 (10.0)	11 (4.7)	
T2	9 (22.5)	81 (34.3)	
T3	18 (45.0)	78 (33.0)	
T4	9 (22.5)	66 (28.0)	0.169
N stage			
N0	6 (15.0)	19 (8.0)	
N1	19 (47.5)	74 (31.4)	
N2	14 (35.0)	125 (53.0)	
N3	1 (2.5)	18 (7.6)	0.047

*Two-sided $\chi 2$ test.

advanced in N stage than patients on IMRT alone (P = 0.047). Therefore, prognostic factors, such as age, gender, cigarette smoking, alcohol use, family history, histologic type, and stage group were further used for building a multivariate Cox model and adjusting the final results.

Survival

The 3-year actuarial rates for OS, MFS, RFS, and DFS were 90.3%, 84.2%, 80.3%, and 69.2% for all of the patients, respectively. The overall mortality rate, distant metastasis rate, relapse rate and rate of patients with relapse or metastasis or both, along with the association between the survivals and treatment for IMRT alone and the addition of chemotherapy to the IMRT arm are shown in **Table 2**. A significant difference was noted in the RFS for patients with or without the addition of chemotherapy (log-rank P = 0.041), with a 3-year RFS rate of 82.0% for chemotherapy plus IMRT and 68.6% for IMRT alone. Patients treated by IMRT alone were at an approximately 2-fold increased risk for occurrence of relapse (HR = 2.13; 95% CI, 1.03−4.40) compared to patients with combination chemotherapy and IMRT. We also showed that freedom from relapse or metastasis or both was 71.1% in the IMRT combined chemotherapy arm and 57.6% in the IMRT alone arm at 3 years, and the survival curves were borderline significantly different (log-rank P = 0.056). A trend toward improved MFS favoring the addition of the chemotherapy arm was observed with a 3-year RFS rate of 84.7% for patients in the combined treatment arm and 81.7% for patients in the IMRT alone arm, but this difference was not significant (HR = 1.78; 95% CI, 0.77−4.12). The OS were not statistically different between the two groups (log-rank P = 0.829).

Table 2. Patterns of disease failure in patients treated with IMRT alone versus combination of IMRT and chemotherapy.

	IMRT plus chemotherapy (n = 236)		IMRT (n = 40)				
Failure Pattern	**Failure No.**	**Failure Rate**	**Failure No.**	**Failure Rate**	**Log rank *P***	**HR (95%CI)***	***P****
Locoregional only	41	14.4	11	27.5	0.04	2.13 (1.03–4.40)	0.04
Distant metastases only	33	14.0	8	20.0	0.28	1.78 (0.77–4.12)	0.18
Locoregional or distant metastases or both	69	29.2	16	40.0	0.06	1.80 (0.10–3.28)	0.05
Death	28	11.9	4	10.0	0.83	1.05 (0.35–3.16)	0.93

*Adjusted for age, gender, cigarette smoking, alcohol use, family history, histologic types, stage group, T stage and N stage in multivariate Cox model.

To determine which combined strategy could provide the greatest additional survival benefit, we compared survival among patients treated with IMRT alone, concurrent chemoradiotherapy, neoadjuvant chemoradiotherapy, and neoadjuvant-concurrent chemoradiotherapy (**Table 3**). Patients treated with concurrent chemoradiotherapy had a significantly better DFS (HR = 2.64; 95% CI, 1.12−6.22; P = 0.03) and a borderline significantly better MFS (HR = 2.98; 95% CI, 0.88−10.10; P = 0.08) than patients treated with IMRT alone (**Fig. 1**). The 3-year OS and RFS were 90.7% and 84.0% for the concurrent chemoradiotherapy group, and 94.7% and 68.6% for the IMRT alone group, respectively, with no significant difference between the two groups (P = 0.25 for OS and P = 0.11 for RFS). Compared with the IMRT alone arm, patients treated with neoadjuvant-concurrent chemoradiotherapy had a similar OS and MFS (P = 0.24 and P = 0.53, respectively), and a significantly better RFS and DFS (HR = 4.03; 95% CI, 1.35−12.05; P = 0.01 for RFS and HR = 2.43; 95% CI, 1.09−5.44; P = 0.03 for DFS; **Fig. 1**). Compared with the concurrent chemoradiotherapy arm, neoadjuvant chemotherapy plus concurrent chemoradiotherapy provided no significant benefit in OS, MFS, and DFS. However, patients in the neoadjuvant-concurrent chemoradiotherapy arm had a borderline significant improvement in RFS (HR = 2.44; 95% CI, 0.90−6.67; P = 0.08). There was no statistically significant difference in the OS, MFS, RFS, and DFS between the patients receiving neoadjuvant chemotherapy plus IMRT and patients in the IMRT alone arm. To validate the beneficial effectsderived from adding the concurrent chemotherapy arm or neoadjuvant-concurrent chemotherapy arm, we also analyzed the data in certain stage group or N stage, including stage III, IV, N1, and N2, in which there are analyzable numbers and events. We did find that concurrent chemoradiotherapy provided a borderline significantly better DFS for patients with stage III (HR = 4.04; 95% CI, 0.96−16.96; P = 0.06) and significantly improvement of DFS for patients with stage IV (HR = 46.02; 95% CI, 2.94−720.98; P = 0.006). Neoadjuvant-concurrent chemoradiotherapy contributed to a borderline significantly better RFS (HR = 8.56; 95% CI, 0.86−85.34; P = 0.07) and a significantly better DFS (HR = 7.49; 95% CI, 1.76−31.77; P = 0.006)for patients with stage IV, and a significantly better RFS and DFS for patients with stage N1 (HR = 7.35; 95% CI, 1.58−34.08; P = 0.01for RFS and HR = 4.33; 95% CI, 1.27−14.81; P = 0.02 for DFS).

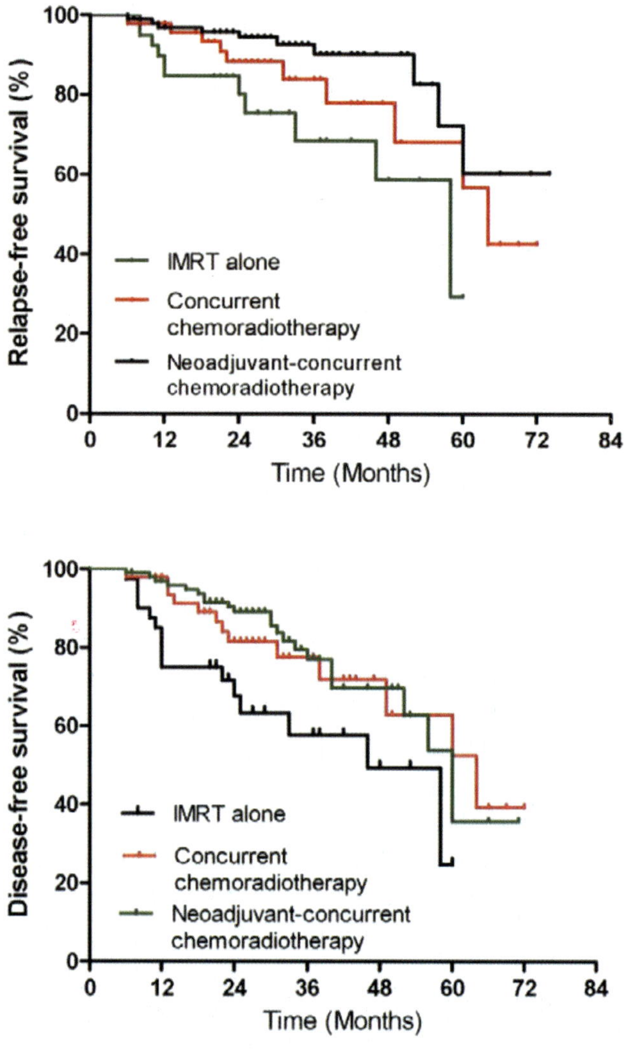

Figure 1. Kaplan-Meier estimates of relapse-free survival and disease-free survival for patients receiving Neoadjuvant-concurrent chemoradiotherapy versus Concurrent chemoradiotherapy versus IMRT alone.

In order to further verify the contribution of combining chemotherapy with IMRT and eliminate the potential impact from confounding chemotherapy regimens on survival, we compared survival among patients treated with IMRT alone, concurrent chemoradiotherapy, and adding neoadjuvant chemotherapy with DF regimen to IMRT and concurrent chemoradiotherapy (**Table 4**). Compared to IMRT alone, neoadjuvant with DF-concurrent chemoradiotherapyprovided a significantly

Table 3. Comparison of survival in patients treated with different treatment strategies.

	Overall survival		Distant metastasis-free survival		Relapse-free survival		Disease-free survival	
	HR (95%CI)*	P*	HR (95%CI)*	P*	HR (95%CI)*	P*	HR (95%CI)*	P*
Concurrent chemoradiotherapy vs IMRT alone	2.48 (0.53–11.68)	0.25	2.98 (0.88–10.10)	0.08	2.23 (0.81–6.13)	0.11	2.64 (1.12–6.22)	0.03
Neoadjuvant-concurrent chemoradiotherapy vs IMRT alone	2.55 (0.54–12.04)	0.24	1.39 (0.49–3.92)	0.53	4.03 (1.35–12.05)	0.01	2.43 (1.09–5.44)	0.03
Neoadjuvent chemoradiotherapy vs IMRT alone	0.286 (0.07–1.10)	0.07	1.62 (0.60–4.40)	0.34	1.62 (0.69–3.80)	0.27	1.38 (0.70–2.75)	0.35
Neoadjuvant-concurrent chemoradiotherapy vs Concurrent chemoradiotherapy	1.64 (0.46–5.82)	0.44	1.02 (0.31–3.33)	0.98	2.44 (0.90–6.67)	0.08	1.23 (0.58–2.60)	0.59

*Adjusted for age, gender, cigarette smoking, alcohol use, family history, histologic types, stage group, T stage and N stage in multivariate Cox model.

better RFS and DFS (HR = 4.37; 95% CI, 1.37−14.00; P = 0.01for RFS and HR = 2.70; 95% CI, 1.16−6.30; P = 0.02 for DFS) and a similar OS and MFS (P = 0.10 and P = 0.31, respectively). There was no significant difference in the OS, MFS, RFS, and DFS between the patients receiving neoadjuvant chemotherapy with DF plus IMRT and the IMRT alone arm. Comparingneoadjuvant chemotherapy with miscellaneouschemotherapy regimens,neoadjuvant chemotherapy with DF regimen contributed to a similarsurvival benefit. However, a significant OS improvement was found favoring the addition of the neoadjuvant chemotherapy with DF regimen to concurrent chemoradiotherapy over concurrent chemoradiotherapy alone (HR = 13.37; 95% CI, 1.24−144.29; P = 0.03).

To identify which factors affected patient outcome, we performed univariate and multivariate analyses to evaluate the prognostic value of age, gender, cigarette smoking, alcohol use, family history, WHO histology, stage group, T stage, and N stage (**Table 5**). The results showed that compared to patients with stage II NPC, patients with stages IV and III were at an approximately 11- and 4-fold increased risk of death (HR = 11.05; 95% CI, 1.63−74.92; P = 0.01 for stage IV and HR = 4.54; 95% CI, 0.76−27.30; P = 0.09 for stage III; **Fig. 2**), respectively. Alcohol consumption was a negative prognostic factor for OS, with P values <0.001 based on univariate analysis (**Fig. 3**) and P = 0.06 based on multivariate analysis, respectively. Advanced N stage was associated with the occurrence of distant metastasis and MFS (HR = 2.79; 95% CI, 1.30−5.97; P = 0.02; **Fig. 4**). There was no significant association between the remaining predictors (age, gender, smoking status, family history of cancer, histology, and T stage) and the survival, recurrence, or metastasis rates based on univariate and multivariate analyses.

Discussion

IMRT has yielded remarkable advances compared to conventional radiotherapy in target conformity, increased radiation dose in the target volume, and sparing of surrounding normal organs at risk [14,15]. The utilization of IMRT is particularly valuable in patients with NPC because the nasopharynx area is complex and surrounded by a number of critical normal structures, including the brain, brain stem, spinal cord, optic pathway, middle and inner ear, parotid glands, and temporomadibular joint, and IMRT yields a concave dose distribution to avoid organs at risk and thus permit the irradiation of patients with complex-shaped tumors in locations which are difficult to access. The clinical applications of IMRT in patients with NPC demonstrated that this radiation technique could improve tumor control [5,7], reduce locoregional and regional failure, provide better survival and quality of life [16], and significantly enhance the therapeutic ratio. In addition, IMRT could maximize protection of normal structures and reduce and delay the onset of acute toxicity [17]. Consequently, IMRT is widely used in treating NPC and has been adopted as the standard of care in many centers that treat patients with NPC.

Conventional radiotherapy combined with chemotherapy was formerly the standard treatment modality for locoregionally advanced NPC [18,19]. The Intergroup-0099 Study first revealed that the addition of cisplatin-based concurrent and adjuvant chemotherapy to conventional radiotherapy could contribute to improvement of event-free survival and OS [9]. Subsequent randomized trials confirmed the survival benefit provided by adding chemotherapy to conventional radiotherapy [20,21]. In clinical practice, cisplatin-based chemotherapy in concurrence with conventional radiotherapy has also proved its superiority to conventional radiotherapy alone for the treatment of locoregion-

Table 4. Survival by treatment arm with DF regimen as neoadjuvant chemotherapy.

	Overall survival		Distant metastasis-free survival		Relapse-free survival		Disease-free survival	
	HR (95%CI)*	P*	HR (95%CI)*	P*	HR (95%CI)*	P*	HR (95%CI)*	P*
Neoadjuvant with DF-concurrent chemoradiotherapy vs IMRT alone	6.72 (0.70–64.14)	0.10	1.78 (0.58–5.45)	0.31	4.37 (1.37–14.00)	0.01	2.70 (1.16–6.30)	0.02
Neoadjuvent chemoradiotherapy with DF vs IMRT alone	0.27 (0.06–1.31)	0.10	1.98 (0.67–5.84)	0.21	1.63 (0.62–4.28)	0.32	1.58 (0.76–3.29)	0.22
Neoadjuvant with DF-concurrent chemoradiotherapy vs Concurrent chemoradiotherapy	13.37 (1.24–144.29)	0.03	1.92 (0.31– 11.77)	0.48	2.32 (0.60–8.99)	0.22	1.45 (0.56–3.70)	0.44

*Adjusted for age, gender, cigarette smoking, alcohol use, family history, histologic types, stage group, T stage and N stage in multivariate Cox model.

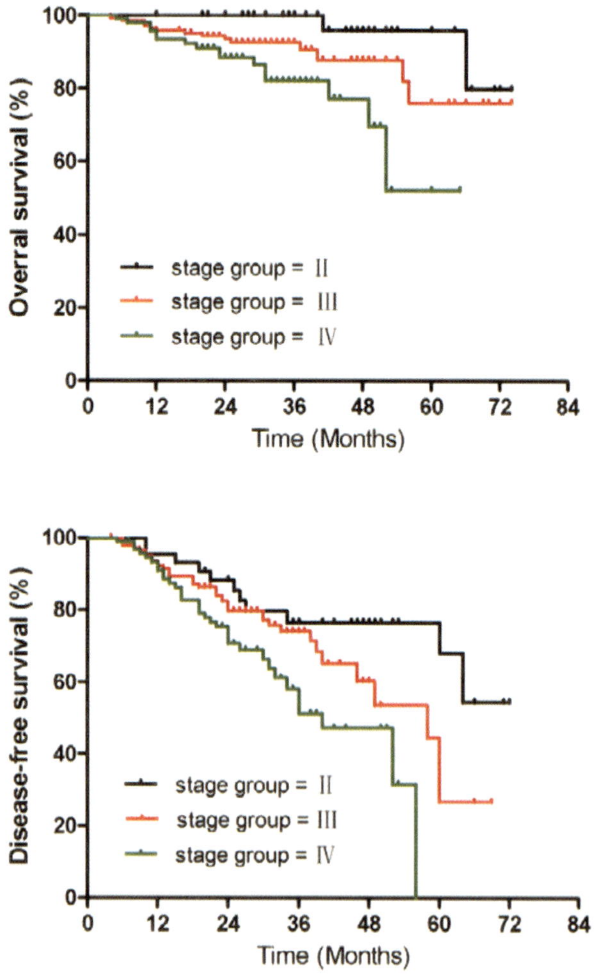

Figure 2. Kaplan-Meier estimates of Overral survival and disease-free survival for patients receiving with stage group being II versus III versus IV.

ally advanced NPC [21]. However, the contribution of adding chemotherapy to radiation has not been confirmed when conventional radiotherapy is replaced with IMRT [10,11]. No significant survival benefit with chemotherapy over IMRT alone

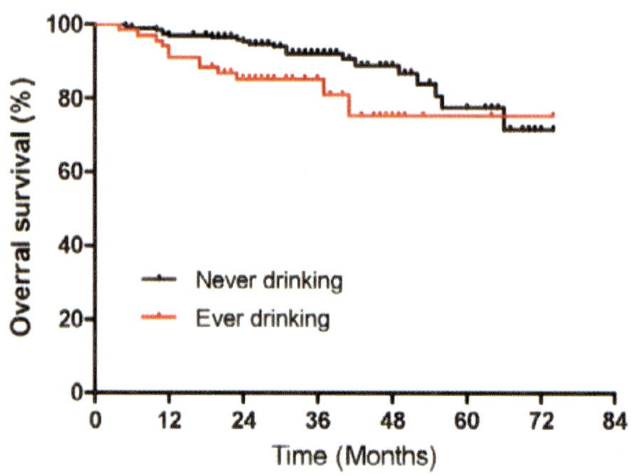

Figure 3. Kaplan-Meier estimates of overall survival of patients with alcohol drinking versus without alcohol drinking.

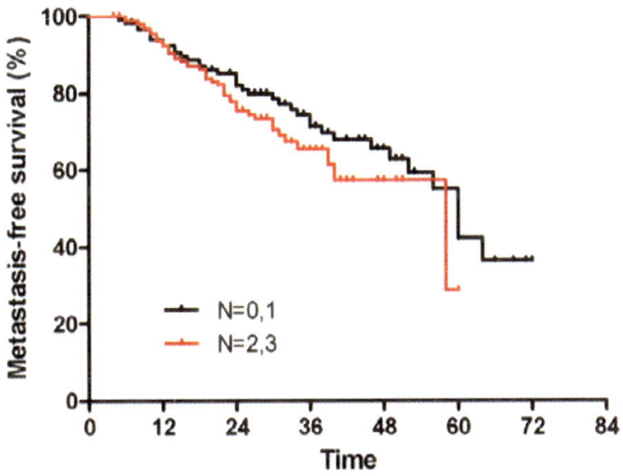

Figure 4. Kaplan-Meier estimates of metastasis-free survival for patients with N stage being 1 or 2 versus 3 or 4.

was demonstrated primarily by achieving a higher local tumor control rate or less metastasis or both in locoregionally advanced NPC patients.

In the current retrospective cohort study, we first reported significant improvement of RFS and borderline significantly elevated DFS favoring the IMRT plus chemotherapy arm for patients with locoregionally advanced NPC in the Cox model adjusted for the prognostic factors. Further analyses demonstrated that the survival improvement of RFS and DFS were indeed from the addition of concurrent chemotherapy and neoadjuvant-concurrent chemotherapy, not from the addition of neoadjuvant chemotherapy. Our findings confirmed the survival benefit with concurrent chemotherapy-based treatment over radiation alone when conventional radiotherapy is replaced with IMRT, although it is inconsistent with the previous comparison between IMRT with and without chemotherapy. There are only three retrospective studies comparing the survival of IMRT alone and IMRT combined with chemotherapy [10,11,12]. A study conducted in China and Singapore observed 107 patients with stage IIb NPC to compare IMRT alone and IMRT combined with various strategies of chemotherapy, including neoadjuvant, concurrent and adjuvant chemotherapy, and found no significant difference in disease control and survival rates in patients treated with or without chemotherapy of any schedule [11]. Another retrospective study assigned 370 patients with locoregionally advanced NPC to compare IMRT with or without concurrent chemotherapy and revealed no significant improvement in local control and rates of OS, MFS, and DFS [10]. However, in the current study adjuvant chemotherapy and neoadjuvant chemotherapy were applied in patients at the discretion of radiation oncologists, which could confound the contribution of the concurrent chemotherapy to IMRT [10]. Su et al.[12] also demonstrated that patients with locoregionally advanced NPC had similar OS, MFS, and DFS when treated by IMRT-based modalities, including IMRT alone, chemoradiotherapy, adjuvant chemoradiotherapy, concurrent chemoradiotherapy, neoadjuvant-concurrent chemoradiotherapy, and concurrent-adjuvant chemoradiotherapy. Nevertheless, in their studies, patients received treatment based on the selection criteria that patients with poor conditions would be treated by IMRT alone and patients with more advanced N stage would receive more chemotherapy. Therefore, we presume that the reason for failing to find a significant improvement in survival with chemotherapy over IMRT alone in previous studies could probably be attributed to the early cancer stage of patients, confounding of other treatment regimens, and treatment selection to patients, thus the addition of chemotherapy to IMRT might contribute to a significant improvement in survival in a well-designed study. Our presumption, which is partly supported by the previous study conducted by Su et al. [12] in which patients with a more advanced N stage because of receiving additional chemotherapy, had similar treatment outcomes to patients with a less advanced N stage who received less chemotherapy. Nevertheless, to validate our presumption regarding the efficacy of chemotherapy and the best strategy for combined treatment, larger, well-designed studies with balanced prognostic factors should be conducted in other patient populations with locoregionally advanced NPC.

Indeed, our findings are biologically plausible. First, cisplatin can enhance radiation-induced cell killing and sensitize the radiation [22,23,24], and it has been verified that radiosensitivity

Table 5. Effect of prognostic factors on survival in multivariable analyses.

	Overall survival		Distant metastasis-free survival		Relapse-free survival		Disease-free survival	
	HR (95%CI)*	P*	HR (95%CI)*	P*	HR (95%CI)*	P*	HR (95%CI)*	P*
Gender, Female vs Male	0.94 (0.38–2.34)	0.89	1.24 (0.56–2.76)	0.60	0.90 (0.44–1.80)	0.76	0.95 (0.55–1.65)	0.87
Age, >50y vs ≤50 y	0.88 (0.42– 1.85)	0.74	1.30 (0.69–2.47)	0.42	0.87 (0.48–1.57)	0.64	1.11 (0.70–1.75)	0.66
Smoking status, Ever vs Never	1.05 (0.44–2.49)	0.91	0.93 (0.45–1.93)	0.84	1.32 (0.69–2.55)	0.41	1.08 (0.64–1.81)	0.77
Drinking status, Ever vs Never	2.17 (0.96–4.91)	0.06	1.74 (0.85-3.56)	0.13	0.88 (0.43–1.80)	0.73	1.09 (0.63–1.88)	0.75
Stage group, III vs II	4.54 (0.76–27.30)	0.09	1.62 (0.29–9.05)	0.58	1.06 (0.33–3.40)	0.92	1.05 (0.40–2.73)	0.92
Stage group, IV vs II	11.05 (1.63–74.92)	0.01	2.91 (0.48–17.82)	0.25	1.44 (0.40–5.21)	0.58	1.69 (0.59–4.83)	0.33
Family history, Yes vs No	1.48 (0.64–3.45)	0.36	0.95 (0.43–2.12)	0.91	0.92 (0.43–2.00)	0.84	0.92 (0.51–1.66)	0.77
Histology, 2 vs 1	1.93 (0.41–9.02)	0.40	1.33 (0.38–4.66)	0.66	0.75 (0.33–1.73)	0.50	0.87 (0.42–1.79)	0.70
Histology, 3vs 1	1.57 (0.33–7.53)	0.57	1.45 (0.40–5.29)	0.57	0.58 (0.24–1.44)	0.24	0.74 (0.35–1.60)	0.45
T stage, T3–T4 vs T1–T2	0.71 (0.25–2.02)	0.52	1.82 (0.74–4.49)	0.20	1.44 (0.57–3.64)	0.44	1.64 (0.83–3.24)	0.16
N stage, N2–N3 vs N0–N1	0.83 (0.34–2.00)	0.67	2.79 (1.30–5.97)	0.01	0.85 (0.44–1.67)	0.64	0.16	

*Adjusted for age, gender, cigarette smoking, alcohol use, family history, histologic types, stage group, T stage and N stage in multivariate Cox mode.

in head and neck cancer can be enhanced by chemotherapy *in vivo* [25], which is why concurrent, but not neoadjuvant chemotherapy, can contribute to the improvement in survival. Second, NPC is not only radiosensitive, but also chemosensitive [6,9]. Chemotherapy should be able to improve survival through decreasing the tumor burden, eradicating distant micrometastases, and reducing disease failure. Finally, chemotherapy could reduce hypoxia in the primary site and metastatic lymph nodes by shrinking the tumor size, which could increase radiosensitivity and increase disease control [26,27].

We also first explored the prognostic value of some carcinogenic factors, including cigarette smoking, alcohol use, and family history of cancer, and showed that alcohol use was a prognostic factor predictive of OS. The underlying biological mechanism of how alcohol use influences the association of survival with the treatment strategy in NPC patients is not clear. We speculate that alcohol consumption, as a risk factor for the etiology of NPC [28], has been reported to influence the histologic distribution of NPC [29,30,31] and thereby impact the prognosis. Another reason for alcohol use associated with poor prognosis might be that regular alcohol use will lead to poor liver function and elevated LDH, which are negative prognosticators for OS, DFS, and DMFS for NPC patients [32]. Nevertheless, to confirm the prognostic value for patients with locoregionally advanced NPC, larger well-designed clinical trials should be conducted in different populations and involve more risk factors to adjust the association.

As a retrospective analysis, the current study had limitations. First, because patients were only included in our study when the selection criteria were met, a selection bias might have occurred. However, such a selection bias most likely has a minimal impact on our result because only a small proportion of patients were excluded and there was still a large study population for the present analysis. Second, the current study was a non-randomized cohort comparison, which might have resulted in selection bias and imbalance between the two groups. Nevertheless, in this study the groups were shown to be well-matched for prognostic factors, except N stage. By contrast, the combined treatment group had more patients with advanced disease, and might have resulted in a survival benefit gained from the combined modality of treatment underestimated by the log-rank test. However, after adjustment with prognostic factors, the potential impact from confounding factors on the hazard ratio might be minimized. Another possible source of bias in the current study might result from the insufficient follow-up and small number of patients studied, which may result in an inadequate number of events needed for analysis and limit the assessment of long-term results of combined modality therapy. Therefore, larger studies with an extended follow-up are needed to confirm these findings in patients with NPC.

In summary, our study provides evidence that IMRT combined with concurrent chemotherapy or neoadjuvant-concurrent chemoradiotherapy resulted in an improvement in DFS or RFS for patients with locoregionally advantage NPC compared to IMRT alone. In addition, our study was the first to determine the prognostic value of some carcinogenic factors, such as smoking status, alcohol use, and family history of cancer, and showed that alcohol consumption was a prognostic factor for OS. This study could be of value to guide effective individualized treatmen for patients with NPC and may be helpful to guide effective individualized treatment. In an attempt to further reveal the contribution of chemotherapy to IMRT and evaluate the long-term results of combined modality therapy, we will recruit more patients to our program and lengthen the follow-up in the future.

Author Contributions

Conceived and designed the experiments: XJ. Performed the experiments: DH CX XF Y. Zhou. Analyzed the data: XJ CX. Contributed reagents/materials/analysis tools: XF Y. Zheng. Wrote the paper: XJ.

References

1. Chinese Center for Disease Control and Prevention (2010) 2008 cause of death database of Chinese National Disease Surveillance System. 57–58.
2. National Cancer Institute (2008) Nasopharynx. Seer program: 92–95.
3. Ng WT, Lee MC, Hung WM, Choi CW, Lee KC, et al. (2011) Clinical outcomes and patterns of failure after intensity-modulated radiotherapy for nasopharyngeal carcinoma. Int J Radiat Oncol Biol Phys 79: 420–428.
4. Lu H, Yao M (2008) The current status of intensity-modulated radiation therapy in the treatment of nasopharyngeal carcinoma. Cancer Treat Rev 34: 27–36.
5. Kam MK, Teo PM, Chau RM, Cheung KY, Choi PH, et al. (2004) Treatment of nasopharyngeal carcinoma with intensity-modulated radiotherapy: the Hong Kong experience. Int J Radiat Oncol Biol Phys 60: 1440–1450.
6. Tham IW, Hee SW, Yeo RM, Salleh PB, Lee J, et al. (2009) Treatment of nasopharyngeal carcinoma using intensity-modulated radiotherapy-the national cancer centre singapore experience. Int J Radiat Oncol Biol Phys 75: 1481–1486.
7. Lai SZ, Li WF, Chen L, Luo W, Chen YY, et al. (2011) How does intensity-modulated radiotherapy versus conventional two-dimensional radiotherapy influence the treatment results in nasopharyngeal carcinoma patients? Int J Radiat Oncol Biol Phys 80: 661–668.
8. Lee AW, Lin JC, Ng WT (2012) Current management of nasopharyngeal cancer. Semin Radiat Oncol 22: 233–244.
9. Al-Sarraf M, LeBlanc M, Giri PG, Fu KK, Cooper J, et al. (1998) Chemoradiotherapy versus radiotherapy in patients with advanced nasopharyngeal cancer: phase III randomized Intergroup study 0099. J Clin Oncol 16: 1310–1317.
10. Lin S, Lu JJ, Han L, Chen Q, Pan J (2010) Sequential chemotherapy and intensity-modulated radiation therapy in the management of locoregionally advanced nasopharyngeal carcinoma: experience of 370 consecutive cases. BMC Cancer 10: 39.
11. Tham IW, Lin S, Pan J, Han L, Lu JJ, et al. (2010) Intensity-modulated radiation therapy without concurrent chemotherapy for stage IIb nasopharyngeal cancer. Am J Clin Oncol 33: 294–299.
12. Su SF, Han F, Zhao C, Huang Y, Chen CY, et al. (2011) Treatment outcomes for different subgroups of nasopharyngeal carcinoma patients treated with intensity-modulated radiation therapy. Chin J Cancer 30: 565–573.
13. Ferlito A (1993) The World Health Organization's revised classification of tumours of the larynx, hypopharynx, and trachea. Ann Otol Rhinol Laryngol 102: 666–669.
14. Miles EA, Clark CH, Urbano MT, Bidmead M, Dearnaley DP, et al. (2005) The impact of introducing intensity modulated radiotherapy into routine clinical practice. Radiother Oncol 77: 241–246.
15. Kam MK, Leung SF, Zee B, Chau RM, Suen JJ, et al. (2007) Prospective randomized study of intensity-modulated radiotherapy on salivary gland function in early-stage nasopharyngeal carcinoma patients. J Clin Oncol 25: 4873–4879.
16. Fang FM, Chien CY, Tsai WL, Chen HC, Hsu HC, et al. (2008) Quality of life and survival outcome for patients with nasopharyngeal carcinoma receiving three-dimensional conformal radiotherapy vs. intensity-modulated radiotherapy-a longitudinal study. Int J Radiat Oncol Biol Phys 72: 356–364.
17. Laskar S, Bahl G, Muckaden M, Pai SK, Gupta T, et al. (2008) Nasopharyngeal carcinoma in children: comparison of conventional and intensity-modulated radiotherapy. Int J Radiat Oncol Biol Phys 72: 728–736.
18. Langendijk JA, Leemans CR, Buter J, Berkhof J, Slotman BJ (2004) The additional value of chemotherapy to radiotherapy in locally advanced nasopharyngeal carcinoma: a meta-analysis of the published literature. J Clin Oncol 22: 4604–4612.
19. Lee N, Xia P, Quivey JM, Sultanem K, Poon I, et al. (2002) Intensity-modulated radiotherapy in the treatment of nasopharyngeal carcinoma: an update of the UCSF experience. Int J Radiat Oncol Biol Phys 53: 12–22.
20. Lee AW, Tung SY, Chua DT, Ngan RK, Chappell R, et al. (2010) Randomized trial of radiotherapy plus concurrent-adjuvant chemotherapy vs radiotherapy alone for regionally advanced nasopharyngeal carcinoma. J Natl Cancer Inst 102: 1188–1198.
21. Wee J, Tan EH, Tai BC, Wong HB, Leong SS, et al. (2005) Randomized trial of radiotherapy versus concurrent chemoradiotherapy followed by adjuvant chemotherapy in patients with American Joint Committee on Cancer/International Union against cancer stage III and IV nasopharyngeal cancer of the endemic variety. J Clin Oncol 23: 6730–6738.
22. Rosier JF, Beauduin M, Bruniaux M, de Bast M, de Coster B, et al. (1999) The effect of 2′-2′ difluorodeoxycytidine (dFdC, gemcitabine) on radiation-induced

cell lethality in two human head and neck squamous carcinoma cell lines differing in intrinsic radiosensitivity. Int J Radiat Biol 75: 245–251.
23. Teicher BA, Ara G, Chen YN, Recht A, Coleman CN (1998) Interaction of tomudex with radiation in vitro and in vivo. Int J Oncol 13: 437–442.
24. Begg AC, van der Kolk PJ, Dewit L, Bartelink H (1986) Radiosensitization by cisplatin of RIF1 tumour cells in vitro. Int J Radiat Biol Relat Stud Phys Chem Med 50: 871–884.
25. Fields MT, Eisbruch A, Normolle D, Orfali A, Davis MA, et al. (2000) Radiosensitization produced in vivo by once- vs. twice-weekly 2′2′-difluoro-2′-deoxycytidine (gemcitabine). Int J Radiat Oncol Biol Phys 47: 785–791.
26. Yu MC, Mo CC, Chong WX, Yeh FS, Henderson BE (1988) Preserved foods and nasopharyngeal carcinoma: a case-control study in Guangxi, China. Cancer Res 48: 1954–1959.
27. Nordsmark M, Overgaard M, Overgaard J (1996) Pretreatment oxygenation predicts radiation response in advanced squamous cell carcinoma of the head and neck. Radiother Oncol 41: 31–39.
28. Ji X, Zhang W, Xie C, Wang B, Zhang G, et al. (2011) Nasopharyngeal carcinoma risk by histologic type in central China: impact of smoking, alcohol and family history. Int J Cancer 129: 724–732.
29. Vaughan TL, Shapiro JA, Burt RD, Swanson GM, Berwick M, et al. (1996) Nasopharyngeal cancer in a low-risk population: defining risk factors by histological type. Cancer Epidemiol Biomarkers Prev 5: 587–593.
30. Zhu K, Levine RS, Brann EA, Gnepp DR, Baum MK (1995) A population-based case-control study of the relationship between cigarette smoking and nasopharyngeal cancer (United States). Cancer Causes Control 6: 507–512.
31. Levine PH, Pocinki AG, Madigan P, Bale S (1992) Familial nasopharyngeal carcinoma in patients who are not Chinese. Cancer 70: 1024–1029.
32. Zhou GQ, Tang LL, Mao YP, Chen L, Li WF, et al. (2012) Baseline serum lactate dehydrogenase levels for patients treated with intensity-modulated radiotherapy for nasopharyngeal carcinoma: a predictor of poor prognosis and subsequent liver metastasis. Int J Radiat Oncol Biol Phys 82: e359–365.

Feasibility of Intensity-Modulated and Image-Guided Radiotherapy for Functional Organ Preservation in Locally Advanced Laryngeal Cancer

Nam P. Nguyen[1]*, Alexander Chi[2], Michael Betz[3], Fabio Almeida[4], Paul Vos[5], Rick Davis[1], Benjamin Slane[1], Misty Ceizyk[1], Dave Abraham[1], Lexie Smith-Raymond[1], Michelle Stevie[1], Siyoung Jang[6], Steven Gelumbauskas[1], Vincent Vinh-Hung[3]

1 Department of Radiation Oncology, University of Arizona, Tucson, Arizona, United States of America, **2** Department of Radiation Oncology, University of West Virginia, Morgantown, West Virginia, United States of America, **3** Department of Radiation Oncology, University Hospitals of Geneva, Geneva, Switzerland, **4** Southwest PET/CT Institute, Tucson, Arizona, United States of America, **5** Department of Biostatistics, East Carolina University, Greenville, North Carolina, United States of America, **6** Department of Radiation Oncology, University of Pittsburgh, Pittsburgh, Pennsylvania, United States of America

Abstract

Purpose: The study aims to assess the feasibility of intensity-modulated and image-guided radiotherapy (IMRT, and IGRT, respectively) for functional preservation in locally advanced laryngeal cancer. A retrospective review of 27 patients undergoing concurrent chemoradiation for locally advanced laryngeal cancers (8 IMRT, 19 IGRT) was undertaken. In addition to regular clinical examinations, all patients had PET imaging at 4 months and 10 months after radiotherapy, then yearly. Loco-regional control, speech quality and feeding-tube dependency were assessed during follow-up visits.

Results: At a median follow-up of 20 months (range 6–57 months), four out of 27 patients (14.8%) developed local recurrence and underwent salvage total laryngectomy. One patient developed distant metastases following salvage surgery. Among the 23 patients who conserved their larynx with no sign of recurrence at last follow-up, 22 (95%) reported normal or near normal voice quality, allowing them to communicate adequately. Four patients (14.8%) had long-term tube feeding-dependency because of severe dysphagia (2 patients) and chronic aspiration (2 patients, with ensuing death from aspiration pneumonia in one patient).

Conclusions and Clinical Relevance: Functional laryngeal preservation is feasible with IMRT and IGRT for locally advanced laryngeal cancer. However, dysphagia and aspiration remain serious complications, due most likely to high radiation dose delivery to the pharyngeal musculatures.

Editor: Chulso Moon, Johns Hopkins University, United States of America

Funding: The authors have no support or funding to report.

Competing Interests: The authors have declared that no competing interests exist.

* E-mail: namphong.nguyen@yahoo.com

Introduction

Locally advanced laryngeal cancer was traditionally treated with total laryngectomy followed by postoperative radiotherapy given the high risk of loco-regional recurrences [1]. However, the presence of a stoma following total laryngectomy is often associated with chronic airway irritation and coughing, sleep difficulties and poor cosmesis [2–4]. Additionally, resection of large tumors and neck dissection may result in substantial chronic postoperative pain [5,6]. In an attempt to improve patient quality of life, the Veterans Administration Laryngeal Study (VALG) first investigated the feasibility of an organ-preservation approach, achieving a 64% rate of larynx preservation with induction chemotherapy followed in responders by definitive radiotherapy, while maintaining a survival rate comparable to that seen in laryngectomized patients [7]. The Radiation Therapy Oncology Group (RTOG) 91–11 Study subsequently demonstrated an even higher rate of laryngeal preservation with concurrent chemoradiation rather than induction chemotherapy followed by radiotherapy alone at least for patients with T3 disease [8]. While the exclusion of patients with T4 lesions from RTOG 91-11 left it unclear whether laryngeal preservation with concurrent chemoradiation was feasible for all patients with locally advanced laryngeal cancer for functional laryngeal preservation, later studies confirmed the feasibility of such an approach for T4 disease as well [9,10]. Nevertherless, persistent concerns remain about the functional consequences of delivering curative radiation doses to the larynx and pharyngeal musculature, with the risk of ensuing chronic edema and fibrosis, leading to voice alteration and chronic dysphagia and potentially defeating the purpose of laryngeal preservation [11,12]. The traditional treatment for locally advanced laryngeal cancer has been two lateral fields matched with an anterior supraclavicular field. This three-dimensional (3-D) radiotherapy technique did not allow sparing of normal tissues which received the same tumor dose. Xerostosmia secondary to radiation related destruction of the parotid glands, osteoradionecrosis secondary to high mandibular dose, and hearing loss from cochlea damage, are common sequellaes of 3-D conformal radiotherapy (3-DRT) leading to poor patient quality of life [13–15]. Recently, intensity-modulated (IMRT) and image-guided radiotherapy (IGRT) have been introduced in the treatment of head and neck cancer to decrease treatment toxicity by improving normal tissue sparing [16–18]. Rapid dose fall off away from the target allows significant sparing of the normal organs at risk for complications and potentially improves patient quality of life with these new radiotherapy techniques. The simultaneously integrated boost (SIB) technique of IMRT and IGRT also allows selective dose assignment to different target levels with the tumor receiving the highest dose and subclinical disease treated to a lower dose, thus allows more control of the radiation dose received by the normal organs adjacent to the target. Preliminary dosimetric studies of laryngeal cancer also demonstrated improved dose conformality of IMRT compared to 3-DRT, potentially leading to improved tumor control if the tumor dose can also be increased with the integrated boost technique [19–20]. However, the advantages of IMRT and IGRT may also be negated because of possible marginal miss if the tumor volume is not clearly defined [21]. Thus, accurate pre-treatment imaging such as positron emission tomography (PET) scans is almost mandatory for laryngeal cancer because of its superior tumor delineation compared to CT scans [22]. Following radiotherapy, high dose to the larynx for tumor control often lead to severe laryngeal edema which may be interpreted as tumor recurrence. The ability of PET scans and PET-CT to distinguish tumor recurrence from laryngeal edema and fibrosis also make it an ideal tool for patient follow-up to avoid unnecessary laryngeal biopsies which may cause chondronecrosis [23–24]. We investigate in this retrospective study the feasibility and potential benefit of IMRT and IGRT for anatomic and functional organ preservation in combination when FDG-PET has been used to guide target volume felineation, and post treatment surveillance. Table 1 illustrates the potential benefits and possible pitfalls of IMRT and IGRT compared to 3-D conformal radiotherapy.

Materials and Methods

The medical records of 27 patients undergoing curative radiotherapy for locally advanced laryngeal cancers at the University of Arizona Radiation Oncology Department were retrospectively reviewed following institutional review board (IRB) approval. The University of Arizona IRB waived the patient consent requirement because of the retrospective nature of the study limited to chart reviews. The patient information was de-identified to protect patient confidentiality. Eight patients were treated with the whole field (WF) IMRT technique on the Elekta linear accelerator (6 MV photons) with 7 to 9 radiation beams from February 2007 to December 2008. Following installation of the helical Tomotherapy unit in December 2008, 19 patients were treated with the WF IGRT technique. Prior to treatment, each patient was simulated in the supine position with a head and neck aquaplast mask for treatment immobilization. A computed tomography (CT) scan with and without intravenous (IV) contrast for treatment planning was performed in the treatment position. The head and neck areas from the vertex to the mid thorax were scanned with a slice thickness of 3 mm CT scan with IV contrast was employed to outline the tumor and grossly enlarged cervical lymph node for target volume delineation. Radiotherapy planning was performed on the CT scan without contrast to avoid possible interference of contrast density on radiotherapy isodose distributions. Diagnostic positron emission tomography (PET)-CT scan planning for tumor imaging was also incorporated with CT planning. A 0.5 cm bolus material was placed on any area of the skin involved by the tumor and on any palpable cervical lymph nodes. Patients treated on Tomotherapy also had 0.5 cm bolus over the thyroid cartilage to prevent possible underdosing of the larynx. Normal organs at risk for complication were outlined for treatment planning (spinal cord, brain stem, bilateral cochlea, mandible, parotid glands, bilateral eyes, and oral cavity). Radiation therapy dose was similar for patients in both groups using the integrated boost technique to decrease treatment toxicity. The tumor and grossly enlarged lymph nodes (CTV1) on CT scan with a margin (PTV1) were treated to 70 Gy in 35 fractions (2 Gy/fraction). The margins were 5 mm to 1 cm all around CTV1 depending on anatomic location. The areas at high risk-PTV2 (at least 1 cm around gross tumor and pathologic cervical lymph nodes) and low risk -PTV3 (subclinical regional lymph nodes with 5 mm margins) for tumor spread were treated respectively to 63 Gy and 56 Gy in 35 fractions, respectively. Minimal target coverage was 95% of the prescribed dose for all targets with at least 99% of the prescribed dose delivered to gross tumor and involved cervical lymph nodes. The lymph nodes in the ipsilateral neck including the retropharyngeal lymph nodes were treated to the base of skull if there was any cervical lymph node enlargement (or PET-positive lymph nodes). Contralateral uninvolved lymph nodes were treated prophylactically with the C1 vertebrae as the superior border. In cases of bilateral cervical lymph node involvement, the bilateral neck was treated to the base of skull to avoid any marginal miss. Mean dose to the parotid was kept below 2600 cGy if there was no ipsilateral cervical lymph node enlargement. Dose constraints for other normal organs at risk (OAR) for complications were: spinal cord (45 Gy), brain stem (50 Gy), optic chiasm (45 Gy), mandible (70 Gy to less than 30% of the mandible).

Concurrent chemoradiation was recommended for all patients. The type of chemotherapy regimen was left at the discretion of the medical oncologist depending on patient functional status and co-

Table 1. Potential advantages and pitfalls of intensity-modulated radiotherapy (IMRT) and image-guided radiotherapy (IGRT) compared to 3-dimentional conformal radiotherapy (3-D CRT).

	IMRT, IGRT	3-D CRT
Advantages:	Sparing of normal organs because of rapid dose fall	No sparing
	Tumor dose escalation possible because of different dose levels within the target volume	No dose escalation
	Visualization of tumor shrinkage feasible for IGRT allowing re-planning during radiotherapy	No visualization
Pitfalls:	Marginal miss if tumor not properly contoured leading to local recurrences.	Unlikely

morbidities. Prophylactic percutaneous gastrostomy (PEG) feeding-tube placement was also recommended for all patients prior to treatment given expected weight loss secondary to acute toxicity including mucositis and dysgueusia. Weekly complete blood count (CBC) and blood chemistry work-ups were performed during chemoradiation. Treatment breaks and weight loss were recorded during chemoradiation. Acute and long-term toxicities were graded according to Radiotherapy Oncology Group (RTOG) group criteria severity scale (http://ctep.cancer.gov).

After treatment, all patients had follow-up visits at one month, then, every three months thereafter. Clinical and direct laryngoscopic examination were performed at each follow up visit. PET scan, or PET-CT imaging was performed at four months and ten months, then yearly after treatment. All PET-positive areas were biopsied to detect recurrence and total salvage laryngectomy (TL) with bilateral neck dissection (BND) carried out, if biopsy was positive. Voice quality (ability to conduct a normal conversation over the phone or ability to communicate without difficulty at work) was assessed at each follow-up visit. Patient ability to resume normal oral feeding and feeding-tube dependency was also evaluated at each visit.

Survival analysis was analyzed using Kaplan-Meier estimation.

Results

We identified 27 patients with loco-regionally advanced invasive squamous cell carcinoma of the larynx treated at the University of Arizona Radiation Oncology department from 2007 to 2010. Median age at diagnosis was 63 years-old (range: 52–84 years-old). There were 25 males and 2 females. Seventeen patients had stage III, nine had stage IVA, and one had stage IVB disease. Twenty six patients received concurrent chemoradiation, while one patient who declined concurrent chemotherapy received radiotherapy alone. Table 2 summarizes patient characteristics. Table 3 summarizes radiation dose to the larynx and other head and neck organs. Figure 1 illustrates the dose-volume histogram of a patient with a T3N0M0 supraglottic laryngeal cancer treated with IGRT demonstating the feasibility of this new technique of radiotherapy to spare the normal head and neck organs from excessive radiation.

Chemotherapy consisted of cisplatin (P) 30 mg/m2 intravenously (IV) weekly in 12 patients and cisplatin 100 mg IV on day 1, 22, and 43 of radiotherapy in 11 patient. Four patients had induction chemotherapy with taxotere (T) 75 mg/m2 IV, cisplatin 100 mg/m2 IV followed by 5-fluorouracil (F) 1000 mg/m2 for four days, repeated every three weeks for two cycles, followed during radiotherapy by carboplatin IV weekly with an area under the curve of 1.5.

At a median follow-up of 20 months (6–57 months), four patients developed local recurrence and underwent salvage TL and BND. One of the four patients was the patient who declined chemotherapy, and who in addition was poorly compliant during radiotherapy despite repeated staff warnings with a two-week treatment break. Two of the three patients with local recurrence developed distant metastases following salvage TL. The third is still free of disease 30 months after treatment. The fourth just completes his surgery for salvage. All recurrences were detected on PET imaging, and proven by biopsy. In two patients with a subglottic recurrence and a second base of tongue primary, respectively, endoscopic examination was normal, with PET imaging leading to confirmation of recurrence. Another patient developed localized non-small cell lung cancer which was discovered on PET imaging and treated with stereotactic body radiotherapy. Three patients died at 11 to 14 months after treatment. The causes of death was stroke, second lung primary, and aspiration pneumonia, each respectively in one patient. The 2-year and 3-year survival is estimated to be 80% and 62.3% respectively for the whole group.

Twenty patients (74%) developed grade 3–4 toxicity during treatment, mainly mucositis (16 patients) and hematologic toxicity (4 patients). Two patient developed aspiration pneumonia, requiring brief intubation in one patient during the sixth week of radiotherapy. While all patients completed radiotherapy, fifteen (55%) had treatment breaks ranging from one to 29 days (median: 7 days) because of grade 3–4 toxicity. Median weight loss, despite prophylactic gastrostomy tube placement, was 9 pounds (0–25 pounds). Chemotherapy was not administered, or not administered according to the protocol in nine patients (33%). In addition to the patient declining chemotherapy, seven had schedule modifications due to side-effects during treatment. The patient receiving induction TPF developed bowel obstruction after two cycles, requiring discontinuation of the third cycle. The same patient subsequently developed pancytopenia (white blood cells: 1300, hemoglobin: 8 g/dl, platelets: 83,000) during chemoradiation requiring discontinuation of carboplatin after week 6 of radiotherapy.

Among patients for whom a standard cisplatin regimen of 100 mg/m2 on days 1, 22, and 43 was planned, one patient required a dose reduction to 80 mg/m2 for the first two cycles, and did not receive the third cycle because of aspiration pneumonia. Another patient also did not receive the third cycle because of neutropenia (white blood cells: 1,000). Another patient had cisplatin dose reduction to 75 mg/m2 after the second cycle because of renal dysfunction (Cr: 1.5, BUN: 36). Among patients receiving weekly cisplatin, two patients had protocol violations: cisplatin was delayed at week 6 in one patient because of neutropenia (white blood cells: 1,500) and discontinued after week 5 in another because of aspiration pneumonia. However, all patients completed the intended dose of radiotherapy despite treatment break.

At last follow-up, 22 of the 23 patients without recurrence reported normal or near normal voice quality, allowing them to communicate effectively at work or over the phone. The remaining patient reported persistent hoarseness and voice weakness, and had still been unable to work full time 12 months after treatment. His follow-up visits confirmed chronic laryngeal edema on endoscopic, with no sign of recurrence on PET imaging at 4 and 10 months after treatment. Among the entire group of 25 patients, four (16%) were still dependent on tube feedings at 6 to 16 months after treatment, due to severe dysphagia in 2 patients, and chronic aspiration in the other 2. Chemotherapy regimens in these four patients were weekly cisplatin in 2 patients, three-weekly cisplatin in one patient, and induction TPF followed by concurrent weekly carboplatin in one patient. The patient who received TPF/carboplatin finally died of aspiration pneumonia with no sign of recurrence 6 months after treatment. Table 4 summarizes acute and late toxicities following treatment for the whole group.

Discussion

To our knowledge, this is the first study looking at functional laryngeal preservation following chemoradiation for locally advanced laryngeal cancer with IMRT and IGRT. Even though our patient number was small and the follow-up relatively short, the anatomic laryngeal preservation rate we observed was similar to that reported in the RTOG 91-11 study, at 89% if we exclude the patient who declined chemotherapy and was non-compliant during radiotherapy. Most patients in the RTOG 91-11 had T2-

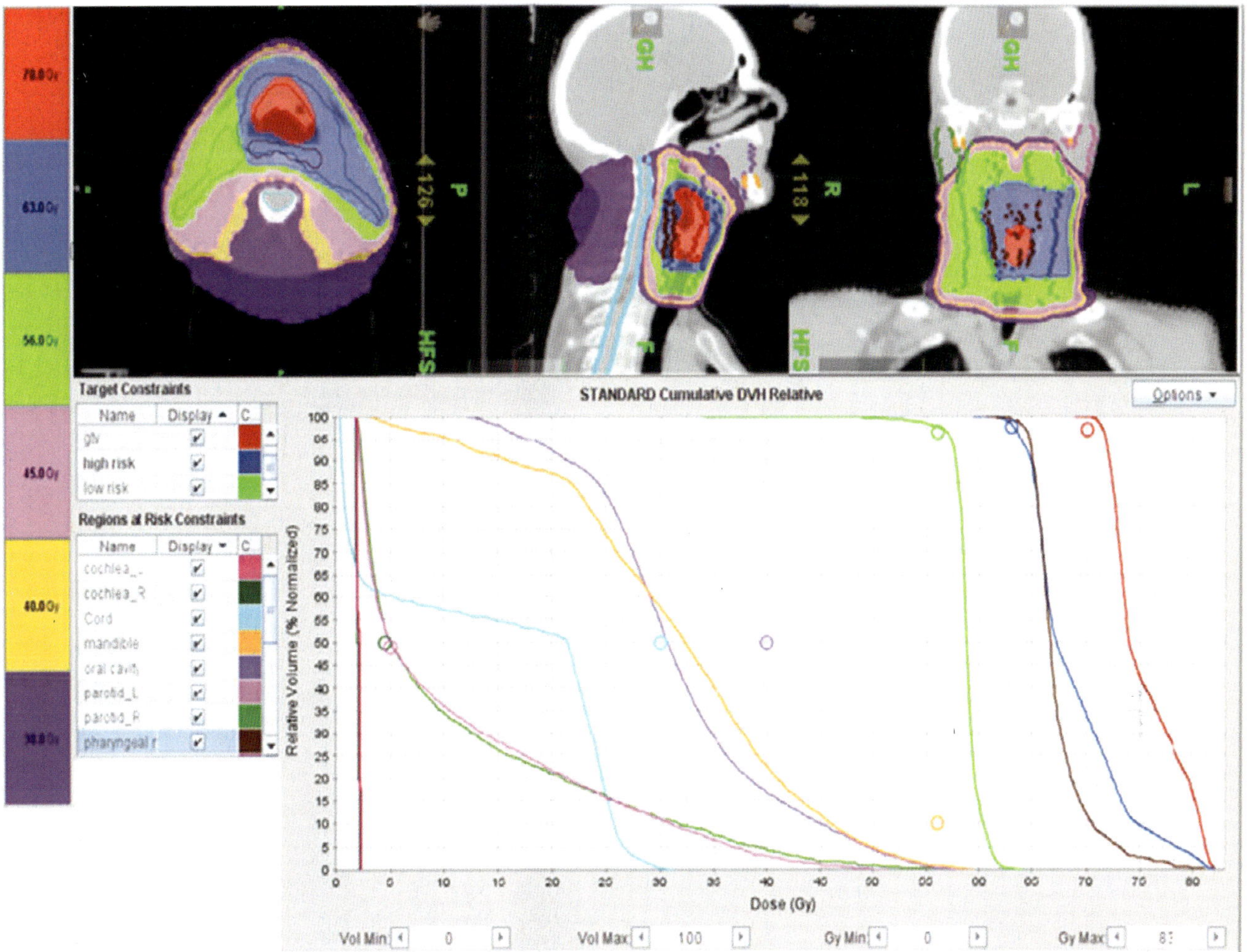

Figure 1. Dose-volume .histogram in a patient with T3N0M0 supraglottic laryngeal cancer illustrating the potential of image-guided radiotherapy to deliver a high radiation dose to the gross tumor while sparing the radiosensitive normal organs. Mean tumor dose: 75.4 Gy; mean right parotid dose (light green):11.4 Gy; mean left parotid dose (violet): 11.3 Gy; mean right (dark green) and left (pink) cochlea dose: 2 Gy; maximum mandibular dose (orange): 59.5 Gy; maximum spinal cord dose (light blue): 31.2 Gy. The radiation dose to these normal structures was well below the threshold for normal tissue damage and could potentially improve the patient quality of life after treatment. The red color illustrated radiation dose (70 Gy) to the gross tumor volume (gtv) while the dark blue and green color demonstrated radiation dose to the high risk area (63 Gy) and low risk area (56 Gy) respectively. The brown color illustrated radiation dose to the pharyngeal muscles which was high (mean 67 Gy) because of the close proximity to the gross tumor and may explain the high rate of dysphagia following radiotherapy for locally advanced laryngeal cancer.

T3 disease because it was thought that patients with T4 disease would have a non functional larynx following treatment [8]. Of note, six of the patients in our study had T4 disease and would thus have been excluded from concurrent chemoradiation in the RTOG study. All of these patients had no sign of recurrence at 11 to 45 months after treatment demonstrating the feasibility of organ preservation with IMRT and IGRT in T4 disease. For instance, one patient had disease invading the soft tissue of the neck and producing acute airway compression requiring emergency tracheostomy. The tumor shrank significantly during treatment allowing removal of the tracheostomy tube after treatment (Figure 2). The patient recovered his voice following treatment and, was able to resume his work without any difficulty with communication. PET imaging following treatment appeared in our patient group to be an effective follow-up strategy, detecting recurrence in two patients with normal endoscopic examination, thus confirming other studies reporting that PET imaging after radiotherapy for laryngeal cancer is helpful in detecting disease recurrence or second primaries, and thereby making laryngeal preservation therapy more feasible without compromising survival [23–25]. No patient with a negative PET scan in our study had disease recurrence, thus corroborating the accuracy of PET scan described in the literature [26]. In fact, in addition to the benefits provided by IMRT and IGRT, we feel that the excellent voice preservation observed in our patients, may in part be due to the avoidance of unnecessary biopsies in patients with negative PET imaging, reducing the edema and scarring frequently observed following laryngeal irradiation. In the recent past, laryngeal biopsy has been recommended in patients with edema persisting beyond six months following radiotherapy for laryngeal cancer [27]. However, recurrence is frequently submucosal and not visualized on direct laryngoscopic examinations and negative biopsy results requiring repeat procedures are common increasing the risk of chondritis and laryngeal necrosis [28,29]. As reported in several

Table 2. Patient characteristics.

	IGRT	IMRT	Total
Patient No	19	8	27
Age			
Median	60	68	63
Range	52–78	60–84	52–84
Sex			
Male	17	8	25
Female	2	0	2
Squamous histology	19	8	27
Sites			
Glottis	5	6	11
Supraglottis	14	2	16
Stages			
III	11	6	17
IVA	7	2	9
IVB	1	0	1
T stages			
T1	0	2	2
T2	5	2	7
T3	9	3	12
T4	5	1	6
Neck nodes			
N0	12	4	16
N1	4	3	7
N2	3	1	4
Treatment			
Radiotherapy alone	1	0	1
Chemoradiation	18	8	26

IGRT: Image-guided radiotherapy; IMRT: Intensity-modulated radiotherapy.

studies, PET imaging has an excellent negative predicting value after treatment, and a negative PET exam in the presence of persistent laryngeal edema after radiotherapy is a strong argument that such edema is benign and not due to local recurrence. Because of the retrospective nature of the study, we did not generally have stroboscopy data available to assess vocal cord mobility. However, only one patient complains of hoarseness and weakness of his voice preventing him from having a full time job as he works as a salesman. He had chronic laryngeal edema which did not improve over time.

The rate of severe chronic dysphagia and aspiration we observed during and after treatment remains high and corroborated RTOG 91-11 data [8]. Among 172 patients randomized to concurrent chemoradiation, 77% of the patients developed severe grade 3–4 toxicity, 5% died from treatment toxicity, and 9% did not complete the intended dose of radiotherapy (70 Gy). At one year, 3% of these patients could not swallow at all, and 23% could only tolerate liquids or soft food. Our study acute grade 3–4 mucositis and late toxicity remained significant with concurrent chemoradiation despite the use of IMRT, an observation corroborated in other studies of IMRT in laryngeal cancers [30,31]. Lee et al [30] reported a 35% rate of grade 3 mucositis and laryngitis in 31 patients with laryngeal and hypopharyngeal cancers undergoing concurrent chemoradiation with IMRT with six patients (19%) remaining dependent on long-term tube feedings. In another study of IMRT for laryngeal and hypopharyngeal cancer, eight out of 36 patients (25%) who had PEG tubes inserted before or during radiotherapy remained tube dependent more than 12 months after treatment. Given the close proximity of the pharyngeal musculature, severe dysphagia and aspiration remains unavoidable with the delivery of curative radiation doses to the larynx. Caglar et al demonstrated that the aspiration risk following IMRT for head and neck cancer was proportional to the volume of the inferior pharyngeal constrictor muscles receiving >50 Gy [32]. While it is thus not surprising that aspiration and long-term feeding-tube dependency remain prevalent after IMRT for laryngeal cancer, the aspiration risk is significantly lower following IMRT than following conventional radiotherapy with two lateral fields and a supraclavicular fields. Nguyen et al reported a 54% aspiration rate after concurrent chemoradiation for locally advanced laryngeal cancer with conventional radiotherapy [33]. In another study, 84% of the patients with definitive conventional radiotherapy for laryngeal cancer reported chronic aspiration [34]. Of note, aspiration after radiotherapy for head and neck cancer is often silent and can cause death from aspiration pneumonia if undetected [35,36]. Compared to conventional radiotherapy, IMRT and IGRT provide more homogeneous dose coverage of target volume and steeper dose gradients, potentially decreasing the radiation dose to the pharyngeal muscles and thereby decreasing the aspiration rate [37]. Nonetherless, severe dysphagia and aspiration remain significantly high with IMRT and IGRT for locally advanced laryngeal cancer. Following treatment, swal-

Table 3. Dose distribution in Gray (Gy) to the larynx and other head and neck organs.

	Mean (range)	Max (range)
Larynx	72.5 (70.5–76.7)	76.1 (71.9–82.2)
Spinal cord		39.1 (28.9–44.6)
Mandible	37.9 (23–56.1)	64 (46.4–74.8)
Right TMJ	12.8 (1.6–41)	34.9 (2.1–46.6)
Left TMJ	9.7 (1.8–23)	22.4 (2.3–44.7)
Right parotid	27.7 (10–40.7)	
Left parotid	32.4 (14.4–40.5)	
Right cochlea	9.4 (1–35)	11.9 (1.9–44.9)
Left cochlea	8.9 (1–35.9)	17.5 (1–47.1)

TMJ: Temporo-mandibular joint.

Table 4. Acute and late toxicities following intensity-modulated and image-guided radiotherapy for 27 patients with locally advanced laryngeal cancer.

Acute	Late
Grade 3–4 mucositis (16)	Long-term tube feedings (4)
Grade 3–4 hematologic toxicity (4)	Aspiration pneumonia (1)
Aspiration pneumonia (2)	
Bowel obstruction (1)	
Herpes Zoster (1)	

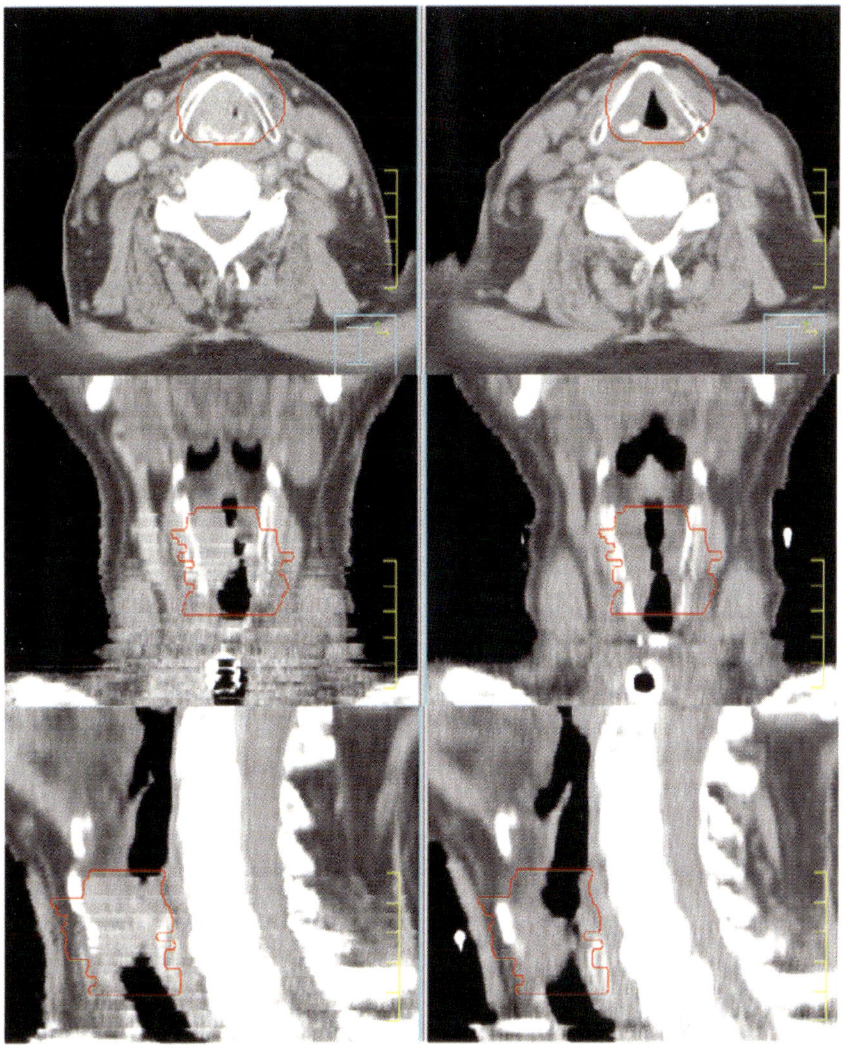

Figure 2. Illustrating the effectiveness of intensity-modulated and image-guided radiotherapy to achieve local control in T4 laryngeal cancer. The tumor invaded the thyroid cartilage and soft tissue of the neck and produced acute airway obstruction requiring emergency tracheostomy. A repeat CT scan at 40 Gy demonstrated significant shrinkage of the tumor allowing removal of the tracheostomy tube after treatment. The patient is disease-free 45 months after treatment and conserve a normal voice allowing him to work part-time after retirement.

lowing therapy should be initiated early within four to six weeks if dysphagia or aspiration are present [38]. Another possible investigation is the use of Amifostine, a radiation protector, which has been proven to decrease late dysphagia following radiotherapy for head and neck cancer [39]. Amifostine should be considered in future prospective trials to investigate whether it can reduce aspiration rate [39].

The limitations of the present study include its retrospective nature, the small number of patients, the short follow-up, and the absence of a matched controlled group treated with 3-D conformal technique. However, it demonstrates the feasibility of modern radiotherapy techniques including IMRT and IGRT for anatomic and functional laryngeal preservation in patients with locally advanced laryngeal cancers. Further prospective studies with larger patient numbers should be performed with these techniques, in order to try confirm their positive impact on patient quality of life.

Conclusions

New radiotherapy techniques such as IMRT and IGRT may be effective for anatomic and functional laryngeal preservation in patients with locally advanced laryngeal carcinoma. However, severe dysphagia and aspiration still remain limiting factors for surviving patients most likely secondary to excessive radiation dose to the pharyngeal muscles. Clinicians should be alerted about the risk of aspiration pneumonia for proper management.

Author Contributions

Conceived and designed the experiments: NPN AC MB FA PV RD BS MC DA LSR MS SJ SG VVH. Performed the experiments: NPN AC. Analyzed the data: NPN AC MB FA PV RD BS MC DA LSR MS SJ SG VVH. Contributed reagents/materials/analysis tools: PV. Wrote the paper: NPN AC MB FA PV RD BS MC DA LSR MS SJ SG VVH. Figures: PV SJ FA.

References

1. Tupchong L, Scott CB, Blitzer PH, Marcial VA, Lowry LD, et al. (1991) Randomized study of preoperative versus postoperative radiation therapy in advanced head and neck carcinoma: long-term follow-up of RTOG study. Int J Radiat Oncol Biol Phys 20:21–28.
2. DeSanto LW, Olsen KD, Perry WC, Rohe DE, Keith RL (1995) Quality of life after surgical treatment of cancer of the larynx. Ann Otol Rhinol Laryngol 104:763–769.
3. Deshmane VH, Parikh HK, Pinni S, Parikh DM, Rao RS (1995) Laryngectomy: a quality of life assessment. Indian J Cancer 32:121:130.
4. Hilgers FJ, Ackerstaff AH, Aaronson NK, Schouwenburg PF, Van Zandwijk N(1990) Physical and psychosocial consequences of total laryngectomy. Clin Otolaryngol 15:421–425.
5. Kuntz AL, Weymuller EA (1999) Impact of neck dissection on quality of life. Laryngoscope 8:1334–1338.
6. Rogers SN, Lowe D, Brown JS, Vaughan ED (1999) The University of Washington head and neck cancer measure as a predictor of outcome following primary surgery for oral cancer. Head Neck 21:394–401.
7. Department of Veterans Affairs Laryngeal Cancer Study Group (1991) Induction chemotherapy plus radiation compared to surgery plus radiation in patients with advanced laryngeal cancer: The department of veterans affair laryngeal cancer study group (1991). N Engl J Med 324:1685–1690.
8. Forastiere AA, Goepfert H, Maor M, et al. (2003) Concurrent chemotherapy and radiotherapy for organ preservation in advanced laryngeal cancer. N Engl J Med 349:2091–2098.
9. Lefebvre JL, Rolland F, Tesselaar M, Bardet E, Leemans CR, et al. (2009) Phase III randomized trial on larynx preservation comparing sequential and alternating chemotherapy and radiotherapy. J Nat Cancer Inst 101:142–152.
10. Posner MR, Norris CM, Wirth LJ, Shin DM, Cullen KJ, et al. (2009) Sequential therapy for the locally advanced larynx and hypopharyngeal cancer subgroup in TAX 324: survival, surgery, and organ preservation. Ann Oncol 20:921–927
11. Sanguineti G, Adapala P, Endres EJ, Brack C, Fiorino C, et al. (2007) Dosimetric predictors of laryngeal edema. Int J Radiat Oncol Biol Phys 68:741–749.
12. Nguyen NP, Moltz CC, Frank C, Vos P, Millar C, et al. (2007) Aspiration rate following nonsurgical therapy for laryngeal cancer. ORL 69:116–120.
13. Braaksma MMJ, Wijers OB, van Sornsen de Koste JR, van der Est H, Schmitz PI, et al. (2003) Optimisation of conformal radiation therapy by intensity-modulation: cancer of the larynx and salivary function. Radiother Oncol 66:291–302.
14. Zevallos JP, Mallen MJ, Lam CY, Karam-Hage M, Blalock J, et al. (2009) Complications of radiotherapy in laryngopharyngeal cancer. Effects of a smoking cessation program. Cancer 115:4636–4644.
15. Liberman PHP, Schultz C, Gomez VSG, Carvalho AL, Pelizzon AC, et al. (2004) Auditory effects after organ preservation protocol for laryngeal/hypopharyngeal carcinomas. Arch Otolaryngol Head Neck Surg 130:1265–1268.
16. Nguyen NP, Vock C, Chi A, Ewell L, Vos P, et al. (2012) Effectiveness of intensity-modulated and image-guided radiotherapy to spare the mandible from excessive radiation. Oral Oncol 48:653–657
17. Nguyen NP, Smith-Raymond L, Vinh-Hung V, Sloan D, Davis R, et al. (2011) Feasibility of Tomotherapy to spare the cochlea from excessive radiation in head and neck cancer. Oral Oncol 47:900–904
18. Nguyen NP, Vos P, Vinh-Hung V, Ceizyk M, Smith-Raymond L, et al. (2012) Feasibility of image-guided radiotherapy based on helical tomotherapy to reduce contralateral parotid dose in head and neck cancer. BMC Cancer, epublication.
19. Penagaricano JA, Ratanatharathorn V, Papanikolaou N, Yan Y (2004) Intensity-modulated radiation therapy reduces the dose to the normal tissue in T2N0M0 squamous cell carcinoma of the glottic larynx. Dosimetry 29:254–257.
20. Dogan N, King S, Emami B, Mohideen N, Mirkovic N, et al. (2003) Assessment of different IMRT delivery methods on target coverage and normal tissue sparing. Int J Radiat Oncol Biol Phys 57:1480–1491.
21. Chen AM, Farwell DG, Luu Q, Chen LM, Vijayakumar S, et al. (2011) Marginal misses after postoperative intensity-modulated radiotherapy for head and neck cancer. Int J Radiat Oncol Biol Phys 80:1423–1429.
22. Gordin A, Daitzchman M, Doweck I, Yefremov N, Golz A, et al. (2006) Fluorodeoxyglucose-Positron emission Tomography/Computed Tomography imaging in patients with carcinoma of the larynx: diagnostic accuracy and impact on management. Laryngoscope 116:273–278.
23. Salaun PY, Abgral R, Querellou S, Couturier O, Valette G, et al. (2007) Does 18fluoro-fluorodeoxyglucose positron emission tomography improve recurrence detection in patients treated for head and neck squamous cell carcinoma with negative clinical follow-up? Head Neck 29:1125–1130.
24. Oe A, Kawabe J, Torii K, Kawamura E, Kotani J, et al. (2006) Detection of local residual tumor after laryngeal cancer treatment using FDG-PET. Ann Nucl Med 21:9–13.
25. Brouwer J, de Bree R, Comans EFI, Akarriou M, Langendijk JA, et al. (2008) Improved detection of recurrent laryngeal tumor FDG-PET as initial method. Radiother Oncol 87:217–220.
26. van Hooren ACG, Brouwer J, de Bree R, Hoekstra OS, Leemans CR, et al. (2009) The cost effectiveness of FDG-PET in selecting patients with suspicion of recurrent laryngeal carcinoma after radiotherapy for direct laryngoscopy. Eur Arch Otorhinolaryngol 266:1441–1448.
27. Ward PD, Calcaterra TC, Kagan AR (1975) The enigma of post-radiation edema and residual or recurrent carcinoma of the larynx and pyriform fossa. Laryngoscope 85:522–529.
28. Brouwer J, bogar EJ, de Bree R, Langendijk JA, Castelijns JA, et al. (2004) Detecting recurrent laryngeal carcinoma after radiotherapy: room for improvement. Eur Arch Otorhinolaryngol 261:417–422.
29. Zbaren P, Caversaccio M, Thoeny HC, Nuyens M, Curshmann J, et al. (2006). Radionecrosis or tumor recurrence after radiation of laryngeal hypopharyngeal carcinomas. Otolaryngol Head Neck Surg 135:838–843.
30. Lee NY, O'Meara W, Chan K, Della-Bianca C, Mechalakos JG, et al. (2007) Concurrent chemotherapy and intensity-modulated radiotherapy for locoregionally advanced laryngeal and hypopharyngeal cancers. Int J Radiat Oncol Biol Phys 60:459–468.
31. Studer G, Peponi E, Kloeck S, Dossenbach T, Huber G, et al. (2010) Surviving hypopharynx-larynx carcinoma in the era of IMRT. Int J Radiat Oncol Biol Phys 77:1391–1396.
32. Caglar HB, Tishler RB, Othus M, Burke E, Li Y, et al. (2008) Dose to larynx predicts for swallowing complications after intensity-modulated radiotherapy. Int J Radiat Oncol Biol Phys 72:1110–1118.
33. Nguyen NP, Moltz CC, Frank C, Vos P, Millar C, et al. (2007) Aspiration rate following nonsurgical therapy for laryngeal cancer. ORL 69:116–120.
34. Hutcheson KA, Barringer DA, Rosenthal DI, May AH, Roberts DB, et al. (2008) Swallowing outcomes after radiotherapy for laryngeal carcinoma. Arch Otolaryngol Head Neck Surg 134:178–183.
35. Nguyen NP, Moltz CC, Frank C, Millar C, Smith HJ, et al. (2007) Effectiveness of the cough reflex in patients with aspiration following radiation for head and neck cancer. Lung 185:243–248.
36. Nguyen NP, Smith HJ, Dutta S, Alfieri A, North D, et al. (2007) Aspiration occurrence during chemoradiation for head and neck cancer. Anticancer Res 27:1669–1672.
37. Clark CH, Bidmead MA, Mubata CD, Harrington KJ, Nutting CM (2004) Intensity-modulated radiotherapy improves target coverage, spinal cord sparing and allows dose escalation in patients with locally advanced cancer of the larynx. Radiother Oncol 70:189–198.
38. Nguyen NP, Moltz CC, Frank C, Smith HJ, Nguyen PD, et al. (2007) Impact of swallowing therapy on aspiration rate following treatment for locally advanced head and neck cancer. Oral Oncol 43:352–357.
39. Buntzel J, Glatzel M, Mucke R, Micke O, Bruns F (2007) Influence of amifostine on late radiation-toxicity in head and neck cancer—a follow-up study. Anticancer Res 2007;27:1953–1956.

14

Feasibility of Tomotherapy-Based Image-Guided Radiotherapy for Locally Advanced Oropharyngeal Cancer

Nam P. Nguyen[1]*, Misty Ceizyk[1], Paul Vos[2], Michael Betz[3], Alexander Chi[4], Fabio Almeida[5], Rick Davis[1], Benjamin Slane[1], Steven Gelumbauskas[1], Lexie Smith-Raymond[1], Dave Abraham[1], Michelle Stevie[1], Siyoung Jang[1], Vincent Vinh-Hung[6]

1 Department of Radiation Oncology, University of Arizona, Tucson, Arizona, United States of America, **2** Department of Biostatistics, East Carolina University, Greenville, North Carolina, United States of America, **3** Hirslanden Radiation Oncology Institute, Lausanne, Switzerland, **4** Department of Radiation Oncology, West Virginia University, Morgantown, West Virginia, United States of America, **5** Southwest PET-CT Institute, Tucson, Arizona, United States of America, **6** Department of Radiation Oncology, University Hospitals of Geneva, Geneva, Switzerland

Abstract

Purpose: The study aims to assess the feasibility of tomotherapy-based image-guided (IGRT) radiotherapy for locally advanced oropharyngeal cancer. A retrospective review of 33 patients undergoing concurrent chemoradiation for locally advanced oropharyngeal cancers was conducted. Radiotherapy planning, treatment toxicity and loco-regional control were assessed.

Results: At a median follow-up of 32 months (6–47 months), no patient developed loco-regional recurrence. Two patients (6%) developed distant metastases. Grade 3–4 acute toxicity was respectively 72% and 25% for mucositis and gastrointestinal toxicity. Two patients (6%) had long-term dependence on tube feedings. Dose-volume histogram demonstrated excellent target volume coverage and low radiation dose to the organs at risk for complications.

Conclusions and clinical relevance: IGRT provides excellent loco-regional control but acute toxicity remains significant and needs to be addressed in future prospective trials. The feasibility of Tomotherapy to decrease radiation dose to the normal tissues merits further investigations.

Editor: Kevin Camphausen, NIH, United States of America

Funding: The authors have no support or funding to report.

Competing Interests: The authors have declared that no competing interest exists.

* E-mail: NamPhong.Nguyen@yahoo.com

Introduction

The prevalence of oropharyngeal cancer is steadily rising in the United States despite a reduction of other head and neck cancers [1]. The increase in oropharyngeal cancers is mainly observed in young patients and related to human papilloma virus (HPV) 16 which may reach epidemic proportion [2]. Most patients with oropharyngeal malignancyare frequently diagnosed at advanced stages because the submucosal spread of the tumor making it difficult to detect clinically despite patient's symptoms [3]. Locally advanced oropharyngeal cancers can be treated with either surgery followed by postoperative radiation or concurrent chemoradiation with similar survival [4]. Resection of the tongue base or soft palate is frequently associated with significant morbidity because of the crucial role of these organs in speech and deglutition [5,6]. In addition, neck dissection, often bilateral, may induce severe pain because of nerve damage which may decrease patient quality of life [7]. Thus, concurrent chemoradiation is frequently selected over surgery for patients with locally advanced oropharyngeal cancers because of anatomic organ preservation [8]. However, chemoradiation is associated with significant toxicity, mainly grade 3–4 mucositis and hematologic toxicity, and long-term dysphagia because of damage to the pharyngeal muscles [9,10]. New radiotherapy technique such as intensity-modulated radiotherapy (IMRT) has been introduced to decrease treatment toxicity in oropharyngeal cancers with promising preliminary results despite a short follow-up [11]. Image-guided radiotherapy (IGRT) is a new technique of IMRT delivery which combines the sharper dose fall off of IMRT and precise target irradiation [12]. The feasibility of IGRT has not been fully investigated in locally advanced oropharyngeal cancer and prompt us to conduct this retrospective study.

Materials and Methods

The medical records of 33 patients undergoing radiotherapy for locally advanced oropharyngeal cancers at the University of Arizona Radiation Oncology department were retrospectively reviewed following institutional review board (IRB) approval from the University of Arizona. The University of Arizona IRB waived the requirement for patient consent because of the retrospective nature of the study limited to charts review. Patient information

Table 1. Patient characteristics.

Patient Number		33
Age	Median	61
	Range	39–84
Sex	Male	31
	Female	2
Histology	Squamous	33
Tumor Sites	Tonsils	19
	Base of Tongue	13
	Soft palate	1
Stages	III	7
	IVA	19
	IVB	5
	IVC	2
T stages	T1	5
	T2	11
	T3	10
	T4	7
Neck nodes	N0	2
	N1	11
	N2	17
	N3	3
Treatment	Radiotherapy alone	1
	Postoperative chemoradiation	5
	Chemoradiation	27
Smoking history	>50-pack year history	31
Follow-up (months)	Median	28
	Range	6–43

Table 2. Dose distribution to target volume and to critical organs at risk for complications following image-guided radiotherapy for head and neck cancer.

PTV1	Mean	97.1%
	Range	95–99%
PTV2	Mean	96.9%
	Range	95–99%
PTV3	Mean	96.3%
	Range	95–99%
Spinal cord	Maximum	36.7 Gy
	Range	28.9–42 Gy
Brain stem	Maximum	44.5 Gy
	Range	35.7–50.2 Gy
Right parotid	Mean	39 Gy
	Range	18.4–65.4 Gy
Left parotid	Mean	37.6 Gy
	Range	19.6–63.8 Gy
Larynx	Mean	24.5 Gy
	Range	17.3–45.5 Gy
Right cochlea	Mean	6.9 Gy
	Range	3.6–14.3 Gy
Left cochlea	Mean	8.7 Gy
	Range	4–28.4 Gy
Mandible	Maximum	70.4 Gy
	Range	64.8–74.6 Gy
	Mean	47.3 Gy
	Range	38.8–60 Gy

PTV1: target volume receiving 66 to 70 Gy; PTV2: target volume receiving 59.6 to 63 Gy; PTV3: target volume receiving 54 to 56 Gy; Gy: gray.

was de-identified to protect patient confidentiality. All patients were treated with the whole field IGRT technique on the helical Tomotherapy unit from December 2008 to February 2011. Prior to treatment, each patient was simulated in the supine position with a head and neck aquaplast mask for treatment immobilization. A computed tomography (CT) scan with and without intravenous (IV) contrast for treatment planning was performed in the treatment position. The head and neck areas from the vertex to the mid thorax were scanned with a slice thickness of 3 mm CT scan with IV contrast was employed to outline the tumor and grossly enlarged cervical lymph node for target volume delineation. Radiotherapy planning was performed on the CT scan without contrast to avoid possible interference of contrast density on radiotherapy isodose distributions. Diagnostic positron emission tomography (PET)-CT scan planning for tumor imaging was also incorporated with CT planning when available for tumor imaging. A 0.5 cm bolus material was placed on any area of the skin involved by the tumor and on any palpable cervical lymph nodes. Normal organs at risk for complication were outlined for treatment planning (spinal cord, brain stem, bilateral cochlea, mandible, parotid glands, bilateral eyes, and oral cavity).

For patients with definitive chemoradiation, the tumor and grossly enlarged lymph nodes (CTV1) on CT scan with a margin (PTV1) were treated to 70 Gy in 35 fractions (2 Gy/fraction). The margins were 5 mm to 1 cm all around CTV1 depending on anatomic location. The areas at high risk-PTV2 (at least 1 cm around gross tumor and pathologic cervical lymph nodes) and low risk -PTV3 (subclinical regional lymph nodes with 5 mm margins) for tumor spread were treated respectively to 63 Gy and 56 Gy in 35 fractions, respectively. Patients undergoing postoperative chemoradiation were treated to 66 Gy, 59.4 Gy, and 54 Gy in 33 fractions to PTV1, PTV2, and PTV3 respectively. Indications for postoperative chemoradiation were positive margins and/or extra-capsular lymph nodes invasion. Minimal target coverage was 95% of the prescribed dose for all targets with at least 99% of the prescribed dose delivered to gross tumor and involved cervical lymph nodes. The lymph nodes in the ipsilateral neck including the retropharyngeal lymph nodes were treated to the base of skull if there was any cervical lymph node enlargement (or PET-positive lymph nodes). Contralateral uninvolved lymph nodes were treated prophylactically with the C1 vertebrae as the superior border of the radiation field. In case of bilateral cervical lymph node involvement, both sides of the neck were irradiated including the base of skull to avoid any marginal miss. Mean dose to the parotid was kept below 2600 cGy if there was no ipsilateral cervical lymph node enlargement. Dose constraints for other normal organs at risk (OAR) for complications were: spinal cord (45 Gy), brain stem (50 Gy), optic chiasm (45 Gy), mandible (70 Gy to less than 30% of the mandible).

Concurrent chemoradiation was recommended for all patients. The type of chemotherapy regimen was left at the discretion of the medical oncologists depending on patient functional status and comorbidities. Prophylactic percutaneous gastrostomy tubes feedings placement was recommended for all patients prior to radiotherapy because of the expected weight loss secondary to chemoradiation-induced mucositis. Weekly complete blood count (CBC) and blood chemistry to assess renal function were performed during chemoradiation. Treatment breaks and weight loss were recorded during chemoradiation. Acute and long-term toxicities were graded according to Radiotherapy Oncology Group (RTOG) group severity scale (http://ctep.cancer.gov).

All patients had a follow-up visit one month and regularly three months following treatment. Clinical examination and direct endoscopic exam were performed at each follow-up to detect recurrent disease. A PET scan or PET-CT scan were performed four months, ten months and yearly after treatment if there was no evidence of disease. PET positive areas were biopsied to detect recurrence and surgery and/or chemotherapy were carried out for salvage if the biopsy demonstrated disease recurrence. Patient ability to resume normal oral feeding and dependency on tube feedings was also evaluated at each visit.

Survival data was analyzed using Kaplan-Meier estimation.

Results

We identified 33 patients with invasive squamous cell carcinoma of the oropharynx treated at the University of Arizona Radiation Oncology department from 2007 to 2011.

Median age at diagnosis was 61 years-old (range: 39-83 years-old). There were 31 males and 2 female. There was 7 stage III, 19 stage IVA, 5 stage IVB and two stage IVC. Treatment consisted of: radiotherapy alone (1), postoperative chemoradiation (5), and definitive concurrent chemoradiation (27). The patient who had radiotherapy alone did not have chemotherapy because of significant co-morbidity with recurrent pneumonia prior to treatment. Except for two patients, all patients had a smoking history. Three patients had HPV 16 testing because of their young age and absence of smoking history. Two of these three patients were HPV 16 positive. Radiotherapy technique consisted of WF IGRT on the helical Tomotherapy unit. Table 1 summarizes patient characteristics. Table 2 summarizes radiation dose distributions among various OAR and to PTV1-3.

Chemotherapy consisted of cisplatin (P) 30 mg/m2 intravenously (IV) weekly (21) and cisplatin 100 mg IV on day 1, 22, and 43 of radiotherapy (7). One patient had carboplatin IV weekly with an area under the curve (AUC) of 1.5 because poor kidney function. Three patient had induction chemotherapy with taxotere (T) 75 mg/m2 IV, cisplatin 100 mg/m2 IV followed by 5-fluorouracil (F) 1000 mg/m2 for four days, repeated every three weeks for three cycles followed four weeks later by carboplatin IV weekly with an area under the curve of 1.5 during radiotherapy. One patient had cetuximab IV 400 mg/m2 followed by 250 mg/m 2 weekly during radiotherapy because of concern that he may not tolerate conventional chemotherapy.

At a median follow-up of 32 months (6–47 months), no patient developed loco-regional recurrence. The two stages IVc patients had lung metastases on diagnosis. They had induction chemotherapy followed by concurrent chemoradiation. The lung metastases initially responded to induction chemotherapy but recurred four to six months respectively after chemoradiation requiring adjuvant chemotherapy and stereotactic body radiotherapy. One patient developed hematuria after chemoradiation. He was diagnosed to have locally advanced bladder cancer and died from the bladder cancer. The 3-year survival is estimated to be 92% for the whole group.

Twenty-four patients (72%) developed grade 3-4 toxicity mucositis. Six patients (25%) had grade 3–4 nausea and vomiting requiring IV fluid for hydration.

The patient who had recurrent pneumonia prior to radiotherapy continued to have pneumonia during treatment and required multiple hospital admissions.

Two patients did not complete radiotherapy. One patient decided against medical advice to discontinue treatment at 48 Gy because of grade 4 mucositis. One patient was involved in a car accident and treatment was stopped at 68 Gy. Eighteen patients (54%) had treatment breaks ranging from three to 28 days (median: 3 days) because of grade 3–4 toxicity. Median weight loss was 16 pounds (0–40 pounds).

Chemotherapy was not administered according to the protocol in six patients (18%).

One patient did not receive chemotherapy because of recurrent pneumonia prior to treatment and the concern for chemotherapy-induced immunosuppression. The patient who had induction TPF had 25% TPF dose reduction after the first cycle of chemotherapy because of neutropenia. Among patients who had weekly cisplatin 30 mg/m2, one patient developed acute tubular necrosis after the first week of chemotherapy which required its replacement with carboplatin, another patient had cisplatin on hold during week 5 because of severe vomiting. The patient who had weekly carboplatin did not receive carboplatin after week 5 because of severe weight loss and PEG tube malfunction.

For the whole group of 33 patients, two (6%) had prolonged tube feedings at 21 months and 29 months respectively because of severe dysphagia and dysgueusia. They were able to discontinue tube feedings afterward. One patient (3%) had soft tissue mucosal ulceration which resolved with antibiotics and oral hygiene.

Discussion

To our knowledge, this is the first study looking at the feasibility of chemoradiation for locally advanced oropharyngeal cancer with tomotherapy-based IGRT and PET imaging. Even though the patient number is small with a relatively short follow-up, all patients achieved clinical and PET proven loco-regional control. We include two patients who had lung metastases at diagnosis because they were in remission following induction chemotherapy and required radiotherapy for local control. Even though the lung metastases recurred after chemoradiation, they did not have loco-regional failure even though they both had large size primaries and neck nodes (T4,N3). Even though we lacked information on HPV 16 status in most patients, the majority of the patients had a history of heavy smoking which conferred a poor prognosis. Tomotherapy is able to deliver a high radiation dose with rapid fall off. In addition, pre-treatment megavolt (MV) CT performed before treatment and re-positioning to compensate for body motion and tumor shrinkage decreased the risk of marginal miss [13–17].

As we reported previously, the study mean laryngeal and cochlea dose remained consistently low [16,18]. Low dose to the larynx may reduce the risk of laryngeal edema and preserve voice quality. Decreased cochlea dose may decrease the risk of hearing loss and potentially improve patient quality of life because of the proven ototoxicity of cisplatin-based chemotherapy. The mean parotid dose was high because most of the patients presented with cervical lymph node metastases at diagnosis. It is our policy not to spare the ipsilateral parotid gland in case of neck node involvement because of the risk recurrence in the peri-parotid area [19]. As a result, loco-regional control was excellent despite locally advanced disease. For instance, Figure 1 illustrated a

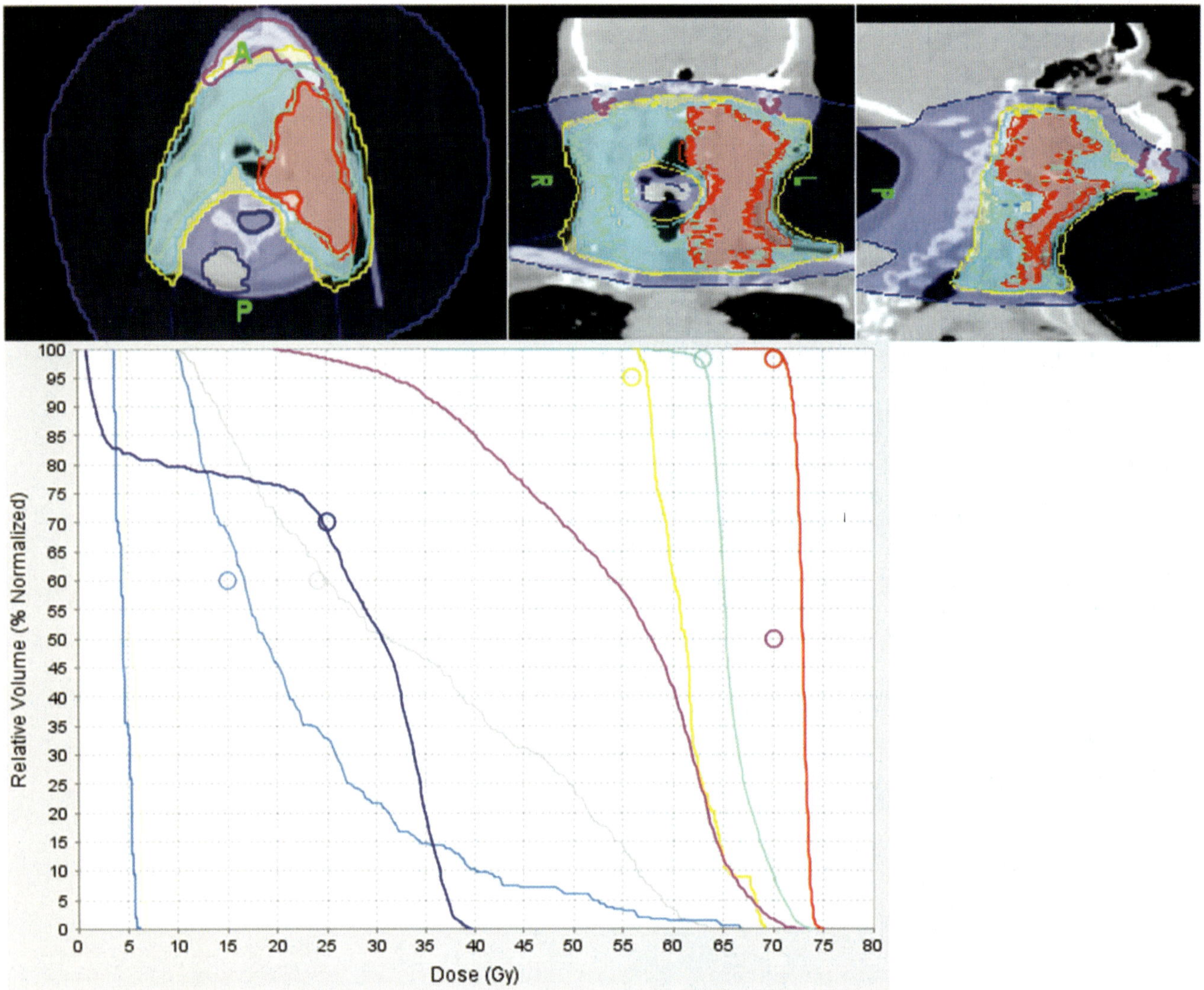

Figure 1. Illustration of the effectiveness of Tomotherapy to deliver high radiation dose to the gross tumor and cervical lymph nodes while sparing adjacent normal structures. The patient had locally advanced base of the tongue cancer (T4) associated with massive cervical metastases (N3) and lung metastases at diagnosis. Following induction chemotherapy which resulted in resolution of the lung metastases, he had concurrent chemoradiation for local control and achieved a complete response of the gross tumor and lymph nodes on post-treatment PET-CT. The lung metastases recurred after treatment and were treated with adjuvant chemotherapy and consolidation stereotactic body radiotherapy. The patient is currently on remission two years after the treatment with no long-term complications except for xerostomia because of low radiation dose to the normal organs. The parotid glands could not be spared because of the close proximity to the gross lymph nodes and areas at high risk for disease.Red line: gross tumor and cervical lymph nodes treated to 70 Gy; green line: area at high risk for disease treated to 63 Gy; pink line: mandibular dose (mean: 56 Gy), gray line: pharyngeal muscles dose (mean: 33.6 Gy); gray-blue line: laryngeal dose (mean: 22.5 Gy); navy blue line: spinal cord dose (max: 39.4 Gy); light blue line: right cochlea dose: (mean: 4.5 Gy); light brown line: left cochlea dose: (mean: 5.3 Gy).

patient with a T4N3M1 (IVc) base of tongue carcinoma who presented with lung metastases at diagnosis. Following induction chemotherapy with TPF, the patient underwent concurrent chemoradiation with complete resolution of the gross tumor and cervical lymph nodes on follow-up PET-CT. The lung metastases were treated with adjuvant chemotherapy and stereotactic body irradiation. The patient is currently on remission two years after treatment with no long-term complications because of the low dose of radiation to the normal tissues. Even though the study follow-up is relatively short, PET-CT following treatment allows us to detect disease recurrence or second primaries effectively [20–23]. Indeed, the patient who had biopsy-proven bladder cancer was diagnosed on PET-CT. PET-CT may also have predictive prognostic value. In a study of 80 head and neck cancer patients who underwent radiotherapy and were monitored with PET-CT, the patients who had a negative PET-CT within six months of treatment completion had a 2-year disease-free survival of 93% [20]. The high accuracy rate of PET-CT in predicting survival benefit for patients who were disease-free by PET criterias following radiotherapy or chemoradiation for head and neck cancer was also corroborated in other studies [21–23]. Thus, we feel confident that the excellent loco-regional control observed in our study may be maintained with a longer follow-up.

We observe a high rate of grade 3–4 mucositis and gastrointestinal toxicity during treatment. The combination of chemotherapy and radiation for locally advanced oropharyngeal cancer is frequently associated with significant acute toxicity because of the large volume of normal tissues irradiated even with IMRT

[11,24]. However, the acute toxicity frequently resolved by four to six weeks after chemoradiation. We have a special team of dietitians, speech pathologists, and home health nurses who monitored patients closely during and after treatment because of the significant weight loss secondary to mucositis. Only two patients (6%) became dependent on long-term tube feedings because chronic dysphagia and dysgueusia. They eventually recovered andhad removal of the feedings tubes. If we look at the long-term toxicity of patients with locally advanced oropharyngeal cancer treated with concurrent chemotherapy and conventional radiotherapy, up to 37% of the patients had prolonged tube feedings after treatment because of severe dysphagia or aspiration [9]. Long-term dependence on feeding tubes was also observed in 14% of the patients treated with IMRT and chemotherapy for oropharyngeal cancer [11]. Even with a special IMRT technique designed to reduce irradiation to the larynx and pharyngeal muscles which are critical structures for swallow, four out of 76 patients (5%) still experienced significant dysphagia one year following chemoradiation for oropharyngeal cancer [25].

Thus, our treatment complications profile compares favorably with other studies on oropharyngeal cancers and may improve further in the future as we acquire more experience with this new technique of radiotherapy. We also consider the administration of amifostine, a radiation protector, during chemoradiation for oropharyngeal cancers in the future to reduce the severity of mucositis and long-term dysphagia [26,27].

The limitations of the present study include the retrospective nature of the study, the small number of patients, the lack of HPV 16 information on most patients, and the relatively short follow-up. We do not have a matched cohort of oropharyngeal cancer patients treated with the conventional radiotherapy technique because these patients did not have a dose-volume histogram for comparison. However, our study demonstrates the feasibility of tomotherapy treatment for local control in patients with locally advanced oropharyngeal cancers with acceptable toxicity. Further prospective studies with a large number of patients should be performed with tomotherapy to assess the impact of this new technique on patient quality of life because of the unique ability of Tomotherapy to decrease radiation dose to the normal tissues.

Conclusions

Tomotherapy-based IGRT provides excellent loco-regional control and in patients with locally advanced oropharyngeal carcinoma with acceptable long-term toxicity. However, acute toxicity, mainly mucositis remains significant and should be taken into consideration in future prospective trials.

Author Contributions

Performed statistical analysis: PV. Conceived and designed the experiments: NPN MC PV MB AC FA RD BS SG LSR DA MS SJ VVH. Performed the experiments: NPN MC. Analyzed the data: NPN MC PV MB AC FA RD BS SG LSR DA MS SJ VVH. Wrote the paper: NPN MC PV MB AC FA RD BS SG LSR DA MS SJ VVH.

References

1. Shiboski CH, Schmidt BL, Jordan RC (2005) Tongue and tonsil carcinoma. Increasing trends in the U.S. population ages 20–44 years. Cancer 103:1843–1849.
2. Nguyen NP, Chi A, Nguyen LM, Ly BH, Karlsson U, et al. (2010) Human papillomavirus-associated oropharyngeal cancer: a new clinical entity. Q J Med 103:229–236.
3. Jemal A, Siegel R, Ward E, Hao Y, Xu J, et al. (2008) Cancer statistics, 2008. CA Cancer J Clin 58:71–96.
4. Soo KC, Tan EH, Wee J, Lim D, Tai BC, et al. (2005) Surgery and adjuvant radiotherapy vs concurrent chemoradiotherapy in stage III/IV nonmetastatic squamous cell carcinoma of the head and neck: a randomized comparison. Br J Cancer 93:279–286.
5. Lauciello FR, Vergo T, Schaaf NG, Zimmerman R (1980) Prosthodontic and speech rehabilitation after partial and complete glossectomy. J Prosthet Dent 43:204–211.
6. Pauloski BR, Rademaker AW, Logemann JA, McConnell FM, Heiser MA, et al. (2004) Surgical variables affecting swallowing in patients treated for oral/oropharyngeal cancer. Head Neck 26:625–636.
7. Kuntz AL, Weymuller EA (1999) Impact of neck dissection on quality of life. Laryngoscope 8:1334–1338.
8. Parsons JT, Mendenhall WM, Stringer SP, Amdur RJ, Hinerman RW, et al. (2002) Squamous cell carcinoma of the oropharynx: surgery, radiation therapy, or both. Cancer 94:2967–2980.
9. Nguyen NP, Vos P, Smith HJ, Ly BH, Karlsson U, et al. (2007) Concurrent chemoradiation for locally advanced oropharyngeal cancer. Am J Otolaryngol 28:3–8.
10. Nguyen NP, Frank C, Moltz CC, Vos P, Smith HJ, et al. (2009) Analysis of factors influencing aspiration risk following chemoradiation for oropharyngeal cancer. Br. J Radiol 82:675–680.
11. de Arruda FF, Puri DR, Zhung J, Narayana A, Wolden S, et al. (2006) Intensity-modulated radiation therapy for the treatment of oropharyngeal carcinoma: The Memorial Sloan Kettering center experience. Int J Radiat Oncol Biol Phys 64:363–373.
12. Lee TF, Fang FM, Chao PJ, Su TJ, Wang LK, et al. (2008) Dosimetric comparisons of helical tomotherapy and step-and-shoot intensity-modulated radiotherapy in nasopharyngeal carcinoma. Radiother Oncol 89:89–96.
13. Jacob V, Bayer W, Astner ST, Kneschaurek P (2010) A planning comparison of dynamic IMRT for different collimator leaf thickness with helical tomotherapy and RapidArc for prostate and head and neck tumors. Strahlenther Onkol 186:502–510.
14. Murthy V, Master Z, Gupta T, Ghosh-Laskar S, Buddrukkar A, et al. (2010) Helical tomotherapy for head and neck squamous cell carcinoma: Dosimetric comparison with linear accelerator-based step-and-shoot IMRT. J Cancer Res Treat 6:194–198.
15. Chen AM, Lee NY, Yang CC, Liu T, Naravan S, et al. (2010) Comparison of intensity-modulated radiotherapy using helical tomotherapy and segmental multileaf collimator-based techniques for nasopharyngeal carcinoma: dosimetric analysis incorporating quality assurance guidelines from RTOG 0225. Technol Cancer Res Treat 9:291–298.
16. Nguyen NP, Ceizyk M, Vos P, Vinh-Hung V, Davis R, et al. (2010) Effectiveness of image-guided radiotherapy for laryngeal sparing in head and neck cancer. Oral Oncol 46:283–286.
17. Ulrich S, Sterzing F, Nill S, Schubert K, Herfarth KK, et al. (2009) Comparison of arc-modulated cone beam therapy and helical tomotherapy for three different types of cancer. Med Phys 36:4702–4710.
18. Nguyen NP, Smith-Raymond L, Vinh-Hung V, Sloan D, Davis R, et al. (2011) Feasibility of Tomotherapy to save the cochlea from excessive radiation in head and neck cancer. Oral Oncol 47:414–419.
19. Cannon DM, Lee NY (2008) Recurrence in region of spared parotid gland afterdefinitive intensity-modulated radiotherapy for head and neck cancer. Int J Radiat Oncol Biol Phys 70:660–665.
20. Salaun PY, Abgral R, Querellou S, Couturier O, Valette G, et al. (2007) Does 18-fluorodeoxyglucose positron emission tomography improve recurrence detection in patients treated for head and neck squamous cell carcinoma with negative clinical follow-up? Head Neck 29:1125–1130.
21. Malone JP, Gerberi MAT, Vasireddy S, Hughes LF, Rao K, et al. (2009) Early prediction of response to chemoradiotherapy for head and neck cancer. Arch Otolaryngol Head Neck Surg;135:1119–1125.
22. Yao M, Smith RB, Graham MM, Hoffman HT, Tan H, et al. (2005) The role of FDG PET in management of neck metastases from head and neck cancer after definitive radiotherapy treatment. Int J Radiat Oncol Biol Phys 63:991–999.
23. Ong SC, Schoder H, Lee NY, Patel SG, Carlson D, et al. (2008) Clinical utility of 18F-FDG PET/CT in assessing the neck after concurrent chemoradiotherapy for locoregionally advanced head and neck cancer. J Nucl Med 49:532–540.
24. Daly ME, Le QT, Maxim PG, Loo BW, Kaplan MJ, et al. (2010) Intensity-modulated radiotherapy in the treatment of oropharyngeal cancer: clinical outcomes and pattern of failure. Int J Radiat Oncol Biol Phys 76:1339–1346.
25. Feng FY, Kim HM, Lyden TH, Haxer MJ, Worden FP, et al. (2010) Intensity-modulated chemoradiotherapy aiming to reduce dysphagia in patients with oropharyngeal cancer: clinical and functional results. J Clin Oncol 28:2732–2738.
26. Buntzel J, Glatzel M, Mucke R, Micke O, Bruns F (2007) Influence of amifostine on late radiation-toxicity in head and neck cancer—a follow-up study. Anticancer Res 27:1953–1956.
27. Buntzel J, Kuttner K, Frolich D, Glatzel M (1998) Selective cytoprotection withamifostine in concurrent radiochemotherapy for head and neck cancer. Ann Oncol 9:505–509.

15

Delayed Contrast Extravasation MRI for Depicting Tumor and Non-Tumoral Tissues in Primary and Metastatic Brain Tumors

**Leor Zach[1,6], David Guez[2], David Last[2], Dianne Daniels[2,6], Yuval Grober[3], Ouzi Nissim[3], Chen Hoffmann[4,6], Dvora Nass[5], Alisa Talianski[1], Roberto Spiegelmann[3,6], Zvi R. Cohen[3,6], Yael Mardor[2,6]*

1 Oncology Institute, Sheba Medical Center, Ramat-Gan, Israel, **2** Advanced Technology Center, Sheba Medical Center, Ramat-Gan, Israel, **3** Neurosurgery Department, Sheba Medical Center, Ramat-Gan, Israel, **4** Radiology Institute, Sheba Medical Center, Ramat-Gan, Israel, **5** Pathology Institute, Sheba Medical Center, Ramat-Gan, Israel, **6** Sackler Faculty of Medicine, Tel-Aviv University, Tel-Aviv, Israel

Abstract

The current standard of care for newly diagnosed glioblastoma multiforme (GBM) is resection followed by radiotherapy with concomitant and adjuvant temozolomide. Recent studies suggest that nearly half of the patients with early radiological deterioration post treatment do not suffer from tumor recurrence but from pseudoprogression. Similarly, a significant number of patients with brain metastases suffer from radiation necrosis following radiation treatments. Conventional MRI is currently unable to differentiate tumor progression from treatment-induced effects. The ability to clearly differentiate tumor from non-tumoral tissues is crucial for appropriate patient management. Ten patients with primary brain tumors and 10 patients with brain metastases were scanned by delayed contrast extravasation MRI prior to surgery. Enhancement subtraction maps calculated from high resolution MR images acquired up to 75 min after contrast administration were used for obtaining stereotactic biopsies. Histological assessment was then compared with the pre-surgical calculated maps. In addition, the application of our maps for prediction of progression was studied in a small cohort of 13 newly diagnosed GBM patients undergoing standard chemoradiation and followed up to 19.7 months post therapy. The maps showed two primary enhancement populations: the slow population where contrast clearance from the tissue was slower than contrast accumulation and the fast population where clearance was faster than accumulation. Comparison with histology confirmed the fast population to consist of morphologically active tumor and the slow population to consist of non-tumoral tissues. Our maps demonstrated significant correlation with perfusion-weighted MR data acquired simultaneously, although contradicting examples were shown. Preliminary results suggest that early changes in the fast volumes may serve as a predictor for time to progression. These preliminary results suggest that our high resolution MRI-based delayed enhancement subtraction maps may be applied for clear depiction of tumor and non-tumoral tissues in patients with primary brain tumors and patients with brain metastases.

Editor: Tao Jiang, Beijing Tiantan Hospital, Capital Medical University, China

Funding: This research is supported by the Kamin program of the Israeli Ministry of Industry and Commerce. The funders had no role in study design, data collection and analysis, decision to publish, or preparation of the manuscript.

Competing Interests: Leor Zach, David Guez, David Last, Dianne Daniels and Yael Mardor are authors on a pending patent titled VESSEL FUNCTION MAPS (Oct 2011).

* E-mail: yael.mardor@sheba.health.gov.il

Introduction

MRI is considered the gold standard imaging modality for the central nervous system. Although MR images provide high resolution and good sensitivity standard MR sequences still suffer of low specificity especially in the case of brain tumors during or after treatment. Tumor progression, inflammation and infection can induce similar changes in enhancement which are impossible to differentiate. Treatment related changes, including radiotherapy-induced changes, add another level of complexity to the interpretation of the brain images which remains challenging notwithstanding the increased utilization of advanced imaging methodologies. Previous studies suggest that nearly half of glioblastoma multiforme (GBM) patients with radiological deterioration after standard chemoradiation do not suffer from tumor recurrence but from pseudoprogression induced by the treatment [1–8]. Treatment decision, as whether to operate on a patient with radiographic deterioration, continue chemoradiation or change to another non-surgical treatment is a daily struggle involving interdisciplinary teams of neurosurgeons, neuro-oncologists and neuro-radiologists which are often unable to reach unanimous interpretation of the patient's status. Therefore, reliable distinction between these conditions is essential for appropriate patient management and for appropriate patient selection for clinical trials [9–13].

It has been previously suggested [14–16] that the histological tumor fraction (i.e., tumor burden) comprises a subcomponent of the total enhancement seen on contrast-enhanced MRI and represents a potentially useful predictor of survival in patients with recurrent brain tumors. In fact, studies suggest that histological quantification of tumor burden provides more meaningful prognostic information than simply reporting the presence of tumor [17–18].

Brain metastases are the most common intracranial tumor in adults, occurring in approximately 10% to 30% of adult cancer patients. It is believed that the annual incidence is rising (due to better treatment of systemic disease and improved imaging modalities). The prognosis of patients diagnosed with brain metastases is generally poor.

Stereotactic radiosurgery (SRS) is a radiotherapy technique which permits the delivery of a single large dose of radiation to the tumor while minimizing irradiation of adjacent normal tissue. It is applied to treat both benign and malignant tumors as well as for vascular lesions and functional disorders. Among the reported complications of SRS is radiation-induced necrosis which, similarly to pseudoprogression, can be difficult to differentiate both clinically and radiologically from recurrent tumor at the treatment site. The incidence of radiation induced necrosis may vary between 5% to 11% according to the volume of the treated lesion and the applied dose [19].

The difficulty in interpretation of these post treatment images prevents appropriate treatment in nearly half of treated GBM patients and 5–11% of treated brain metastases patients [1–8,19]. The ability to clearly differentiate tumor from non-tumoral tissues is crucial for appropriate patient management in GBM and brain metastases as well as in other brain tumors undergoing surgery, chemotherapy and/or radiation therapy.

Conventional MRI is currently unable to provide reliable distinction between tumor progression and treatment effects such as pseudoprogression and radiation necrosis [9–11]. MRS can distinguish residual or recurrent tumors from pure treatment-related necrosis, but not from mixed necrosis and tumor tissue [20]. Diffusion weighted MRI (DWMRI) and diffusion-tensor MRI has also been assessed for differentiating tumor/necrosis after RT [21–26], however, the specificity of DWMRI is less than MRS. It has been suggested that combining DWMRI with MRS may improve the differentiation [27]. FDG-PET has been shown to be useful in differentiating necrosis from recurrence, but the reported sensitivity and specificity of FDG PET in the brain are low [28]. There is limited, but increasing evidence that PET with amino acid tracers may contribute to the differentiation between treatment-related necrosis from tumor recurrence [29]. Whether these techniques will also allow a reliable distinction between pseudoprogression and real progression is yet to be determined.

A number of fast acquisition MRI techniques have been applied to study microvasculature parameters in this context. The two most commonly used methods are dynamic contrast-enhanced MRI (DCE MRI) and dynamic susceptibility-weighted contrast MRI (DSC MRI) [30–32]. DCE MRI measures the changes in T1 relaxation associated with disrupted BBB following contrast administration using parameters such as fractional blood volume (fBV) and permeability (Kps or Ktrans). DSC MRI uses echo planar sequences with a rapid bolus of gadolinium-based contrast agents to assess changes in T2* within the vasculature and interstitial space. Typical calculated parameters are the relative peak height (rPH), relative cerebral blood volume (rCBV) and the percentage recovery (%REC) or recirculation factor (RF).

Parametric maps that are derived from DCE and DSC data have been proposed as noninvasive methods for assessing response to therapy. Treatment induced changes typically shows decreased rCBV, whereas recurrence shows high rCBV [33–39]. Still, most of these studies show some degree of overlap between the two disease entities. DSC was recently applied by Gahramanov et al [40] which demonstrated the feasibility for differentiating pseudoprogression from real tumor progression using ferumoxytol. Narang et al [41] applied DCE to a cohort of 29 patients with gliomas and brain metastasis suspected for treatment-induced necrosis or recurrent/progressive tumor and demonstrated the feasibility of predicting real progression. Barajas et al [42] applied DSC MRI for differentiating tumor progression from radiation necrosis in GBM patients undergoing external beam radiation therapy. Their analysis showed that rPH and rCBV were significantly higher in patients with recurrent GBM than in patients with radiation necrosis while the %REC values were significantly lower.

Using fast acquisition techniques has the disadvantages of low spatial resolution and high sensitivity to susceptibility artifacts. Due to these limitations, significant results are mostly obtained by averaging over the entire enhancing lesion while important information regarding the location and shape of small active tumor regions may be limited. This effect stands out especially in the case of GBM, where psuedoprogression hardly ever describes a status with no residual tumor (unlike the case of brain metastases and radiation necrosis where complete tumor resolution is more likely to occur), as we know that the vast majority of all GBM patients, including those experiencing pseudoprogression, eventually recur.

More encouraging results were obtained using delayed T1-weighted MRI (T1-MRI) permeability methods, which image beyond the first pass circulation of contrast, sometimes as long as 10–15 min. Hazle et al were able to reliably distinguish between recurrence, radiation necrosis, and a combination of both factors [43]. They found that radiation necrosis and tumor enhance at different rates, enabling significant differentiation between recurrent tumor, radiation necrosis and mixed radiation necrosis and tumor ($p<0.001$). Diehn et al [44] showed that using intra-tumoral and peri-tumoral MRI information it was possible to predict activation of hypoxia and proliferation gene-expression programs, respectively. Furthermore, the intratumoral distribution of gene-expression patterns was found to predict patient outcome.

In the current study we apply a novel methodology based on delayed contrast extravasation MRI for calculating delayed enhancement subtraction maps, depicting unique temporal enhancement characteristics with high resolution and high sensitivity to subtle BBB disruption [45]. In order to confirm the application of our maps for differentiating tumor tissues from non tumoral tissues we compared pre-surgical maps of patients with primary or metastatic brain tumors with histological assessment of resected tissue samples.

Materials and Methods

Patients and Treatment

The study was conducted after approval of the local ethics committee at Sheba Medical Center. Written informed consent was obtained from all patients.

Ten patients with primary brain tumors and 10 patients with brain metastases were recruited prior to surgery and scanned by conventional and delayed contrast extravasation MRI. In all 20 patients pre-surgical delayed enhancement subtraction maps were compared with histological findings. In addition, the application of our maps for prediction of progression was studied in a small cohort of 13 newly diagnosed GBM patients undergoing standard chemoradiation and followed up to 19.7 months post therapy.

Table 1. Biopsied samples and map characteristics.

Sample #	Patient #	delayed enhancement population	Histological description	Tumor type
1	1	Mixed regions of red, blue and green populations	One cellular region consisted of small cells with no mitoses. Proliferation was seen in 5% of the cells by Ki67 staining, implying active tumor. Other regions showed post radiation changes. One region was of brain parenchyma with no obvious abnormalities	GBM post chemoradiation
2	1	Cortical region of blue population and deeper white matter region of red population	Subcortical infiltrating zone of active tumor with rare mitosis and a deeper, white matter region of post radiation changes. Ki67 staining of the active tumor zone showed proliferation in 3–5% of the cells	GBM post chemoradiation
3	1	Region of blue population	Active tumor consisting of a hypercellular area of small cells. Ki67 staining showed proliferation in 10–12% of the cells	GBM post chemoradiation
4	1	Mixed regions of blue and red populations	Regions of active tumor consisting of a hypercellular area of small cells and regions of post radiation changes. Ki67 staining in the active tumor region showed proliferation in 10–12% of the cells	GBM post chemoradiation
1	4	Region of red population	Radiation necrosis	GBM post chemoradiation
2	4	Cortical region of blue population and white matter region of red population	Cortical region shows active tumor accumulating focally beneath the meninges. Focal proliferation of blood vassals and palisading necrosis are identified as well. Most of the deeper white matter region show radiation necrosis	GBM post chemoradiation
1	11	Region of blue population	Highly cellular tumor with small regions of tumor necrosis with and without pseudo palisading regions of proliferating blood cells	Secondary GBM post chemoradiation
2	11	Region of blue population	Highly cellular tumor	Secondary GBM post chemoradiation
3	11	Region of blue population	Highly cellular tumor with small regions of tumor necrosis with and without pseudo palisading regions of proliferating blood cells	Secondary GBM post chemoradiation
4	11	Region of blue population	Highly cellular tumor with large proliferating vessels and small regions of tumor necrosis with palisading regions of proliferating blood cells	Secondary GBM post chemoradiation
1	13	Region of blue population	Tumor consisting of atypical cells, mitoses and proliferating vessels	Newly diagnosed GBM
1	14	Region of blue population	Tumor consisting of atypical cells and numerous mitoses	GBM post chemoradiation
2	14	Border between a red region and a blue region	A region of necrosis with scanty nuclear dust and a region of tumor with pleomorphism and small regions of palisading necrosis	GBM post chemoradiation
1	16	Border between a red region and a blue region	Necrotic region including necrotic blood vessels and nuclear dust and a cellular tumor region with atypical cells, mitoses and vascular proliferation	Newly diagnosed GBM
2	16	Region of blue population	Tumor region with small foci of palisading necrosis	Newly diagnosed GBM
1	17	Region of blue population	Highly cellular tumor with small necrotic foci	Newly diagnosed GBM
1	19	Region of blue population	Regions of high cellularity and of low cellularigy typical of oligodendroglioma tumors	Newly diagnosed analplastic oligodendroglioma
1	20	Region of red population on the border of a blue population	Mostly necrotic tissue including necrotic blood vessels. Small foci of tumor are present	Newly diagnosed analplastic oligodendroglioma
2	20	Region of blue population on the border of a red population	Most of the tissue is tumor. One small area of necrosis at the periphery of the section	Newly diagnosed analplastic oligodendroglioma
3	20	Region of blue population on the border of surrounding brain	Mostly tumor tissue bordered by brain tissue infiltrated by tumor	Newly diagnosed analplastic oligodendroglioma
1	21Metastasis #1	Sample taken from a blue region bordered by a green region on one side and a red region on the other	A sample showing a region of morphological active tumor bordered by normal cerebellum tissue on one side and necrotic tissue on the other	Sample taken from NSCLC cerebellar brain metastasis
2	21Metastasis #1	Sample taken from a red region bordered by a blue region	A sample showing a large necrotic region borders by tumor	Sample taken from NSCLC cerebellar brain metastasis

Table 1. Cont.

Sample #	Patient #	delayed enhancement population	Histological description	Tumor type
1	27	Mixed area of blue and red regions	A mixture of active tumor regions and necrotic regions	Sample taken from NSCLC cortical brain metastasis
2	27	Blue region with small red foci on the border of surrounding brain	Several small samples of active tumor, tumor necrosis and edematous brain	Sample taken from NSCLC cortical brain metastasis
1	29	Red region on the border of surrounding brain	Radiation induced gliotic brain tissue	Sample taken from breast cerebellar brain metastasis
2	29	Mixed blue and red region on the border of surrounding brain	cerebral tissue and mixed regions of tumor and radiation necrosis	Sample taken from breast cerebral brain metastasis
3	29	Mixed blue, green and red regions	tumor, cerebral tissue and radiation necrosis with ecstatic blood vessels	Sample taken from breast cerebral brain metastasis
4	29	A red region bordered by surrounding brain on one side and a blue region on the other	Gliotic brain and radiation necrosis with a small tumor mass	Sample taken from breast cerebral brain metastasis
1	30	Red region surrounded by a blue rim	small regions of tumor (~30% of the sample) within larger region of necorosis (~70% of the sample)	Sample taken from breast cortical brain metastasis
2	30	Blue region on the border of surrounding brain	small tumoral region on the border of normal cortex	Sample taken from breast cortical brain metastasis
3	30	Blue region on the border of surrounding brain	Highly cellular tumor adjacent to normal cortex	Sample taken from breast cortical brain metastasis
4	30	Red region bordered by small blue region on one side and surrounding brain on the other	mostly necrosis with small foci of tumor and adjacent normal brain	Sample taken from breast cortical brain metastasis

List of 32 biopsied samples, delayed enhancement subtraction map characteristics and histological evaluation of 9 patients with primary brain tumors and 4 patients with brain metastases.

Primary Brain Tumors Group

The primary brain tumor patients consisted of 8 patients with histologically confirmed glioblastoma (World Health Organization [WHO] grade IV astrocytoma) of which 3 were newly diagnosed patients, 4 progressed following chemoradiation (60 Gy in 30 daily fractions, 5 days a week, with concomitant daily temozolomide of 75 mg/m^2 for 42 days. Chemoradiation was followed by adjuvant temozolomide of 150–200 mg/m^2 daily for 5 days every 28 days.) and one patient with secondary GBM was recruited 2 years after resection of an Anaplastic Astrocytoma (WHO grade III tumor) and chemoradiation. Two patients with newly diagnosed Anaplastic Oligodendrioma (WHO grade III tumor) were recruited as well.

The mean age of this group of patients was 58.6±3.6 with a range of 37–80. Nine of the 10 patients were men.

Brain Metastases Group

The brain metastases patients consisted of 4 patients with breast cancer metastases, 4 with non small cell lung cancer (NSCLC) metastases, 1 with malignant melanoma metastases and 1 patient with adenoid cystic carcinoma metastases. All patients were treated with a single dose of 18–20 Gy (to the 80% isodose line) LINAC based SRS 13.1±2.9 months prior to resection.

The mean age of this group of patients was 50.2±4.0 with a range of 30–67. Four of the 10 patients were men.

Newly Diagnosed GBM Group

In an attempt to explore additional possible applications of our calculated maps, 13 newly diagnosed GBM patients were scanned by conventional and delayed extravasation MRI 3–4 weeks after chemoradiation and every 2 months thereafter. Patients with clinical deterioration underwent additional MRI exams at the discretion of the physician. These patients were followed for 2–19.7 months. Eight of the later have progressed while 5 remained progression free.

The mean age of this group of patients was 54.3±4.1 with a range of 28–72. Eight of the 13 patients were men.

Inclusion criteria for all patients included WHO performance status of 2 or less and adequate hematologic, renal, and hepatic function. Exclusion criteria included contraindications to MRI and stable condition to undergo an MRI exam.

MRI Data Acquisition

MR images were acquired using a clinical General Electric 3.0 T MRI machine (GE Medical Systems, Waukesha, WI, USA) with the HD12 operating system, gradients intensity of up to 4.3 Gauss/cm and the standard GE phased array head-coil. MR sequences included T2* perfusion-weighted MRI (PWI), Fast spin-echo T2-weighted MRI, T2 FLAIR and echo-planar diffusion-weighted MRI (DWMRI). High resolution spin-echo T1-weighted MR images (T1-MRIs) were acquired before and at 3 time points after contrast injection: 2.6±0.1 min (immediately after the PWI sequence), 15.4±0.4 min and 75.3±0.7 on average. These times are referred to as the 2 min, 15 min and 75 min time points throughout the text. In order to minimize the burden on the patients, they were scanned up to 30 min after contrast injection, and were then asked to return for a short scan 75 min after contrast injection. T1-MRI was acquired with TE/TR = 22/240 ms, field of view 26×19.5 cm, 5/0.5 mm slice thickness and 512×512 pixels. A standard single dose (0.2 ml/Kg) of Gd-DOTA (Dotarem, 0.5 mmol/mL, Guerbet, 95943 Roissy CdG Cedex, France) was injected intravenously using an automatic injection system 6 seconds after starting the PWI sequence.

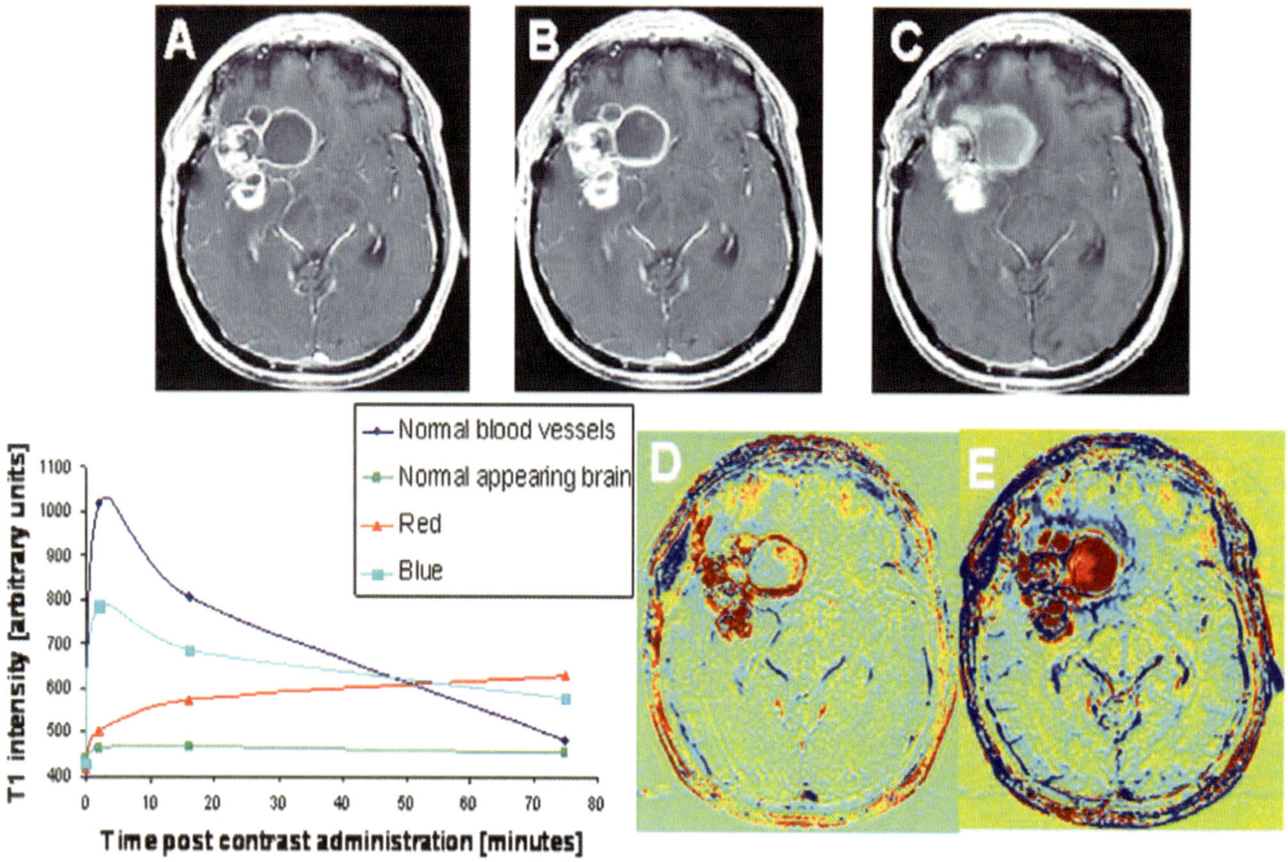

Figure 1. Enhancement subtraction maps. Examples of axial high resolution T1-weighted MR images acquired 2 min (A), 15 min (B) and 75 min (C) after contrast administration in a patient (#3) with newly diagnosed GBM undergoing standard chemoradiation are shown. Subtraction maps were calculated from the data acquired at 2 and 15 min (D) and 2 and 75 min (E) post contrast administration. Blue regions represent fast clearance of the contrast agent from the tumor while red regions represent slow accumulation of the contrast in the tissue. It can be seen that abnormal enhancement patterns in the 75 min map are depicted more clearly and over larger regions than in the 15 min map. The signal intensity of regions with different enhancement patterns as a function of time post contrast administration is shown in the plot. It can be seen that the red and blue components of the tumor enhance and decay at different rates.

MRI Data Analysis

All image analysis was performed using MatLab (version R2006b, The MathWorks, Inc. Natick, MA, US).

The overall goal of the analysis was to obtain delayed subtraction maps, where the T1-MRIs of the 1st series post contrast were subtracted from the T1-MRIs of later series. These maps depict spatial distribution of contrast accumulation/clearance in the tissue, blood vessels and CSF. For example, in case of normal blood vessels, due to clearance of contrast agent from the blood system, there is no increase in contrast accumulation in the late scans; therefore, the subtraction maps show negative values (blue in the maps). The signal decay of the blood vessels is faster than that of the tissue (where the signal is averaged over the tissue and microvasculature), therefore, blood vessels have lower values than tissue. In case of contrast accumulation, i.e. regions where contrast clearance is slower than contrast accumulation, the maps show positive values (red in the maps).

In order to increase the sensitivity to small changes it was essential to perform image pre-processing consisting of corrections for intensity variations and whole body image registration.

Correcting for intensity variations. Signal intensity homogeneity throughout the image and between slices depends on various parameters including: strength and homogeneity of the static magnetic field, oscillating excitation field, gradients, sensitivity of the receiving coil and various parameters of the sampled tissue. An intensity correction was performed on each image separately by calculating an intensity variation map consisting of the large scale intensity variations. The later map was then subtracted from the original image.

Rigid body and elastic/local registration. Rigid body registration was performed using least squares approach and 6 parameter (rigid body) spatial transformation with the SPM5 (Statistical parametric mapping) MatLab routine (an academic software kit by "Wellcome Trust Centre for Neuroimaging"). Since head movements affected the magnetic fields thus inducing distortions in the MRIs, it was necessary to add local/elastic registration. The registration was performed by dividing each slice to a grid of 20×20 mm volumes. Each square volume was allowed to move freely in x-y-z till the sum of the absolute values of the intensity difference between the 2 time points reached a minimum. The resulting three 3D translation matrices were smoothed using circular smearing and interpolated to obtain translation values per pixel. These high resolution matrices were then applied to register T1-MRIs of the second time point to the location of the first time point.

Subtraction maps. Following the pre-processing, subtraction maps were calculated by simply subtracting the processed images

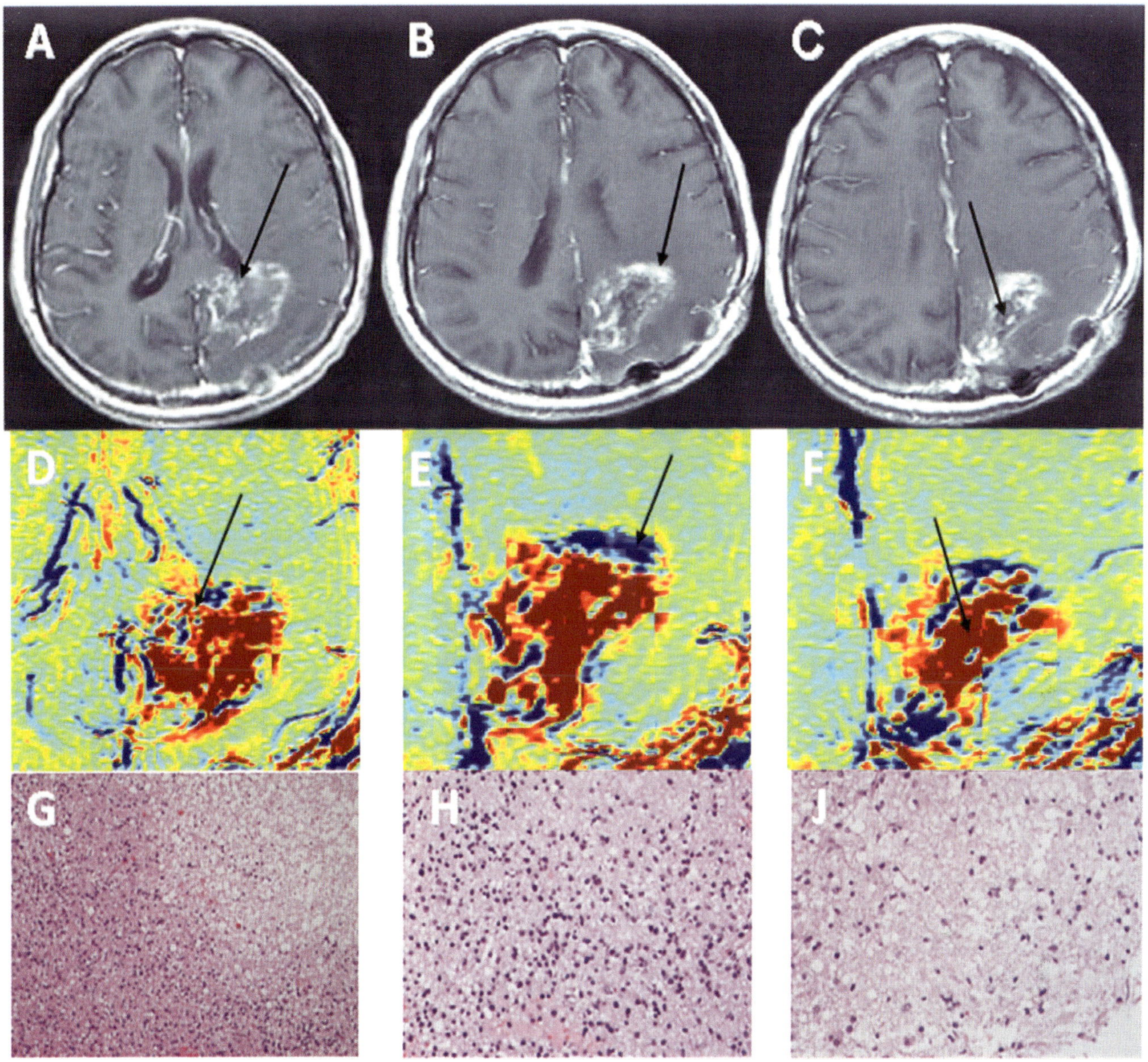

Figure 2. Histological determination of tumor and non-tumoral components – GBM. Examples of contrast-enhanced T1-weighted MRI (A–C), enhancement subtraction maps calculated from the 2 and 75 min data (D–F) and H&E stained histological samples of a rapidly growing lesion in patient #1 with newly diagnosed GBM undergoing standard chemoradiation are shown. Data was acquired prior to surgery, 6 months after initiation of treatment. Samples were taken from a mixed blue and red region (A, D, arrows), a blue region (B, E, arrows) and a red region (C, F, arrows). Histological analysis reveals mixed regions of tumor and necrosis (G, magnification ×200), hypercellular tumor (H, magnification ×400) and radiation necrosis (J, magnification ×400), respectively.

of the series acquired 2 min after the contrast injection from a series acquired later on.

Enhancing lesion volume. The enhancing portion of the lesions, depicted on conventional contrast-enhanced MRI, was calculated from the spin-echo contrast-enhanced T1-MRIs acquired 2 min after contrast injection. Regions of interest (ROIs) were defined over the entire enhancing region in each slice. A threshold, determined from intensity distribution histograms of the tumor and surrounding regions, was applied to the ROIs to include only enhancing portions of the tumor. The number of pixels in the enhancing portions of the ROIs were counted and multiplied by the volume of a single pixel. The resulting volume was referred to as the state of the art parameter for assessment of tumor volume [12].

Histology

A total of 32 stereotactic tissue samples and 8 resected lesions acquired from 10 patients with primary brain tumors and 10 patients with brain metastases were histologically examined and compared with our delayed enhancement subtraction maps. Stereotactic locations for tissue samples were determined prior to surgery using the calculated subtraction maps which were co-registered to the conventional T1-MRIs, for 9 patients with primary brain tumors (20 tissue samples) and 4 patients with metastatic tumors (12 tissue samples) (Table 1). Existence/absence

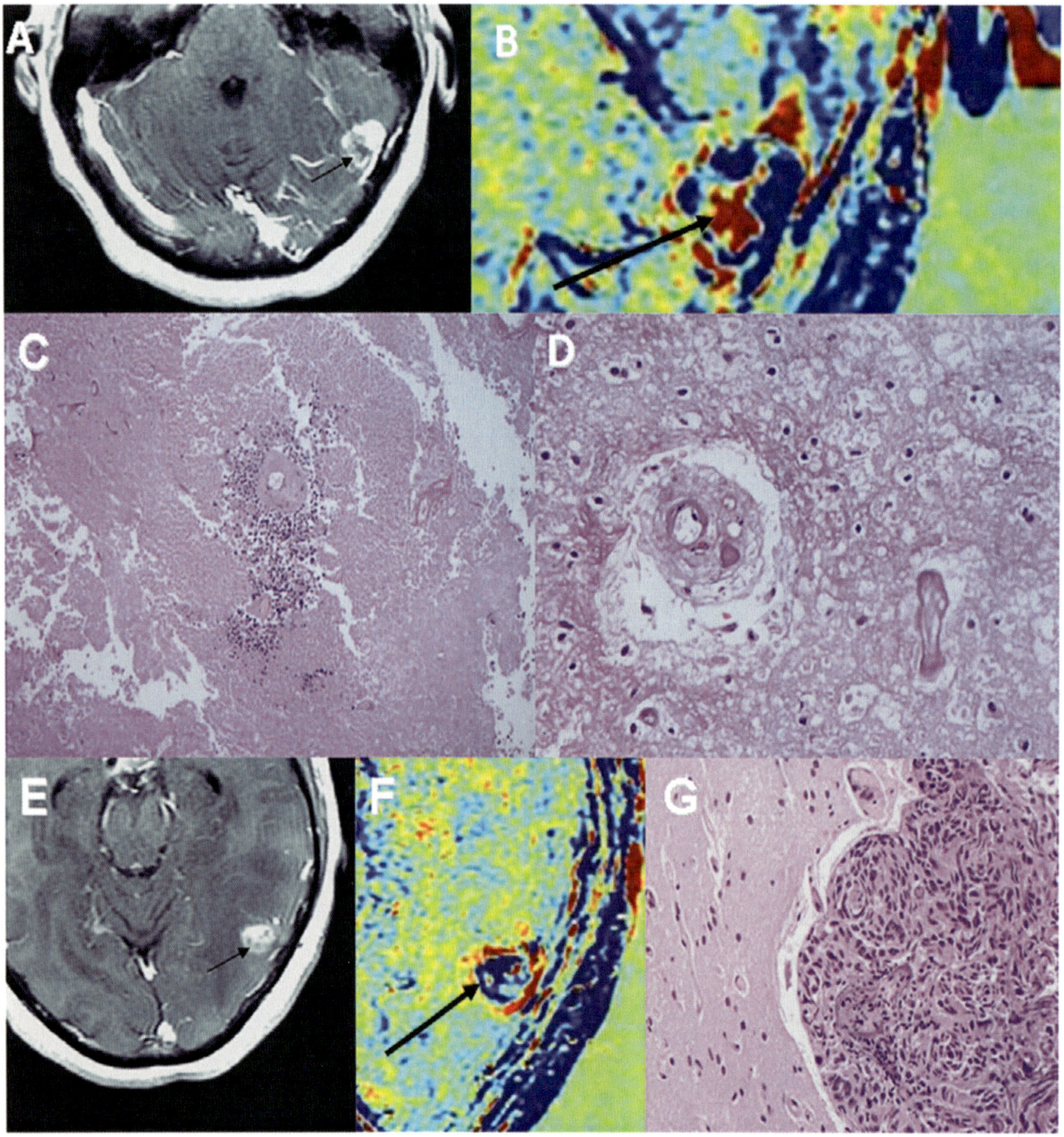

Figure 3. Histological determination of tumor and non-tumoral components – brain metastases. Examples of contrast-enhanced T1-weighted MRI (A, E), enhancement subtraction maps calculated from the 2 and 75 min data (B, F) and H&E stained histological samples (C, D, G) of a cortical breast cancer brain metastasis of patient #30, 2 years post radiosurgery, are shown. Sample #4 taken from a red region marked by arrows in A and B shows a small tumor foci, surrounding a viable blood vessel, within a larger region of necrosis (magnification x100). An example of necrotic blood vessels within the necrotic region (x400) is shown in D. Sample #3 taken from a blue region on the border of normal brain marked by arrows in E and F shows a highly cellular tumor adjacent to normal cortex (G, x200).

of morphologically active tumor in the histological analysis of 8 metastatic tumors acquired from 7 patients was compared with the pre-surgical maps as well (Table 2). Eight additional samples were obtained from one GBM patient, chosen by the neurosurgeon during surgery as representative samples (patient #3, Table 2).

All samples were marked by the neurosurgeon during resection and then fixed and stained by H&E according to the routine hospital procedure.

Histological interpretation was performed by the hospital neuro-pathologist. Morphologically active tumor was defined as demonstrating one or more of the following characteristics: hyper

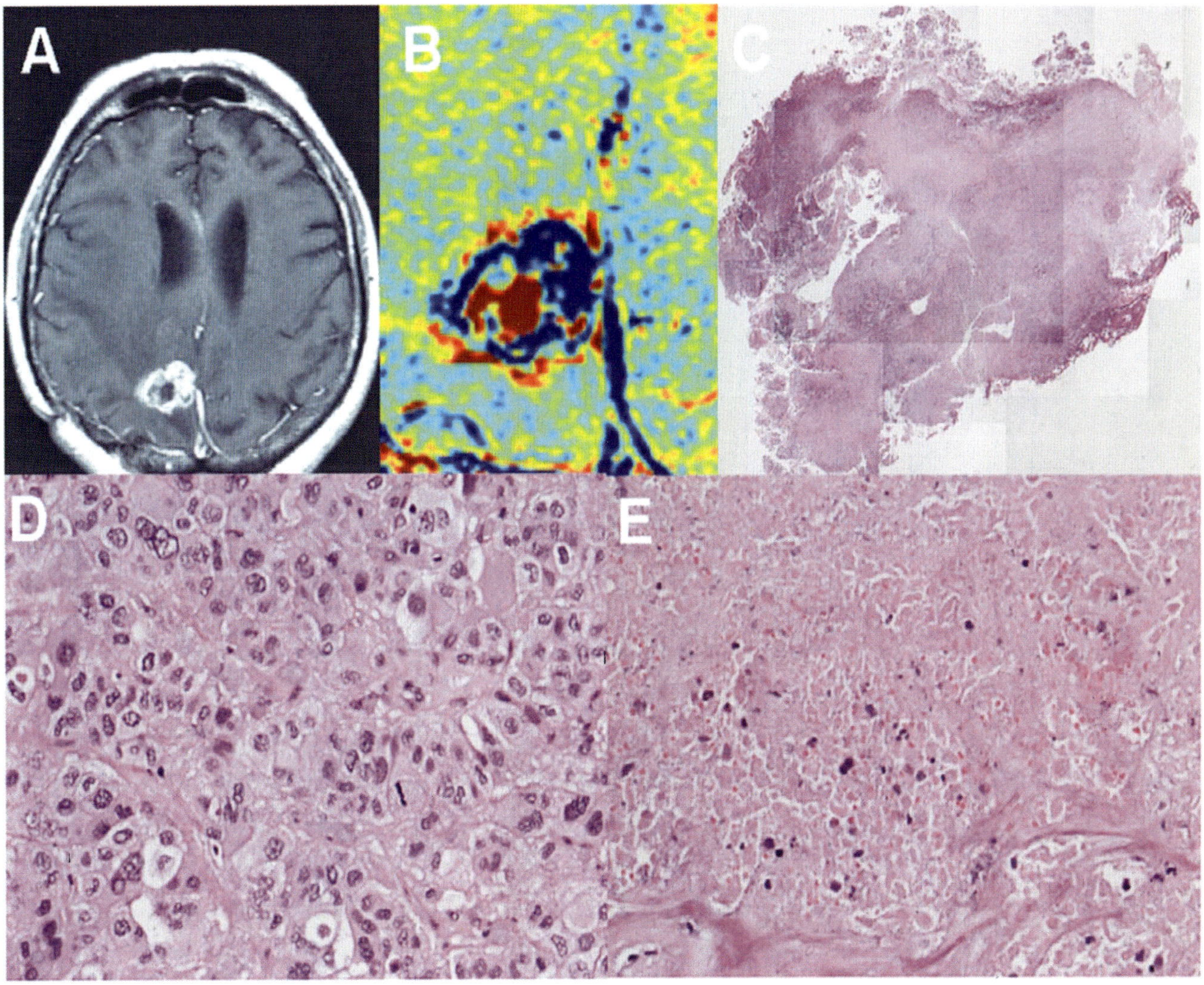

Figure 4. Histological determination of tumor and non-tumoral components – brain metastases. Examples of contrast-enhanced T1-weighted MRI (A), enhancement subtraction map calculated from the 2 and 75 min data (B), macro H&E stained histological sample (C, magnification x20), tumor region from a peripheral region of the sample (D, magnification x400) and radiation necrosis from the central region of the sample (E, magnification x400) of a medial NSCLC brain metastasis of patient #23 (metastasis #1), 1 year post radiosurgery, are shown. The metastasis was resected unblock and marked by the neurosurgeon to enable comparison with the MRI data. H&E staining shows a large central necrotic region surrounded by a rim of morphologically active tumoral tissue, in agreement with the subtraction map. It is also possible to see part of a necrotic blood vessel in the region of radiation necrosis (E) and scattered blood cells in the tissue.

cellularity, small cells, mitosis, high Ki67, pseudo-palisading necrosis and vascular proliferation.

Non-tumoral abnormal tissue was defined as demonstrating one or more of the following characteristics: radiation changes including large, widely spaced atypical astrocytes, blood vessels hyalinization, fibrinoid material in vessels, proliferating small vessels and non palisading tumor necrosis.

Progression (GBM Patients Only)

Disease progression was diagnosed using standard MRI sequences. Each case was presented to the hospital tumor board, consisting of a neuro-oncologist, a neurosurgeon and a neuro-radiologist. The physicians were blinded to the delayed enhancement subtraction maps so that progression was diagnosed according to the RANO (revised Mcdonald's) criteria. When disease progression was determined, the patient's treatment was changed (surgery or Bevacizumab). The time from the first MRI follow-up to disease progression is listed for all patients in Table 3. In those patients with no disease progression, the time of the last follow-up was listed.

Time to Progression (TTP) (GBM Patients Only)

TTP was defined as the time from the end of chemoradiation till progression was determined.

Tumor Growth Rate (GBM Patients Only)

The feasibility of applying the delayed enhancement subtraction maps for prediction of TTP was demonstrated by studying the correlation between initial tumor growth rate and TTP. Initial tumor growth was calculated as $(V-Vo)/Vo$, where V was the tumor volume at the second follow-up and Vo was the tumor volume calculated from the first follow-up MRI (3 weeks after the end of treatment). Initial tumor growth rate was calculated by

Table 2. Non-biopsied tumors histology and map characteristics.

Patient #	delayed enhancement population	Histological description*	Tumor type
3	Overall enhancing lesion consists of 71% blue population and 22% red population	Cellular tumor with many mitoses and regions of "geographic necrosis". In some regions of the tumor it is also possible to see proliferative blood vesselsSome regions surrounding the tumor (not in all slices and not all around the tumor) depict brain tissue infiltrated by a small number of tumor cells. The main findings in these regions around the tumor are abnormal proliferation of blood vessels and many histiocytes	GBM post chemoradiation
21 Metastasis #2	lesion consisting of blue (58%) regions and red (31%) regions	Metastatic carcinoma showing squamoid features with extensive areas of tumor necrosis	NSCLC cortical brain metastasis
22	lesion consisting of blue (56%) regions and red (35%) regions	Several samples showing regions of tumor and regions of radiation necrosis. Significant cauterize artifacts are noticed as well	Adenoid Cystic Carcinoma Cortical brain metastasis
23 Metastasis #1	Metastasis consisting of a central red (42%) region surrounded by a thick blue rim (47%)	Central slice shows a large necrotic region surrounded by significant regions of morphologically active tumor	NSCLC mediall brain metastasis Pathology report addressing metastases resected unblock
23 Metastasis #2	lesion consisting of blue (56%) regions and red (33%) regions	Morphologically active tumor is present in the histological samples	NSCLC cortical brain metastasis
24	lesion consisting of a large blue (56%) region surrounded by a red rim (34%)	Active tumor was found	Melanoma midline brain metastasis
25	lesion consisting of a blue central region (61%) surrounded by a red (33%) region	Active tumor was found	Breast cortical brain metastasis
26	lesion consisting of thin blue rim (40%) within a larger red (51%) mass	Large mass of radiation necrosis. Small foci of active tumor were found after ki67 staining	Breast peri-ventricular brain metastasis
28	lesion is mostly red (53%) with small elongated blue regions (27%)	Mostly necrotic samples with small foci of active tumor	NSCLC medial brain metastasis

List of tumors with no stereotactic biopsies, delayed enhancement subtraction map characteristics and histological evaluation of 1 patient with primary brain tumor and 7 patients with brain metastases.
*Pathology report is based on all samples obtain from the neurosurgeons unrelated to the pre-surgical maps.

dividing the tumor growth by the time that passed between the first and second MRI follow-ups.

Statistical Methods

Results for averaging over a group of values are presented as average±standard error. Correlations were assessed by performing t tests and calculating two-tailed p-values, unless otherwise stated. Prediction of TTP was assessed using the logrank test [46]. In view of the small number of patients involved, the p-values were calculated based on the permutation distribution [47]. In this method one calculates the logrank statistic for each possible allocation of the patients to the two predictor groups "high" and "low" preserving the number of patients in each group, and then calculates the p-value as the proportion of allocations that yield a logrank statistic equal to or higher than the one observed with the study data.

Results

Delayed Enhancement Subtraction Maps

Enhancement subtraction maps were calculated using the data acquired 15 (15 min maps) and 75 min (75 min maps) after contrast injection. Two primary enhancement patterns were found in our maps: One characterized by slower contrast clearance than contrast accumulation at the delayed time point relative to the 2 min time point (positive signal, colored red in our maps) and the other by faster clearance than accumulation (negative signal, colored blue in our maps). Normal brain regions, due to the intensity variation correction, had an average value of zero (green). Examples of 15 and 75 min maps are shown in Figure 1. It can be seen that the fast (blue) region in the 75 min map is depicted more clearly and over larger regions than in the 15 min map. Examples of the signals intensities of the fast and slow regions as a function of time after contrast injection are shown as well, demonstrating the different rates of contrast accumulation and clearance of these regions.

Histology, Tumor Versus Non Tumoral Tissues

Thirty two stereotactic samples acquired from 9 patients with primary brain tumors and 4 patients with brain metastases undergoing surgery were compared with our pre-surgery calculated maps. The samples were taken from fast (blue) regions according to the maps, slow (red) regions, and regions consisting of mixed fast and slow components. Histological evaluation confirmed for all samples the discrimination between fast regions, determined to consist of morphologically active tumor, and slow regions, consisting of non-tumoral tissues. Regions consisting of both fast and slow components in the maps consisted of tumor and non-tumoral tissues in the histological samples (Figures 2, 3, 4, Table 1).

Patient #3 (Table 2) with a newly diagnosed GBM underwent a second resection 6 months after chemoradiation due to clinical deterioration. The patient died 10 days post-surgery. The maps calculated from his last MRI scan, showed that the fast component

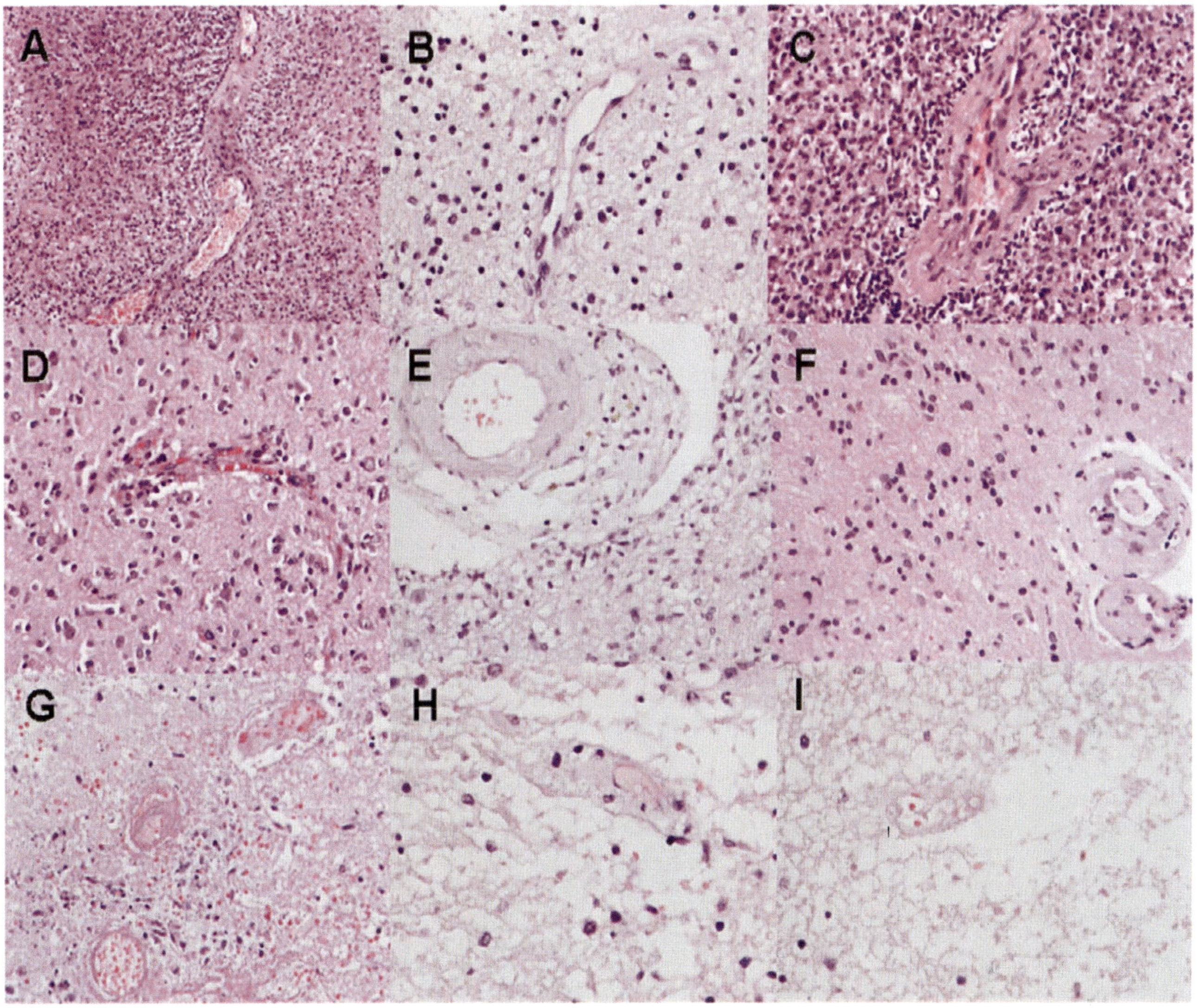

Figure 5. Vessel morphology. Examples of vessel morphology sampled from regions appearing blue in the maps of patients with primary brain tumors are shown in images A–F. Vessels from regions appearing red in the maps are shown in G–I. Samples D and G were taken from patient #4. Samples B, E, H and I were taken from patient #1. A and C were taken from patient #11 and F was taken from patient #13. It can be seen that the samples obtained from blue regions in the maps (A–F) present swollen endothelial cells, dilated lumen, peri-vascular dense fibrous tissue and glomeruloid lumen. Samples taken from red regions in the maps show different stages of vessel necrosis. The vessels shown in G show early necrosis, with scattered blood cells surrounding the necrotic vessels, while the vessels in H and I show later stages of vessel necrosis. The silhouette is reserved and there are residual red blood cells but the endothelial cells are necrotic.

reached 71±3% of the enhancing lesion volume. Histological analysis was performed for 8 samples taken from 2 main regions of the lesion. In both regions the tumor load was estimated by the neuro-pathologist to cover ~70% of the examined samples, in agreement with our calculated maps.

Eight additional metastases acquired from 7 patients, showed a fast component in our maps and were confirmed by histology to consist of morphologically active tumor (Figures 3, 4, Table 2).

Histology, Blood Vessels

In an attempt to find a morphological explanation for the difference between the vessels function of fast and slow regions in our maps, we examined the morphological appearance of blood vessels in these regions. Typical fast population vessel morphology consisted of proliferating endothelial cells, dilated lumen, peri vascular fibrosis and glomeruloid vessels. The outline of the vessels lumens in these regions seemed to be undamaged. Vessels in the slow regions, on the other hand, presented different stages of vessel necrosis with significantly damaged lumens. In most vessels a silhouette of the vessel wall could still be recognized, but only rarely residual endothelial cells could still be detected. In some cases scattered blood cells were seen in various distances from the necrotic vessel. Examples are shown in Figures 3, 4, 5.

Significance of Long Delays

The volumes and intensities of the fast population, calculated from the 75 min maps, were found to be significantly different then those calculated from the 15 min maps (data calculated from 30 MRI exams of the 30 recruited patients): $r=0.91$, $p<0.0001$ and $r=0.79$, $p<0.0001$, respectively (Wilcoxon matched-pairs signed-ranks test). The average ratio between the volumes of the fast population calculated from the 75 min maps and the volumes

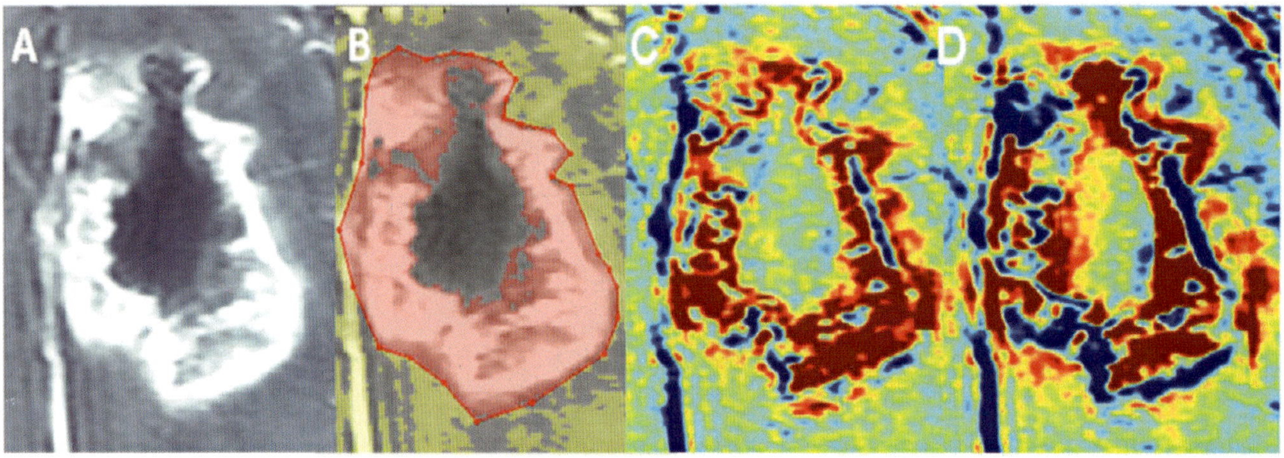

Figure 6. Enhancing lesion volume. Contrast-enhanced T1-weighted MRI without (A) and with (B) a mask selecting the enhancing portion of a GBM tumor (patient #4) are shown. The enhancing lesion volume was calculated from the pixels marked pink in (B). Enhancement subtraction maps calculated at 15 min (C) and 75 min (D) demonstrate the contributions of the red/non-tumor and blue/tumor contributions to the enhancing lesion volume.

calculated from the15 min maps was 2.0 ± 0.3 and the average ratio between the intensities of the fast population at the two time points was 1.8 ± 0.1, suggesting increased sensitivity to tumor tissues at the longer delays. There was no significant difference in this increased sensitivity between the primary brain tumors and the brain metastases groups.

Correlation with Conventional MRI

The volume of the fast population was found to correlate significantly with the enhancing lesion volume (representing the conventional tumor volume): $r=0.94$, $p<0.0001$ (based on 30 acquired MRI exams). According to our maps, in this cohort of patients $48.4\pm1.9\%$ (on average) of the enhancing lesion on conventional MRI **did not** represent morphologically active tumor (Figure 6). For example, according to our maps only 55%, 38%, 39%, 56% and 83% of the enhancing lesions presented in Figures 1, 2, 6, 7A and 7D respectively, consisted of the fast population. There was no significant difference in the average percentage of the fast population between the primary brain tumors and the brain metastases groups.

Significant correlation was also found between fast population volume×intensity and rCBV calculated from PWI ($r=0.69$, $p<0.005$), suggesting that rCBV may be a dominant characteristic of the fast population. Still, the relatively low r value implies that there may be other contributions to the fast component. Examples of agreement and disagreement between the vessel function maps and rCBV are shown in Figure 7.

Correlation with TTP (GBM Patients) – Preliminary Results

In an attempt to explore the feasibility of applying our maps for predicting time to progression 13 newly diagnosed patients were followed by conventional and delayed-contrast extravasation MRI. The follow-up periods of each patient are listed in Table 3. Four parameters were studied as possible predictors for progression: Initial fast volume, initial enhancing volume, initial fast growth rate and initial enhancing growth rate. Kaplan-Meier curves of TTP in patients above and below the median of each predictor are shown in Figure 8. The p values were calculated with the log rank test using the permutation distribution. It can be seen that the initial fast growth rate provides a near-significant difference between the two groups of patients, in contrast to the other predictors, suggesting that this predictor may be a candidate for prediction of TTP. A larger study consisting of more patients and longer follow-ups is required in order to assess the application of our maps for this purpose.

Examples of Progression and Pseudoprogression in GBM Patients Post Chemoradiation

Within the cohort of GBM patients with follow-up, for 7 of the 8 progressing patients, progression was determined in the first MRI follow-up in which significant increase in the fast component volume was noticed. For one patient progression was determined 5 weeks after the increase in the fast component. While an increase in the fast component preceded progression in all patients, significant increase of the enhancing lesion volume was not necessarily followed by progression. An example of a patient who experienced significant increase in the enhancing lesion volume 4.2 months post treatment but remained progression free for an additional 7.4 months is shown in Figure 9A, B, C. An example of a patient who experienced significant increase in the fast volume 6.5 months post treatment (with no significant increase in the enhancing lesion volume) is shown in Figure 9D, E, F. This patient was determined to progress 6.5 months post treatment and underwent surgery.

Discussion

GBM is the most common and most aggressive type of primary brain tumor in humans. The current standard of care for newly diagnosed GBM is surgical resection (when possible) followed by radiotherapy with concomitant and adjuvant temozolomide chemotherapy. The rate of early treatment induced radiological changes which mimic tumor progression – pseudoprogression - increased significantly since the addition of chemotherapy to the treatment regimen. Due to the increasing occurrence of brain metastases and the expending use of radiosurgery to treat them, the rate of treatment-induced radiation necrosis is rising as well. Conventional MR imaging is currently unable to provide reliable distinction between tumor recurrence and treatment effects.

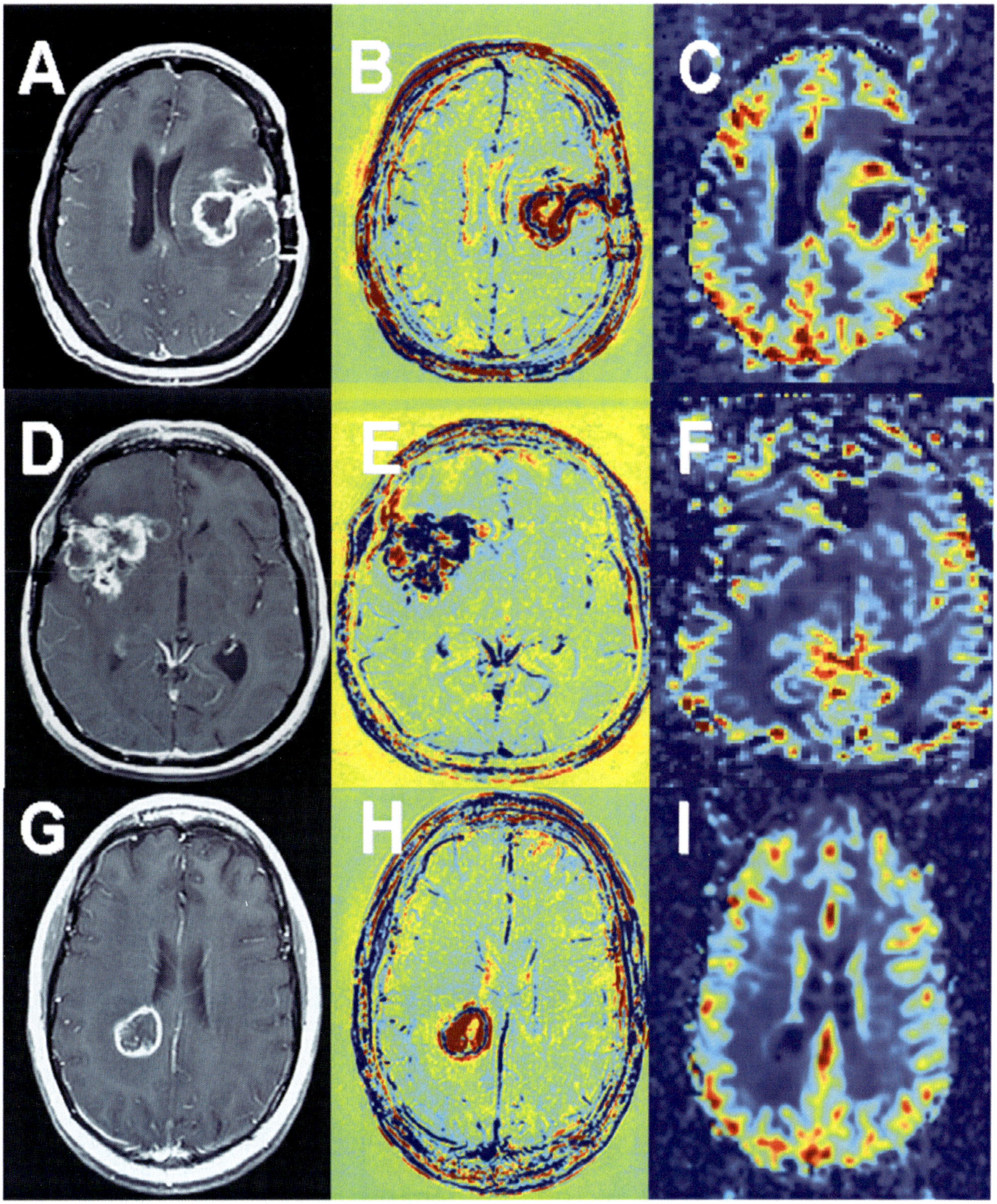

Figure 7. Comparison with rCBV. Contrast-enhanced T1-weighted MRI (A, D, G), enhancement subtraction maps (B, E, H) and rCBV maps (C, F, I) of patients # 6 (A–C), #3 (D–F) and #26 (G–I) are shown. Patient #6 (GBM) shows a blue rim surrounding the surgery site, representing morphologically active tumor, in agreement with high rCBV values in the corresponding rCBV map. Patient #3 (GBM) is a contradicting example, showing a massive lesion dominated by the blue population in the subtraction maps (confirmed by histology to consist of ~70% morphologically active tumor), in contrast to low rCBV values in the corresponding rCBV map. Patient #26 (breast cancer brain metastases) shows a thin rim of the blue populations in our maps in agreement with a thin rim of increased rCBV values. The advantages of our vessel function maps over rCBV acquired using DSC in means of high resolution, high sensitivity to contrast and minimum sensitivity to susceptibility artifacts can be seen.

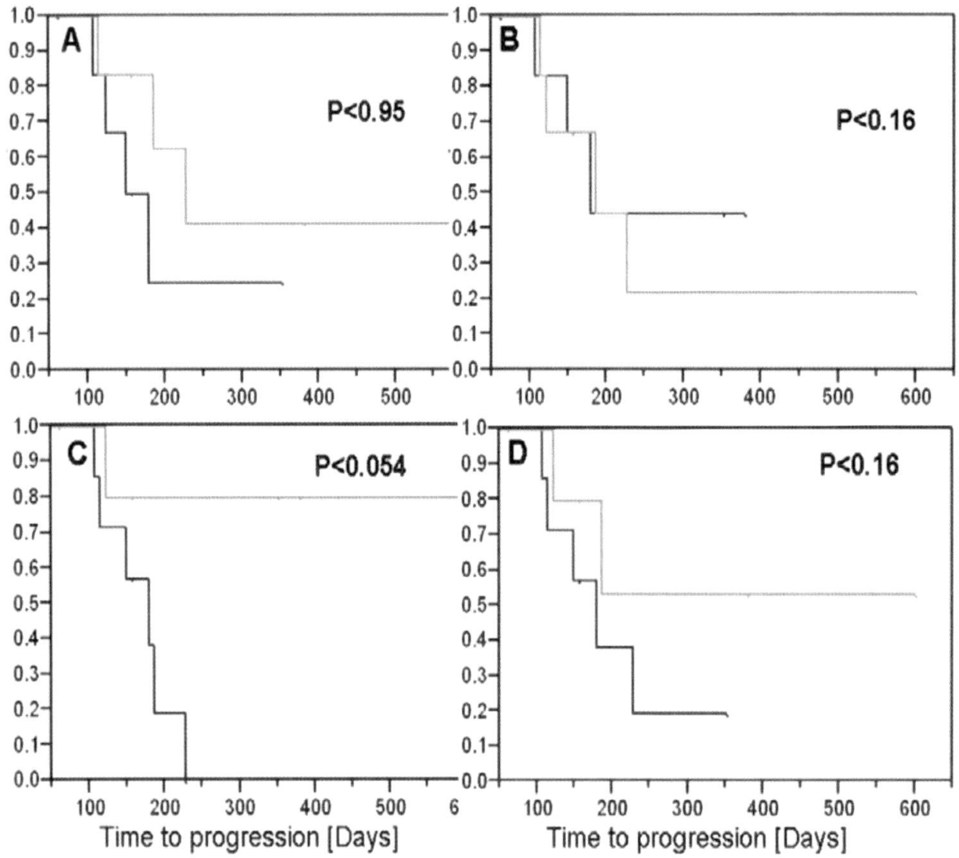

Figure 8. Correlation with time to progression. The correlation between the late enhancement subtraction maps and time to progression was studied in a small cohort of 13 GBM patients post chemoradiation. Kaplan-Meier curves of time to progression in patients above and below the median of four predictors are shown: Initial fast volume (A), initial enhanced volume (B), initial fast growth rate (C) and initial enhanced growth rate (D). The curves are plotted for each predictor for patients above (black) and below (gray) the median. It can be seen that the initial fast growth rate predictor provides a near-significant difference between the two groups of patients, suggesting this predictor may be a candidate for prediction of time to progression.

Clinically, this question has important consequences; therefore, a reliable distinction between these conditions is crucial.

A significant advantage of using the delayed enhancement and clearance rates instead of the commonly studied early rates (DCE and DSC) is the ability to apply sequences with lower temporal resolution, such as high resolution spin-echo T1-MRI. These sequences nearly completely avoid susceptibility artifacts while providing high signal-to-noise ratios, high resolution and high sensitivity to contrast variations. By measuring the clearance of the contrast agent from the tissue at these long delays it is reasonable to assume that the sensitivity to physiological parameters is increased, providing additional information unattainable when using short acquisition times. This assumption is supported by the two fold increase in sensitivity to tumoral (fast) tissue obtained by increasing the delay from 15 to 75 minutes. In this context it is important to note that the patients are not held in the scanner for these long times. The patients are scanned for 30 min post contrast injection and then asked to return for an additional short scan of the 75 min point.

Recent PWI studies suggest that high rCBV values are associated with tumor recurrence and low values with treatment effects. Still, up to date, there are no published studies supporting consensuses regarding which PWI-based analytic method best estimates histological tumor fraction as a predictor of progression or overall survival in GBM patients post treatment [17]. Our preliminary results show significant correlation of the fast component with high rCBV values, suggesting that rCBV may be a dominant characteristic of this population. Still, in some patients we observed low rCBV values in fast regions of the subtraction maps. This may be explained by distortion of the PW images in this population of post-surgery patients due to close vicinity of the tumor to surgical screws. Distortion may also be induced by hemorrhages which are frequent in these tumor types. In some cases the contradiction between our maps, depicting a blue component representing morphologically active tumor (confirmed histologically), and low rCBV values may be explained by the low resolution of the PW images impeding the sensitivity to small tumoral regions in contrast to the high resolution/sensitivity of our maps. On the other hand, these contradicting cases may imply existence of other contributions to the fast component, such as increased vessel permeability. A study designed to mathematically model the signal time curves for determining the dominant factors contributing to the different enhancement populations is ongoing.

The most pronounced effect depicted in the delayed enhancement subtraction maps is the clear differentiation between fast and slow populations, where the terms fast and slow refer to the clearance rate of the contrast agent between the early time point (2 min) and the delayed time point (75 min). The common feature of vessels morphology in the fast regions was found to be the

Table 3. Newly diagnosed GBM cohort.

Patient #	1ST Surgery	2nd Surgery	Samples compared with histology	Time to progression [months]	Treatment at progression
1	GTR	STR	4	7.5	Surgery+Bevacizumab
2	GTR	–	–	Not reached (19.7)	–
3	GTR	GTR	8	6.5	surgery
4	GTR	GTR	2	6.2	Surgery+Bevacizumab
5	STR	–	–	3.6	Bevacizumab
6	GTR	GTR	–	11.6	Surgery+ Bevacizumab
7	GTR	–		Not reached) 12.5	–
8	STB		–	Died from unrelated disease (3)	–
9	STB	–		Not reached (5.2)	–
10	GTR		–	5.0	Bevacizumab
12	STB	–		4.1	Bevacizumab
15	GTR		–	3.6	Bevacizumab
18	GTR	–		Not reached (5.2)	–

List of newly diagnosed GBM patients with post chemoradiation treatment follow-up.
*Column #2: Patients were diagnosed with GBM prior to initiation of chemoradiation by histological analysis of either gross tumor resection (GTR), sub-total resection (STR) or stereotactic biopsy samples (STB).
*Column #4: Stereotactic samples were taken from locations determined using the late enhancement subtraction maps calculated from the pre-surgical MRIs.
*Column #5: In cases where progression was not reached, the duration of follow-up is listed in parenthesis.

undamaged vessels lumens, while vessels in the slow regions presented significantly damaged lumens. Therefore, one explanation for the difference between the 2 populations may be that vessels in the fast regions provide efficient contrast clearance from the tissue, while the damaged lumens in the slow regions are unable to clear the accumulating contrast efficiently, resulting in contrast accumulation.

The association between the fast/slow components of the maps and tumor/non-tumoral tissues as determined by histological analysis is currently based on 32 biopsy samples obtained from 9 patients with primary brain tumors and 4 patients with brain metastases. Additional confirmation was obtained from 1 GBM patient and 8 metastases resected from 7 patients. These data suggest that our subtraction maps, calculated from delayed contrast extravasation MRI, enable clear differentiation between tumor and non-tumoral tissues in various types of brain tumors. Additional data is needed to establish the reliability of this conclusion. This study is ongoing.

The manner of which our maps may be applied for differentiating progression from pseudoprogression in GBM patients post chemoradiation was demonstrated in Figure 9. In our maps, progression is reflected by a significant increase in the fast component of the enhancing lesion while pseudoprogression is reflected by an increase in the slow component with no significant increase in the fast component. Therefore, using our maps in routine MRI follow-up may aid the physician in determining progression versus pseudoprogression in patients presenting an increase in the enhancing lesion on T1-MRI. An increase in the fast component volume, suggesting progression, implies that a change in the current therapy should be employed. No significant increase in the fast volume component, suggesting pseudoprogression, implies that the patient is responding to the current therapy and thus continuation is preferred, if possible.

The maps may be applied in a similar manner to patients following SRS. Patients with growing volumes of the slow component would be recommended for follow-up, if possible, while patients with growing volumes of the fast component would be recommended for treatment such as surgery or repeated SRS.

Due to improved treatment protocols and extended survival early and late radiation-induced neuro-toxicity of patients with brain tumors undergoing radiation-based therapies has become a major concern and efforts to minimize unnecessary exposure of surrounding normal brain without compromising treatment efficacy are of increasing interest [48–49]. The ability of our maps to depict morphologically active tumor regions with high resolution may thus be applied for optimizing radiation treatment planning by localizing the treatment to the fast/blue regions in our maps. This methodology may be similarly applied in the post surgery scenario to enable differentiation between post surgical changes and tumor remnants thus allowing depicting and treating residual tumor post surgery.

High resolution depiction of tumoral tissues may also be beneficial in the planning of surgical resections, especially in the case of close proximity to functionally eloquent brain regions. In these cases determination of the exact extent of the tumor might be crucial for the decision whether microsurgical tumor removal might be warranted. Our maps may also be applied for guiding stereotactic biopsies for molecular classification of the tumor. In this case our maps may aid in preventing the acquisition of biopsies with a high amount of necrosis or out of the infiltration zone with 'contamination' of the specimen by normal brain tissue, both potentially leading to false-negative results [50].

Novel approaches for local drug delivery including injections, infusions, trans-nasal delivery, convection enhanced delivery, local BBB disruption and various types of polymeric implants may also benefit from the application of our maps for planning and monitoring the treatments.

Increased tumor vascularity has been shown to correlate with both shortened survival and higher grade of malignancy in gliomas. Consequently, anti-angiogenic agents such as Bevacizumab, a monoclonal antibody targeting vascular endothelial growth factor, are now commonly employed to treat progressive

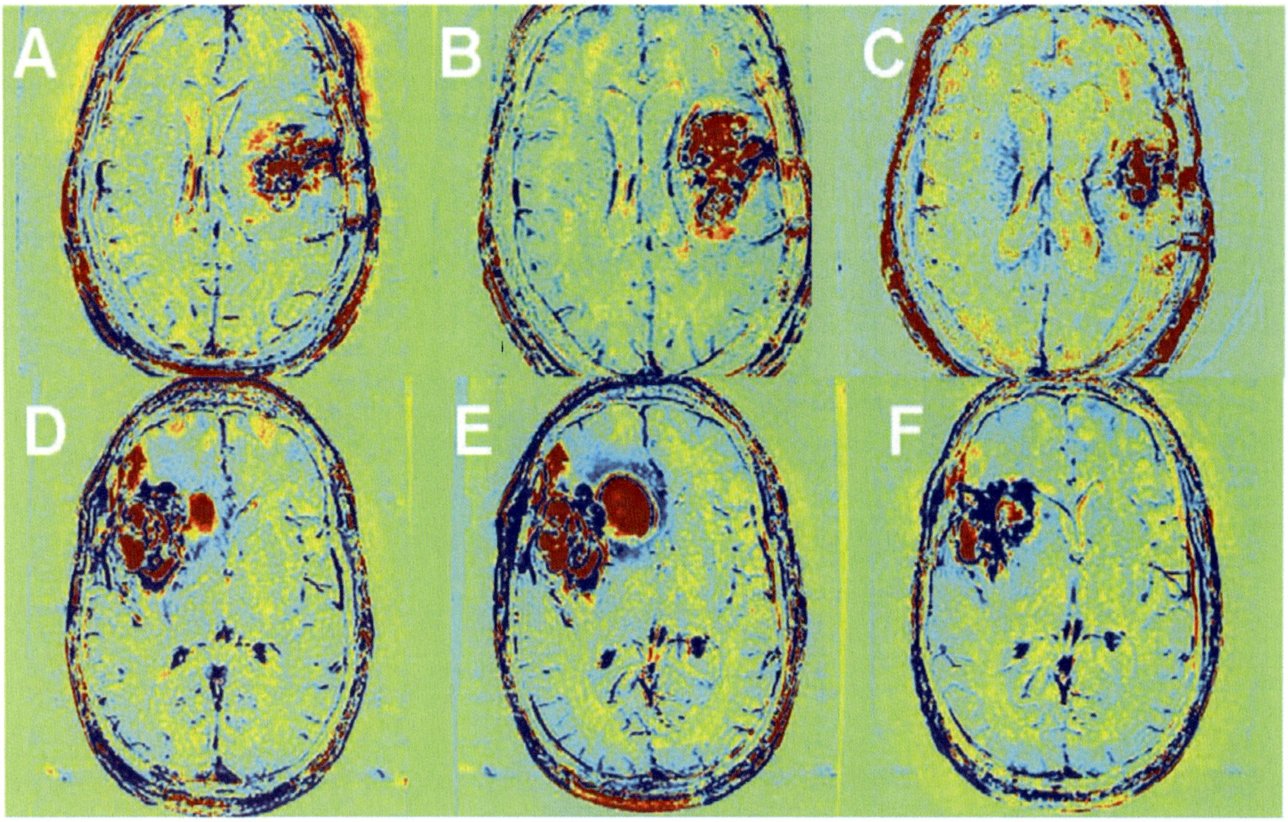

Figure 9. Examples of progression and pseudoprogression in GBM patients post chemoradiation. Late enhancement subtraction maps of a patient (#6) with significant increase in the enhancing lesion due to increase in the red volume (A–C) and a patient (#3) with significant increase in the blue component (D–F) with minor changes in the enhancing volume are shown. In the first example, the total enhancing volume has increased by 34% from 3 weeks (A) to 4.2 months (B) post chemoradiation, and then decreased to 33% below the initial volume (C) 9 months post treatment. The blue volume slightly increased by 6% in the first 4 months (A, B) and then significantly decreased to 47% below the initial volume at 9 months (C) while the red volume increased by 51% in the first 4.2 months (A, B) and decreased to 13% above the initial volume by 9 months (C). This patient progressed 11.6 months post treatment. In the second example, the total enhancing volume has increased by 16% from 3 weeks (D) to 2.5 months (E) and then remained 17% above the initial volume (F) 6.5 months post treatment. The blue volume slightly increased by 2% in the first 2.5 months (D,E) and then significantly increased to 57% above the initial volume at 6.5 months (F) while the red volume increased by 39% in the first 2.5 months (D, E) and decreased to 61% below the initial volume by 6.5 months (F). This patient progressed 6.5 months post treatment when he was referred to surgery.

malignant gliomas. The wide-spread use of these agents has added a layer of complexity to the evaluation and characterization of malignant gliomas as these agents have been shown to rapidly and markedly decrease contrast enhancement on contrast-enhanced T1-MRI [51–54]. We have recently initiated a study in which our subtraction maps are applied to recurrent GBM patients treated by Bevacizumab in an attempt to provide improved depiction of the tumor thus enabling better patient follow-up and understanding of Bevacizumab mechanism of action in GBM patients.

As up to 45% of suspected low-grade gliomas turn out to be high grade gliomas, histological diagnosis is mandatory before any therapeutic decision [55]. As even these partially anaplastic lesions may not display contrast enhancement on conventional contrast-enhanced T1-MRI, additional imaging information is warranted. We hope that the high sensitivity of our maps may provide additional valuable information for delineation of the tumor borders as well as for targeting stereotactic biopsies.

Additional studies are required in order to assess the reliability of these applications.

In summary, the difficulty in interpretation of post treatment images prevents appropriate treatment in nearly half of treated GBM patients and a significant number of patients with brain metastases. The presented results demonstrate the feasibility for a straightforward application of our high resolution delayed enhancement subtraction maps in the daily clinical scenario. The ability to clearly differentiate tumor from non-tumoral tissues may provide the physician with a clear understanding of the patient current situation thus enabling improved patient management.

Acknowledgments

The authors thank our patients and their families for participating in this important study. We thank Prof Zvi Ram for many productive discussions and Sharona Salomon and Shoshana Farfuri for their invaluable help in managing the regulatory aspects of the study.

Author Contributions

Conceived and designed the experiments: LZ YG YM. Performed the experiments: LZ DG DL DD YG ON CH DN RS ZRC YM AT. Analyzed the data: LZ DG DL DD YG ON DN YM. Wrote the paper: LZ DG DL DD YM.

References

1. Fink J, Born D, Chamberlain MC (2011) Pseudoprogression: Relevance with respect to treatment of high-grade gliomas. Curr Treat Opt in Oncol 12: 240–252.
2. Brandsma D, Stalpers L, Taal W, Sminia P, van den Bent MJ (2008) Clinical features, mechanisms, and management of pseudoprogression in malignant gliomas. Lancet Oncol 9: 453–461.
3. Chamberlain MC, Glantz MJ, Chalmers L, Van Horn A, Sloan AE (2007) Early necrosis following concurrent Temodar and radiotherapy in patients with glioblastoma. J Neurooncol 82: 81–83.
4. Taal W, Brandsma D, de Bruin HG, Bromberg JE, Swaak-Kragten AT, et al. (2008) Incidence of early pseudoprogression in a cohort of malignant glioma patients treated with chemoirradiation with temozolomide. Cancer 113: 405–410.
5. Stupp R, Mason WP, van den Bent MJ, Weller M, Fisher B, et al. (2005) European Organization for Research and Treatment of Cancer Brain Tumor and Radiotherapy Groups, National Cancer Institute of Canada Clinical Trials Group. Radiotherapy plus concomitant and adjuvant temozolomide for glioblastoma. N Engl J Med 352: 987–996.
6. de Wit MC, de Bruin HG, Eijkenboom W, Sillevis Smitt PA, van den Bent MJ (2004) Immediate post-radiotherapy changes in malignant glioma can mimic tumor progression. Neurology 63: 535–537.
7. Chaskis C, Neyns B, Michotte A, De Ridder M, Everaert H (2009) Pseudoprogression after radiotherapy with concurrent temozolomide for high-grade glioma: clinical observations and working recommendations. Surg Neurol 72: 423–428.
8. Brandsma D, van den Bent MJ (2009) Pseudoprogression and pseudoresponse in the treatment of gliomas. Curr Opin Neurol 22: 633–638.
9. Young RJ, Gupta A, Shah AD, Graber JJ, Zhang Z, et al. (2011) Potential utility of conventional MRI signs in diagnosing pseudoprogression in glioblastoma, Neurology 76: 1918–1924.
10. Jahangiri A, Aghi MK (2012) Pseudoprogression and treatment effect. Neurosurg Clin N Am 23: 277–287.
11. Rane N, Quaghebeur G (2012) CNS effects following the treatment of malignancy. Clin Radiol 67: 61–68.
12. Wen PY, Macdonald DR, Reardon DA, Cloughesy TF, Sorensen AG, et al. (2010) Updated response assessment criteria for high-grade gliomas: response assessment in neuro-oncology working group, J Clin Oncol 28: 1963–1972.
13. Van den Bent M, Volgelbaum M, Wen P, Macdonald DR, Chang SM (2009) Endpoint assessment in gliomas: novel treatments limit the usefulness of the classical Macdonald criteria. J Clin Oncol 27: 2905–2908.
14. Forsyth PA, Kelly PJ, Cascino TL, Scheithauer BW, Shaw EG, et al. (1995) Radiation necrosis or glioma recurrence: is computer-assisted stereotactic biopsy useful? J Neurosurg 82: 436–444.
15. Perry A, Schmidt RE (2006) Cancer therapy-associated CNS neuropathology: an update and review of the literature. Acta Neuropathol 111: 197–212.
16. Kim JH, Bae Kim Y, Han JH, Cho KG, Kim SH, et al. (2012) Pathologic Diagnosis of Recurrent Glioblastoma: Morphologic, Immunohistochemical, and Molecular Analysis of 20 Paired Cases. Am J Surg Pathol 36: 620–628.
17. Hu LS, Eschbacher JM, Heiserman JE, Dueck AC, Shapiro WR, et al. (2012) Reevaluating the imaging definition of tumor progression: perfusion MRI quantifies recurrent glioblastoma tumor fraction, pseudoprogression, and radiation necrosis to predict survival. Neuro Oncol May 17 [Epub ahead of print].
18. Tihan T, Barletta J, Parney I, Lamborn K, Sneed PK, et al. (2006) Prognostic value of detecting recurrent glioblastoma multiforme in surgical specimens from patients after radiotherapy: should pathology evaluation alter treatment decisions? Hum Pathol 37: 272–282.
19. Shaw E, Scott C, Souhami L, Dinapoli R, Kline R, et al. (2000) Single dose radiosurgical treatment of recurrent previously irradiated primary brain tumors and brain metastases: final report of RTOG protocol 90–05. Int J Radiat Oncol Biol Phys 47: 291–298.
20. Rock JP, Scarpace L, Hearshen D, Gutierrez J, Fisher JL, et al. (2004) Associations among MRS, ADC, and image-guided histopathology with special attention to radiation necrosis. Neurosurgery 54: 1111–1117.
21. Chan YL, Yeung DK, Leung SF, Chan PN (2003) DWMRI in radiation-induced cerebral necrosis. ADC in lesion components. J Comput Assist Tomogr 27: 674–680.
22. Zeng QS, Li CF, Zhang K, Liu H, Kang XS, et al. (2007) Multivoxel 3D proton MR spectroscopy in the distinction of recurrent glioma from radiation injury. J Neurooncol 84: 63–69.
23. Stadnik TW, Chaskis C, Michotte A, Shabana WM, van Rompaey K, et al. (2001) Diffusion-weighted MR imaging of intracerebral masses: comparison with conventional MR imaging and histologic findings. AJNR Am J Neuroradiol 22: 969–976.
24. Lu S, Ahn D, Johnson G, Law M, Zagzag D, et al. (2004) Diffusion-tensor MR imaging of intracranial neoplasia and associated peritumoral edema. Radiology 232: 221–228.
25. Matsusue E, Fink JR, Rockhill JK, Ogawa T, Maravilla KR, et al. (2010) Distinction between glioma progression and post-radiation change by combined physiologic MR imaging. Neuroradiology 52: 297–306.
26. Xu JL, Li YL, Lian JM, Dou SW, Yan FS, et al. (2010) Distinction between postoperative recurrent glioma and radiation injury using MR diffusion tensor imaging. Neuradiology 52: 1193–1199.
27. Ricci PE, Karis JP, Heiserman JE, Fram EK, Bice AN, et al. (1998) Differentiating recurrent tumor from radiation necrosis: time for re-evaluation of PET? Am J Neuroradiol 19: 407–413.
28. Tsuyuguchi N, Takami T, Sunada I, Iwai Y, Yamanaka K, et al. (2004) Methionine positron emission tomography for differentiation of recurrent brain tumor and radiation necrosis after stereotactic radiosurgery–in malignant glioma. Ann Nucl Med 18: 291–296.
29. Nelson SJ (2011) Assessment of therapeutic response and treatment planning for brain tumors using metabolic and physiological MRI. NMR Biomed 24: 734–749.
30. Lacerda S, Law M (2009) Magnetic resonance perfusion and permeability imaging in brain tumors. Neuroimaging Clin N Am 19: 527–557.
31. Mills SJ, Soh C, O'Connor JP, Rose CJ, Buonaccorsi G, et al. (2010) Enhancing fraction in glioma and its relationship to the tumoral vascular microenvironment: a dynamic contrast-enhanced MR imaging study. Am J Neuroradiol 31: 726–731.
32. Barboriak DP, MacFall JR, Viglianti BL, Dewhirst MW (2008) Comparison of three physiologically-based pharmacokinetic models for the prediction of contrast agent distribution measured by dynamic MR imaging. J Magn Reson Imaging 27: 1388–1398.
33. Aronen HJ, Perkiö J (2002) Dynamic susceptibility contrast MRI of gliomas. Neuroimaging Clin N Am 12: 501–523.
34. Covarrubias DJ, Rosen BR, Lev MH (2004) Dynamic magnetic resonance perfusion imaging of brain tumors. Oncologist 9: 528–537.
35. Sugahara T, Korogi Y, Tomiguchi S, Shigematsu Y, Ikushima I, et al. (2000) Posttherapeutic intraaxial brain tumor: the value of perfusion-sensitive contrast-enhanced MRI for differentiating tumor recurrence from nonneoplastic contrast-enhancing tissue. Am J Neuroradiol 21: 901–909.
36. Hu LS, Baxter LC, Smith KA, Feuerstein BG, Karis JP, et al. (2009) Relative cerebral blood volume values to differentiate highgrade glioma recurrence from posttreatment radiation effect: direct correlation between image-guided tissue histopathology and localized dynamic susceptibility-weighted contrast-enhanced perfusion MR imaging measurements. AJNR 30: 552–558.
37. Gasparetto EL, Pawlak MA, Patel SH, Huse J, Woo JH, et al. (2009) Posttreatment recurrence of malignant brain neoplasm: accuracy of relative cerebral blood volume fraction in discriminating low from high malignant histologic volume fraction. Radiology 250: 887–896.
38. Mangla R, Singh G, Ziegelitz D, Milano MT, Korones DN, et al. (2010) Changes in relative cerebral blood volume 1 month after radiation temozolomide therapy can help predict overall survival in patients with glioblastoma. Radiology 256: 575–584.
39. Kim YH, Oh SW, Lim YJ, Park CK, Lee SH, et al. (2010) Differentiating radiation necrosis from tumor recurrence in highgrade gliomas: assessing the efficacy of 18F-FDG PET, 11C-methionine PET and perfusion MRI. Clin Neurol Neurosurg 112: 758–765.
40. Gahramanov S, Raslan AM, Muldoon LL, Hamilton BE, Rooney WD, et al. (2011) Potential for differentiation of pseudoprogression from true tumor progression with dynamic susceptibility-weighted contrast-enhanced Magnetic resonance imaging using ferumoxytol vs gadoteridol: A pilot study. Int J Radiat Oncol Biol Phys 79: 514–523.
41. Narang J, Jain R, Arbab AS, Mikkelsen T, Scarpace L, et al. (2011) Differentiating treatment-induced necrosis from recurrent/progressive brain tumor using nonmodel-based semiquantitative indices derived from dynamic contrast-enhanced T1-weighted MR perfusion, Neuro-Oncol 13: 1037–1046.
42. Barajas RF Jr, Chang JS, Segal MR, Parsa AT, McDermott MW, et al. (2009) Differentiation of recurrent glioblastoma multiforme from radiation necrosis after external beam radiation therapy with dynamic susceptibility weighted contrast-enhanced perfusion MR imaging. Radiology 253: 486–496.
43. Hazle JD, Jackson EF, Schomer DF, Leeds NE (1997) Dynamic imaging of intracranial lesions using FSE imaging: differentiation of brain tumors and treatment effects. J Magn Reson Imaging 7: 1084–93.
44. Diehn M, Nardini C, Wang DS, McGovern S, Jayaraman M, et al. (2008) Identification of noninvasive imaging surrogates for brain tumor gene-expression modules. Proc Natl Acad Sci U S A 105: 5213–5238.
45. Israeli D, Tanne D, Daniels D, Last D, Shneor R, et al. (2011) The Application of MRI for Depiction of Subtle Blood Brain Barrier Disruption in Stroke. Int J Biol Sc 7: 1–8.
46. Peto R, Peto J (1972) Asymptotically efficient rank invariant test procedures. J Roy Stat Soc Series A 135: 195–206.
47. Moses L (1952) Non-parametric statistics for psychological research. Psychol Bull 49: 122–143.
48. Rane N, Quaghebeur G (2012) CNS effects following the treatment of malignancy. Clin Radiol 67: 61–68.
49. Abe E, Aoyama H (2012) The role of whole brain radiation therapy for the management of brain metastases in the era of stereotactic radiosurgery. Curr Oncol Rep 14: 79–84.
50. Tonn JC, Thon N, Schnell O, Kreth FW (2012) Personalized surgical therapy. Ann Oncol 23: Suppl 10: x28–x32.

51. Russell SM, Elliott R, Forshaw D, Golfinos JG, Nelson PK, et al. (2009) Glioma vascularity correlates with reduced patient survival and increased malignancy. Surg Neurol 72: 242–246.
52. Batchelor TT, Sorensen AG, di Tomaso E, Zhang WT, Duda DG, et al. (2007) AZD2171, a pan-VEGF receptor tyrosine kinase inhibitor, normalizes tumor vasculature and alleviates edema in glioblastoma patients. Cancer Cell 11: 83–95.
53. Varallyay CG, Muldoon LL, Gahramanov S, Wu YJ, Goodman JA, et al. (2009) Dynamic MRI using iron oxide nanoparticles to assess early vascular effects of antiangiogenic versus corticosteroid treatment in a glioma model. J Cereb Blood Flow Metab 29: 853–860.
54. Vredenburgh JJ, Desjardins A, Herndon JE 2nd, Dowell JM, Reardon DA, et al. (2007) Phase II trial of bevacizumab and irinotecan in recurrent malignant glioma. Clin Cancer Res 13: 1253–1259.
55. Kunz M, Thon N, Eigenbrod S, Hartmann C, Egensperger R et al. (2011) Hot spots in dynamic (18)FET-PET delineate malignant tumor parts within suspected WHO grade II gliomas. Neuro-oncol 13: 307–316.

16

Interobserver Reproducibility of Diffusion-Weighted MRI in Monitoring Tumor Response to Neoadjuvant Therapy in Esophageal Cancer

Robert M. Kwee[1,2]*, Alexander K. Dik[1], Meindert N. Sosef[3,4], Ralph C. M. Berendsen[5], Sander Sassen[1], Guido Lammering[6], Ruud Clarijs[7], Liekele E. Oostenbrug[8], Rachel L. G. M. Blom[9], Roy F. A. Vliegen[1]

1 Department of Radiology, Atrium Medical Center Parkstad, Heerlen, The Netherlands, **2** Department of Radiology, Maastricht University Medical Center, Maastricht, The Netherlands, **3** Department of Surgery, Atrium Medical Center Parkstad, Heerlen, The Netherlands, **4** Surgical Collaborative Network Limburg, Limburg, The Netherlands, **5** Department of Medical Physics, Atrium Medical Center Parkstad, Heerlen, The Netherlands, **6** Department of Radiation Oncology, MediClin Robert-Janker-Clinic, Bonn, Germany, **7** Department of Pathology, Atrium Medical Center Parkstad, Heerlen, The Netherlands, **8** Department of Internal Medicine and Gastroenterology, Atrium Medical Center Parkstad, Heerlen, The Netherlands, **9** Department of Surgery, Academic Medical Center, Amsterdam, The Netherlands

Abstract

Objective: To investigate the reproducibility of diffusion-weighted magnetic resonance imaging (DW-MRI) in assessing tumor response early in the course of neoadjuvant chemoradiotherapy in patients with operable esophageal cancer.

Methods: Eleven male patients (mean age 54.8 years) with newly diagnosed esophageal cancer underwent DW-MRI before and 10 days after start of chemoradiotherapy. Reproducibility of apparent diffusion coefficient (ADC) measurements by manual (freehand) and semi-automated volumetric methods was assessed.

Results: Interobserver reproducibility for the assessment of mean tumor ADC by the manual measurement method was good, with an ICC of 0.69 (95% CI, 0.36 to 0.85; $P = 0.001$). Interobserver reproducibility for the assessment of mean tumor ADC by the semi-automated volumetric measurement method was very good, with an ICC of 0.96 (95% CI, 0.91 to 0.98; $P < 0.001$).

Conclusion: Semi-automated volumetric ADC measurements have higher reproducibility than manual ADC measurements in assessing tumor response to chemoradiotherapy in patients with esophageal adenocarcinoma.

Editor: Domenico Coppola, H. Lee Moffitt Cancer Center & Research Institute, United States of America

Funding: These authors have no support or funding to report.

Competing Interests: The authors have declared that no competing interests exist.

* E-mail: rmkwee@gmail.com

Introduction

Esophageal cancer is a disease with a poor prognosis and high mortality. There were an estimated 482,000 new cases and 407,000 patients died of the disease worldwide in 2008 [1]. Preoperative chemoradiotherapy has shown to improve survival compared with surgery alone [2,3]. However, not all patients benefit from preoperative chemoradiotherapy. In the Chemoradiotherapy for Oesophageal Cancer Followed by Surgery Study trial, as much as 39% of patients had no histopathological tumor regression (tumor regression defined as <10% viable tumor cells in the resected specimen) [3]. Yet, toxicity due to chemotherapy occurs in 11%–90% and there is a risk of radiation-induced complications [3,4]. In patients who respond insufficiently, inefficient neoadjuvant therapy should be discontinued, and surgery should not be delayed. On the other hand, patients who respond favorably may benefit from additional preoperative treatment and surgery may be delayed or even refrained from. Therefore, there is a need for a method which can differentiate responders from nonresponders early in the course of neoadjuvant treatment. Studies investigating the value of Fluorine 18 (^{18}F) fluorodeoxyglucose positron emission tomography (^{18}F FDG PET) in assessing response to neoadjuvant treatment show heterogeneous results [5]. Diffusion-weighted magnetic resonance imaging (DW-MRI) may be an attractive alternative to ^{18}F FDG PET, because patients do not need to fast before the examination, no exogenous contrast material is required, and acquisition time is much shorter. Therefore, the objective of the present study was to investigate the reproducibility of DW-MRI in assessing tumor response early in the course of neoadjuvant chemoradiotherapy in patients with operable esophageal cancer. In addition, we also investigated the potential of DW-MRI in differentiating responders from nonresponders in a limited number of patients.

Materials and Methods

Patient selection

Patients with newly diagnosed esophageal cancer who were referred to our hospital, which is a regional referral center for the treatment of esophageal cancer, were eligible for inclusion. Only

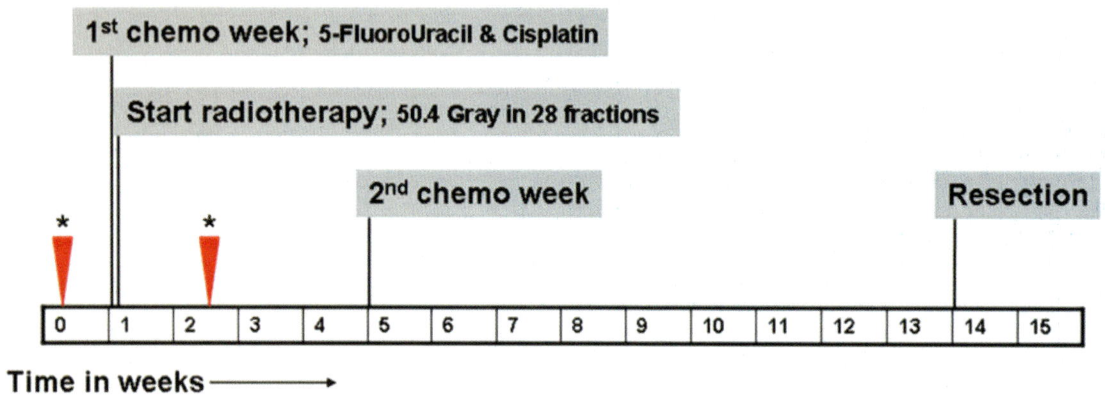

Figure 1. Timing of neoadjuvant therapy, surgery, and MRI (timing of MRI scans is indicated by asterisks and arrowheads).

patients who were considered operable and who underwent preoperative chemoradiotherapy were eligible for inclusion. Neoadjuvant therapy regimen and timing are displayed in Figure 1. Patients who already started neoadjuvant therapy before inclusion and patients with standard contraindications for MRI [6] were excluded. This study was approved by the institutional review board of our hospital (Medisch Ethische Toetsingscommissie Atrium-Orbis-Zuyd). All patients gave written informed consent.

MRI protocol and image review

All MRI scans were performed on one 1.5 Tesla scanner (MAGNETOM Avanto, Siemens AG, Healthcare Sector, Erlangen, Germany). For signal reception, a total of 12 elements of an anteriorly placed body matrix coil and a posteriorly placed spine matrix coil (total imaging matrix system, Siemens AG, Healthcare Sector, Erlangen, Germany), were used. Sagittal and transverse T2-weighted images and DW images were obtained under free breathing so that the entire tumor was imaged. Scan parameters are displayed in Table 1. Total imaging time, including acquisition of scout images, was 10 minutes and 4 seconds. Patients underwent two MRI scans. The first MRI scan was performed within 2 weeks before start of neoadjuvant therapy; the second MRI scan was performed on the 10th day after initiation of neoadjuvant therapy. Time interval between the two scans varied from 12 to 21 days.

Quantitative apparent diffusion coefficient (ADC) measurements of the primary esophageal tumor, before and after initiation of neoadjuvant therapy, were performed using a manual and a semi-automated volumetric method, as described below.

Table 1. Details of the MRI protocol.

Scan parameters	T2-weighted TSE	T2-weighted TSE	Single-shot SE-EPI DWI with STIR
Imaging plane	Coronal	Transverse	Transverse
TR (ms)	4350	3230	3400
TE (ms)	118	98	78
Turbo factor	13	16	Epifactor 150
Echo spacing (ms)	10.7	10.9	0.7
Bandwidth (Hz/pixel)	201	222	1628
NSA	2	2	6
B-value (s/mm^2)	NA	NA	0, 300, 1000
No. of slices	26	48	26
FOV (mm)	250	280	380
Matrix size	256	512	192
Slice thickness (mm)	3.0	4.0	4.0
Voxel size (mm)	1.2×1.0×3.0	0.8×0.5×4.0	2.0×2.0×4.0
Acquisition time (minutes)	02:08	04:23	03:14

DWI: diffusion-weighted imaging.
EPI: echo planar imaging.
FOV: field of view.
NA: not applicable.
NSA: number of signal averages.
SE: spin-echo.
STIR: short TI inversion recovery.
TSE: turbo spin-echo.

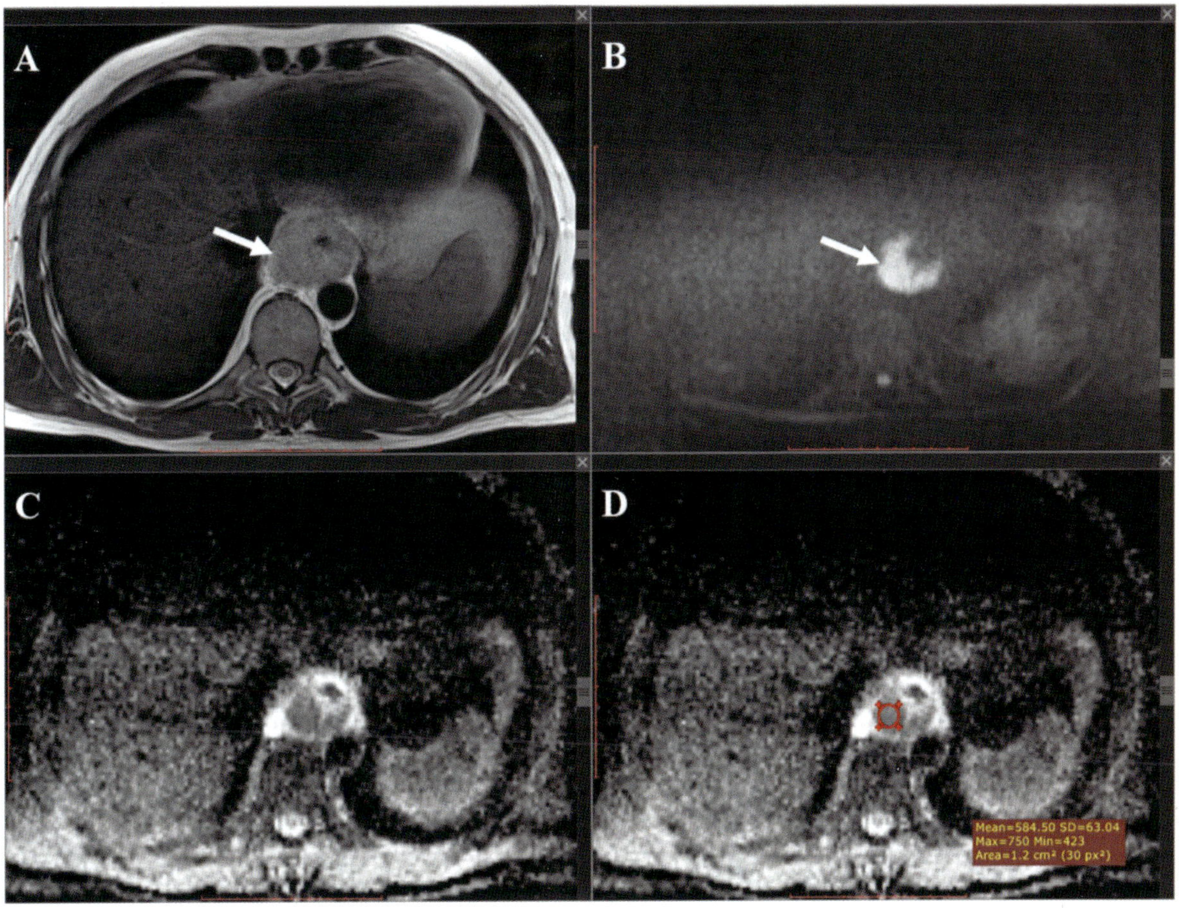

Figure 2. Manual measurement method. T2-weighted (A) and b1000 DW (B) images, and corresponding ADC map (C and D). An esophageal tumor can be depicted as thickening of the esophageal wall (arrow in (A) with high signal intensity on the corresponding b1000 DW image (arrow in B) and low signal intensity on the corresponding ADC map (arrow in C). An ROI was manually drawn in the tumor on the ADC map (red circular region in D) to calculate the tumor ADC value.

For the manual method, measurements were performed on a Picture Archiving and Communications System (Sienet Magic v50 2004, Siemens, Germany). For each tumor, 2 circular regions of interest (ROIs) were manually drawn on the ADC images, which corresponded to the location of the primary tumor on the coregistered transverse T2-weighted and DW images. Subsequently, mean ADC value of the 2 ROIs (corrected for ROI size) was calculated. Figure 2 gives an example. Measurements were performed by a board-certified radiologist with 13 years of experience in cross-sectional imaging (R.F.A.V.), who was blinded to the histopathological results. To assess interobserver reproducibility, measurements were also performed by a fourth-year radiology resident (S.S.) who was blinded to the results of the first reader and to the histopathological results. For further statistical analyses, the average value of the two readers was used.

For the semi-automated volumetric method, measurements were performed using a dedicated open source image processing package (Fiji [7]), based on ImageJ (Rasband, National Institute of Mental Health, Bethesda, USA). The healthy esophagus does not show any high signal on DW-MRI [8]. Therefore, any high signal in the esophagus that exceeded the signal intensity of the surrounding background (lung or air) was considered positive for the presence of tumor. A visually set threshold was applied to the b1000 DW images to generate strictly black and white images, with all the white pixels representing tumor. An image filter called "Particle Analyser" then constructed groups of pixels, i.e. ROIs. Only ROIs which were located around the primary tumor were manually selected and copied to the coregistered ADC maps. ADC values of the ROIs in each slice were assessed, resulting in a volumetric measurement. Mean ADC value of the entire tumor was then calculated. Figure 3 gives an example. Measurements were performed by a fifth-year radiology resident (A.K.D.), who was blinded to the histopathological results. To assess interobserver reproducibility, measurements were also performed by a third-year radiology resident (R.M.K.) who was blinded to the results of the first reader and to the histopathological results. For further statistical analyses, the average value of the two readers was used.

Histopathological response assessment

The surgical specimens were examined by experienced pathologists and scored according to the tumor regression grade scoring system (TRG) as described by Mandard et al. [9]. TRG was quantified in five grades: TRG 1 (complete regression) showed absence of residual cancer and fibrosis extending through the different layers of the esophageal wall; TRG 2 was characterized by the presence of rare residual cancer cells scattered through the fibrosis; TRG 3 was characterized by an increase in the number of residual cancer cells, but fibrosis still predominated; TRG 4 showed residual cancer outgrowing fibrosis; and TRG 5 was

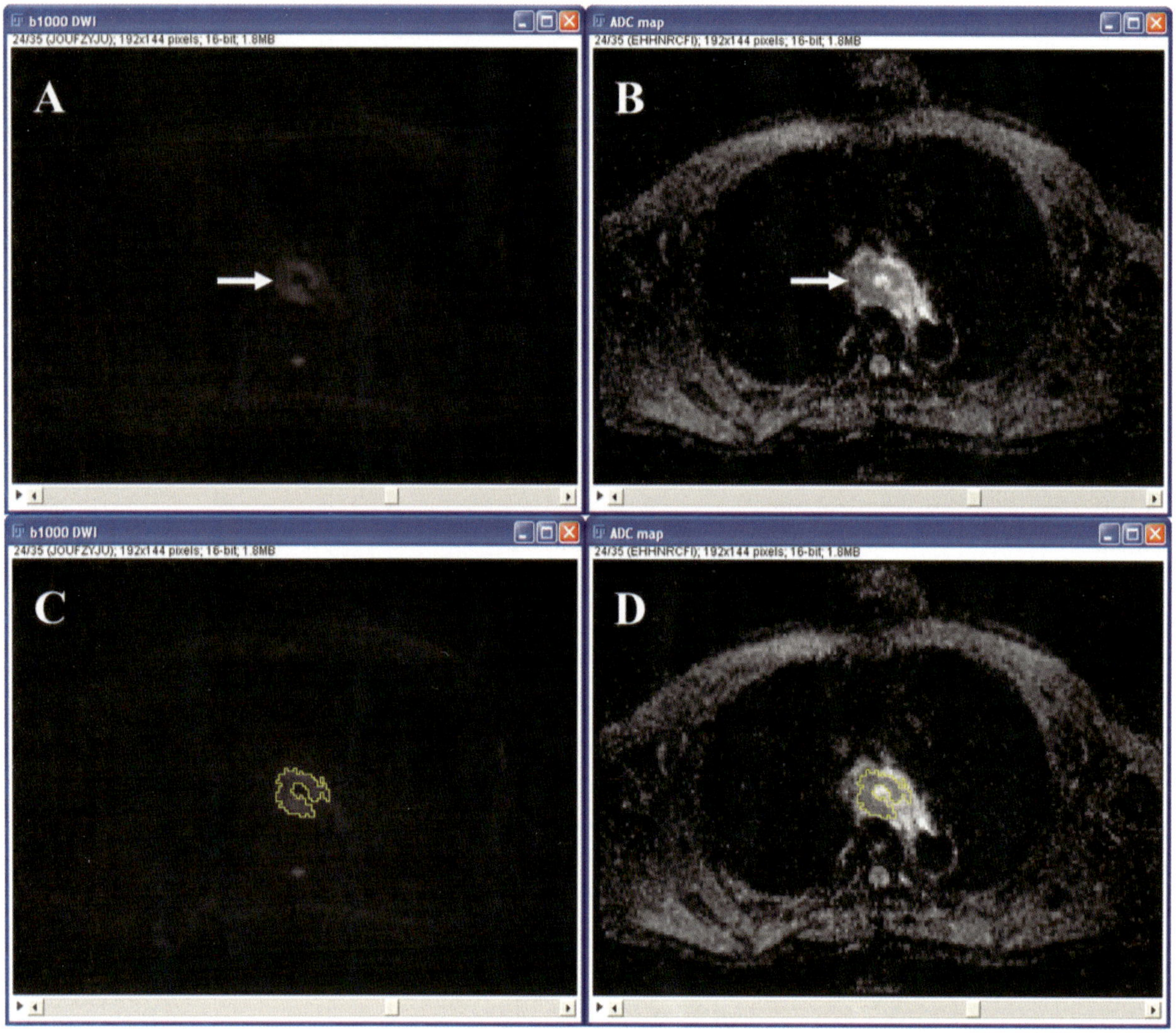

Figure 3. Semi-automated measurement method. B1000 DW image (A and C) and corresponding ADC map (B and D). An esophageal tumor can be depicted as an area of high signal intensity centrally at the b1000 DW image (arrow in A) and as an area of low signal intensity centrally at the corresponding ADC map (arrow in B). After visually selecting a threshold, the software automatically placed an ROI (area bordered by a yellow line in C) around the tumor at the b1000 DW image, which was then copied to the corresponding ADC map (D) to calculate the tumor ADC value.

characterized by absence of regressive changes [9]. TRG score was considered the reference standard for tumor response, with TRG scores 1–2 defined as responding and TRG scores 3–5 defined as nonreponding to neoadjuvant chemoradiotherapy.

Statistical analysis

Statistical analyses were performed by using Statistical Package for the Social Sciences software, version 18.0 (SPSS Inc, Chicago, IL, USA), and MedCalc software (MedCalc, Mariakerke, Belgium). The intraclass correlation coefficient (ICC) was calculated and Bland-Altman plots [10] were constructed to determine interobserver variation in assessing tumor ADC values by the manual and semi-automated volumetric method. Accordingly, agreement in ADC measurements between the manual and semi-automated volumetric method was also determined. ICC values <0.20, 0.21–0.40, 0.41–0.60, 0.61–0.80, and 0.81–1.00 were considered to indicate poor, fair, moderate, good, and very good agreement, respectively. Differences in mean pretreatment ADC and percentage change in ADC between patients with (TRG grade 1–2) and without (TRG grade 3–5) tumor response were assessed by the Mann-Whitney U test and graphically displayed by boxplots. This was done both for the manual and semi-automated volumetric ADC measurements. Correlations between mean pretreatment tumor ADC and TRG score, and correlations between percentage change in mean tumor ADC after start of neoadjuvant therapy and TRG score, were assessed by Pearson rank correlation tests. This was also done both for the manual and semi-automated volumetric measurement methods. Very weak, weak, moderate, strong, and very strong correlation were defined as Pearson ρ's of 0–0.19, 0.20–0.39, 0.40–0.59, 0.60–0.79, and 0.80–1.00, respectively. Scatter plots were constructed to graphically display the correlations. All levels of statistical significance were set at 0.05.

Results

Between February 2010 and July 2012, 105 patients with newly diagnosed esophageal cancer were referred to our hospital. Sixty of these patients were considered operable, of which 17 were

Table 2. Tumor type, initial clinical tumor stage, whether or not undergoing 1st/2nd MRI scan, visibility of tumor at DWI scan, results of histopathological analysis, and tumor response to neoadjuvant therapy for all patients.

Patient no.	Tumor type	Initial clinical tumor stage		Patient undergoing 1st/2nd MRI scan	Tumor visible at 1st/2nd DWI scan	Histopathological analysis of resected specimen, TRG score	Tumor response to neoadjuvant therapy (TRG score 1 or 2)
		T	**N**				
1	Adenocarcinoma	2	1	yes/yes	yes/yes	1	yes
2	Adenocarcinoma	3	1	yes/yes	yes/yes	1	yes
3	Adenocarcinoma	4	2	yes/yes	yes/yes	4	no
4	Adenocarcinoma	2	1	yes/yes	yes/yes	4	no
5	Adenocarcinoma*	3	3	yes/yes	yes/yes	4	no
6	Adenocarcinoma	3	3	yes/yes	yes/yes	4	no
7	Adenocarcinoma	3	1	yes/yes	yes/yes	3	no
8	Squamous cell carcinoma	3	1	yes/yes	yes/yes	1	yes
9	Adenocarcinoma*	3	2	yes/yes	no/no	3	no
10	Adenocarcinoma	2	2	yes/yes	no/no	3	no
11	Adenocarcinoma	2	1	yes/yes	no/no	3	no
12	Adenocarcinoma	3	1	yes/no	yes/NA	2	yes
13	Adenocarcinoma	3	1	yes/no	yes/NA	Death before surgery	
14	Adenocarcinoma	1	1	yes/no	yes/NA	Not operated: scapula metastasis detected at ^{18}F FDG PET/CT after neoadjuvant therapy	
15	Adenocarcinoma	4	3	yes/yes	yes/yes	Not operated: liver metastases detected at first MRI scan	
16	Adenocarcinoma	3	0	yes/yes	yes/yes	Not operated: scapula metastasis detected at ^{18}F FDG PET/CT after neoadjuvant therapy	
17	Adenocarcinoma	3	1	yes/yes	yes/yes	Peritoneal metastases discovered at surgery; tumor not resected	

*: Some degree of signet ring cell differentiation was encountered.
NA: not applicable.

Table 3. Average and standard deviations (SDs) of mean tumor ADC before and after start of chemoradiotherapy and average percentage change in mean tumor for the manual and semi-automated methods.

	Manual method*	Semi-automated method*
Average and SD of mean ADC value before start of chemoradiotherapy ($*10^{-3}$ mm^2/s)	0.913±0.170	1.029±0.262
Average and SD of mean ADC value after start of chemoradiotherapy ($*10^{-3}$ mm^2/s)	1.257±1.015	1.102±0.280
Average percentage change between first and second MRI scan	32.9±15.0	10.7±12.3

* The average value of two readers was used.

prepared to participate in the present study. All 17 included patients were men, with a mean age of 54.8 years (range 40–71 years). Their characteristics are displayed in Table 2. All tumors were located in the distal third of the esophagus. There were 16 adenocarcinomas and one squamous cell carcinoma. In two adenocarcinomas some degree of signet ring cell differentiation was encountered. Initial clinical tumor stage, based on ^{18}F FDG PET/CT and endoscopic ultrasonography findings, varied from cT1N1 to cT4aN3. Of the 17 included patients, three did not undergo the second MRI scan, because of illness during chemoradiotherapy ($n = 2$) and because not showing up ($n = 1$). Two of these patients were not operated on because of death before surgery and because ^{18}F FDG PET/CT after neoadjuvant therapy revealed distant metastases. Two other patients were also not operated on because ^{18}F FDG PET/CT after neoadjuvant therapy also revealed distant metastases and because liver metastases were detected at the first MRI scan, respectively. In one patient, no tumor was resected because peritoneal metastases were discovered peroperatively. Eventually, there were 11 patients who underwent two preoperative MRI scans (before and during neoadjuvant therapy) and surgical resection of the tumor.

Of the aforementioned 11 patients, 3 had a tumor which was not visible on the DW images. These 3 patients were only included in the manual measurement method, because their tumors could be seen on the coregistered T2-weighted images from which an ROI could be copied to the location of the tumor on the ADC images. Tumor ADC values obtained by manual and semi-automated volumetric measurements before and after start of chemoradiotherapy and percentage change are displayed in Table 3. Interobserver reproducibility for the assessment of mean tumor ADC by the manual measurement method was good (see Figure 4), with an ICC of 0.69 (95% CI, 0.36 to 0.85; $P = 0.001$). Interobserver reproducibility for the assessment of mean tumor ADC by the semi-automated volumetric measurement method was very good (see Figure 5), with an ICC of 0.96 (95% CI, 0.91 to 0.98; $P<0.001$). Agreement between the manual and semi-automated volumetric method for measurement of mean tumor ADC was good (see Figure 6), with an ICC of 0.73 (95% CI, 0.39 to 0.88; $P<0.001$). There were no significant differences in mean pretreatment ADC and ADC change between patients with and without tumor response, neither for the manual (Figure 7A and B) nor for semi-automated volumetric method (Figure 8A and B). We

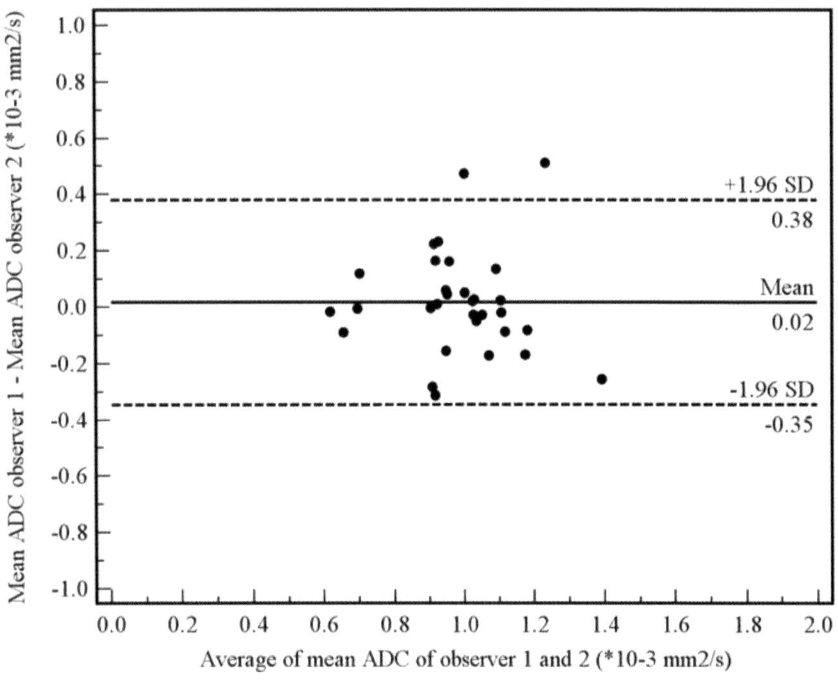

Figure 4. Interobserver reproducibility using the manual measurement method. Measurements from both the first and second MRI scan were included in this analysis. Bland-Altman plot shows the difference between measurements of two observers (R.F.A.V. and S.S.) against the average measurement, with mean absolute difference (continuous line) and 95% CI of the mean difference (dashed lines).

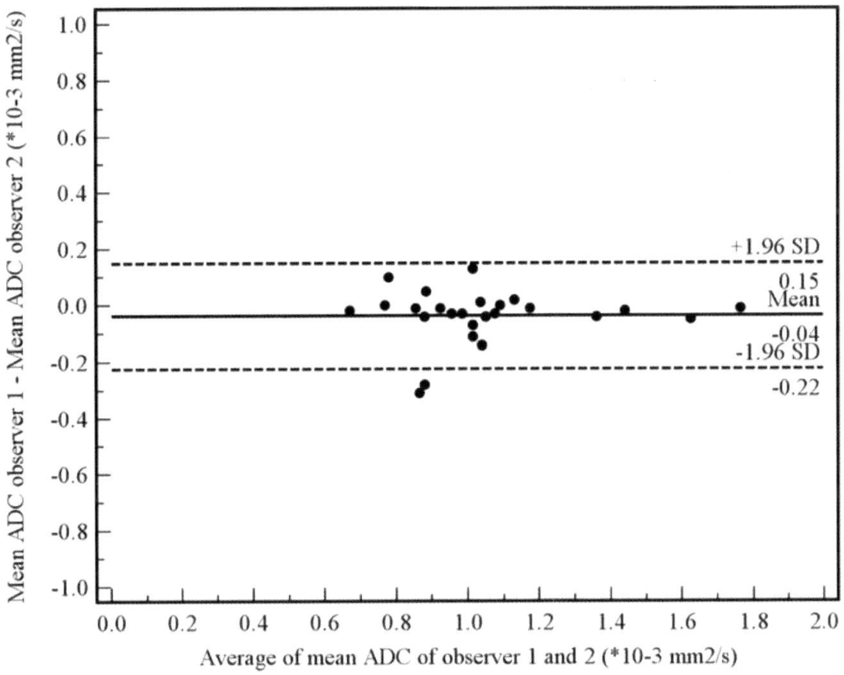

Figure 5. Interobserver reproducibility using the semi-automated measurement method. Measurements from both the first and second MRI scan were included in this analysis. Bland-Altman plot shows the difference between measurements of two observers (A.D.K. and R.M.K.) against the average measurement, with mean absolute difference (continuous line) and 95% CI of the mean difference (dashed lines).

also did not find a correlation between mean pretreatment tumor ADC and TRG score, neither for the manual nor for the semi-automated volumetric measurement method (Figure 9A and B). We also did not find a correlation between change in mean tumor ADC between the first and second MRI scan and TRG score, neither for the manual nor for semi-automated volumetric method

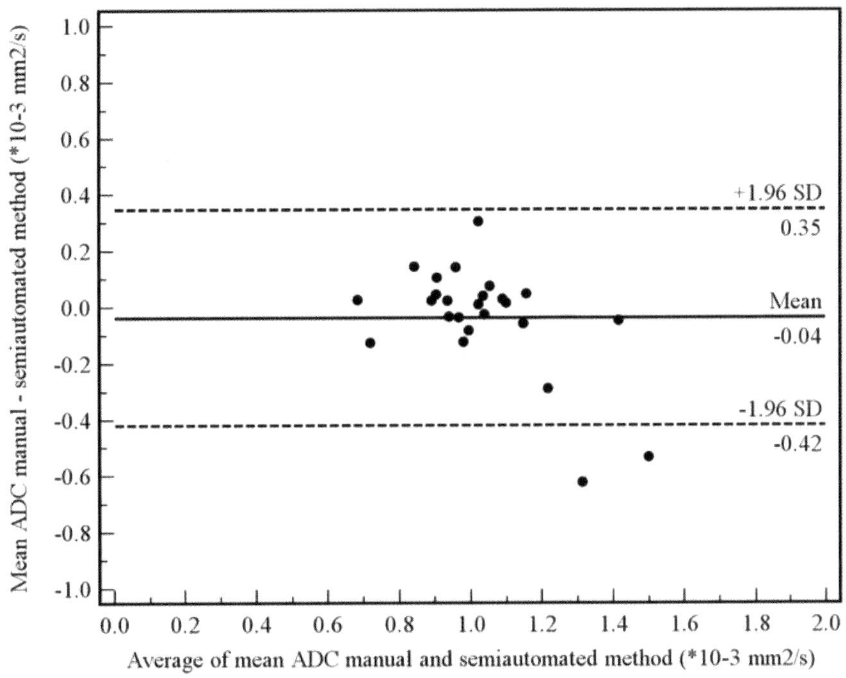

Figure 6. Agreement between the manual and semi-automated method in measuring mean tumor ADC. Measurements from both the first and second MRI scan were included in this analysis. Bland-Altman plot shows the difference between the manual and semi-automated measurements against the average measurement, with mean absolute difference (continuous line) and 95% CI of the mean difference (dashed lines).

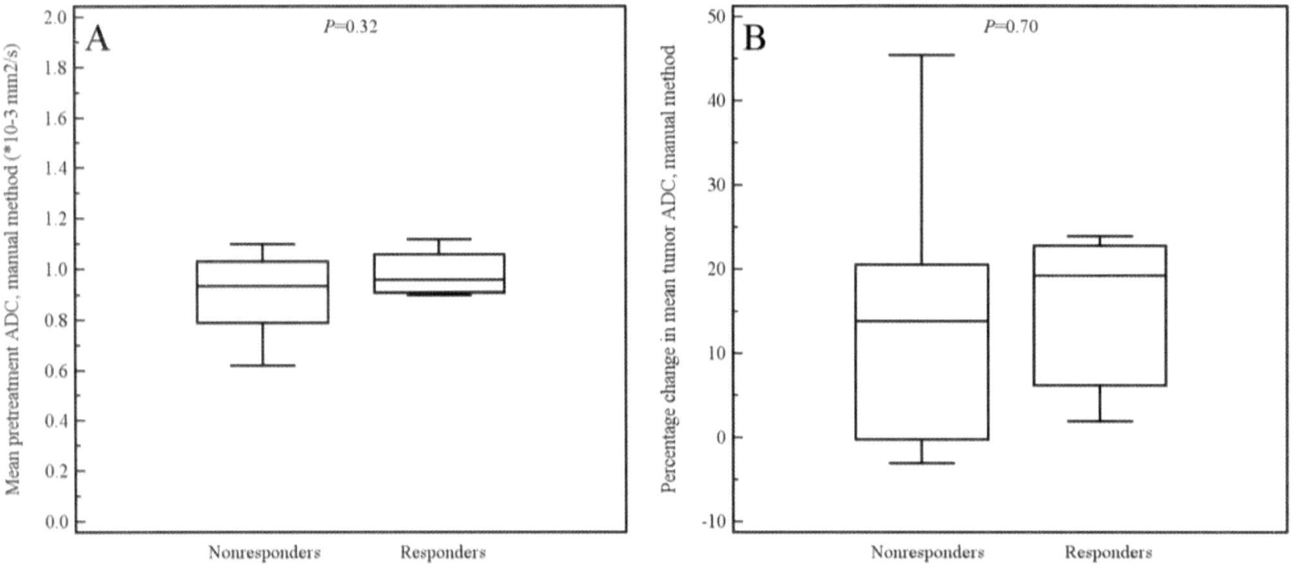

Figure 7. Box plots show the distribution of mean pretreatment ADC values (A) and percentage change in ADC value (B), as measured by the manual method, for patients with and without tumor response.

(Figure 10A and B). Of note, the interested reader who wishes to see all original data may contact the corresponding author.

Discussion

As diffusion within tumors is impeded by the presence of cellular membranes and macromolecular structures, treatment with chemotherapy and radiation therapy can result in the loss of cell membrane integrity which can be detected as an increase in mean tumor ADC [11]. DW-MRI for monitoring neoadjuvant therapy has already been applied in a wide variety of cancer types and organ sites, including the liver, breast, bone, soft tissue tumors, cervical tumors, head and neck tumors, as well as rectal cancer [11]. To date, there are only few published studies investigating the clinical value of DW-MRI in evaluating esophageal cancer. An initial study by Sakurada et al. [8] in 24 patients showed that DW-MRI only has a limited role in detecting esophageal cancer and nodal staging. Another study in 123 patients with esophageal squamous cell cancer found that ADC values of primary tumors were lower as clinical T and N stages were more advanced [12]. Aoyagi et al. [13] showed that tumors with lower ADC values had more stromal collagen and higher amount of vascular endothelial growth receptor expression (a marker for tumor neoangiogenesis). A study by the same research group [14], in 80 patients with esophageal squamous cell carcinoma who were treated with chemoradiotherapy, showed that higher mean pretreatment tumor

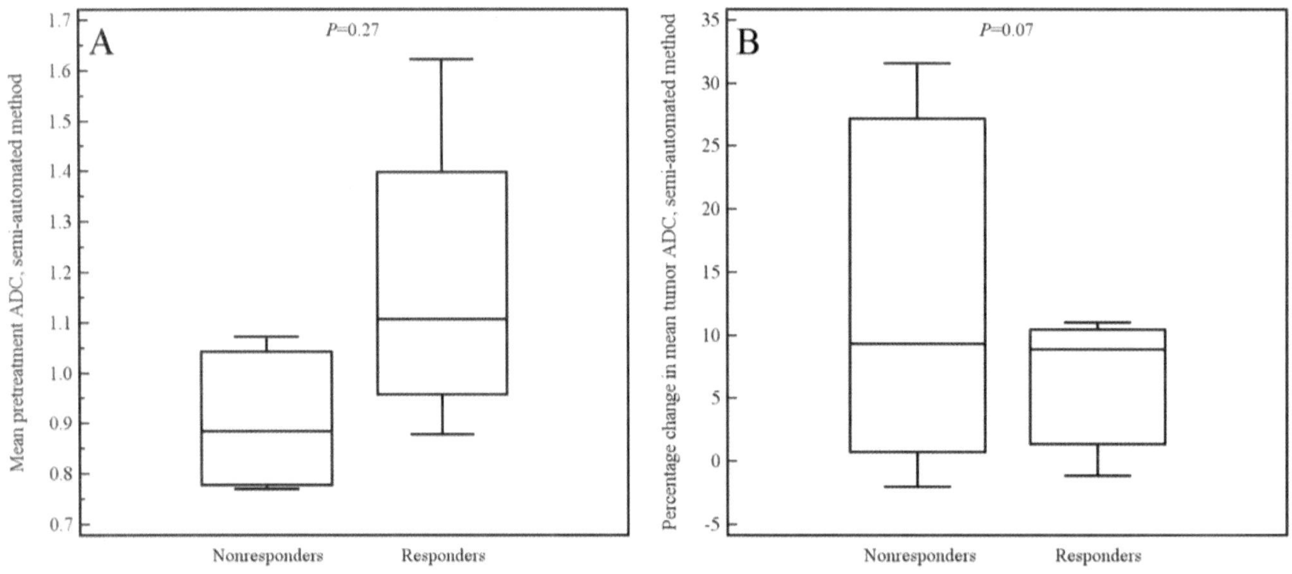

Figure 8. Box plots show the distribution of mean pretreatment ADC values (A) and percentage change in ADC value (B), as measured by the semi-automated method, for patients with and without tumor response.

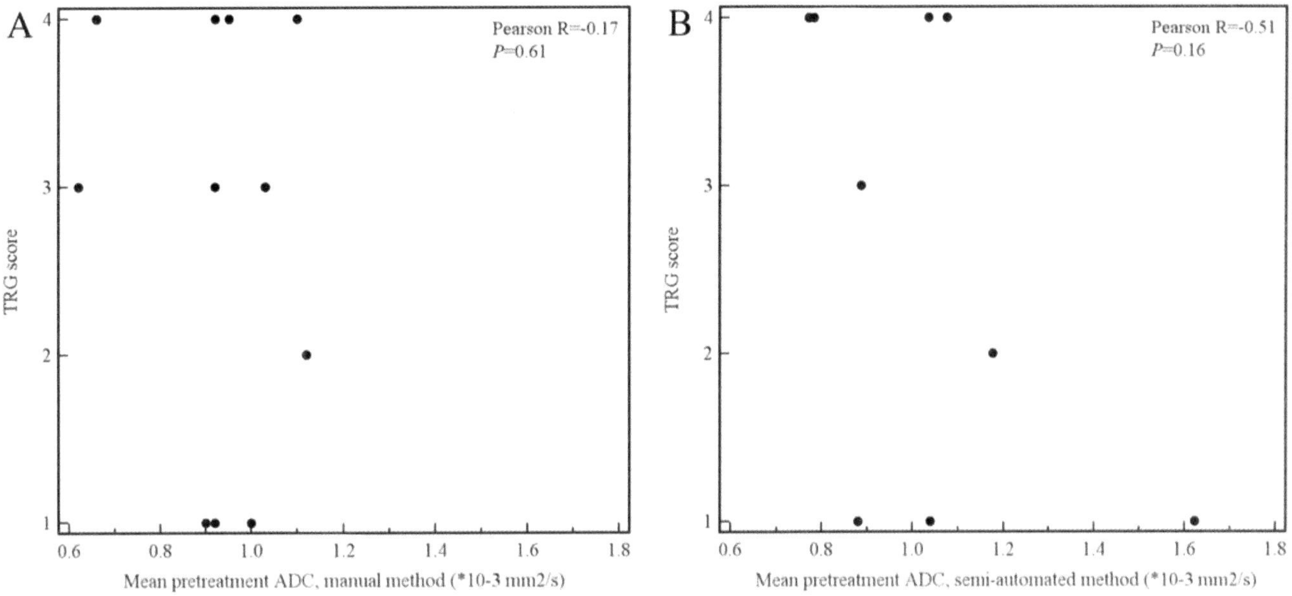

Figure 9. Scatter plots of mean pretreatment tumor ADC value (x-axis) and TRG score (y-axis), both for the manual (A) and semi-automated measurements (B).

ADC values were associated with longer overall survival. However, the association between change in tumor ADC value after start of chemoradiotherapy and overall survival was not investigated [14]. Sun et al. [15] assessed tumor ADC values before and after start of radiotherapy in 12 patients with esophageal cancer. They showed that patients with a higher increase in tumor ADC value had longer overall survival [15]. However, patients from their study [15] did not receive concurrent chemotherapy and radiotherapy, which is now the standard treatment [2,3]. In addition, in both Aoyagi et al.'s study [14] and Sun et al.'s study [15], no correlation between ADC measurements and histopathological tumor response or disease-free survival was performed. To our knowledge, our study is the first to perform serial DW-MRI in assessing tumor response to neoadjuvant chemoradiotherapy in patients with operable esophageal cancer.

The deep location of the esophagus, movement related to respiration, peristalsis and cardiac motion, and the presence of local field inhomogeneities caused by susceptibility changes at tissue interface make DW-MRI of esophageal cancer challenging. There are no established protocols for performing DW-MRI of esophageal cancer. The final scanning protocol we used was based

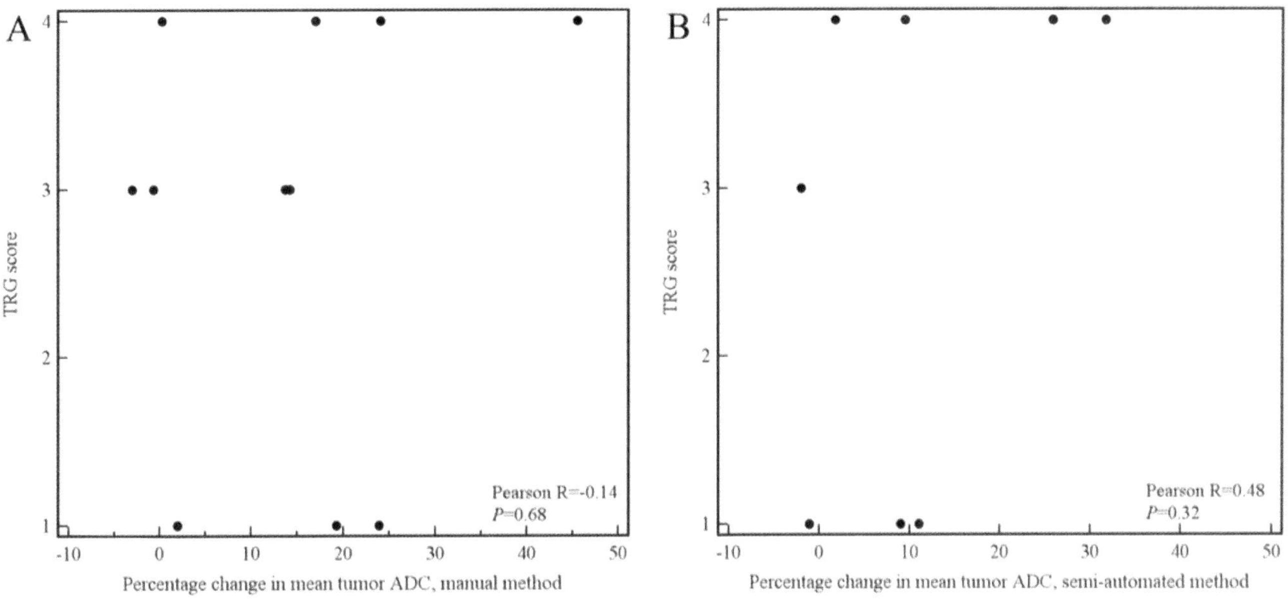

Figure 10. Scatter plots of percentage change in mean tumor ADC value between the first and second MRI scan (x-axis) and TRG score (y-axis), both for the manual (A) and semi-automated measurements (B).

on our experience in the use of DW-MRI in other tumors (such as rectal cancer), published literature [8,12], and test scanning in cooperation with the medical physics department. In three patients of our study (two with initial T2 disease and one with initial T3 disease), the primary tumor could not be detected on the DW-images. This is in conformity with Sakurada et al.'s study [8], where the primary tumor could not be detected in as much as 50.6%. In their study [8], the majority of early esophageal cancers (T1 and T2 tumors) were not detected, while almost all of the T3 and T4 tumors were detected. Thus, it is likely that the low detection rate of DW-MRI is due to the relatively small size of early cancers. Imaging at higher field strength, the use of stronger and faster gradients, and the use of more sophisticated multichannel coils (which enable accelerated parallel imaging) can improve spatial resolution and may increase visibility of smaller esophageal cancers.

We showed that reproducibility of semi-automated volumetric ADC measurements was higher than that of ADC measurements based on the manual placement of ROIs on two slices. This may be expected, as the semi-automated volumetric measurement method leaves less room for variation; the only manual steps to be undertaken are selection of a threshold and selection of ROIs which are within tumor.

In addition, heterogeneity within a tumor may require analysis of the entire tumor volume to obtain reproducible results. Accordingly, a previous study in rectal cancer patients also showed that ADC values obtained from the entire tumor volume were more reproducible than ADC values obtained from an ROI on a single slice or small sample ROIs [16]. Improvements to MRI scanner hardware, as described above, can enhance the resolution of MRI images which may further improve reproducibility of tumor ADC value measurements. A voxel-based analytical method, where changes in individual voxels can be monitored [11], may also improve reproducibility and may provide more reliable results. However, such an approach is challenging, since the esophagus is not a rigid and fixed structure, making spatial registration of DW images obtained before and after start of neoadjuvant therapy difficult.

In the present study, there were 12 and 9 patients for whom pretreatment ADC values (as assessed by the manual and semi-automated volumetric method, respectively) could be correlated to histopathological tumor response. We did not find a significant difference in mean pretreatment tumor ADC between responders and nonresponders. There were 11 and 8 patients for whom change in tumor ADC (as assessed by the manual and semi-automated volumetric method, respectively) could be correlated to histopathological tumor response. As expected, average mean tumor ADC, as measured by both manual and semi-automated methods, increased after neoadjuvant therapy (see Table 3). However, we found no significant difference in change in mean tumor ADC between responders and nonresponders. Although there may truly be no difference, sample size may have been insufficient to detect a significant correlation. Yet, the scatter plots also did not show any trend in relation to TRG score.

The present study has several limitations. First, as already addressed, our study population was relatively small. Most patients who were eligible for inclusion did not want to participate in our study, because they were already facing a difficult time with frequent visits to the hospital and radiation therapy clinic ahead. Because of the low statistical power of the present study, a false-negative result (type II error) cannot be excluded. Further research is needed to confirm or refute our findings. Second, we included mainly patients with adenocarcinoma, which is the most frequent type of esophageal cancer in the Western World [17]. The use of DW-MRI in assessing tumor response to neoadjuvant therapy in patients with squamous cell carcinoma needs to be further investigated. Third, we only performed one MRI scan after start of neoadjuvant therapy. In all patients, this MRI scan was obtained at the 10th day after start of neoadjuvant therapy. This may have been too early or too late to demonstrate significant effect of neoadjuvant treatment. If scanning is performed too early or too late, there may be a decrease in tumor ADC due to either cell swelling or due to the formation of tumor fibrosis, respectively. Future studies need to perform serial DW-MRI scans after start of neoadjuvant therapy to assess whether there is an optimal time point at which change in mean tumor ADC should be assessed. Fourth, we only correlated ADC measurements to histopathological tumor response. The correlation between ADC measurements and clinical endpoints, such as disease-free and overall survival, was not investigated. However, it has been shown that histopathological tumor response after neoadjuvant therapy is strongly related to disease-free and overall survival in patients with esophageal cancer [9,18–20].

In conclusion, the results of the present study show that semi-automated volumetric ADC measurements have higher reproducibility than manual ADC measurements in monitoring response to neoadjuvant chemoradiotherapy in patients with esophageal adenocarcinoma. Our results, although they should be interpreted with care because of small sample size, suggest that pretreatment tumor ADC and change in tumor ADC 10 days after start of chemoradiotherapy do not correlate to tumor response.

Author Contributions

Conceived and designed the experiments: RMK AKD MNS RCMB SS GL RC LEO RLGMB RFAV. Performed the experiments: RMK AKD SS GL RC RFAV. Analyzed the data: RMK AKD RFAV. Wrote the paper: RMK AKD. Revising the article critically for important intellectual content: MNS RCMB SS GL RC LEO RLGMB RFAV.

References

1. Ferlay J, Shin HR, Bray F, Forman D, Mathers C, et al. (2008) Estimates of worldwide burden of cancer in 2008: GLOBOCAN 2008. Int J Cancer 127:2893–2917.
2. Sjoquist KM, Burmeister BH, Smithers BM, Zalcberg JR, Simes RJ, et al. (2011) Australasian Gastro-Intestinal Trials Group. Survival after neoadjuvant chemotherapy or chemoradiotherapy for resectable oesophageal carcinoma: an updated meta-analysis. Lancet Oncol 12:681–692.
3. van Hagen P, Hulshof MC, van Lanschot JJ, Steyerberg EW, van Berge Henegouwen MI, et al; CROSS Group (2012) Preoperative chemoradiotherapy for esophageal or junctional cancer. N Engl J Med 366:2074–2084.
4. Malthaner RA, Collin S, Fenlon D (2006) Preoperative chemotherapy for resectable thoracic esophageal cancer. Cochrane Database Syst Rev 3:CD001556.
5. Kwee RM (2010) Prediction of tumor response to neoadjuvant therapy in patients with esophageal cancer with use of 18F FDG PET: a systematic review. Radiology 254:707–717.
6. MRIsafety.com. Available: http://www.mrisafety.com. Accessed 2013 Oct 5.
7. Schindelin J, Arganda-Carreras I, Frise E, Kaynig V, Longair Mr, et al. (2012) Fiji: an open-source platform for biological-image analysis. Nat Methods 9:676–682.
8. Sakurada A, Takahara T, Kwee TC, Yamashita T, Nasu S, et al. (2009) Diagnostic performance of diffusion-weighted magnetic resonance imaging in esophageal cancer. Eur Radiol 19:1461–1469.
9. Mandard AM, Dalibard F, Mandard JC, Marnay J, Henry-Amar M, et al. (1994) Pathologic assessment of tumor regression after preoperative chemoradiotherapy of esophageal carcinoma. Clinicopathologic correlations. Cancer 73:2680–2686.
10. Bland JM, Altman DG (1986) Statistical methods for assessing agreement between two methods of clinical measurement. Lancet 1:307–310.
11. Thoeny HC, Ross BD (2010) Predicting and monitoring cancer treatment response with diffusion-weighted MRI. J Magn Reson Imaging; 32:2–16.

12. Aoyagi T, Shuto K, Okazumi S, Shimada H, Nabeya Y, et al. (2010) Evaluation of the clinical staging of esophageal cancer by using diffusion-weighted imaging. Exp Ther Med 1:847–852.
13. Aoyagi T, Shuto K, Okazumi S, Hayano K, Satoh A, et al. (2012) Apparent diffusion coefficient correlation with oesophageal tumour stroma and angiogenesis. Eur Radiol 22:1172–1177.
14. Aoyagi T, Shuto K, Okazumi S, Shimada H, Kazama T, et al. (2011) Apparent diffusion coefficient values measured by diffusion-weighted imaging predict chemoradiotherapeutic effect for advanced esophageal cancer. Dig Surg 28:252–257.
15. Sun YS, Cui Y, Tang L, Qi LP, Wang N, et al. (2011) Early evaluation of cancer response by a new functional biomarker: apparent diffusion coefficient. AJR Am J Roentgenol 197:W23–29.
16. Lambregts DM, Beets GL, Maas M, Curvo-Semedo L, Kessels AG, et al. (2011) Tumour ADC measurements in rectal cancer: effect of ROI methods on ADC values and interobserver variability. Eur Radiol 21:2567–2574.
17. Enzinger PC, Mayer RJ (2003) Esophageal cancer. N Engl J Med 349:2241–2252.
18. Ancona E, Ruol A, Santi S, Merigliano S, Sileni VC, et al. (2001) Only pathologic complete response to neoadjuvant chemotherapy improves significantly the long term survival of patients with resectable esophageal squamous cell carcinoma: final report of a randomized, controlled trial of preoperative chemotherapy versus surgery alone. Cancer 91:2165–2174.
19. Donington JS, Miller DL, Allen MS, Deschamps C, Nichols FC 3rd, et al. (2003) Tumor response to induction chemoradiation: influence on survival after esophagectomy. Eur J Cardiothorac Surg 24:631–636.
20. Chirieac LR, Swisher SG, Ajani JA, Komaki RR, Correa AM, et al. (2005) Posttherapy pathologic stage predicts survival in patients with esophageal carcinoma receiving preoperative chemoradiation. Cancer 103:1347–1355.

17

Prognostic Nomograms for Predicting Survival and Distant Metastases in Locally Advanced Rectal Cancers

Junjie Peng[1,2]ⁱ, Ying Ding[3]ⁱ, Shanshan Tu[4], Debing Shi[1,2], Liang Sun[5], Xinxiang Li[1,2], Hongbin Wu[1,2], Sanjun Cai[1,2]*

1 Department of Colorectal Surgery, Fudan University Shanghai Cancer Center, Shanghai, China, **2** Department of Oncology, Shanghai Medical College, Fudan University, Shanghai, China, **3** Department of Biostatistics, University of Pittsburgh, Pittsburgh, Pennsylvania, United States of America, **4** Department of Statistics, University of Pittsburgh, Pittsburgh, Pennsylvania, United States of America, **5** School of Science and Technology, Georgia Gwinnett College, Atlanta, Georgia, United States of America

Abstract

Aim: To develop prognostic nomograms for predicting outcomes in patients with locally advanced rectal cancers who do not receive preoperative treatment.

Materials and Methods: A total of 883 patients with stage II–III rectal cancers were retrospectively collected from a single institution. Survival analyses were performed to assess each variable for overall survival (OS), local recurrence (LR) and distant metastases (DM). Cox models were performed to develop a predictive model for each endpoint. The performance of model prediction was validated by cross validation and on an independent group of patients.

Results: The 5-year LR, DM and OS rates were 22.3%, 32.7% and 63.8%, respectively. Two prognostic nomograms were successfully developed to predict 5-year OS and DM-free survival rates, with c-index of 0.70 (95% CI = [0.66, 0.73]) and 0.68 (95% CI = [0.64, 0.72]) on the original dataset, and 0.76 (95% CI = [0.67, 0.86]) and 0.73 (95% CI = [0.63, 0.83]) on the validation dataset, respectively. Factors in our models included age, gender, carcinoembryonic antigen value, tumor location, T stage, N stage, metastatic lymph nodes ratio, adjuvant chemotherapy and chemoradiotherapy. Predicted by our nomogram, substantial variability in terms of 5-year OS and DM-free survival was observed within each TNM stage category.

Conclusions: The prognostic nomograms integrated demographic and clinicopathological factors to account for tumor and patient heterogeneity, and thereby provided a more individualized outcome prognostication. Our individualized prediction nomograms could help patients with preoperatively under-staged rectal cancer about their postoperative treatment strategies and follow-up protocols.

Editor: Keping Xie, The University of Texas MD Anderson Cancer Center, United States of America

Funding: This work was supported by the grants from Shanghai Municipal Commission of Health and Family Planning Program KJ201204. The funders had no role in study design, data collection and analysis, decision to publish, or preparation of the manuscript.

Competing Interests: The authors have declared that no competing interests exist.

* Email: caisanjun@gmail.com

ⁱ These authors contributed equally to this work.

Background

Colorectal cancer is the most commonly diagnosed gastrointestinal malignancy in the world. As most of patients with rectal cancer present with locally advanced disease at diagnosis, neoajuvant chemoradiation is the standard recommendation to improve patients' outcomes including quality of life. Compared to colon cancer, treatment is more heterogeneous in rectal cancer. In real clinical practice, approximately 20–50% of patients with stage II–III rectal cancer in North America receive definitive surgery prior to adjuvant treatment [1,2], and the proportion is even higher in Asia [3]. The reasons for not giving neoadjuvant therapy may be multifarious. Although neoadjuvant chemoradiotherapy (CRT) has been confirmed to improve local control for locally advanced rectal cancer, its efficacy in preventing distant metastases and improving OS remains controversial [4]. Because preoperative CRT is associated with increased complications compared to surgery alone, we sought to characterize patients with locally advanced rectal cancer who were adequately treated with surgery followed by adjuvant chemotherapy[5–7].

Currently, the TNM stage system from the American Joint Commission on Cancer (AJCC) and the International Union Against Cancer [8,9] is the most reliable prognostic system for all stages of rectal cancer patients with or without preoperative treatment [10,11]. However, TNM staging does not integrate demographic features like age, or other pathological features like histopathology, perineural invasion, or tumor location, into a patient's outcome prediction. More individualized outcome prediction models could help physicians advise patients about personalized treatment strategies and follow-up protocols.

Developing a nomogram for prognosis or treatment prediction has been considered helpful in individualized medicine and successful applications have been utilized in many malignancies[12–15]. This statistically based tool provides a predicted probability of a specific outcome, using a combined set of proven or potential prognostic factors. Recently, a nomogram was developed to predict outcomes of locally advanced rectal cancers with preoperative radiotherapy or CRT [16]. However, due to changes in pathological features after preoperative treatment, this nomogram only applies to patients who receive preoperative treatment. Our study was designed to develop prognostic nomograms for patients with locally advanced rectal cancer who did not receive preoperative treatment.

Materials and Methods

Ethics

A retrospective study was conducted at the Fudan University Shanghai Cancer Center. This study was approved by the Fudan University Shanghai Cancer Center Institutional Ethics Committee. According to hospital routine, patients are asked to provide a written informed consent after their admission that their clinical and outcome information will be used in future scientific studies. Patients' records and follow-up information were anonymized and de-identified prior to analysis. The institutional Ethics Committee approved the exception of informed consent if informed consent could not be obtained due to patients' death or lost of follow-up in our institutional database.

Patient Population

All patients with AJCC stage II–III (restaged according to 7th Edition) [8] rectal cancers were collected from the institutional colorectal cancer database. The statistical analyses were performed for patients operated between 1986 and 2005 (N = 833), whose tumors were located within 15 cm from anal verge. Patients who met one of the following criteria were excluded: (1) received preoperative treatment, (2) synchronous distant metastases, (3) surgery without curative intent, and (4) complete loss of follow-up after surgery.

An independent group of patients with stage II–III rectal cancer (N = 84) who were operated between January 2006 and June 2007 were selected for validation (Table 1).

Follow-up

According to institutional follow-up protocol, all patients were asked to follow-up every 3–6 months after surgery in the first 3 years, and 6–12 months thereafter in the next two years. Follow-up information was recorded in the database. A minimum follow-up of 60 months was required for the patients who are alive in the validation dataset so that their 5-year survival status is known. The primary endpoint is the overall survival (OS) time. Local recurrence (LR) time and distant metastases (DM) time are the secondary endpoints. The LR time was calculated from the time of surgery to the time when cancer recurrence was determined in the pelvis or anastomosis by physical examination, colonoscopy, or imaging studies. The DM time was defined from the time of surgery to the identification of distant recurrence. There were three times of massive follow-up for all off-records patients via mail or telephone in1996, 2002, and 2007.

Statistical Model Creation

Kaplan-Meier plots and log-rank tests were performed for each potential predictive variable for the primary endpoint OS and the secondary endpoints LR and DM. Cox proportional hazards (PH) model was performed to develop the predictive model for OS. All decisions with respect to the grouping of the categorical variables and categorizing the continuous variables were made before modeling. These predictive models were the basis for the nomograms and the estimated probabilities of interest (e.g., 5-year OS) were calculated and presented in the nomograms.

Model Validation

Each nomogram went through two validation procedures: internal validation using the study patients for the model creation and external validation using the independent validation patients. For each outcome variable, the predicted probability from the nomogram was compared with the actual status (e.g., alive or dead 5 years from surgery) for these uncensored observations. In addition, the Harrell's concordance index (c-index) was calculated for each nomogram [17]. This index calculates the proportion of all usable patient pairs in which the predictions and the outcomes are concordant and has a similar interpretation to that of the AUC. All the above validation analyses were performed for the study patient data and the independent validation data.

All the statistical analyses were performed using R 3.0.1.

Results

Outcomes and survival analyses

Of the 833 patients with locally advanced rectal cancer in training group, 267 patients (32%) experienced local recurrence and/or distant metastases, and 263 patients (31.5%) died of cancer or other reasons up to our last follow-up. Of those alive, median follow-up time was 51 months. The 5-year LR, DM, OS probabilities (estimated using Kaplan-Meier method) for all patients were 22.3%, 32.7% and 63.8%, respectively.

Demographic and clinicopathologic variables that potentially predict OS, LR and DM were collected, including age, gender, tumor location, preoperative carcinoembryonic antigen level (CEA), tumor differentiation, tumor histopathology, number of metastatic lymph nodes, number of total sampled lymph nodes, lymphovascular invasion, perineural invasion, T classification, N classification and adjuvant treatment. For each outcome variable (LR, DM, and OS), univariate analysis identified statistically significant predictors in the demographic features, clinical features, pathological features and treatment modalities. 5-year local control, distant control and overall survival rates were provided for every category of each predictor with p-values obtained from the Log-rank tests (Table 1).

Nomograms

For the development of nomograms, all patients in the main dataset were included (N = 833), and the nomograms were validated using the external dataset (N = 84). Two nomograms for overall survival and distant metastases were successfully developed (Figure 1). The predictors included in the nomograms are gender, age (< = 49, 50–69, > = 70), tumor location (<5 cm, 5 cm-10 cm, >10 cm), adjuvant chemotherapy (No/Yes), adjuvant chemoradiotherapy (No/Yes), T classification (T1–T2, T3, T4), N classification (N0, N1a, N1b, N2a, N2b), CEA (< = 5, >5) and ratio of metastatic lymph nodes. Table 2 presents the hazard ratio (HR) with 95% CI and the pvalue for each predictor, and the c-index for the main dataset and the external dataset respectively. For OS prediction, the c-index was 0.76 in external validation, with a 95% CI of 0.67 to 0.86. Similarly, for DM prediction, the c-index was 0.73 (95% CI, 0.63–0.84). However, the nomogram for local recurrence prediction was not developed because of the poor c-index value in external validation (c-index, 0.6; 95% CI, 0.45–0.75).

Table 1. Characteristics of all patients with locally advanced rectal cancer and outcomes for 833 patients in training group.

Variable	Training Group							Validation Group
	No. (%)	Local Control		Distant Control		Overall Survival		No. (%)
	(n = 833)	5 Year	P-value	5 Year	P-value	5 Year	P-value	(n = 84)
Demographic Variables								
Gender								
Male	490 (58.8)	0.770	0.423	0.637	0.006	0.608	0.008	50 (59.5)
Female	343 (41.2)	0.787		0.725		0.682		34 (40.5)
Age, years								
< = 49	262 (31.4)	0.738	0.354	0.649	0.191	0.609	0.097	29 (34.5)
50–69	432 (51.9)	0.802		0.699		0.668		50 (59.5)
> = 70	139 (16.7)	0.772		0.637		0.604		5 (6.0)
Clinical Variables								
Tumor location								
Low (<5 cm)	181 (21.7)	0.656	<0.001	0.638	0.221	0.563	0.011	26 (31.0)
Mid (5cm, 10 cm)	570 (68.5)	0.806		0.677		0.651		54 (64.3)
High (>10 cm)	82 (9.8)	0.846		0.719		0.715		4 (4.8)
CEA								
< = 5	406 (48.7)	0.817	0.005	0.696	0.073	0.660	0.062	67 (79.8)
>5	427 (51.3)	0.740		0.650		0.616		17 (20.2)
Pathological Variables								
Pathology								
Adenocarcinoma	683 (82.0)	0.773	0.947	0.683	0.184	0.653	0.128	79 (94.0)
MAC or SRC	150 (18.0)	0.792		0.625		0.574		5 (6.0)
Tumor grade								
Low-intermediate grade	708 (85.0)	0.788	0.119	0.681	0.272	0.643	0.356	65 (77.4)
High grade	125 (15.0)	0.713		0.630		0.612		19 (22.6)
pT classification								
T1	13 (1.6)	0.587	0.003	0.539	0.002	0.539	0.001	0 (0)
T2	93 (11.2)	0.83		0.711		0.676		3 (3.6)
T3	351 (42.1)	0.836		0.756		0.725		81 (86.4)
T4	376 (45.1)	0.714		0.589		0.550		0 (0)
pN classification								
N0	324 (38.9)	0.837	<0.001	0.774	<0.001	0.775	<0.001	14 (16.7)
N1a	142 (17.1)	0.753		0.699		0.683		13 (15.5)
N1b	152 (18.2)	0.793		0.638		0.539		24 (28.6)
N2a	112 (13.4)	0.734		0.581		0.548		18 (21.4)

Table 1. Cont.

Variable	Training Group							Validation Group
	No. (%)	Local Control		Distant Control		Overall Survival		No. (%)
	(n = 833)	5 Year	P-value	5 Year	P-value	5 Year	P-value	(n = 84)
N2b	103 (12.4)	0.619		0.451		0.396		15 (17.8)
Lymphovascular invasion								
Yes	178 (21.4)	0.780	0.956	0.610	0.139	0.547	0.019	42 (50.0)
No	655 (78.6)	0.776		0.691		0.666		42 (50.0)
Perineural invasion								
Yes	111 (13.3)	0.698	0.076	0.544	0.003	0.515	0.002	34 (41.5)
No	722 (86.7)	0.787		0.692		0.656		50 (58.5)
No. of metastatic lymph nodes								
=0	324 (38.9)	0.775	<0.001	0.837	0.002	0.774	<0.001	14 (16.7)
>=1	509 (61.1)	0.552		0.735		0.606		70 (83.3)
Treatment Variables								
Surgery type								
AR	494 (59.3)	0.832	<0.001	0.689	0.087	0.660	0.012	51 (60.7)
APR	339 (40.7)	0.697		0.649		0.607		33 (39.3)
Adjuvant treatment								
No treatment	252 (30.3)	0.676	<0.001	0.662	0.332	0.633	0.670	16 (19.0)
CT only	277 (33.3)	0.781		0.698		0.663		25 (29.8)
CRT only	123 (14.8)	0.822		0.718		0.612		3 (3.6)
CRT plus CT	181 (21.7)	0.905		0.697		0.628		40 (47.6)

Note: Tumor location was determined the distance from anal verge by preoperative colonoscopy or digital examination.
Abreviations: pT stage, pathological T stage; pN stage, pathological N stage; CEA, carcinoembryonic antigen; MAC, mucinous adenocarcinoma; SRC, signet ring cell carcinoma; AR, anterior resection; APR, abdominoperineal resection; CT, chemotherapy; CRT, chemoradiotherapy.

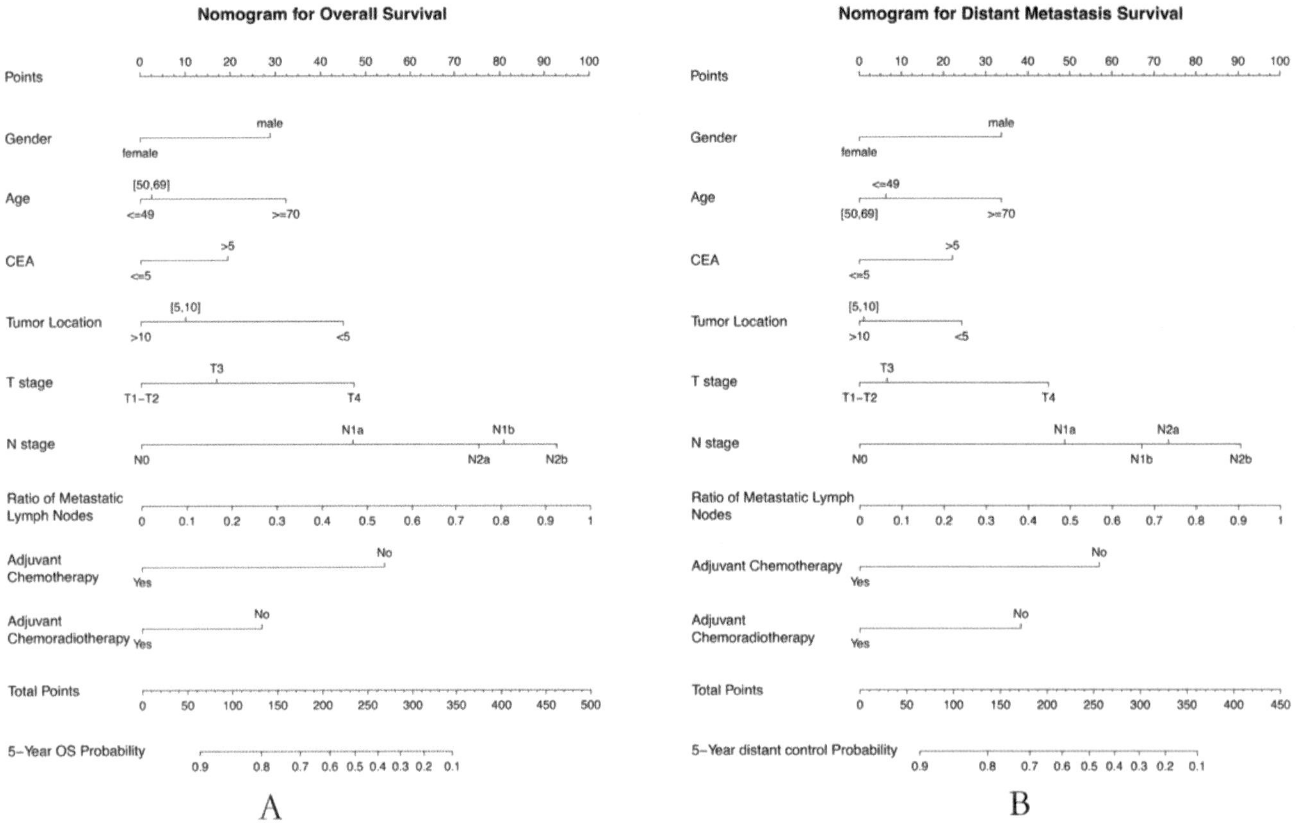

Figure 1. Nomograms developed for predicted 5-year overall survival (A) and distant control survival (B). Each variable value is assigned a score, and the sum of scores is converted to a probability of observed events in the lowest scale.

Predicted events within each AJCC stage classification

Within each AJCC stage (7th Edition), the 5-year OS rates were 82.2% (stage IIA), 70.2% (stage IIB–C), 70.1% (stage IIIA), 57.0% (stage IIIB) and 44.8% (stage IIIC); and the 5-year DM rates were 19.8% (stage IIA), 28.7% (stage IIB–C), 28.1% (stage IIIA), 34.9% (stage IIIB), and 52.0% (stage IIIC), respectively. The Kaplan-Meier survival probability curves by AJCC stage were plotted for OS and DM in Figure 2. The overall log-rank tests for testing whether the survival curves are the same among all AJCC stage groups are significant for both OS and DM ($p<0.001$).

Based on our developed nomograms, the predicted probability of 5-year overall survival and distant control for each patient was computed, and the corresponding histograms were produced by AJCC stage classification from stage IIA to stage IIIC, respectively (Figure 3). The histograms showed that even within the same AJCC stage category, there are still a substantive amount of variability in terms of the predicted 5-year OS and DM-free probabilities, while in average the later stage patients have a smaller probabilities compared to earlier stage patients for both survival outcomes. Greater variations were observed for later stage patients (stage IIIB and IIIC) than earlier stage patients (stage IIA to IIIC) in terms of both 5-year OS and DM-free predicted probabilities.

Discussion

In current study, for AJCC stage II–III (7th edition) rectal cancers without neoadjuvant treatment, we have developed prognostic monograms with independent validation samples for predicting OS and DM, based on demographic, clinicopathological and adjuvant treatment information. Our models were developed using a 20-year period institutional database; during that time, neoadjuvant RT or CRT was not well applied in China. Our predictive models are helpful to support decision-making in clinical practice and follow-up protocols, especially in patients with rectal cancer who are preoperatively under-staged and undergo surgical resection first.

The purpose of treatment in rectal cancer is to potentially improve symptoms through local control, increase chance of cure, or prolong survival. Although the German Rectal Cancer Study Group established the significant improvements in local control and toxicity for patients with locally advanced rectal cancer treated with preoperative CRT [4], long-term follow-up and other clinical trials didn't show benefit in overall survival and distant control for patients undergoing preoperative CRT[18–21]. A variety of factors ultimately influence a patient's decision to receive preoperative CRT, such as proximal tumor location, suboptimal preoperative staging methods, inaccessible facilities for optimal radiotherapy, patient preference, and/or financial considerations. The potential benefits of receiving preoperative CRT must be carefully evaluated with the potential risks. Currently, there is no nationwide or international report about the accurate proportion of preoperative CRT in locally advanced rectal cancer. The US National Cancer Database (NCDB) reported that in 2008, 41% of patients with stage I–II rectal cancer received proctocolectomy with chemotherapy or radiotherapy, in which 80% of chemotherapy, which is mainly accompanied by radiotherapy, was delivered preoperatively. However, the percentage of preoperative CRT in stage II–III rectal cancer was not reported [2]. In Canada, only an average of 45% of stage II–III rectal cancers treated in 2007–2008

Table 2. Multivariate analyses of 5-year outcomes: the final predictors for developing the nomograms.

Variable	Cox PH Regression			Nomogram	
	HR	95% CI	*p*-value	C-index	95% CI
Distant Metastases					
Gender					
Male vs Female	1.42	[1.07,1.88]	0.014		
Age (years)					
50–69 vs <=49	0.94	[0.69,1.27]	0.672		
>=70 vs <=49	1.33	[0.92,1.93]	0.134		
Tumor location					
Mid ([5 cm, 10 cm]) vs Low (<5 cm)	0.79	[0.58,1.07]	0.122		
High (>10 cm) vs Low (<5 cm)	0.78	[0.46,1.31]	0.344		
Adjuvant chemotherapy					
Yes vs No	0.55	[0.41,0.74]	<0.0001		
Adjuvant chemoradiotherapy					
Yes vs No	0.67	[0.50,0,90]	0.008	Training Data: 0.68	[0.64,0.72]
pT classification				Validation Data:0.73	[0.63,0.83]
T3 vs T1–T2	1.07	[0.66,1.72]	0.781	Ten-fold Cross	
'T4' vs 'T1–T2'	1.59	[1.03,2.47]	0.038	Validation	
pN classification				(Training Data): 0.65	
'N1a' vs 'N0'	1.66	[1.05,2.62]	0.031		
'N1b' vs 'N0'	2.00	[1.23,3.27]	0.005		
'N2a' vs 'N0'	2.14	[1.21,3.80]	0.009		
'N2b' vs 'N0'	2.56	[1.23,5.32]	0.012		
CEA					
>5 vs <=5	1.26	[0.96,1.64]	0.093		
LNR					
Continuous*	1.11	[1.02,1.20]	0.013		
Overall Survival					
Gender					
Male vs Female	1.37	[1.06, 1.78]	0.017		
Age (years)					
50–69 vs <=49	1.03	[0.77,1.36]	0.854		
>=70 vs <=49	1.42	[1.00,2.02]	0.049		
Tumor location					
Mid ([5 cm, 10 cm]) vs Low (<5cm)	0.68	[0.52, 0.90]	0.007		
High (>10 cm) vs Low (<5 cm)	0.61	[0.37, 1.01]	0.053		
Adjuvant chemotherapy					
Yes vs No	0.56	[0.42, 0.73]	<0.0001		
Adjuvant chemoradiotherapy					
Yes vs No	0.75	[0.57, 0.98]	0.033	Training data: 0.70	[0.66, 0.73]
pT stage				Validation data: 0.76	[0.67, 0.86]
'T3' vs 'T1–T2'	1.20	[0.77, 1.87]	0.414	Ten-fold Cross	
'T4' vs 'T1–T2'	1.68	[1.11,2.52]	0.013	Validation	
pN stage				(Training Data): 0.67	
'N1a' vs 'N0'	1.67	[1.08, 2.59]	0.021		
'N1b' vs 'N0'	2.42	[1.54, 3.79]	0.00012		
'N2a' vs 'N0'	2.28	[1.33, 3.91]	0.0028		
'N2b' vs 'N0'	2.75	[1.40, 5.44]	0.0035		
CEA					
>5 vs <=5	1.24	[0.96, 1.59]	0.097		

Table 2. Cont.

Variable	Cox PH Regression			Nomogram	
	HR	95% CI	*p*-value	C-index	95% CI
LNR					
Continuous*	1.12	[1.03, 1.20]	0.0046		

Note: The concordance index (c-index) for the training and external validation are given for the nomogram as a performance measure; Tumor location was determined the distance from anal verge by preoperative colonoscopy or digital examination.
*LNR was analyzed as a continuous variable.
Abbreviations: HR, hazard ratio; PH, proportional hazards; c-index, concordance index; CEA, carcinoembryonic antigen; LNR, metastatic lymph nodes ratio.

were reported to undergo preoperative RT or CRT in a Canadian nationwide cancer performance report [1,22]. In Asian countries, much lower percentage of stage II–III rectal cancers undergo preoperative RT or CRT, as most surgeons in Asia do not usually recommend preoperative CRT for clinical T2 or T3 rectal cancers [3]. The wide variation in indications and clinical applications of neoadjuvant RT or CRT reflect the complexity of the disease, which should alert international rectal cancer expert organizations as well as health-care administrators. Therefore, in current clinical circumstance, there are still a great number of patients with locally advanced rectal cancer receiving curative surgical treatment prior to RT or CRT. Our study will help rectal cancer patients and physicians to pursue more individualized postoperative treatment according to their risks of disease control and survival expectations.

With the wide utilization of neoadjuvant CRT in clinical practice and randomized clinical trials, several studies focused on the outcome prediction in patients with combined modality treatment. Recently, a prediction nomogram was developed to predict local recurrence, distant metastases, and survival for patients with locally advanced rectal cancer treated with long-course chemoradiotherapy (CRT) followed by surgery in five European phase III clinical trials [16]. Postoperative ypT stage and ypN stage were most relevant to overall survival. However, as downstaged by preoperative CRT, the two most important prognostic factors (ypT and ypN classfications) could not be well applied to patients treated with curative surgery prior to adjuvant treatment. Otherwise, the decision of neoadjuvant CRT mainly relies on preoperative staging of the primary tumor. The accuracy of T and N stage by preoperative MRI or endorectal ultrasound varies, especially in N stage. A number of patients with locally advanced rectal cancer will be under-staged preoperatively and undergo surgery first. The postoperative treatment and outcome prediction for this group of patients are currently lacking. Moreover, although perioperative CRT or CT has been proved to be effective in rectal cancer, in real clinical circumstance, there are still a part of patients with locally advanced rectal cancer undergoing surgery alone. According to a large-scale population-based study through the California Cancer Registry, there were still 33% and 18.6% of patients with stage II and stage III rectal cancer undergoing surgery alone from the year 1994 to 2008 [23]. Similarly, 57.4% and 13.0% of patients with stage II and stage III rectal cancer underwent surgery alone in our study. Currently, we are lacking of studies in defining characteristics of patients who

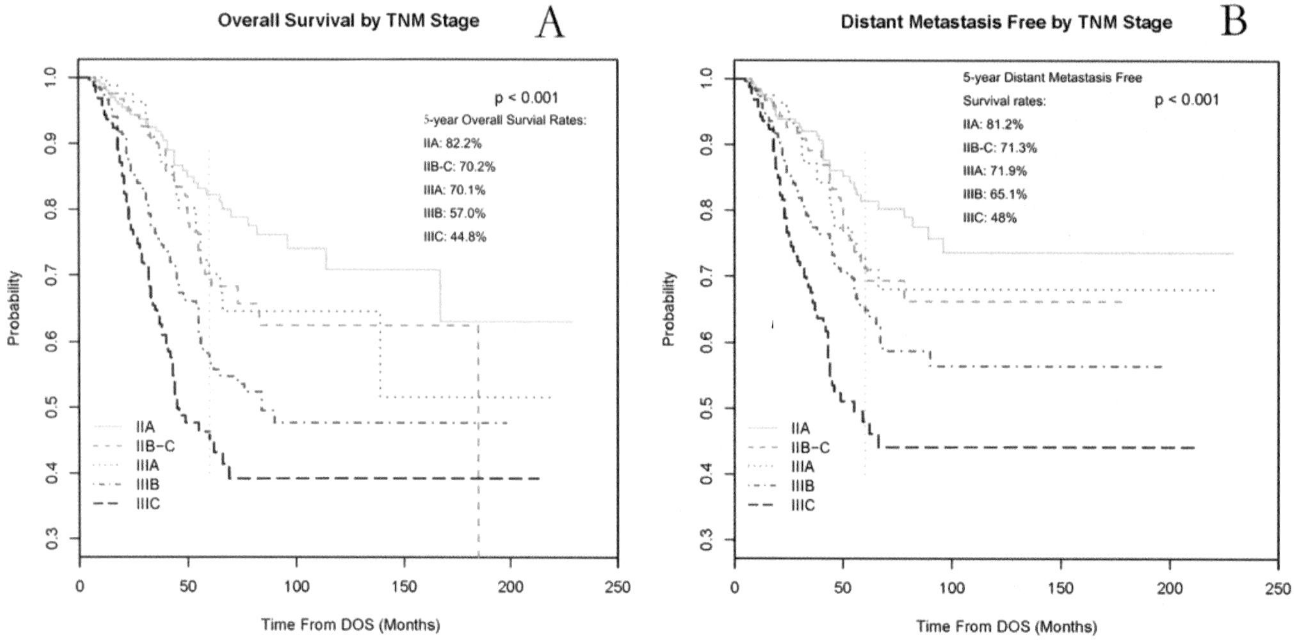

Figure 2. The overall survival (A) and distant metastases free (B) Kaplan-Meier probability curves within each stage (AJCC 7th Edition) classification in locally advanced rectal cancer.

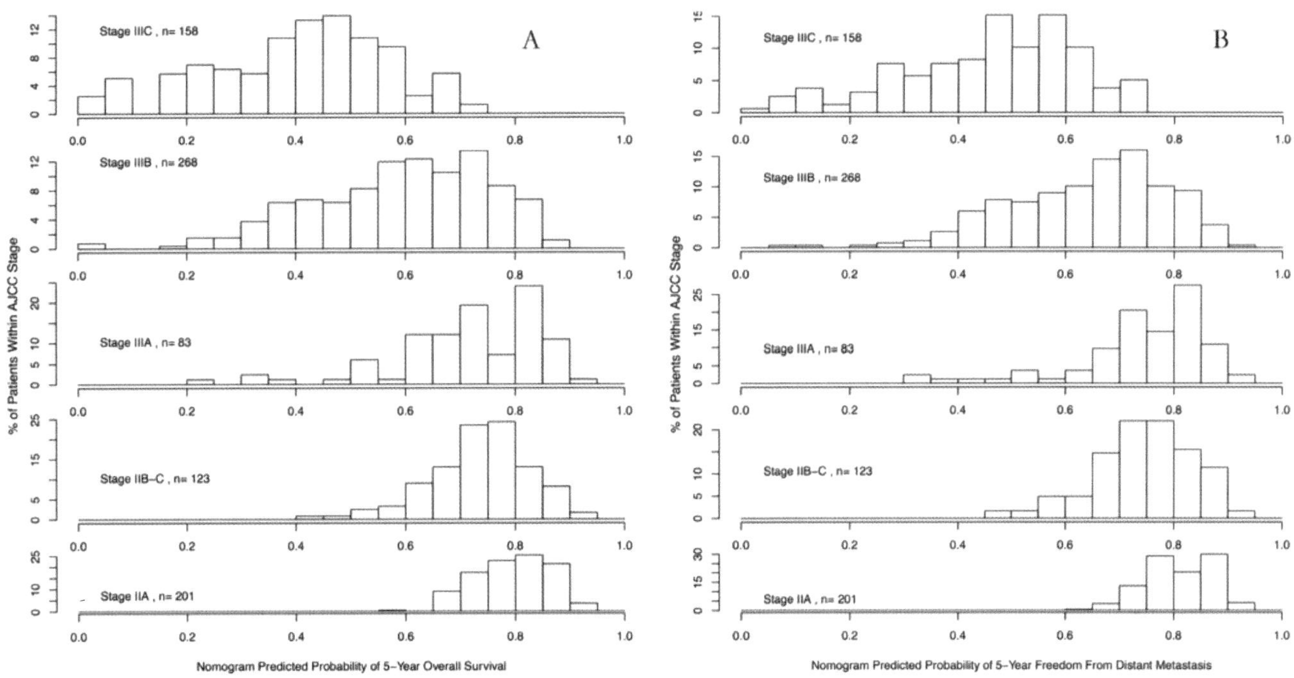

Figure 3. Histogram of nomogram-predicted 5-year overall survival rate (A) and distant control rate (B) within each subgroup of the 7th edition of American Joint Committee on Cancer (AJCC) stage.

have good outcomes without neoadjuvant therapy, particularly with surgery alone. Our nomogram provides a helpful tool for identifying patients with good outcomes if they were preoperatively under-staged and underwent surgery first. Meanwhile, as preoperative CRT contributed small improvements in overall survival and distant metastases, our study provided helpful tools and comparable dataset for predicting patients' distant control and overall survival in locally advanced rectal cancer with multiple treatment modalities.

The goal of our study is to develop monograms to predict overall survival and distant metastases for patients without preoperative treatment. To our knowledge, using the 7th edition of AJCC staging system was the first predicting model for OS and distant control in rectal cancer (Figure 2), especially in Asian patients who were less represented in the AJCC stage system. Similar survival differences among different AJCC stage categories were observed in our patient cohort, as compared with Surveillance, Epidemiology, and End Results (SEER) population-based data [24]. Postoperative T stage and N stage were still most significant factors to predict OS and DM rates. However, from the predicted outcomes based on our nomograms, heterogeneities in the risk of death and distant metastases still largely existed within each sub-category stage from stage IIA to stage IIIC. Specifically, from the histograms in Figure 3, the variability of predicted OS and DM rates was observed greater in patients in stage IIIB and IIIC than patients in stage IIA–IIIA. This suggests that the prediction value of OS and DM may be better in patients with stage IIIB and IIIC rectal cancer when adding these demographic and clinicopathological variables which were not included in TNM staging system; while for patients with stage IIA to IIIA, molecular markers (eg. microsatellite instability, loss of heterozygosity, etc.), rather than adding more clinicopathological variables, may be benefit to further improve the accuracy of outcome prediction. By integrating important demographic and clinicopathological features, our nomogram helped further individualize the outcome prediction based on current TNM staging system. More personalized postoperative treatment may be utilized for preoperatively under-staged patients with rectal cancer in the same AJCC stage.

In addition to the TN stage, metastatic lymph nodes ratio (LNR) was reported to be a reliable prognostic factor both in colon and rectal cancer[25–28]. However, utilization LNR in clinical practice is relatively difficult, as optimal cut-off of the continuous LNR value has not been established. We also found LNR was one of most important prognostic factors for predicting DM and OS, in addition to patients' N stage. LNR was treated as a continuous variable in our predicting nomograms, which contributed to improve the performance of our model in predicting patients' survival outcomes. Data from the five European trials found small but statistical significant improvement in distant control for patients with neoadjuvant CRT [16]. A recent meta-analysis of 21 randomized controlled trials from 1975 to 2011 concluded that adjuvant 5-Fu-based chemotherapy was beneficial for rectal cancer patients in improving overall survival and disease-free survival [29]. However, the benefit of adjuvant chemotherapy after combined treatment of rectal cancer is still not well defined in single randomized trials [4,19,21]. In our patient cohort, we only found improvements in local control in patients with any adjuvant treatment, compared with no adjuvant treatment. Further clinical trials are needed to explore the effect of adjuvant chemotherapy (single agent or combination) in improving distant control and overall survival.

Currently, there are emerged debates about adding adjuvant radiotherapy to node positive patients who receive surgical treatment first because of under-staged disease by preoperative imaging. Although randomized clinical trials proved the improvement of local control in node positive rectal cancer [30,31], the risks of treatment toxicities and decremented quality of life limited its clinical use [32,33]. A predicted nomogram for local recurrence including demographic and clincopathological variables may help physicians to choose patients who may benefit more from adjuvant radiotherapy. In our study, improved local control was observed in patients with any adjuvant treatment in univariate analysis, and the most optimal local control were observed in patients with adjuvant chemoradiotherapy followed by chemotherapy (Table 2). Unfortunately, our study was not able to develop a reliable nomogram for predicting local recurrence. Treatment variations in adjuvant setting, heterogeneous data, lacking of statistical power, less events in the validation group may be attributed to this. Further studies are needed to develop a reliable predictive model for local recurrence in preoperatively under-staged patients.

As a retrospective study, there are other limitations: detailed regimens of adjuvant chemotherapy could not be clearly provided for each patient; techniques of radiotherapy are changing over the 20 years; detailed information of recurrence may be unclear for part of patients, as well as loss of follow-up problems. However, our study still provides a valuable tool to help clinicians manage under-staged patients with rectal cancer who undergo surgery first. Further study is needed to provide optimal postoperative treatment for these patients.

Conclusions

The prognostic nomograms integrated demographic and clinicopathological factors to account for tumor and patient heterogeneity, and thereby provided a more individualized outcome prognostication than that by the AJCC staging system alone. Our individualized prediction nomograms could help physicians counsel and advise patients about their personalized treatment strategies and follow-up protocols, especially in patients with preoperatively under-staged rectal cancer.

Author Contributions

Conceived and designed the experiments: JP SC. Performed the experiments: DS XL HW. Analyzed the data: LS YD ST SC. Contributed reagents/materials/analysis tools: XL HW. Wrote the paper: JP YD.

References

1. Rahal R, Forte T, Lockwood G, Klein-Geltink J, Bryant H (2012) Recently published indicators allow for comparison of radiation treatment rates relative to evidence-based guidelines for rectal cancer. Current oncology 19: 175–176.
2. Database NC American College of Surgeons Commission on Cancer, 2008 Data Submission.
3. Hyodo I, Suzuki H, Takahashi K, Saito Y, Tanaka S, et al. (2010) Present status and perspectives of colorectal cancer in Asia: Colorectal Cancer Working Group report in 30th Asia-Pacific Cancer Conference. Japanese journal of clinical oncology 40 Suppl 1: i38–43.
4. Sauer R, Becker H, Hohenberger W, Rodel C, Wittekind C, et al. (2004) Preoperative versus postoperative chemoradiotherapy for rectal cancer. The New England journal of medicine 351: 1731–1740.
5. Lai LL, Fuller CD, Kachnic LA, Thomas CR Jr (2006) Can pelvic radiotherapy be omitted in select patients with rectal cancer? Seminars in oncology 33: S70–74.
6. Peeters KC, van de Velde CJ, Leer JW, Martijn H, Junggeburt JM, et al. (2005) Late side effects of short-course preoperative radiotherapy combined with total mesorectal excision for rectal cancer: increased bowel dysfunction in irradiated patients–a Dutch colorectal cancer group study. Journal of clinical oncology : official journal of the American Society of Clinical Oncology 23: 6199–6206.
7. Tepper JE, O'Connell M, Niedzwiecki D, Hollis DR, Benson AB 3rd, et al. (2002) Adjuvant therapy in rectal cancer: analysis of stage, sex, and local control–final report of intergroup 0114. Journal of clinical oncology : official journal of the American Society of Clinical Oncology 20: 1744–1750.
8. Edge S, Byrd DR, Compton CC, Fritz AG, Greene FL, et al. (2010) AJCC Cancer Staging Manual (7th Edition). New York: Springer.
9. Green FL, Page DL, Fleming ID, Fritz A, Balch CM, et al. (2002) AJCC Cancer Staging Manual (6th edition). Chicago, IL, American Joint Committee on Cancer.
10. Capirci C, Valentini V, Cionini L, De Paoli A, Rodel C, et al. (2008) Prognostic value of pathologic complete response after neoadjuvant therapy in locally advanced rectal cancer: long-term analysis of 566 ypCR patients. International journal of radiation oncology, biology, physics 72: 99–107.
11. Quah HM, Chou JF, Gonen M, Shia J, Schrag D, et al. (2008) Pathologic stage is most prognostic of disease-free survival in locally advanced rectal cancer patients after preoperative chemoradiation. Cancer 113: 57–64.
12. Gronchi A, Miceli R, Shurell E, Eilber FC, Eilber FR, et al. (2013) Outcome Prediction in Primary Resected Retroperitoneal Soft Tissue Sarcoma: Histology-Specific Overall Survival and Disease-Free Survival Nomograms Built on Major Sarcoma Center Data Sets. Journal of clinical oncology : official journal of the American Society of Clinical Oncology.
13. Meretoja TJ, Strien L, Heikkila PS, Leidenius MH (2012) A simple nomogram to evaluate the risk of nonsentinel node metastases in breast cancer patients with minimal sentinel node involvement. Annals of surgical oncology 19: 567–576.
14. Wang Y, Li J, Xia Y, Gong R, Wang K, et al. (2013) Prognostic nomogram for intrahepatic cholangiocarcinoma after partial hepatectomy. Journal of clinical oncology : official journal of the American Society of Clinical Oncology 31: 1188–1195.
15. Giordano A, Egleston BL, Hajage D, Bland J, Hortobagyi GN, et al. (2013) Establishment and validation of circulating tumor cell-based prognostic nomograms in first-line metastatic breast cancer patients. Clinical cancer research : an official journal of the American Association for Cancer Research 19: 1596–1602.
16. Valentini V, van Stiphout RG, Lammering G, Gambacorta MA, Barba MC, et al. (2011) Nomograms for predicting local recurrence, distant metastases, and overall survival for patients with locally advanced rectal cancer on the basis of European randomized clinical trials. Journal of clinical oncology : official journal of the American Society of Clinical Oncology 29: 3163–3172.
17. Harrell FE Jr, Lee KL, Mark DB (1996) Multivariable prognostic models: issues in developing models, evaluating assumptions and adequacy, and measuring and reducing errors. Statistics in medicine 15: 361–387.
18. Gray R, Barnwell J, McConkey C, Hills RK, Williams NS, et al. (2007) Adjuvant chemotherapy versus observation in patients with colorectal cancer: a randomised study. Lancet 370: 2020–2029.
19. Bosset JF, Collette L, Calais G, Mineur L, Maingon P, et al. (2006) Chemotherapy with preoperative radiotherapy in rectal cancer. The New England journal of medicine 355: 1114–1123.
20. Sebag-Montefiore D, Stephens RJ, Steele R, Monson J, Grieve R, et al. (2009) Preoperative radiotherapy versus selective postoperative chemoradiotherapy in patients with rectal cancer (MRC CR07 and NCIC-CTG C016): a multicentre, randomised trial. Lancet 373: 811–820.
21. Sauer R, Liersch T, Merkel S, Fietkau R, Hohenberger W, et al. (2012) Preoperative versus postoperative chemoradiotherapy for locally advanced rectal cancer: results of the German CAO/ARO/AIO-94 randomized phase III trial after a median follow-up of 11 years. Journal of clinical oncology : official journal of the American Society of Clinical Oncology 30: 1926–1933.
22. Canadian Partnership Against Cancer (2011) The 2011 Cancer System Performance Report. Toronto, ON: CPAC.
23. Cho MM, Morgan JW, Knutsen R, Oda K, Shavlik D, et al. (2013) Outcomes of Multimodality Therapies for Patients With Stage II or III Rectal Cancer in California, 1994–2009. Diseases of the colon and rectum 56: 1357–1365.
24. Gunderson LL, Jessup JM, Sargent DJ, Greene FL, Stewart A (2010) Revised tumor and node categorization for rectal cancer based on surveillance, epidemiology, and end results and rectal pooled analysis outcomes. Journal of clinical oncology : official journal of the American Society of Clinical Oncology 28: 256–263.
25. Ferri M, Lorenzon L, Onelli MR, La Torre M, Mercantini P, et al. (2013) Lymph node ratio is a stronger prognotic factor than microsatellite instability in colorectal cancer patients: Results from a 7 years follow-up study. International journal of surgery.
26. Lu YJ, Lin PC, Lin CC, Wang HS, Yang SH, et al. (2013) The Impact of the Lymph Node Ratio is Greater than Traditional Lymph Node Status in Stage III Colorectal Cancer Patients. World journal of surgery 37: 1927–1933.
27. Greenberg R, Itah R, Ghinea R, Sacham-Shmueli E, Inbar R, et al. (2011) Metastatic lymph node ratio (LNR) as a prognostic variable in colorectal cancer patients undergoing laparoscopic resection. Techniques in coloproctology 15: 273–279.
28. Peng J, Xu Y, Guan Z, Zhu J, Wang M, et al. (2008) Prognostic significance of the metastatic lymph node ratio in node-positive rectal cancer. Annals of surgical oncology 15: 3118–3123.
29. Petersen SH, Harling H, Kirkeby LT, Wille-Jorgensen P, Mocellin S (2012) Postoperative adjuvant chemotherapy in rectal cancer operated for cure. The Cochrane database of systematic reviews 3: CD004078.
30. Tveit KM, Guldvog I, Hagen S, Trondsen E, Harbitz T, et al. (1997) Randomized controlled trial of postoperative radiotherapy and short-term time-scheduled 5-fluorouracil against surgery alone in the treatment of Dukes B and C rectal cancer. Norwegian Adjuvant Rectal Cancer Project Group. The British journal of surgery 84: 1130–1135.
31. Fisher B, Wolmark N, Rockette H, Redmond C, Deutsch M, et al. (1988) Postoperative adjuvant chemotherapy or radiation therapy for rectal cancer: results from NSABP protocol R-01. Journal of the National Cancer Institute 80: 21–29.

18

Development and Validation of a Prediction Model for Tube Feeding Dependence after Curative (Chemo-) Radiation in Head and Neck Cancer

Kim Wopken[1]*, Hendrik P. Bijl[1], Arjen van der Schaaf[1], Miranda E. Christianen[1], Olga Chouvalova[1], Sjoukje F. Oosting[3], Bernard F. A. M. van der Laan[4], Jan L. N. Roodenburg[5], C. René Leemans[6], Ben J. Slotman[2], Patricia Doornaert[2], Roel J. H. M. Steenbakkers[1], Irma M. Verdonck-de Leeuw[6], Johannes A. Langendijk[1]

1 Department of Radiation Oncology, University of Groningen, University Medical Center Groningen, Groningen, the Netherlands, **2** Department of Radiation Oncology, VU University Medical Center, Amsterdam, the Netherlands, **3** Department of Medical Oncology, University of Groningen, University Medical Center Groningen, Groningen, the Netherlands, **4** Department of Otolaryngology/Head and Neck Surgery, University of Groningen, University Medical Center Groningen, Groningen, the Netherlands, **5** Department of Oral and Maxillofacial Surgery, University of Groningen, University Medical Center Groningen, Groningen, the Netherlands, **6** Department of Otolaryngology-Head and Neck Surgery, VU University Medical Center, Amsterdam, the Netherlands

Abstract

Background: Curative radiotherapy or chemoradiation for head and neck cancer (HNC) may result in severe acute and late side effects, including tube feeding dependence. The purpose of this prospective cohort study was to develop a prediction model for tube feeding dependence 6 months ($TUBE_{M6}$) after curative (chemo-) radiotherapy in HNC patients.

Patients and Methods: Tube feeding dependence was scored prospectively. To develop the multivariable model, a group LASSO analysis was carried out, with $TUBE_{M6}$ as the primary endpoint (n = 427). The model was then validated in a test cohort (n = 183). The training cohort was divided into three groups based on the risk of $TUBE_{M6}$ to test whether the model could be extrapolated to later time points (12, 18 and 24 months).

Results: Most important predictors for $TUBE_{M6}$ were weight loss prior to treatment, advanced T-stage, positive N-stage, bilateral neck irradiation, accelerated radiotherapy and chemoradiation. Model performance was good, with an Area under the Curve of 0.86 in the training cohort and 0.82 in the test cohort. The $TUBE_{M6}$-based risk groups were significantly associated with tube feeding dependence at later time points ($p<0.001$).

Conclusion: We established an externally validated predictive model for tube feeding dependence after curative radiotherapy or chemoradiation, which can be used to predict $TUBE_{M6}$.

Editor: Richard E. Burney, University of Michigan, United States of America

Funding: This work was supported by the Dutch Cancer Society (grant no. RUG 2008-3983). The funders had no role in study design, data collection and analysis, decision to publish, or preparation of the manuscript.

Competing Interests: B. Slotman has received travel support and honorarium from Varian medical systems and BrainLAB AG. All remaining authors have declared no conflicts of interest. The Department of Radiation Oncology of the University of Groningen, University Medical Center Groningen has research agreements with Philips, Elekta, RaySearch and Mirada.

* E-mail: k.wopken@umcg.nl

Introduction

Patients with head and neck cancer (HNC) often receive intensive anticancer treatment such as radiotherapy as single modality or in combination with chemotherapy and/or targeted agents such as cetuximab. Many patients may have severe difficulties maintaining adequate nutritional intake prior to treatment. This is caused by local tumor growth, which leads to swallowing dysfunction, trismus, odynophagia, dysgeusia and aspiration. In addition, anticancer therapy causes severe side effects such as acute mucositis and xerostomia inducing swallowing dysfunction. After completing such therapy, a substantial proportion of patients without baseline swallowing dysfunction ultimately develop persistent or even progressive swallowing dysfunction. In some cases they require tube feeding for a long period of time [1].

Recently it was shown that swallowing dysfunction has a major impact on health-related quality of life [2]. With grade III–IV swallowing dysfunction according to the RTOG Late Radiation Morbidity Scoring System, the most important general dimensions of health-related quality of life were moderately to severely affected. Moreover, swallowing dysfunction has been associated with psychological distress not only in patients themselves, but also in their spouses [3]. These results demonstrate that swallowing dysfunction in general, and tube feeding dependence in particular, are clinically relevant long-term side effects after curative (chemo-) radiotherapy.

Moreover, high-intensity treatment regimens have resulted in improved survival, but with higher rates of tube feeding dependence in these survivors [4,5]. The prevalence of patients with long-term tube feeding dependence is therefore expected to increase.

Previous studies have shown that the dose to the larynx and pharyngeal musculature in radiotherapy treatment of HNC is associated with the risk of long-term swallowing dysfunction [6–8] and are considered swallowing organs at risk. Advanced radiation delivery techniques such as intensity modulated radiotherapy (IMRT) have been used to reduce the radiation dose to the swallowing organs at risk [9]. Promising results have been reported on the use of swallowing exercises before and during treatment to reduce the risk of persisting swallowing dysfunction after curative (chemo-) radiation [10,11]. Thus, predictive models that can identify patients at increased risk of tube feeding dependence after curative (chemo-) radiotherapy before starting treatment would allow selection of suitable candidates for preventive strategies, such as swallowing sparing IMRT and/or preventive swallowing exercises.

Therefore, the main purpose of this study was to develop a prediction model for tube feeding dependence after curative (chemo-) radiotherapy in HNC based on pretreatment characteristics that can be used to improve selection of patients, prior to treatment, for these preventive measures and/or support decision making with regard to the treatment strategy in an early stage (e.g. definitive radiotherapy versus primary surgery). This prediction model was validated in an external and independent prospective cohort to further support its general applicability.

Material and Methods

Ethics statement

All patients were subjected to a prospective data registration program in which complications and treatment results in terms of local control and survival are prospectively assessed. This is done within the framework of routine clinical practice in which outcome and complications are systemically scored as part of a quality assurance program. All data obtained and used for this study has been anonymized.

The (Dutch) Medical Research Involving Human Subjects Act is not applicable to data collection as part of routine clinical practice and use of these data for scientific papers regarding the quality assurance program. Only research that is within the scope of the Medical Research Involving Human Subjects Act needs approval from an (accredited) ethics committee. Therefore, the hospital ethics committee (the Medisch Ethische Toetsingscommissie; METc) concluded that data collection by this program is regarded as part of routine patient care and granted us a waiver from needing ethical approval for the conduct of this study.

In the Netherlands a patient of course has to give his/her consent for the collection of the extra data on behalf of the quality assurance program and the use of these data for scientific papers regarding the quality assurance program. However, according to Dutch legislation, consent is free of form, and verbal consent is sufficient. Therefore, patients were asked to participate in this quality assurance program and asked for permission to use their data for the program and scientific papers regarding the program. Refusal of participation was recorded in their medical record.

Patients

The population of this prospective cohort study was composed of 610 consecutive patients with carcinoma of the mucosal surfaces of the larynx, oropharynx, oral cavity, hypopharynx and nasopharynx, who received curative radiotherapy with or without chemotherapy or cetuximab. Data from patients treated at our hospital were used to develop the prediction model (training cohort: 427 patients), while data from patients treated at another hospital were used to externally validate the model (test cohort: 183 patients).

Baseline weight loss was defined as the percentage of total body weight lost during the 6 months prior to radiation, with 1 to 10% weight loss defined as moderate and more than 10% defined as severe weight loss.

As we were primarily interested in radiation-induced swallowing dysfunction, patients that used a feeding tube at baseline were excluded from this analysis (RTOG grade 3–4). Moreover, patients had to be free of local recurrence or distant metastases at the time of assessment of swallowing dysfunction.

Treatment

All patients were treated either with conventional 3D conformal radiotherapy (3D-CRT) or IMRT. The dose to the parotid glands was reduced as much as possible. In the cohorts included in this analysis, no dose constraints for the swallowing organs at risk were used.

Patients undergoing concomitant chemoradiotherapy were treated with conventional fractionation (2.0 Gray (Gy) per fraction, 5 times per week up to 70 Gy in 7 weeks). Patients with stage I–II and stage III–IV tumors who were considered ineligible for (chemo-) radiotherapy were treated with accelerated radiotherapy with a concomitant boost technique (2.0 Gy per fraction, 6 times per week up to 70 Gy in 6 weeks). Since 2008, patients with locally advanced (stage III–IV) tumors, for whom chemotherapy was considered infeasible, have been treated with cetuximab using a loading dose of 400 mg/m^2 one week prior to radiotherapy and a weekly dose of 250 mg/m^2 during accelerated radiotherapy (2.0 Gy per fraction, 6 times per week up to 70 Gy in 6 weeks).

In the training cohort, concomitant chemotherapy consisted of cisplatin 100 mg/m^2 on days 1, 22 and 43. In the test cohort, concomitant chemotherapy consisted of 3 cycles of carboplatin (300–350 mg/m^2) on day 1 and 5-fluorouracil (5-FU) on days 1 to 4 as a continuous infusion (600 mg/m^2/24 hours) every 3 weeks.

At both institutions, prophylactic PEG tube placement was standard of care in all patients treated with curative concomitant chemoradiation and patients were instructed to refrain from using the PEG-tube. In patients with significant weight loss ($>$5% weight loss in 1 month or $>$10% in 6 months or BMI $<$18.5 kg/m^2) and/or low nutritional intake (less than half of daily requirements for energy, proteins or fluids) and/or severe swallowing dysfunction prior to treatment, PEG tubes were placed prior to treatment. However, these patients were excluded from the analysis.

Reactive placement of feeding tubes was used for patients with significant weight loss or swallowing dysfunction during treatment; in this situation a nasogastric feeding tube was placed during treatment if swallowing problems were considered temporarily and expected to recover soon. In case of severe swallowing problems early during treatment and/or expected to sustain for a longer period of time, there was a preference for PEG-tube placement.

Follow up schedule and assessments

In both hospitals, acute and late radiation-induced side effects were prospectively assessed according to the RTOG/EORTC Acute and Late Radiation Morbidity Scoring System. Tube feeding dependence was scored separately. For the present analysis, the primary endpoint was tube feeding, either with PEG (percutaneous endoscopic gastrostomy) or nasogastric tube at 6 months after completion of treatment ($TUBE_{M6}$). Patients were considered tube feeding dependent if a feeding tube was present and used because oral intake was limited or impossible.

Definition of risk groups

The total population of the training cohort was divided into three risk groups based on the risk on $TUBE_{M6}$. The division into low, intermediate and high risk groups was arbitrary: patients were considered low risk when the probability for $TUBE_{M6}$ was ≤5%, intermediate risk when this value was >5–15% and high risk for values >15%. To determine whether the model could be extrapolated for the same patients at later time points, the positive and negative predictive values for $TUBE_{M6}$ were calculated at 12, 18 and 24 months.

Statistics

After the regression analysis, the variance inflation factor was calculated to check for high correlations between candidate prognostic variables. There were no high correlations and, therefore, no changes were made to the variables.

For the development of the prediction model the least absolute shrinkage and selection operator (LASSO) method was used, which is a logistic regression analysis with a bound on the absolute magnitude of the regression coefficients [12]. This method includes all variables in the modeling process but only a subset of predictor variables are eventually included in the model, setting the coefficients of variables that have negligible effects to zero. The LASSO method has been successfully applied to build Normal Tissue Complication (NTCP) models for HNC patients [13]. Given the inclusion of categorical variables in the current data, the group-LASSO (variant of LASSO) was used for building the prediction models. The amount of shrinkage was selected by optimizing the Bayesian information criterion (BIC) over the regularization path.

The environment for statistical computing R (R Development Core Team, R: A language and Environment for statistical Computing, Version 2.15, Vienna, 2012) was used to do the calculation. The package 'grpreg' was used to build the group-LASSO model.

For the selected variables x_i and their fitted coefficients β_i, the Normal Tissue Complication Probability (NTCP) is given by:

$$NTCP = \left(1 + e^{-S}\right)^{-1}, \textit{ in which}$$

$$S = \beta_0 + \sum_{i=1}^{n} \beta_i \cdot x_i$$

Model performance was described using different validation measures [14,15]. The discriminating ability of the model was described by the area under the curve (AUC) value based on the Receiver Operating Characteristics curve. The discrimination slope was calculated as the absolute difference between the mean predicted NTCP value for patients with and without the outcome. The calibration of the model reflects the agreement between observed outcomes and predictions. The calibration slope and intercept were calculated as described by Miller et al. [16]. To evaluate whether the model performance measures based on the observed outcomes differed from their expected values, we used Monte-Carlo to generate the expected distributions and calculated p-values. Finally, a Hosmer-Lemeshow test with 10 groups was performed to evaluate the calibration of the model.

Results

Univariate analysis of the training cohort

The training cohort consisted of 427 patients, 77% male and 23% female with a mean age of 62 years. The pretreatment characteristics of the patients are listed in Table 1. Out of 427 patients, 55 (12.9%) were tube feeding dependent at 6 months after completion of treatment. In the univariate analysis, younger age, higher T-classification, higher N-classification, primary tumor site other than the larynx, concomitant chemoradiation, bilateral irradiation, weight loss at baseline and swallowing dysfunction at baseline were significantly associated with $TUBE_{M6}$ (Table 2).

Group-LASSO analysis in training cohort

The LASSO analysis arrived at a multivariable model containing 5 variables with non-zero coefficients: weight loss prior to treatment, T-classification and N-classification, bilateral irradiation of the neck, and treatment modality, including accelerated radiotherapy and chemoradiotherapy (Table 3).

In individual cases, the risk of $TUBE_{M6}$ can be estimated using the following equation:

$$NTCP = \left(1 + e^{-S}\right)^{-1},$$

where $S = -3.69$ + *(T-stage * 1.01)* + *(N-stage * 0.87)* + *(moderate weight loss * 0.82)* + *(severe weight loss * 1.51)* + *(bilateral neck irradiation * 0.35)* + *(accelerated radiotherapy * 0.25)* + *(chemoradiotherapy * 0.41)*

The risk of $TUBE_{M6}$ can also be estimated by using the nomogram (Figure 1). In the training cohort, model performance was excellent, with an AUC of 0.86 The discrimination slope had a value of 0.21. The Hosmer-Lemeshow chi square had a value of 9.35 (p-value 0.3) indicating good agreement between expected and observed rates.

External validation

The test cohort consisted of 183 patients, 73% male and 27% female, with a mean age of 62 years. The training and test cohort differed significantly with regard to T-classification, N-classification, the applied treatment modalities and radiation techniques, and weight loss at baseline (Table 1). Out of 183 patients, 27 (14.8%) were tube feeding dependent at 6 months after completion of treatment. Model performance in the external test cohort was good, with an AUC of 0.82 (Expected: 0.80, 95% CI: 0.72–0.86, p-value: 0.8) and a discrimination slope of 0.20 (Expected: 0.19, 95% CI: 0.13–0.25, p-value 0.6). The calibration graph (Figure S1) illustrates that the observed NTCP-values of $TUBE_{M6}$ in the test cohort are in close proximity of the predicted NTCP-values. The Hosmer-Lemeshow test showed no statistically significant difference between predicted and measured outcomes in the test cohort (Table S1).

Relationship with tube feeding dependence at subsequent time points

The prevalence of tube feeding dependence was 6.9% (23 of 335 patients at risk) at 12 months ($TUBE_{M12}$), 3.6% (9 of 251 patients at risk) at 18 months ($TUBE_{M18}$) and 4.0% (8 of 200 patients at risk) at 24 months ($TUBE_{M24}$). $TUBE_{M6}$ was very predictive for tube feeding dependence at later time points. The negative predictive values of $TUBE_{M6}$ for $TUBE_{M12}$, $TUBE_{M18}$, $TUBE_{M24}$ were 97.1%, 99.1% and 98.9%, respectively, indicating that almost all patients who were not tube feeding dependent at 6 months remained independent at subsequent time points. The positive predictive values of $TUBE_{M6}$ for $TUBE_{M12}$, $TUBE_{M18}$,

Table 1. Pre-treatment charactistics in the training cohort and test cohort.

Variable		Training cohort (n = 427)		Test cohort (n = 183)		P-value
		Number	%	Number	%	
Sex	Male	329	77%	134	73%	p = 0.311
	Female	98	23%	49	27%	
Age	18–65 years	269	63%	117	64%	p = 0.826
	>65 years	158	37%	66	36%	
T-classification	Tis-T1	129	30%	33	18%	p = 0.002
	T2	157	37%	74	40%	
	T3	88	21%	36	20%	
	T4	53	12%	40	22%	
N-classification	N0	291	68%	88	48%	p<0.001
	N1	36	8%	19	10%	
	N2a	9	2%	6	3%	
	N2b	40	9%	16	9%	
	N2c	42	10%	48	26%	
	N3	9	2%	6	3%	
Primary site	Larynx	242	57%	91	50%	p = 0.282
	Oropharynx	103	24%	59	32%	
	Oral cavity	28	7%	10	6%	
	Hypopharynx	33	8%	16	9%	
	Nasopharynx	21	5%	7	4%	
Treatment modality	Conventional radiotherapy	148	35%	12	6%	p<0.001
	Accelerated radiotherapy	204	48%	131	72%	
	Chemoradiation	75	17%	40	22%	
Radiation technique	3D-CRT	379	89%	77	42%	p<0.001
	IMRT	48	11%	106	58%	
Neck irradiation	Primary alone	106	25%	40	22%	p = 0.496
	Primary + ipsilateral neck	33	8%	11	6%	
	Primary + bilateral neck	288	67%	132	72%	
Weigh loss at baseline	No weight loss	320	75%	113	62%	p = 0.002
	Weight loss 1–10%	84	20%	50	27%	
	Weight loss >10%	23	5%	20	11%	
Baseline swallowing	No swallowing problems	338	79%	148	81%	p = 0.601
(grading according to RTOG)	Mild swallowing problems, soft diet	76	18%	32	18%	
	Moderate swallowing problems, liquid diet	13	3%	3	2%	

Abbreviations: 3D-CRT, Three Dimensional Conformal Radiotherapy; IMRT, Intensity-Modulated Radiation Therapy; RTOG, Radiation Therapy Oncology Group.

$TUBE_{M24}$ were 50.0%, 36.8% and 40.0%, respectively, indicating recovery from tube feeding dependence in more than half of the patients.

Discussion

The purpose of the current study was to develop and validate a prediction model for tube feeding dependence 6 months after curative (chemo-) radiotherapy in HNC patients. Such a model could be used in clinical practice to predict which patients are at risk for long-term tube feeding dependence, prior to treatment, and would thus be suitable candidates for preventive measures such as swallowing exercises and/or swallowing sparing IMRT.

In the LASSO analysis, five independent prognostic factors for $TUBE_{M6}$ were identified: advanced T-stage (T3–T4), positive N-stage, weight loss at baseline, bilateral irradiation of the neck, and treatment modality. Model performance in both the training cohort and the test cohort from another hospital was good to excellent, which confirms the generalization ability of the model.

A prediction model as presented in this study is increasingly desirable due to the more aggressive treatment regimens that are being used in HNC, including altered fractionation schedules for radiotherapy, concomitant (chemo-) radiotherapy or both. These intensive cancer treatments have improved loco-regional control and overall survival [17–19] but at the expense of an increase in radiation-induced side effects [20] in particular long-term swallowing dysfunction [21].

Prophylactic feeding tube placement is standard practice in many institutions to avoid treatment interruptions and unplanned

Table 2. Results of the univariate logistic regression analysis with tube feeding dependence at 6 months ($TUBE_{M6}$) as primary endpoint in patients included in the training cohort.

Variable		Univariate analysis		
		Odds ratio	(95% CI)	P-value
Sex	Male	1.00		
	Female	1.61	(0.86–3.00)	p = 0.135
Age	>65 years	1.00		
	18–65 years	2.32	(1.18–4.54)	p = 0.014
T-classification	Tis-T2	1.00		
	T3–T4	10.02	(5.08–19.78)	p<0.001
N-classification	N0	1.00		
	N+	7.67	(4.05–14.50)	p<0.001
Primary site	Larynx	1.00		
	Oral cavity	8.63	(2.92–25.51)	p<0.001
	Oropharynx	8.74	(3.93–19.47)	p<0.001
	Nasopharynx	6.09	(1.70–21.83)	p = 0.006
	Hypopharynx	9.71	(3.52–26.79)	p<0.001
Treatment modality	Conventional radiotherapy	1,00		
	Accelerated radiotherapy	1.77	(0.79–3.99)	p = 0.167
	Chemoradiation	7.72	(3.38–17.67)	p<0.001
Radiation technique	3D-CRT	1.00		
	IMRT	1.67	(0.76–3.67)	p = 0.202
Neck irradiation	Local or unilateral irradiation	1.00		
	Bilateral irradiation	15.45	(3.71–64.39)	p<0.001
Baseline swallowing	Grade 0	1.00		
(grading according to RTOG)	Grade 1–2	3.20	(1.62–6.32)	p = 0.001
Weight loss	No weight loss	1.00		
(baseline)	1–10%	5.66	(2.93–10.94)	p<0.001
	>10%	16.36	(6.42–41.68)	p<0.001

Abbreviations: 3D-CRT, Three Dimensional Conformal Radiotherapy; IMRT, Intensity-Modulated Radiation Therapy; RTOG, Radiation Therapy Oncology Group; CI, Confidence Interval.

hospitalizations because of compromised nutritional intake and/or dehydration [22]; adequate nutrition has been shown to improve tolerance and response rates to (chemo-) radiotherapy [23].

However, others have shown that pretreatment feeding tube placement may lead to increased long-term swallowing dysfunction, longer feeding tube duration and the need for pharyngo-esophageal dilatation [24]. In addition, long-term feeding tube dependence may significantly reduce quality of life after treatment for HNC [22,25]. Terrell *et al.* [26] showed that feeding tube dependence was the strongest clinical predictor of negative effects on health-related quality of life relative to other medical co-morbidities. It was associated with significantly lower scores on 10 out of 12 collective domains in the Medical Outcomes Study Short Form 36-item Health Survey and HNC quality-of-life instruments. As already mentioned, at both institutions, prophylactic PEG tube placement was standard of care in all patients treated with curative concomitant chemoradiation and patients were instructed to refrain from using the PEG-tube. In patients with significant weight loss (>5% weight loss in 1 month or >10% in 6 months or BMI <18.5 kg/m^2) and/or low nutritional intake (less than half of daily requirements for energy, proteins or fluids) and/or severe swallowing dysfunction prior to treatment, PEG tubes were placed prior to treatment. However, these patients were excluded from the analysis.

Chemoradiotherapy was a prognostic factor in the LASSO analysis. It should be stressed that given the fact that all patients receiving concomitant chemoradiation received prophylactic PEG tube placement, the Odds ratio of 1.51 should be considered the results of this preset combination and that no conclusions can be drawn with regard to these two factors separately. However, given this Odds ratio of 1.51 and the Odds ratio of 1.28 found for accelerated radiotherapy (without prophylactic PEG-tube placement), we believe that the contribution of prophylactic PEG tube feeding is probably limited or absent.

The training cohort and test cohort were from two different hospitals with different chemotherapy regimens in each hospital. In the training cohort, cisplatinum was used while in the test cohort 5-FU in combination with carboplatin was used. The model performance in both cohorts was comparable, which indirectly confirms that there will probably be no major difference between the two chemotherapy regimens.

Given that both advanced T-stage (larger tumors) and N-stage and bilateral irradiation of the neck were prognostic factors for feeding tube dependence at 6 months after (chemo-) radiotherapy, it can be hypothesized that the risk of tube feeding dependence is

Table 3. Results of the LASSO analysis with tube feeding dependence at 6 months ($TUBE_{M6}$) as primary endpoint.

Variable	B	95% CI of B	OR	P-value
T-classification				
T3–T4 vs. Tis-T2	1.01	(0.79–1.32)	2.75	p<0.001
N-classification				
N+ vs. N0	0.87	(0.65–1.10)	2.39	p<0.001
Weight loss (baseline)				
1–10% weight loss vs. no weight loss	0.82	(0.65–0.99)	2.27	p<0.001
>10% weight loss vs. no weight loss	1.51	(1.19–1.83)	4.53	p<0.001
Neck irradiation				
Bilateral vs. local/unilateral	0.35	(0.06–0.66)	1.42	p = 0.011
Treatment modality				
Chemoradiation vs. conventional fractionation	0.41	(0.16–0.68)	1.51	p = 0.001
Accelerated fractionation vs. conventional fractionation	0.25	(0.10–0.41)	1.28	p = 0.001
Constant	−3.69	(−4.19–−3.21)		

Abbreviations: OR, Odds Ratio; CI, Confidence Interval; B, model coefficient beta.

related to the radiation dose distribution in the anatomical structures involved in swallowing, such as the pharyngeal constrictor muscles. A number of authors indeed showed a dose-volume-effect relationships of anatomical structures involved in swallowing and swallowing dysfunction after (chemo-) radiotherapy, such as the pharyngeal constrictor muscles [8,27–29].

Accelerated radiotherapy was also an independent prognostic factor for tube feeding dependence. These results are in line with those presented by Overgaard *et al.* who showed that accelerated radiotherapy lead to more frequent and longer persisting confluent mucositis than the conventionally treated group and consequently long-term dysphagia [30]. Another more recent updated study, however, showed that accelerated RT does increase acute but not late morbidity, including dysphagia [31].

In the current study, baseline weight loss was also an independent prognostic factor for tube feeding dependence. This

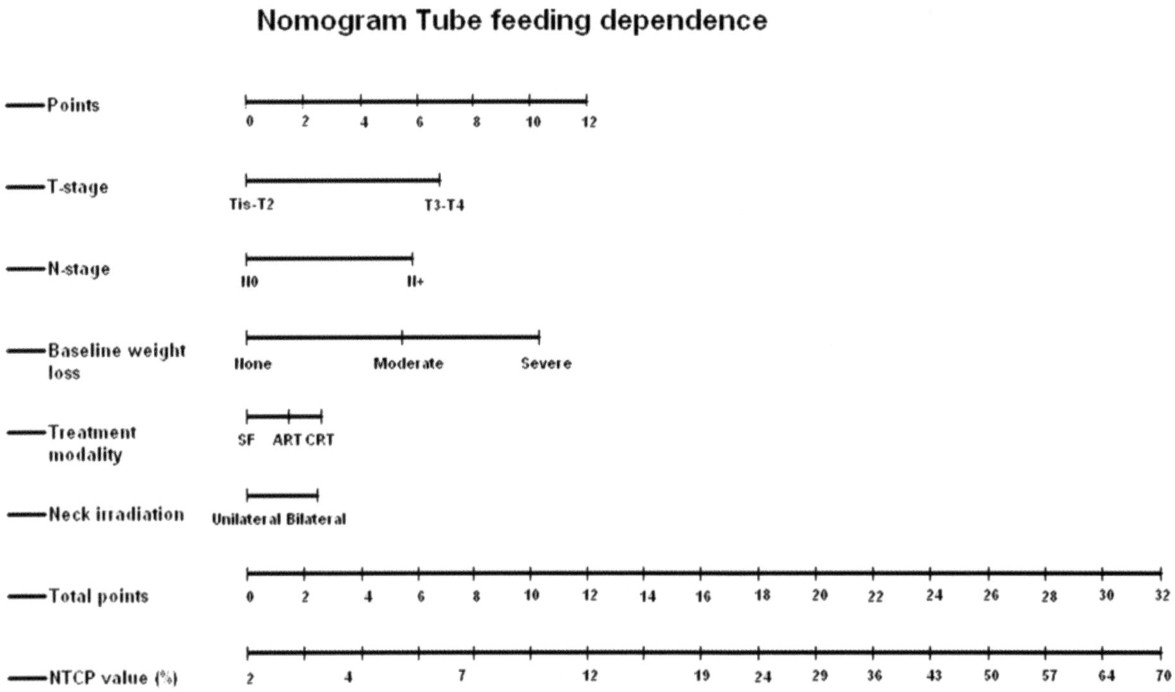

Figure 1. Nomogram for tube feeding dependence to determine normal tissue complication probability (NTCP) values for each individual patient. Abbreviations: SF, conventional radiotherapy; ART, accelerated radiotherapy; CRT, chemoradiation.

is in accordance with a previous report [1] in which baseline weight loss was shown to be an independent prognostic factor for grade 2–4 RTOG swallowing dysfunction at 6 months after treatment. This suggests that a relatively high percentage of baseline swallowing dysfunction is not recognized by radiation oncologists and that swallowing dysfunction is therefore often underreported, even in the case of prospective assessment of toxicity.

From clinical practice we know that the reasons for feeding tube placement are not solely related to swallowing problems, but may be multifactorial. Nausea due to chemotherapy treatment, changes in taste or saliva production and other factors may also necessitate feeding tube placement. We did not directly take these factors into account in this analysis since it was not possible to obtain information about this for each individual patient. This is something, however, that may have influenced feeding tube placement and use in this patient group.

As the main purpose of the current analysis was to develop and validate a multivariable prediction model that can be used to select patients prior to treatment (i.e. during the preparation phase of radiotherapy) for preventive measures, we did not take into account candidate variables related to dose distributions in swallowing organs at risk. This, however, will be investigated in future research.

Our results show that $TUBE_{M6}$ after treatment is predictive for tube feeding dependence at later time points up to 24 months after completion of radiotherapy. This is also in accordance with previous reports [1], which showed that swallowing dysfunction at 6 months after curative (chemo-) radiation is highly predictive for swallowing dysfunction at subsequent time points up to several years after treatment.

Conclusion

The present study is the first to provide an externally validated prediction model for tube feeding dependence after (chemo-) radiation in a population-based cohort of patients with HNC. This model enables clinicians to select patients that have not yet started treatment, based on pretreatment characteristics, who are at greatest risk for tube feeding dependence after treatment, and to implement preventive strategies for them.

Supporting Information

Figure S1 Calibration plots for the predictive model for tube feeding dependence at 6 months ($TUBE_{M6}$) at internal validation (A) and external validation (B).

Table S1 Performance of the prediction model for TUBEM6. Abbreviations: AUC, Area Under Curve; H-L, Hosmer-Lemeshow.

Author Contributions

Conceived and designed the experiments: HPB BJS IMVDL JAL. Analyzed the data: KW AVDS SFO JLNR CRL BJS. Wrote the paper: KW HPB AVDS MEC OC SFO BFAMVDL JLNR CRL BJS PD RJHMS IMVDL JAL. Final approval of manuscript: KW HPB AVDS MEC OC SFO BFAMVDL JLNR CRL BJS PD RJHMS IMVDL JAL. Collection and assembly of data: KW MEC OC BFAMVDL PD RJHMS IMVDL JAL. Provision of study material or patients: BJS JAL.

References

1. Langendijk JA, Doornaert P, Rietveld DH, Verdonck-de Leeuw IM, Leemans CR, et al (2009) A predictive model for swallowing dysfunction after curative radiotherapy in head and neck cancer. Radiother Oncol 90: 189–195.
2. Langendijk JA, Doornaert P, Verdonck-de Leeuw IM, Leemans CR, Aaronson NK, et al (2008) Impact of late treatment-related toxicity on quality of life among patients with head and neck cancer treated with radiotherapy. J Clin Oncol 26: 3770–3776.
3. Verdonck-de Leeuw IM, Eerenstein SE, Van der Linden MH, Kuik DJ, de Bree R, et al (2007) Distress in spouses and patients after treatment for head and neck cancer. Laryngoscope 117: 238–241.
4. Ang KK, Harris J, Garden AS, Trotti A, Jones CU, et al (2005) Concomitant boost radiation plus concurrent cisplatin for advanced head and neck carcinomas: Radiation therapy oncology group phase II trial 99-14. J Clin Oncol 23: 3008–3015.
5. Staar S, Rudat V, Stuetzer H, Dietz A, Volling P, et al (2001) Intensified hyperfractionated accelerated radiotherapy limits the additional benefit of simultaneous chemotherapy—results of a multicentric randomized german trial in advanced head-and-neck cancer. Int J Radiat Oncol Biol Phys 50: 1161–1171.
6. Caglar HB, Tishler RB, Othus M, Burke E, Li Y, et al (2008) Dose to larynx predicts for swallowing complications after intensity-modulated radiotherapy. Int J Radiat Oncol Biol Phys 72: 1110–1118.
7. Eisbruch A, Schwartz M, Rasch C, Vineberg K, Damen E, et al (2004) Dysphagia and aspiration after chemoradiotherapy for head-and-neck cancer: Which anatomic structures are affected and can they be spared by IMRT? Int J Radiat Oncol Biol Phys 60: 1425–1439.
8. Levendag PC, Teguh DN, Voet P, van der Est H, Noever I, et al (2007) Dysphagia disorders in patients with cancer of the oropharynx are significantly affected by the radiation therapy dose to the superior and middle constrictor muscle: A dose-effect relationship. Radiother Oncol 85: 64–73.
9. Feng FY, Kim HM, Lyden TH, Haxer MJ, Worden FP, et al (2010) Intensity-modulated chemoradiotherapy aiming to reduce dysphagia in patients with oropharyngeal cancer: Clinical and functional results. J Clin Oncol 28: 2732–2738.
10. Kotz T, Federman AD, Kao J, Milman L, Packer S, et al (2012) Prophylactic swallowing exercises in patients with head and neck cancer undergoing chemoradiation: A randomized trial. Arch Otolaryngol Head Neck Surg 138: 376–382.
11. Carroll WR, Locher JL, Canon CL, Bohannon IA, McColloch NL, et al (2008) Pretreatment swallowing exercises improve swallow function after chemoradiation. Laryngoscope 118: 39–43.
12. Tibshirani R (1996) Regression shrinkage and selection via the lasso. J R Statist Soc B 58: 267–288.
13. Xu CJ, van der Schaaf A, Schilstra C, Langendijk JA, Van't Veld AA (2012) Impact of statistical learning methods on the predictive power of multivariate normal tissue complication probability models. Int J Radiat Oncol Biol Phys 82: e677–84.
14. Vergouwe Y, Moons KG, Steyerberg EW (2010) External validity of risk models: Use of benchmark values to disentangle a case-mix effect from incorrect coefficients. Am J Epidemiol 172: 971–980.
15. Steyerberg EW, Vickers AJ, Cook NR, Gerds T, Gonen M, et al (2010) Assessing the performance of prediction models: A framework for traditional and novel measures. Epidemiology 21: 128–138.
16. Miller ME, Langefeld CD, Tierney WM, Hui SL, McDonald CJ (1993) Validation of probabilistic predictions. Med Decis Making 13: 49–58.
17. Pignon JP, le Maitre A, Maillard E, Bourhis J, MACH-NC Collaborative Group (2009) Meta-analysis of chemotherapy in head and neck cancer (MACH-NC): An update on 93 randomised trials and 17,346 patients. Radiother Oncol 92: 4–14.
18. Bourhis J, Overgaard J, Audry H, Ang KK, Saunders M, et al (2006) Hyperfractionated or accelerated radiotherapy in head and neck cancer: A meta-analysis. Lancet 368: 843–854.
19. Langendijk JA, Leemans CR, Buter J, Berkhof J, Slotman BJ (2004) The additional value of chemotherapy to radiotherapy in locally advanced nasopharyngeal carcinoma: A meta-analysis of the published literature. J Clin Oncol 22: 4604–4612.
20. Trotti A, Bellm LA, Epstein JB, Frame D, Fuchs HJ, et al (2003) Mucositis incidence, severity and associated outcomes in patients with head and neck cancer receiving radiotherapy with or without chemotherapy: A systematic literature review. Radiother Oncol 66: 253–262.
21. Eisbruch A, Lyden T, Bradford CR, Dawson LA, Haxer MJ, et al (2002) Objective assessment of swallowing dysfunction and aspiration after radiation concurrent with chemotherapy for head-and-neck cancer. Int J Radiat Oncol Biol Phys 53: 23–28.
22. Morton RP, Crowder VL, Mawdsley R, Ong E, Izzard M (2009) Elective gastrostomy, nutritional status and quality of life in advanced head and neck cancer patients receiving chemoradiotherapy. ANZ J Surg 79: 713–718.

23. Salas S, Deville JL, Giorgi R, Pignon T, Bagarry D, et al (2008) Nutritional factors as predictors of response to radio-chemotherapy and survival in unresectable squamous head and neck carcinoma. Radiother Oncol 87: 195–200.
24. Mekhail TM, Adelstein DJ, Rybicki LA, Larto MA, Saxton JP, et al (2001) Enteral nutrition during the treatment of head and neck carcinoma: Is a percutaneous endoscopic gastrostomy tube preferable to a nasogastric tube? Cancer 91: 1785–1790.
25. Nguyen NP, Frank C, Moltz CC, Vos P, Smith HJ, et al (2005) Impact of dysphagia on quality of life after treatment of head-and-neck cancer. Int J Radiat Oncol Biol Phys 61: 772–778.
26. Terrell JE, Ronis DL, Fowler KE, Bradford CR, Chepeha DB, et al (2004) Clinical predictors of quality of life in patients with head and neck cancer. Arch Otolaryngol Head Neck Surg 130: 401–408.
27. Bhide SA, Gulliford S, Kazi R, El-Hariry I, Newbold K, et al (2009) Correlation between dose to the pharyngeal constrictors and patient quality of life and late dysphagia following chemo-IMRT for head and neck cancer. Radiother Oncol 93: 539–544.
28. Christianen ME, Schilstra C, Beetz I, Muijs CT, Chouvalova O, et al (2011) Predictive modelling for swallowing dysfunction after primary (chemo)radiation: Results of a prospective observational study. Radiother Oncol.
29. Dirix P, Abbeel S, Vanstraelen B, Hermans R, Nuyts S (2009) Dysphagia after chemoradiotherapy for head-and-neck squamous cell carcinoma: Dose-effect relationships for the swallowing structures. Int J Radiat Oncol Biol Phys 75: 385–392.
30. Overgaard J, Hansen HS, Specht L, Overgaard M, Grau C, et al (2003) Five compared with six fractions per week of conventional radiotherapy of squamous-cell carcinoma of head and neck: DAHANCA 6 and 7 randomised controlled trial. Lancet 362: 933–940.
31. Mortensen HR, Overgaard J, Specht L, Overgaard M, Johansen J, et al (2012) Prevalence and peak incidence of acute and late normal tissue morbidity in the DAHANCA 6&7 randomised trial with accelerated radiotherapy for head and neck cancer. Radiother Oncol 103: 69–75.

Is There a Benefit in Receiving Concurrent Chemoradiotherapy for Elderly Patients with Inoperable Thoracic Esophageal Squamous Cell Carcinoma?

Peng Zhang[1]9, Mian Xi[1]9, Lei Zhao[1], Jing-Xian Shen[2], Qiao-Qiao Li[1], Li-Ru He[1], Shi-Liang Liu[1], Meng-Zhong Liu[1]*

1 Sun Yat-sen University Cancer Center, State Key Laboratory of Oncology in South China, Collaborative Innovation Center for Cancer Medicine, Department of Radiation Oncology, Cancer Center, Sun Yat-sen University, Guangzhou, People's Republic of China, **2** Sun Yat-sen University Cancer Center, State Key Laboratory of Oncology in South China, Collaborative Innovation Center for Cancer Medicine, Imaging Diagnosis and Interventional Center, Cancer Center, Sun Yat-sen University, Guangzhou, People's Republic of China

Abstract

Background and purpose: The benefit of concurrent chemoradiotherapy (CCRT) in elderly patients with inoperable esophageal squamous cell carcinoma (SCC) is controversial. This study aimed to assess the efficiency and safety of CCRT in elderly thoracic esophageal cancer patients.

Methods and materials: Between January 2002 and December 2011, 128 patients aged 65 years or older treated with CCRT or radiotherapy (RT) alone for inoperable thoracic esophageal SCC were analyzed retrospectively (RT alone, n = 55; CCRT, n = 73).

Results: No treatment-related deaths occurred and no patients experienced any acute grade 4 non-hematologic toxicities. Patients treated with CCRT developed more severe acute toxicities than patients who received RT alone. The 3-year overall survival (OS) rate was 36.1% for CCRT compared with 28.5% following RT alone ($p = 0.008$). Multivariate analysis identified T stage and treatment modality as independent prognostic factors for survival. Further analysis revealed that survival was significantly better in the CCRT group than in the RT alone group for patients $\leq$ 72 years. Nevertheless, the CCRT group had a similar OS to the RT group for patients $>$ 72 years.

Conclusion: Our results suggest that elderly patients with inoperable thoracic esophageal SCC could benefit from CCRT, without major toxicities. However, for patients older than 72 years, CCRT is not superior to RT alone in terms of survival benefit.

Editor: Andreas-Claudius Hoffmann, West German Cancer Center, Germany

Funding: This work was supported by the grant from the Sci-Tech Project Foundation of Guangdong Province (No.42012B031800287). Website: http://www.gdstc.gov.cn. PZ and MX received the funding. The funders provided help in data collection and analysis.

Competing Interests: The authors have declared that no competing interests exist.

* Email: liumengzhong@126.com

9 These authors contributed equally to this work.

Introduction

Esophageal cancer is remains a virulent disease, with a 5-year survival rate of only 17% [1]. The risk of esophageal cancer increases with age, with a mean age at diagnosis of 67 years [2]. The number of elderly patients with esophageal cancers is expected to increase in the near future as the number of elderly people increases.

Surgical resection is the preferred treatment for localized esophageal cancer patients. However, a recent population-based study showed that older patients have less intensive treatment of esophageal cancer including surgery [3]. In addition, the literature states that patients over the age of 70 have relatively high rates of postoperative morbidity and mortality, and 75 years of age is often considered the age limit for surgery [4,5].

For the medically or technically inoperable patients, concurrent chemoradiotherapy (CCRT) is the mainstay of treatment for locally advanced esophageal cancer. The Radiation Therapy Oncology Group (RTOG) trial 85-01 established the superiority of CCRT compared with radiotherapy (RT) alone in esophageal cancer patients. However, the acute toxicity of this regimen was substantial: sixty-four percent of patients treated with CCRT experienced severe or life threatening side effects and only 23% of patients enrolled were aged over 70 [6].

Few studies have focused on elderly patients; therefore, no standard treatment modality has been established for inoperable

Table 1. Patient characteristics.

Characteristic	All patients (n = 128)	Patients with CCRT (n = 73)	Patients with RT alone (n = 55)
Age (years)			
> 72	57 (44.5%)	25 (34.2%)	32 (58.2%)
≤ 72	71 (55.5%)	48 (65.8%)	23 (41.8%)
Sex			
Male	89 (69.5%)	57 (78.1%)	32 (58.2%)
Female	39 (30.5%)	16 (21.9%)	23 (41.8%)
Charlson score			
≥ 1	42 (32.8%)	23(31.5%)	19 (34.5%)
< 1	86 (67.2%)	50 (68.5%)	36 (65.5%)
Pathological grade			
Well differentiated	10 (7.8%)	6 (8.2%)	4 (7.3%)
Moderately differentiated	47 (36.7%)	28 (38.3%)	19 (34.6%)
Poorly/undifferentiated	45 (35.2%)	21 (28.8%)	24 (43.6%)
Unknown	26 (20.3%)	18 (24.7%)	8 (14.5%)
Location			
Upper third	38 (29.7%)	24 (32.9%)	14 (25.4%)
Middle third	69 (53.9%)	38 (52.1%)	31 (56.4%)
Lower third	21 (16.4%)	11 (15.0%)	10 (18.2%)
Primary tumor length			
≤ 5 cm	78 (60.9%)	42 (57.5%)	35 (63.6%)
> 5 cm	50 (39.1%)	31 (42.5%)	20 (36.4%)
T stage			
T1-T2	25 (19.5%)	18 (24.7%)	10 (18.2%)
T3-T4	103 (80.5%)	55 (75.3%)	45 (81.8%)
N stage			
N0	26 (20.3%)	14 (19.2%)	15 (27.3%)
N1	102 (79.7%)	59 (80.8%)	40 (72.7%)
M stage			
M0	78 (60.9%)	40 (54.8%)	38 (69.1%)
M1	50 (39.1%)	33 (45.2%)	17 (30.9%)
Radiation dose (Gy)			
< 60	49 (38.3%)	23 (31.5%)	26 (47.3%)
≥ 60	79 (61.7%)	50 (68.5%)	29 (52.7%)

Abbreviations: CCRT, concurrent chemoradiotherapy; RT, radiotherapy.

esophageal cancer in elderly patients. Several studies have reported the efficacy and toxicity of CCRT in elderly patients with inoperable esophageal cancer, but the results were controversial [7–10]. In addition, the published reports are mainly on small series of patients, making it difficult to carry out reliable analysis. Therefore, we reviewed our institutional experience to evaluate the efficiency and safety of CCRT compared with RT alone in elderly thoracic esophageal cancer patients. We defined an elderly population according to Social Security and Medicare regulations as persons aged 65 years or older.

Patients and Methods

Ethics statement

This study was approved by the institutional review board (IRBs) of Cancer Center, Sun Yat-sen University. Written informed consent was obtained from all the patients in accordance with the regulations of the IRBs.

Patient's inclusion

Esophageal cancer patients treated with RT at Sun Yat-Sen University Cancer Center between January 2002 and December 2011 were retrospectively reviewed. The inclusion criteria were (1) aged 65 years or older at the time of diagnosis; (2) Eastern Cooperative Oncology Group performance status of ≤ 2; (3) histologically conformed as thoracic esophageal squamous carcinoma (SCC); (4) unable or refusing to undergo surgical resection; (5) no prior therapy; (6) no history of concomitant or previous malignancy; (7) complete and retrievable clinical records.

Among 795 esophageal cancer patients treated with RT from 2002 to 2011, 128 patients who fulfilled the criteria were included.

Table 2. Acute toxicity.

CTC Grade	Patients with CCRT (n = 73)					Patients with RT alone (n = 55)				
	0	1	2	3	4	0	1	2	3	4
Anemia	15	26	27	5	0	12	23	19	1	0
Leukocytopenia	9	18	29	12	5	8	24	16	7	0
Thrombopenia	27	23	16	7	0	26	23	6	0	0
Gastrointestinal	26	16	16	15	0	13	19	20	3	0
Skin toxicity	16	26	28	3	0	17	24	13	1	0
Esophagitis	12	30	27	4	0	16	23	14	2	0
Pneumonitis	50	16	5	2	0	39	13	2	1	0

Abbreviations: CCRT, concurrent chemoradiotherapy; RT, radiotherapy.

Patient pretreatment characteristics

The pretreatment work-up included complete history collection, physical examination, computed tomography (CT) scans of the chest and abdomen, barium esophagography, endoscopy, endoscopic ultrasonography, and pulmonary function test. Bone scans were performed if clinically indicated. The 6th edition (2002) of the American Joint Committee on Cancer TNM staging system was used to classify tumors. The Charlson comorbidity index was used to perform analysis of this cohort's comorbidity burden [11].

Treatment details

The majority of patients (102 of 128) received three-dimensional conformal radiotherapy (3DCRT) and other 26 patients were treated with intensity-modulated radiotherapy (IMRT). Gross tumor volume (GTV) was defined as any visible primary tumor on the computerized imaging or endoscopy and included metastatic lymph nodes. Clinical target volume (CTV) was defined as the GTV with superoinferior 3-cm and lateral 2-cm margins. The planning target volume (PTV) was created by adding 1-cm in the superoinferior dimension and 0.8-cm radically to the CTV. Radiotherapy was delivered with 6–8 MV photons using a 1.8–2.0 Gy daily fraction and five fractions per week. The median prescription dose was 60 Gy (range, 46–70 Gy) to PTV in 25–35 fractions administered over 5–7 weeks.

Application of concurrent chemotherapy was performed after careful evaluation of organ function, performance status, and severity of comorbidities. Platinum-based chemotherapy combined with 5-fluorouracil (5-FU) or docetaxel was administered to 73 patients and the remaining 55 patients received RT alone. In the CCRT group, 33 patients received two cycles of docetaxel 60 mg/m^2 and cisplatin75 mg/m^2 delivered on day 1 and 22 of RT with standard premedication [12]. Forty patients were treated with two cycles of 60 mg/m^2 of cisplatin administered on days 1 and 29 and 1000 mg/m^2 of 5-FU administered as a continuous intravenous infusion for 96 hours on days 1–4 and 29–32 [13]. Dose reduction of chemotherapy was considered if any grade 4 hematological toxicities occurred.

Evaluation of response and toxicity

Patients were followed up every three months by physical examination, chest and abdominal CT, barium esophagography, and endoscopy or endoscopic ultrasonography. The clinical tumor response was evaluated 6–8 weeks after completion of RT according to the Response Evaluation Criteria in Solid Tumors (RECIST ver. 1.1). A complete response (CR) was defined as no remnant disease on CT image and pathological CR on endoscopy. The National Cancer Institute Common Toxicity Criteria (version 3.0) was used to score treatment toxicity.

Statistical analysis

The cutoff date of the last follow-up was April 30, 2013 for the censored data analysis. The Kaplan–Meier method was used to calculate overall survival (OS) and progression-free survival (PFS) for each potential prognostic factor, which were measured from the time of diagnosis. The log-rank test was used to test the differences between groups. The χ^2 test was used to compare patients' treatment-related toxicities between subgroups. Cox regression was used to perform multivariate analyses. All statistical analysis was performed using SPSS 16.0 software (SPSS Inc., Chicago, IL, USA). A p value of <0.05 was considered statistically significant.

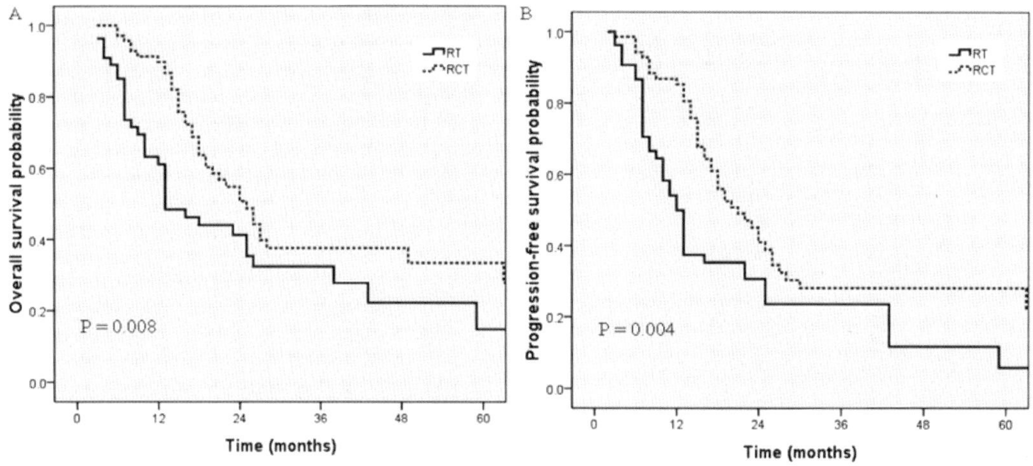

Figure 1. Overall survival (A) and progression-free survival (B) for the CCRT group and the RT alone group in the whole group of patients.

Results

Patients' characteristics

Clinical baseline characteristics are detailed in Table 1. The median age of the 128 patients was 72 years, ranging from 65 to 89 years. Twenty-eight patients (21.9%) had stage I/II disease and forty-nine patients (38.3%) had stage of III disease. Sixteen patients (12.5%) were diagnosed with stage IVa and the remaining 34 (26.6%) were diagnosed with stage IVb. Of the 34 stage IVb patients, except for one patient with liver metastasis and one with sacral bone metastasis, 32 had non-regional lymph nodal metastases. The Charlson score for the majority of patients was 0. Thirty patients (23.4%) had a Charlson score of 1, and 12 patients (9.4%) had a Charlson score ≥ 2. Twenty-three patients (18.0%) had chronic cardiovascular disease, 10 patients (7.8%) had chronic obstructive pulmonary disease, 17 patients (13.3%) had diabetes, and four patients (3.1%) had liver cirrhosis.

Tumor response and toxicity

All patients were evaluated for clinical tumor response. In the CCRT group (n = 73), CR was achieved in 17 (23.3%); partial response (PR) in 34 (46.6%); stable disease (SD) in 19 (26.0%); and progressive disease (PD) in 3 patients (4.1%), yielding an objective response rate of 67.1%. However, in the RT alone group (n = 55), the objective response rate declined to 47.3% (CR = 6 and PR = 20) and eight patients (14.5%) exhibited PD. A significant difference in response rate was observed between the two groups ($p = 0.032$).

All patients were evaluable for toxicity. As shown in Table 2, most treatment-related and documented acute toxicities were grade 1 and 2. No treatment-related deaths occurred and no patients experienced any acute grade 4 non-hematological toxicity. Most common grade 3 and 4 toxicities were leukopenia and gastrointestinal toxicity. Charlson score > 1 versus ≤ 1 did not influence the adverse events of grade 3–4 ($p = 0.474$). Acute grade 3–4 hematological toxicity was identified in 36.9% of the CCRT patients and 14.5% of the RT alone patients ($p = 0.001$). Patients treated with CCRT developed more grade ≥ 2 esophagitis and pneumonitis than patients who received RT alone (52.1% vs. 34.5%, $p = 0.005$).

Survival and prognostic analysis

The median follow-up period was 18.0 months (range, 3.0 to 89.0 months). During follow-up, 66 of the 128 patients (51.6%) relapsed and distant metastasis occurred in 33 patients (25.8%). Cancer was the cause of death in 64 patients (84.2%) among the patients who had died at the time of the current analysis (n = 76).

The 3-year OS and PFS rates for the whole group were 33.2% and 24.1%, respectively. The median OS of all patients was 16.0 months and the median PFS was 15.0 months. As shown in Fig.1, patients who received CCRT had a better OS compared with patients treated with RT alone (36.1% *vs.* 28.5% after 3 years, $p = 0.008$). The 3-year PFS rate of the CCRT group was also significantly higher than that for the RT alone group (27.2% *vs.* 16.3%, $p = 0.004$).

Sex, age, Charlson score, pathological grade, primary esophageal tumor location, tumor length, clinical T stage, clinical N stage, M stage, radiation dose and treatment modality were subjected to univariate analysis (Table 3). The results suggested that several variables were significantly associated with the OS: T stage ($p < 0.001$), M stage ($p = 0.012$), tumor length ($p = 0.039$) and treatment modality ($p = 0.008$). The variables significantly associated with the PFS were: T stage ($p = 0.007$), M stage ($p = 0.031$) and treatment modality ($p = 0.006$).

To identify independent prognostic factors, the factors that were found to be significant on univariate analysis were subjected to multivariate analysis. Multivariate analysis revealed that clinical T stage ($p = 0.002$) and treatment modality ($p = 0.002$) were independent factors affecting OS and PFS in elderly esophageal SCC patients (Table 4).

Subgroup analysis

As the median age of the whole group was 72 years, we subdivided the elderly patients into two groups: > 72 years and ≤ 72 years. As shown in Fig. 2, for patients ≤ 72 years, OS and PFS were significantly better in the CCRT group than in the RT alone group ($p =$ 0.003, 0.042). Median OS was 22.0 months in the CCRT group versus 13.0 months in the RT alone group. Nevertheless, for patients > 72 years, OS and PFS were similar in the two groups ($p = 0.337$, 0.363; Fig. 3).

Among patients who received CCRT, we further evaluated the efficacy of different chemotherapy regimens. Patients in the CCRT group were divided into two groups: those who received a

Table 3. Univariate analysis demonstrating factors associated with OS and PFS.

Factor	No.	OS *p*-value	PFS *p*-value
Sex		0.149	0.774
Male	89		
Female	39		
Age (years)		0.865	0.103
> 72	57		
≤ 72	71		
Charlson score		0.947	0.314
≥ 1	42		
< 1	86		
Pathological grade		0.847	0.683
Well differentiated	10		
Moderately differentiated	47		
Poorly/undifferentiated	45		
Unknown	26		
Location		0.325	0.634
Upper third	38		
Middle third	69		
Lower third	21		
Primary tumor length		0.039	0.169
≤ 5 cm	78		
> 5 cm	50		
T stage		0.000	0.007
T1-T2	25		
T3-T4	103		
N stage		0.804	0.359
N0	26		
N1	102		
M stage		0.012	0.041
M0	78		
M1	50		
Radiation dose (Gy)		0.056	0.226
< 60	49		
≥ 60	79		
Treatment modality		0.008	0.004
CCRT	73		
RT alone	55		

Abbreviations: OS, overall survival; PFS, progression-free survival; CCRT, concurrent chemoradiotherapy; RT, radiotherapy.

docetaxel combined regimen (n = 33) and those who received a 5-FU combined regimen (n = 40). The median OS periods were 21.0 and 17.0 months ($p = 0.013$), and the median PFS periods were 20.0 and 15.0 months ($p = 0.061$), respectively.

Discussion

Based on several clinical trials, CCRT has been the standard treatment for locally advanced esophageal cancer and is superior to RT alone [6]. However, very few studies have investigated CCRT in elderly patients [7–10]. The efficacy and toxicity of CCRT compared with RT alone for elderly patients have not been well documented previously. To clarify this issue, in the present study we compared the efficiency and safety of CCRT with RT alone in elderly patients with advanced thoracic esophageal SCC.

The surgical approach in elderly esophageal cancer patients remains a topic of debate because of the potentially higher rate of post-operative complications [14,15]. Several studies reported that CCRT was an effective treatment with no significant toxicity in elderly esophageal cancer patients [7–10,16–19]. However, Takeuchi et al. reported that an elderly patient group showed a significantly inferior median survival time compared with the nonelderly patient group (14.7 months *vs*. 35.1 months, $P = 0.01$)

Table 4. Multivariate analysis of prognostic factors for patients with elderly esophageal SCC.

Endpoint	Variable	P^a	HR	95% CI for HR
OS	Tumor length	0.220	1.355	0.833–2.204
	T stage	0.002	3.139	1.546–6.371
	M stage	0.073	1.615	0.957–2.727
	Treatment modality	0.002	0.468	0.292–0.750
PFS	T stage	0.014	2.117	1.166–3.844
	M stage	0.032	1.668	1.044–2.665
	Treatment modality	0.001	0.480	0.308–0.747

Abbreviations: CI, confidence interval; HR, hazards ratio; OS, overall survival; PFS, progression-free survival; SCC, squamous cell carcinoma.
[a]P values were calculated using an adjusted Cox proportional hazards model.

[20]. In the current study, patients who received CCRT had a 3-year OS of 37.6%, suggesting that CCRT is an effective treatment modality with a low incidence of severe toxicity for elderly patients.

Up to now, only two studies compared CCRT with RT alone in elderly esophageal cancer patients. Semrau et al. reported 51 patients aged ≥ 70 with inoperable esophageal cancer undergoing RT or CCRT, and revealed that patients treated with CCRT had a 2-year OS rate of 53.3% compared with 16.7% for RT patients ($P = 0.039$) [17]. In the study by Xu et al. [20], median OS for the CCRT group was 17 months, while it was 8 months in the RT group ($P = 0.013$). Consistent with previous reports, our study also revealed that CCRT had a higher response rate and an obvious survival benefit compared with RT alone, without a major increase in adverse events.

In the present study, 24 of 57 (42.1%) of patients aged older than72 years received CCRT, whereas 49 of 71 (69.0%) of patients between 65 and 72 years received CCRT. Given this difference in treatment, we consider our analysis to be a comparison of the treatment outcomes between relatively none-lderly patients (65–72 years old) and elderly patients (> 72 years). In the subgroup analysis, CCRT has a survival benefit compared with RT alone in patients between 65 and 72 years. Nevertheless, for patients > 72 years, OS and PFS were similar in the two groups. This may be partially explained by the poor life expectancy of patients older than 72 years. According to the Life Tables in 2010 in China, the average life expectancy was 74.8 years. The late toxicity of CCRT may be another reason. Marota et al reported that the 2-year cumulative incidence of late cardiopulmonary toxicities of Grade 3 or greater for patients 75 years or older was 29%, compared with 3% for younger patients, thus CCRT was not tolerated by patients older than 75 years [21].

Data on elderly patients who received RT alone are limited. Hishikawa et al. reported the survival within different age groups of esophageal cancer receiving external beam RT and brachytherapy boost, and revealed that the 2-year OS rate of patients aged 70–79 years was 17.2%, which is similar to the patients aged 43–69 years (16.7%). Therefore, the study suggested that RT should be the first choice of treatment for patients > 80 years old [22]. Yamakava et al, reported on 40 cases aged ≥ 80 years treated with RT alone and concluded that RT is a safe and effective treatment for esophageal cancer in patients over 80 years old [23]. In our study, in terms of the limited survival benefit of CCRT over RT, treatment modality should be evaluated on an

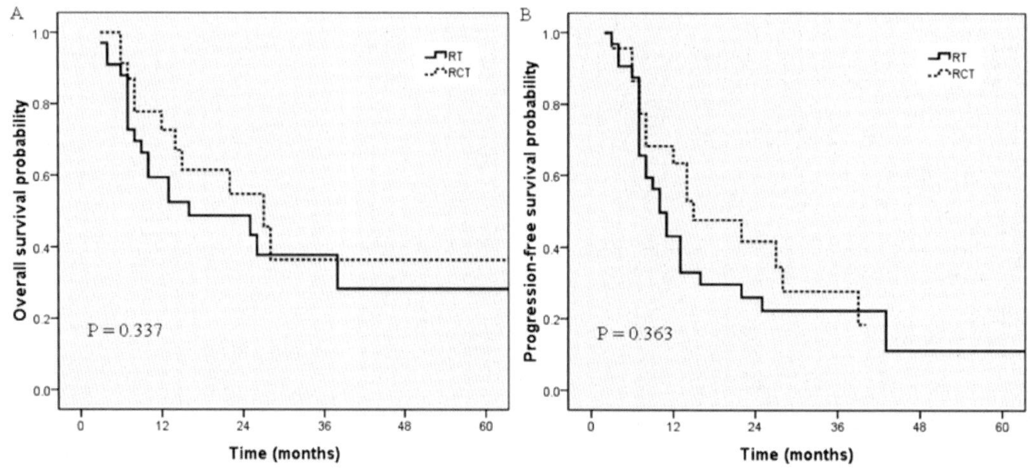

Figure 2. Overall survival (A) and progression-free survival (B) for the CCRT group and the RT alone group in patients older than 72 years.

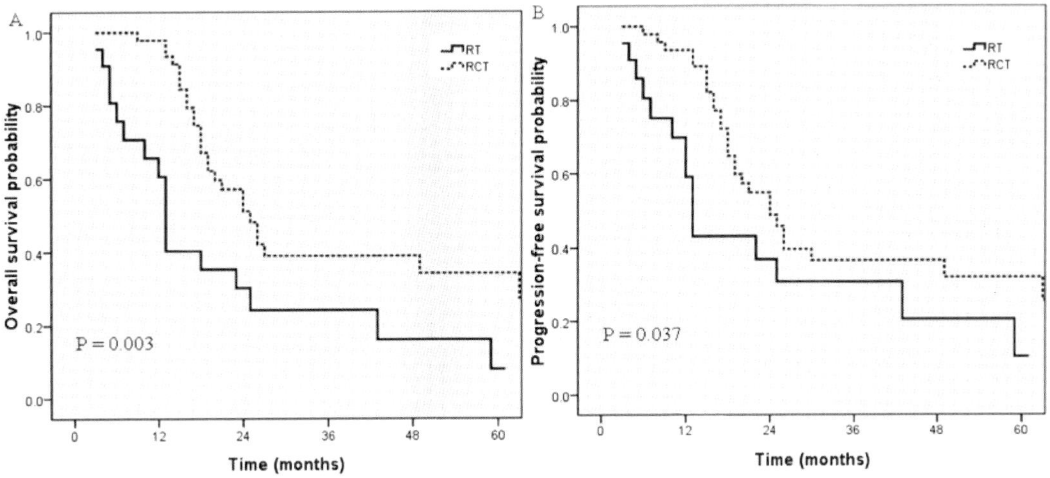

Figure 3. Overall survival (A) and progression-free survival (B) for the CCRT group and the RT alone group in patients between 65 and 72 years old.

individual basis in such cases and RT alone should be a reasonable option for patients in higher age groups.

Numerous studies on patients with advanced esophagogastric cancer suggested that cisplatin-based chemotherapy toxicities did not increase with age [24]. With regard to ≤ grade 3 side effects, it was possible to minimize and make tolerable such adverse events using previously described methods and careful close monitoring. Tougeron et al. reported that 4.6% of elderly patients who received combined chemoradiation experienced a grade 4 hematological toxicity [7]. In the CCRT group of our study, grade 4 hematological toxicities were observed in five patients (6.8%) only, suggesting that documented toxicities were not severe and supportive treatment was manageable. In addition, no treatment-related deaths occurred and no patients experienced any acute grade 4 non-hematologic toxicities. The incidence of severe acute toxicity in our cohort was lower than that reported in previous studies for non-elderly esophageal cancer patients [6,12]. Therefore, cisplatin-based CCRT is a safe treatment option for elderly esophageal SCC patients.

To improve survival for locally advanced esophageal cancer, taxane-based preoperative chemoradiotherapy schedules have been investigated in some exploratory trials. Wu et al compared the efficacy and feasibility of neoadjuvant chemoradiotherapy with docetaxel plus cisplatin or with cisplatin plus 5-FU for local advanced esophageal SCC, and showed that docetaxel plus cisplatin can be well tolerated and achieved a higher pathological complete response rate than cisplatin plus 5-FU (35.1% *vs*. 20.8%, $P=0.048$) [25]. However, there has been no prospective randomized trial to validate the benefit of different concurrent chemotherapy regimens for definitive RT. Hsu et al retrospectively analyzed the effects of paclitaxel-based chemoradiation for esophageal SCC and showed improved local disease compared with the regimen of 5-FU and cisplatin [26]. In the CCRT group in our study, there was a survival advantage for patients who received the docetaxel combined regimen compared with those who received the 5-FU combined regimen; thus, a prospective study addressing this regimen is warranted.

Age as a prognostic factor is still debated and several studies did not show any prognostic significance for age [27,28]. Semrau et al. compared 152 patients aged < 70 years treated with the definitive CCRT protocol and 51 patients aged ≥ 70 with esophageal cancer, and concluded that there was no significant difference in OS in the two groups; however, PFS showed a significant difference in favor of the ≥ 70 years group [17]. However, Takeuchi et al. demonstrated inferior survival in the elderly patient group compared with the non-elderly group. He attributed this to a lower response, a higher mortality from complications, and a lower compliance in the elderly group [20]. Our results showed that age has no bearing on the survival of elderly patients. This may be partially because our study did not include patients treated with best supportive care or endo-esophageal stenting only. The selected population may represent a favorable group of patients suffering from advanced esophageal cancer.

The prognostic value of comorbidity is far from conclusive. Tougeron et al. reported that a Charlson score ≤ 2 is an independent prognostic factor associated with better survival for elderly patients [16]. However, several studies showed that moderate to severe comorbidity are not predictive of survival [8,18]. In our study, a Charlson score ≥ 1 vs. <1 did not influence the incidence of adverse events. No significant association was found between the Charlson comorbidity index and OS or PFS; this may be attributed to the patients' selection bias.

The current study is limited by its retrospective design and the heterogeneity of the concurrent chemotherapy regimens. Considering all the aspects in the study, large-scale prospective clinical trials for elderly esophageal cancer patients are required in the future.

Conclusions

Elderly patients older than 65 years with inoperable thoracic esophageal SCC could benefit from CCRT without major toxicities. However, for patients older than 72 years, CCRT is not superior to RT alone in terms of survival benefit. Further prospective studies are warranted to confirm the results.

Author Contributions

Conceived and designed the experiments: PZ MX MZL. Performed the experiments: PZ MX LZ JXS QQL. Analyzed the data: QQL LRH SLL. Contributed reagents/materials/analysis tools: PZ MX QQL SLL. Contributed to the writing of the manuscript: PZ MX MZL.

References

1. Siegel R, Naishadham D, Jemal A (2013) Cancer Statistics, 2013. CA Cancer J Clin 63: 11–30.
2. Enzinger PC, Mayer RJ (2003) Esophageal cancer. N Engl J Med 349: 2241–2252.
3. Steyerberg EW, Neville B, Weeks JC, Earle CC (2007) Referral patterns, treatment choices, and outcomes in locoregional esophageal cancer: population-based analysis of elderly patients. J Clin Oncol 25: 2389–2396.
4. Kinugasa S, Tachibana M, Yoshimura H, Dhar DK, Shibakita M, et al. (2001) Esophageal resection in elderly esophageal carcinoma patients: improvement in postoperative complications. Ann Thorac Surg 71: 414–418.
5. Law S, Wong KH, Kwok KF, Chu KM, Wong J (2004) Predictive factors for postoperative pulmonary complications and mortality after esophagectomy for cancer. Ann Surg 240: 791–800.
6. Herskovic A, Martz K, al-Sarraf M, Leichman L, Brindle J, et al. (1992) Combined chemotherapy and radiotherapy compared with radiotherapy alone in patients with cancer of the esophagus. N Engl J Med 326: 1593–1598.
7. Tougeron D, Di Fiore F, Thureau S, Berbera N, Iwanicki-Caron I, et al. (2008) Safety and outcome of definitive chemoradiotherapy in elderly patients with oesophageal cancer. Br J Cancer 99: 1586–1592.
8. Anderson SE, Minsky BD, Bains M, Hummer A, Kelsen D, et al. (2007) Combined modality chemoradiation in elderly oesophageal cancer patients. Br J Cancer 96: 1823–1827.
9. Nallapareddy S, Wilding GE, Yang G, Iyer R, Javle M (2005) Chemoradiation is a tolerable therapy for older adults with esophageal cancer. Anticancer Res 25: 3055–3060.
10. Mak RH, Mamon HJ, Ryan DP, Miyamoto DT, Ancukiewicz M, et al. (2010) Toxicity and outcomes after chemoradiation for esophageal cancer in patients age 75 or older. Dis Esophagus 23: 316–323.
11. Reid BC, Alberg AJ, Klassen AC, Samet JM, Rozier RG, et al. (2001) Comorbidity and survival of elderly head and neck carcinoma patients. Cancer 92: 2109–2116.
12. Li QQ, Liu MZ, Hu YH, Liu H, He ZY, et al. (2010) Definitive concomitant chemoradiotherapy with docetaxel and cisplatin in squamous esophageal carcinoma. Dis Esophagus 23: 253–259.
13. Liu H, Lu L, Zhu Q, Hao Y, Mo Y, et al. (2011) Cervical nodal metastases of unresectable thoracic esophageal squamous cell carcinoma Characteristics of long-term survivors after concurrent chemoradiotherapy. Radiother Oncol 99: 181–186.
14. Sabel MS, Smith JL, Nava HR, Mollen K, Douglass HO, et al. (2002) Esophageal resection for carcinoma in patients older than 70 years. Ann Surg Oncol 9: 210–214.
15. Gockel I, Sultanov FS, Domeyer M, Goenner U, Junginger T (2007) Developments in esophageal surgery for adenocarcinoma: a comparison of two decades. BMC Cancer 7: 114.
16. Tougeron D, Hamidou H, Scotté M, Di Fiore F, Antonietti M, et al. (2010) Esophageal cancer in the elderly: an analysis of the factors associated with treatment decisions and outcomes. BMC Cancer 10: 510.
17. Semrau R, Herzog SL, Vallböhmer D, Kocher M, Hölscher A, et al. (2012) Radiotherapy in elderly patients with inoperable esophageal cancer. Is there a benefit? Strahlenther Onkol 188: 226–232.
18. Go SI, Sup Lee W, Hee Kang M, Song HN, Jin Kim M, et al. (2012) Response to concurrent chemoradiotherapy as a prognostic marker in elderly patients with locally advanced esophageal cancer. Tumori 98: 225–232.
19. Xu HY, Du ZD, Zhou L, Yu M, Ding ZY, et al. (2014) Safety and efficacy of radiation and chemoradiation in patients over 70 years old with inoperable esophageal squamous cell carcinoma. Oncol Lett 7: 260–266.
20. Takeuchi S, Ohtsu A, Doi T, Kojima T, Minashi K, et al. (2007) A retrospective study of definitive chemoradiotherapy for elderly patients with esophageal cancer. Am J Clin Oncol 30: 607–611.
21. Morota M, Gomi K, Kozuka T, Chin K, Matsuura M, et al. (2009) Late toxicity after definitive concurrent chemoradiotherapy for thoracic esophageal carcinoma. Int J Radiat Oncol Biol Phys 75: 122–128.
22. Hishikawa Y, Kurisu K, Taniguchi M, Kamikonya N, Miura T (1991) Radiotherapy for carcinoma of the esophagus in patients aged eighty or older. Int J Radiat Oncol Biol Phys 20: 685–688.
23. Yamakawa M, Shiojima K, Takahashi M, Saito Y, Matsumoto H, et al. (1994) Radiation therapy for esophageal cancer in patients over 80 years old. Int J Radiat Oncol Biol Phys 30: 1225–1232.
24. Trumper M, Ross PJ, Cunningham D, Norman AR, Hawkins R, et al. (2006) Efficacy and tolerability of chemotherapy in elderly patients with advanced oesophago-gastric cancer: A pooled analysis of three clinical trials. Eur J Cancer 42: 827–834.
25. Wu S, Chen MY, Luo JC, Wei L, Chen Z (2012) Comparison between docetaxel plus cisplatin and cisplatin plus fluorouracil in the neoadjuvant chemoradiotherapy for local advanced esophageal squamous cell carcinoma. Zhonghua Zhong Liu Za Zhi 34: 873–876.
26. Hsu FM, Lin CC, Lee JM, Chang YL, Hsu CH, et al. (2008) Improved local control by surgery and paclitaxel-based chemoradiation for esophageal squamous cell carcinoma: results of a retrospective non-randomized study. J Surg Oncol 98: 34–41.
27. Lagarde SM, ten Kate FJ, Reitsma JB, Busch OR, van Lanschot JJ (2006) Prognostic factors in adenocarcinoma of the esophagus or gastroesophageal junction. J Clin Oncol 24: 4347–4355.
28. Eloubeidi MA, Desmond R, Arguedas MR, Reed CE, Wilcox CM (2002) Prognostic factors for the survival of patients with esophageal carcinoma in the U.S.: the importance of tumor length and lymph node status. Cancer 95: 1434–1443.

S-1-Based versus Capecitabine-Based Preoperative Chemoradiotherapy in the Treatment of Locally Advanced Rectal Cancer: A Matched-Pair Analysis

Meng Su, Lu-Cheng Zhu, Hang-Ping Wei, Wen-Hua Luo, Rui-Fang Lin, Chang-Lin Zou*

Department of Radiation Oncology and Chemotherapy, The First Affiliated Hospital of Wenzhou Medical University, Wenzhou, China

Abstract

Objective: The aim of this paper was to compare the efficacy and safety of S-1-based and capecitabine-based preoperative chemoradiotherapy regimens in patients with locally advanced rectal cancer through a retrospective matched-pair analysis.

Materials and methods: Between Jan 2010 and Mar 2014, 24 patients with locally advanced rectal cancer who received preoperative radiotherapy concurrently with S-1 were individually matched with 24 contemporary patients with locally advanced rectal cancer who received preoperative radiotherapy concurrently with capecitabine according to clinical stage (as determined by pelvic magnetic resonance imaging and computed tomography) and age (within five years). All these patients performed mesorectal excision 4–8 weeks after the completion of chemoradiotherapy.

Results: The tumor volume reduction rates were 55.9±15.1% in the S-1 group and 53.8±16.0% in the capecitabine group (p = 0.619). The overall downstaging, including both T downstaging and N downstaging, occurred in 83.3% of the S-1 group and 70.8% of the capecitabine group (p = 0.508). The significant tumor regression, including regression grade I and II, occurred in 33.3% of S-1 patients and 25.0% of capecitabine patients (p = 0.754). In the two groups, Grade 4 adverse events were not observed and Grade 3 consisted of only two cases of diarrhea, and no patient suffered hematologic adverse event of Grade 2 or higher. However, the incidence of diarrhea (62.5% *vs* 33.3%, p = 0.014) and hand-foot syndrome (29.2% *vs* 0%, p = 0.016) were higher in capecitabine group. Other adverse events did not differ significantly between two groups.

Conclusions: The two preoperative chemoradiotherapy regimens were effective and safe for patients of locally advanced rectal cancer, but regimen with S-1 exhibited a lower incidence of adverse events.

Editor: John Souglakos, University General Hospital of Heraklion and Laboratory of Tumor Cell Biology, School of Medicine, University of Crete, Greece

Funding: The authors have no support or funding to report.

Competing Interests: The authors have declared that no competing interests exist.

* Email: zcl19670115@163.com

Introduction

Neoadjuvant therapy for locally advanced rectal cancer (LARC) has gained widespread acceptance today. Preoperative radiotherapy (RT) significantly reduced the risk of local recurrence and death from rectal cancer, and the addition of fluoropyrimidine provided further benefits in local control [1–4]. Therefore, fluorouracil-based preoperative chemoradiotherapy (CRT) becomes one of the standard therapy for LARC and oral fluoropyrimidine has gradually taken the place of continuous 5-FU infusion because of its convenience and safety [5].

Capecitabine (Xeloda; Hoffman-La Roche Ltd, Basel, Switzerland) is an oral fluoropyrimidine anticancer agent with substantial activity in colorectal cancer and it has been frequently used in preoperative CRT [6,7]. But diarrhea and hand-foot syndrome were inevitable for mostly patients who used capecitabine.

S-1 (TS-1; Taiho Pharmaceutical, Tokyo, Japan) is another oral fluoropyrimidine anticancer agent, which had similar, and in some cases superior activity, to other active chemotherapies for the treatment of colorectal cancer patients with a promising safety profile [8]. And recently S-1 was applied to preoperative CRT for patients with LARC, which revealed a high efficacy and low incidence of adverse events [9].

Although lots of papers have demonstrated that both oral fluoropyrimidines were effective and safe, doubts still exist about whether S-1 or capecitabine is the better choice when associated with preoperative RT for patients with LARC. Based on this consideration, the aim of this study was to compare the efficacy and safety of S-1-based and capecitabine-based preoperative CRT regimens in patients with LARC through a retrospective matched-pair analysis.

Materials and Methods

Patients

From Jan 2010 to Mar 2014, the medical records of rectal cancer patients were retrospectively reviewed in our hospital. 24

patients with histopathologically confirmed as rectal adenocarcinoma, clinically staged as T3–T4, Tx N+, M0, no history of anticancer therapy, who received preoperative RT concurrently with S-1, were included in this study. For comparison, these patients were individually matched with 24 contemporary patients with histopathologically confirmed as rectal adenocarcinoma, clinically staged as T3–T4, Tx N+, M0, no history of anticancer therapy, who received preoperative RT concurrently with capecitabine. Matching criteria were clinical stage (as determined by pelvic magnetic resonance imaging and computed tomography) and age (within five years). Matching by clinical T stage and N stage was not done in this study because it would have significantly reduced the sample size.

Ethics

This study was approved by the Ethics Committee of the First Affiliated Hospital of Wenzhou Medical University, Wenzhou, China. Written informed consents were obtained from all the patients for publication of this report.

Chemotherapy

Preoperative chemotherapy was delivered throughout the period of pelvic radiation. S-1 and capecitabine were respectively given twice a day in a fixed daily dose of 80 mg/m2 and 825 mg/m2 on days 1 to 14, 22 to 35. The choice of S-1 or capecitabine was determined by the preferences of patients or physicians.

Radiotherapy

The total irradiation dose of 50 Gy was delivered in daily fractions of 2 Gy, five times per week, through a pair of opposed anterior-posterior fields using a 6 MV linear accelerator. The treatment fields were set as follows: The superior border was placed at S1/L5, the inferior border was placed at 3–4 cm below the lowest tumor border or the inferior margin of the obturator foramen, and the lateral borders of the planning target volume were 1.5 cm lateral to the widest bony margin of the true pelvic wall.

Surgery

Surgery was performed 4–8 weeks after the completion of CRT. The total mesorectal excision was the main surgical treatment, and the final choice of low anterior resection or abdominoperineal resection was determined by estimation of surgeon and the will of patient.

Assessment

Tumor responses, including clinical response and pathological response, were evaluated in this paper. The clinical response was determined by assessing the degree of tumor shrinkage. As two assessment instruments of clinical tumor response, magnetic resonance imaging and computed tomography were performed before CRT and 2–7 days before surgery. Tumor volume measurement was based on the Response Evaluation Criteria in Solid Tumors (RECIST) [10].

The pathological responses, including downstaging and tumor regression, were evaluated by examining the resected specimens. Downstaging was determined by comparing the pretreatment clinical stage with the postoperative pathological stage, and the overall downstaging included both T downstaging and N downstaging. Tumor stage was defined according to the 7th edition of the American Joint Committee on Cancer staging manual [11]. The tumor regression grade (TRG) was classified in 5 levels: TRG I (pathological complete response); TRG II (rare residual cancer cells); TGR III (fibrosis outgrowing residual cancer); TGR IV (residual cancer cells outgrowing fibrosis); TGR V (absence of regressive changes) [12]. We defined significant tumor regression (STR) as TRG I/II.

Safety was analyzed by assessing the incidences of adverse events. The adverse event grades were defined according to the Common Terminology Criteria for Adverse Events of the National Cancer Institute, version 3.0 [13].

Statistical analysis

In this matched-pair study, McNemar's chi-square test or Fisher's exact test was used to compare the categorical variables, and the paired *t* test or Wilcoxon signed rank test was used to compare the continuous variables. The Wilcoxon signed rank test was also used to compare the rates of adverse events between the two groups, taking into account the different adverse event grades. Statistical analyses were performed with the Statistical Package for Social Sciences, version 17.0 (SPSS Inc., Chicago, IL, USA). Differences with $p<0.05$ were considered to indicate statistical significance and all statistical tests were two sided.

Result

Patients

24 patients with LARC who received preoperative RT concurrently with S-1 were matched by clinical stage and age with 24 patients with LARC who received preoperative RT concurrently with capecitabine. The baseline characteristics of the patients of two groups were recorded and are showed in Table 1. There was no significant differences between two groups for gender, distance from anal verge, Eastern Cooperative Oncology Group (ECOG) performance states (PS), clinical T classification, clinical N classification, histological differentiation, pre-CRT carcinoembryonic antigen (CEA).

Efficacy

The clinical response and pathological response of two groups are presented in Table 2. The tumor volume reduction rates were 55.9±15.1% (mean ± SD) in S-1 group and 53.8±16.0% in capecitabine group ($p = 0.619$). T downstaging rates were 62.5% for S-1 group and 50.0% for capecitabine group ($p = 0.549$). 70.6% of cN+ patients in S-1 group and 58.8% of cN+ patients in capecitabine group changed into pN- ($p = 0.687$). In S-1 group and capecitabine group, overall downstaging (including T downstaging and N downstaging) rates were 83.3% and 70.8% respectively ($p = 0.508$), and STR (including regression grade I and II) occurred in 33.3% of S-1 patients and 25.0% of capecitabine patients ($p = 0.754$).

Safety

Table 3 presents the treatment-related adverse events which observed among all 48 patients during the period of preoperative CRT. Hand-foot syndrome was only observed in capecitabine group (29.2% *vs* 0%, $p = 0.016$). The incidence of diarrhea was also higher in capecitabine group (62.5% *vs* 33.3%, $p = 0.014$). Except diarrhea and hand-foot syndrome, adverse events did not differ significantly between two groups. Grade 4 adverse events did not occur in either of the groups, and no Grade 2 or higher hematologic adverse event was observed. Besides, only two patients experienced Grade 3 adverse events of diarrhea. Adverse events were mild in two groups, and most of them were relieved after appropriate treatment.

Table 1. Patients' characteristics.

Characteristics	S-1 (n = 24)	Capecitabine (n = 24)	*p*-value
Gender (%)			1.000
Male	19 (79.2)	18 (75.0)	
Female	5 (20.8)	6 (25.0)	
Age (years)			Matched
Mean (SD)	54.8 (10.0)	55.4 (9.8)	
Median (range)	54 (33–80)	54.5 (35–83)	
Distance from anal verge (cm)			0.503
Mean (SD)	5.1 (2.2)	5.5 (1.9)	
Median (range)	5.0 (0.5–10)	6.0 (1–8)	
ECOG PS (%)			0.754
0	14 (58.3)	12 (50.0)	
1	10 (41.7)	12 (50.0)	
Clinical T classification (%)			0.727
cT3	12 (50.0)	14 (58.3)	
cT4	12 (50.0)	10 (41.7)	
Clinical N classification (%)			1.000
cN0	7 (29.2)	7 (29.2)	
cN+	17 (70.8)	17 (70.8)	
Clinical stage (%)			Matched
cStage II	7 (29.2)	7 (29.2)	
cStage III	17 (70.8)	17 (70.8)	
Histological differentiation (%)			0.667
Poorly	5 (20.8)	6 (25.0)	
Moderately	16 (66.7)	13 (54.2)	
Well	3 (12.5)	5 (20.8)	
Pre-CRT CEA (ng/ml) (%)			1.000
≤5	15 (62.5)	14 (58.3)	
>5	9 (37.5)	10 (41.7)	

ECOG PS Eastern Cooperative Oncology Group performance states; *CRT* chemoradiotherapy; *CEA* carcinoembryonic antigen.

Table 2. Clinical and pathologic evaluations of tumor response.

	S-1 (n = 24)	Capecitabine (n = 24)	*p*-value
Tumor shrinkage (%)			0.619
Mean (SD)	55.9 (15.1)	53.8 (16.0)	
Tumor downstage (%)			
T downstaging	15 (62.5)	12(50.0)	0.549
N downstaging*	12 (70.6)	10 (58.8)	0.687
Overall downstaging	20 (83.3)	17 (70.8)	0.508
Tumor regression grade (TRG) (%)			
TRG I/II (STR)	8 (33.3)	6 (25.0)	0.754
TRG III/IV	14 (58.3)	17 (70.8)	0.508
TRG V	2 (8.3)	1 (4.2)	1.000

STR significant tumor regression.
*17 patients in S-1 group and 17 patients in capecitabine group were demonstrated as cN+.

Table 3. Adverse event profiles during treatment.

	S-1 (n = 24)		Capecitabine (n = 24)		*p*-value
	Total (%)	Grade 1/2/3	Total (%)	Grade 1/2/3	
Hematologic					
Leukopenia	5 (20.8)	5/0/0	4 (16.7)	4/0/0	1.000
Neutropenia	4 (16.7)	4/0/0	2 (8.3)	2/0/0	0.688
Anemia	1 (4.2)	1/0/0	1 (4.2)	1/0/0	1.000
Thrombocytopenia	2 (8.3)	2/0/0	0 (0)	0/0/0	0.500
Non-hematologic					
Diarrhea	8 (33.3)	6/2/0	15 (62.5)	7/6/2	0.014
Vomiting	5 (20.8)	4/1/0	9 (37.5)	7/2/0	0.340
AST/ALT	1 (4.2)	1/0/0	1 (4.2)	1/0/0	1.000
Hand-foot syndrome	0 (0)	0/0/0	7 (29.2)	5/2/0	0.016

AST aspartate aminotransferase; *ALT* alanine transaminase.

Surgery

The clinical stage after CRT are showed in Table 4 and did not differ significantly between two groups. All 48 patients underwent radical surgery 4–8 weeks after the completion of chemoradiation. Among them, 38 patients (79.2%) received low anterior resection and 10 patients (20.8%) received abdominoperineal resection. Of the 25 patients who had rectal cancer within 5 cm of the anal verge, 18 patients (72.0%) underwent sphincter preserving surgery. All the patients (100%) had a negative circumferential resection margin.

Postoperative

After surgery, only 1 patient in capecitabine group who received abdominoperineal resection suffered from massive intestinal bleeding and died one month later. No other serious postoperative complications occurred. Of the patients, 47 received fluoropyrimidine-based adjuvant chemotherapy (capecitabine, S-1, FOLFOX or XELOX). Until now, no local recurrence was observed and distant metastasis was only observed in 2 patients of capecitabine group (1 liver metastases, 1 liver and lung metastases). Except 1 patient died of massive intestinal bleeding, all the patients are alive.

Discussion

The short-term aim of treatment for rectal cancer is to achieve complete resection of the tumor, and the long-term aims are to improve overall survival and disease free survival through a high locoregional control and low distant metastasis rate. However, local advanced ones are difficult to reach these goals if receive surgery alone, hence neoadjuvant therapy followed by radical surgery has been introduced to enhance the outcome of LARC [14]. In addition, the neoadjuvant therapy does not increase perioperative complications [15]. According to previous clinical studies, preoperative CRT is superior to preoperative RT by improving pathological response and local control [2–4,16], and it could provide advantages of local control, toxicity, compliance and sphincter preservation rate when compares with postoperative approach [17]. Sphincter preservation is important for LARC patients to preserve a high quality of life.

For years, 5-FU as an essential role in the treatment of rectal cancer has been widely used in CRT. As a radiosensitizer in preoperative CRT, 5-FU usually administered as protracted intravenous infusions. However, protracted intravenous infusions of 5-FU are inconvenient, and patients with central venous catheters are associated with a non-negligible risk of complications such as infection and thrombosis. Nowadays, the quality of life for

Table 4. Clinical stage after chemoradiotherapy.

	S-1 (n = 24)	Capecitabine (n = 24)	*p*-value
Clinical T classification (%)			0.556
cT1–2	11 (45.8)	8 (33.3)	
cT3–4	13 (54.2)	16 (66.7)	
Clinical N classification (%)			0.740
cN0	19 (79.2)	17 (70.8)	
cN+	5 (20.8)	7 (29.2)	
Clinical stage (%)			0.666
cStage I	9 (37.5)	6 (25.0)	
cStage II	10 (41.7)	11 (45.8)	
cStage III	5 (20.8)	7 (29.2)	

cancer patients is increasingly concerned. Therefore, oral fluoropyrimidines such as capecitabine and S-1 have been developed to take the place of intravenous 5-FU. Capecitabine and S-1 are well tolerated which mimic continuous-infusion 5-FU, whilst promising improve patient convenience and quality of life [5,8].

Capecitabine is a fluoropyrimidine carbamate that was rationally designed as an orally administered precursor of 5′-deoxy-5-fluorouridine, which is selectively tumor-activated to the cytotoxic agent 5-FU by exploiting the higher levels of thymidine phosphorylase found in tumor tissues compared with normal tissues [6]. Capecitabine is converted to 5-FU preferentially in tumor tissue via a three-step enzymatic cascade, firstly converted to 5′-deoxy-fluorocytidine by hepatic carboxylesterase in the liver; secondly converted to 5′-deoxy-5-fluorouridine by cytidine deaminase in the liver and tumor tissues; finally converted to 5-FU at the tumor site by the tumor-associated angiogenic factor thymidine phosphorylase, thereby minimizing the exposure of normal tissue to 5-FU [18–20]. In phase II studies, the main toxicities were hand-foot syndrome and diarrhea. The pCR rate was ranging from 12% to 31% and overall downstaging rate was ranging from 59% to 84% [21–23]. The short-term outcomes after preoperative therapy, such as tumor volume reduction, pathological downstaging, toxicity, were similar to 5-FU infusion [7].

S-1 is an oral anticancer drug that combines tegafur (a prodrug that is converted by cells to 5-FU), 5-chloro-2,4-dihydropyrimidine (CDHP) and potassium oxonate in a molar ratio of 1:0.4:1 [8,24]. CDHP is a potent and reversible inhibitor of dihydropyrimidine, thereby prolonging high 5-FU concentration in the circulation [25,26]. Ptassium oxonate is a inhibitor of orotate phosphoribosyltransferase that catalyzes the phosphorylation of 5-FU in the gastrointestinal tract, thereby reducing the gastrointestinal toxic effects of 5-FU [27]. Nakata et al. [28] reported that S-1 could enhance the radiation response of human colon cancer xenografts resistant to 5-FU. In a Phase II study, the rates of pCR, overall downstaging, tumor volume reduction were 22%, 78%, 69±22%, respectively. The adverse events were mild and hand-foot syndrome was not observed [9].

As mentioned above, both S-1 and capecitabine have been used in preoperative CRT for LARC patients, but lack direct comparison between them. According to our knowledge, this is the first study to compare efficacy and safety in patients treated with capecitabine or S-1 in preoperative CRT for LARC using a retrospective matched-pair analysis. In this study, both S-1 group and capecitabine group achieved a high efficacy of tumor responses, and patients in either group could tolerate the treatment-related adverse events. The treatment compliance was extremely high in two groups and all the patients completed the treatment schedule, neither interruption nor dose reduction (including chemotherapy drugs and radiation). Comparison of S-1 group and capecitabine group, the tumor responses such as tumor volume reduction, downstaging and tumor regression did not differ significantly. However, patients treated with capecitabine suffered more adverse events than who treated with S-1. Diarrhea and hand-foot syndrome were mainly discovered in capecitabine group. Thus, patients who treated with capecitabine should pay more money on managing adverse events.

The present study had some limitations. First, the follow-up time was short. Only short-term outcomes were assessed in this study. Overall survival and disease free survival data, as long-term outcomes, need further study to analyze between the two regimens. Second, the number of cases was small and clinical significance was limited. The next step will be to further expand the number of cases. Third, this was a retrospective study. It is advisable to conduct a multicenter randomized controlled study.

Conclusions

The both preoperative CRT regimens were effective and safe for patients of LARC. However, regimen with S-1 had a lower incidence of adverse events. Thus, this retrospective matched-pair study suggested that preoperative CRT with S-1 is a more reasonable choice for LARC.

Supporting Information

Table S1 Baseline characteristics of the rectal cancer patients in two group.

Table S2 The clinical response and pathological response of the rectal cancer patients in two group.

Table S3 The treatment-related adverse events of the rectal cancer patients in two group.

Table S4 The clinical stage after preoperative chemoradiotherapy of the rectal cancer patients in two group.

Author Contributions

Conceived and designed the experiments: CLZ MS. Analyzed the data: MS LCZ. Contributed reagents/materials/analysis tools: MS LCZ WHL HPW RFL. Contributed to the writing of the manuscript: MS.

References

1. Colorectal Cancer Collaborative G (2001) Adjuvant radiotherapy for rectal cancer: a systematic overview of 8,507 patients from 22 randomised trials. Lancet 358: 1291–1304.
2. Ceelen W, Fierens K, Van Nieuwenhove Y, Pattyn P (2009) Preoperative chemoradiation versus radiation alone for stage II and III resectable rectal cancer: a systematic review and meta-analysis. Int J Cancer 124: 2966–2972.
3. Bosset JF, Collette L, Calais G, Mineur L, Maingon P, et al. (2006) Chemotherapy with preoperative radiotherapy in rectal cancer. N Engl J Med 355: 1114–1123.
4. Gerard JP, Conroy T, Bonnetain F, Bouche O, Chapet O, et al. (2006) Preoperative radiotherapy with or without concurrent fluorouracil and leucovorin in T3–4 rectal cancers: results of FFCD 9203. J Clin Oncol 24: 4620–4625.
5. Rich TA, Shepard RC, Mosley ST (2004) Four decades of continuing innovation with fluorouracil: current and future approaches to fluorouracil chemoradiation therapy. J Clin Oncol 22: 2214–2232.
6. Van Cutsem E, Findlay M, Osterwalder B, Kocha W, Dalley D, et al. (2000) Capecitabine, an oral fluoropyrimidine carbamate with substantial activity in advanced colorectal cancer: results of a randomized phase II study. J Clin Oncol 18: 1337–1345.
7. Kim DY, Jung KH, Kim TH, Kim DW, Chang HJ, et al. (2007) Comparison of 5-fluorouracil/leucovorin and capecitabine in preoperative chemoradiotherapy for locally advanced rectal cancer. Int J Radiat Oncol Biol Phys 67: 378–384.
8. Schoffski P (2004) The modulated oral fluoropyrimidine prodrug S-1, and its use in gastrointestinal cancer and other solid tumors. Anticancer Drugs 15: 85–106.
9. Sadahiro S, Suzuki T, Tanaka A, Okada K, Kamijo A, et al. (2011) Phase I/II study of preoperative concurrent chemoradiotherapy with S-1 for locally advanced, resectable rectal adenocarcinoma. Oncology 81: 306–311.
10. Therasse P, Arbuck SG, Eisenhauer EA, Wanders J, Kaplan RS, et al. (2000) New guidelines to evaluate the response to treatment in solid tumors. European Organization for Research and Treatment of Cancer, National Cancer Institute of the United States, National Cancer Institute of Canada. J Natl Cancer Inst 92: 205–216.
11. Edge SB, Byrd DR, Compton CC, Fritz AG, Greene FL, et al. (2010) American Joint Committee on Cancer staging manual. 7th edition. New York: Springer.
12. Mandard AM, Dalibard F, Mandard JC, Marnay J, Henry-Amar M, et al. (1994) Pathologic assessment of tumor regression after preoperative chemor-

adiotherapy of esophageal carcinoma. Clinicopathologic correlations. Cancer 73: 2680–2686.
13. Trotti A, Colevas AD, Setser A, Rusch V, Jaques D, et al. (2003) CTCAE v3.0: development of a comprehensive grading system for the adverse effects of cancer treatment. Semin Radiat Oncol 13: 176–181.
14. van Gijn W, Marijnen CA, Nagtegaal ID, Kranenbarg EM, Putter H, et al. (2011) Preoperative radiotherapy combined with total mesorectal excision for resectable rectal cancer: 12-year follow-up of the multicentre, randomised controlled TME trial. Lancet Oncol 12: 575–582.
15. Ulrich A, Weitz J, Slodczyk M, Koch M, Jaeger D, et al. (2009) Neoadjuvant treatment does not influence perioperative outcome in rectal cancer surgery. Int J Radiat Oncol Biol Phys 75: 129–136.
16. De Caluwe L, Van Nieuwenhove Y, Ceelen WP (2013) Preoperative chemoradiation versus radiation alone for stage II and III resectable rectal cancer. Cochrane Database Syst Rev 2: CD006041.
17. Sauer R, Becker H, Hohenberger W, Rodel C, Wittekind C, et al. (2004) Preoperative versus postoperative chemoradiotherapy for rectal cancer. N Engl J Med 351: 1731–1740.
18. Miwa M, Ura M, Nishida M, Sawada N, Ishikawa T, et al. (1998) Design of a novel oral fluoropyrimidine carbamate, capecitabine, which generates 5-fluorouracil selectively in tumours by enzymes concentrated in human liver and cancer tissue. Eur J Cancer 34: 1274–1281.
19. Ishikawa T, Fukase Y, Yamamoto T, Sekiguchi F, Ishitsuka H (1998) Antitumor activities of a novel fluoropyrimidine, N4-pentyloxycarbonyl-5′-deoxy-5-fluorocytidine (capecitabine). Biol Pharm Bull 21: 713–717.
20. Ishikawa T, Utoh M, Sawada N, Nishida M, Fukase Y, et al. (1998) Tumor selective delivery of 5-fluorouracil by capecitabine, a new oral fluoropyrimidine carbamate, in human cancer xenografts. Biochem Pharmacol 55: 1091–1097.
21. Kim JS, Kim JS, Cho MJ, Song KS, Yoon WH (2002) Preoperative chemoradiation using oral capecitabine in locally advanced rectal cancer. Int J Radiat Oncol Biol Phys 54: 403–408.
22. Kim JC, Kim TW, Kim JH, Yu CS, Kim HC, et al. (2005) Preoperative concurrent radiotherapy with capecitabine before total mesorectal excision in locally advanced rectal cancer. Int J Radiat Oncol Biol Phys 63: 346–353.
23. Krishnan S, Janjan NA, Skibber JM, Rodriguez-Bigas MA, Wolff RA, et al. (2006) Phase II study of capecitabine (Xeloda) and concomitant boost radiotherapy in patients with locally advanced rectal cancer. Int J Radiat Oncol Biol Phys 66: 762–771.
24. Shirasaka T, Shimamato Y, Ohshimo H, Yamaguchi M, Kato T, et al. (1996) Development of a novel form of an oral 5-fluorouracil derivative (S-1) directed to the potentiation of the tumor selective cytotoxicity of 5-fluorouracil by two biochemical modulators. Anticancer Drugs 7: 548–557.
25. Tatsumi K, Fukushima M, Shirasaka T, Fujii S (1987) Inhibitory effects of pyrimidine, barbituric acid and pyridine derivatives on 5-fluorouracil degradation in rat liver extracts. Jpn J Cancer Res 78: 748–755.
26. Takechi T, Nakano K, Uchida J, Mita A, Toko K, et al. (1997) Antitumor activity and low intestinal toxicity of S-1, a new formulation of oral tegafur, in experimental tumor models in rats. Cancer Chemother Pharmacol 39: 205–211.
27. Shirasaka T, Shimamoto Y, Fukushima M (1993) Inhibition by oxonic acid of gastrointestinal toxicity of 5-fluorouracil without loss of its antitumor activity in rats. Cancer Res 53: 4004–4009.
28. Nakata E, Fukushima M, Takai Y, Nemoto K, Ogawa Y, et al. (2006) S-1, an oral fluoropyrimidine, enhances radiation response of DLD-1/FU human colon cancer xenografts resistant to 5-FU. Oncol Rep 16: 465–471.

Comparison of 3D Confromal Radiotherapy and Intensity Modulated Radiotherapy with or without Simultaneous Integrated Boost during Concurrent Chemoradiation for Locally Advanced Head and Neck Cancers

Michael T. Spiotto[1,2]*, Ralph R. Weichselbaum[1,2]

1 Department of Radiation and Cellular Oncology, University of Chicago Medical Center, Chicago, Illinois, United States of America, **2** Department of Radiation Oncology, University of Illinois Hospital and Health Sciences System, Chicago, Illinois, United States of America

Abstract

Objective: Radiotherapy techniques have evolved from 3D conformal radiotherapy (3D-CRT) to intensity modulated radiotherapy (IMRT) where boost fields are delivered either sequentially (IMRTseq) or with a simultaneous integrated boost (IMRT+SIB). Our goal was to compare the outcomes of patients treated with IMRT+SIB to traditional standards.

Methods: We analyzed the efficacy and toxicity of patients treated with concurrent chemoradiation using 3D-CRT, IMRTseq or IMRT+SIB. Between 1993 and 2012, 379 patients with non-metastatic Stage III-IV head and neck squamous cell cancer were treated with concurrent chemoradiation using 3D-CRT (n = 125), IMRTseq (n = 120) and IMRT+SIB (n = 134).

Results: Patients treated with any technique had similar rates of 2y local control, 2y regional control, 2y progression free survival and 2y overall survival. Patients treated with IMRT+SIB had lower rates acute toxicity according to Grade 3 or greater mucositis (3D-CRT: 44.0% vs. IMRTseq: 36.7% vs. IMRT+SIB: 22.4%; $P<.0001$), dermatitis (3D-CRT: 44.0% vs. IMRTseq: 20.0% vs. IMRT+SIB: 7.5%; $P<.0001$) and feeding tube placement during radiotherapy (3D-CRT: 80.0% vs. IMRTseq: 50.8% vs. IMRT+SIB: 44.0%; $P<.0001$) as well as late toxicity as measured by feeding tube use ($P<.0001$) and tracheostomy use ($P<.0001$). On multivariate analysis, IMRT+SIB predicted for less mucositis, dermatitis and feeding tube use compared to 3D-CRT and for less dermatitis compared to IMRTseq.

Conclusions: Compared to 3D-CRT and IMRTseq, IMRT+SIB provided similar outcomes and potentially less toxicity indicating it is a feasible technique for chemoradiation in locally advanced head and neck cancer.

Editor: Kevin Camphausen, NIH, United States of America

Funding: M.T.S. was supported by a grant from the Burroughs Wellcome Career Award for Medical Scientists and the Fanconi Anemia Research Fund. The funders had no role in study design, data collection and analysis, decision to publish, or preparation of the manuscript.

Competing Interests: The authors have declared that no competing interests exist.

* E-mail: mspiotto@radonc.uchicago.edu

Introduction

Over the last 20 years, the delivery of radiotherapy to different cancer sites has changed dramatically, especially for squamous cell carcinomas of the Head and Neck (HNSCCs) region [1–4]. HNSCC patients were classically treated with three dimensional conformal radiotherapy (3D-CRT) where increasing radiation doses were delivered to higher risk areas of disease using sequential radiotherapy plans to treat smaller boost fields, which was also known as a "shrinking-field approach". Patients often experienced severe acute and late toxicities including mucositis, dermatitis and xerostomia. As intensity modulated radiotherapy (IMRT) was implemented, the improved high-dose conformality reduced the dose to normal tissues and offered the potential to minimize radiation toxicity while maintaining similar rates of control [2,4–6]. Still, IMRT plans often relied on this sequential treatment design (IMRTseq). Consequently, using IMRTseq and 3D-CRT plans, each risk area received the same dose per fraction that usually did not exceed 2 Gy in order to minimize acute toxicity.

By contrast, IMRT treatment planning enables the simultaneous delivery of individualized dose levels to distinct at risk areas within a single treatment fraction [1,3]. The advantages to IMRT+SIB includes increased planning efficiency and decreased planning uncertainty as radiation dose can be accounted for in a single plan. In addition, IMRT+SIB, escalates the dose per fraction delivered to the gross disease in order to potentially improve tumor control. Several groups have reported their single and multi-institutional experience in using IMRT+SIB [7–12]. However, it remains unclear how IMRT+SIB compares to previous radiation planning techniques such as IMRTseq or 3D-CRT when treating advanced HNSCC patients with chemoradiation. First, the increased dose per fraction may unintentionally increase acute toxicity as has been described in other altered fractionation series [13,14]. When coupled with concurrent chemotherapy, the added toxicity may result in chemotherapy dose modifications that impact treatment efficacy [15]. By contrast, the decreased fractional dose delivered to lower risk nodal groups may also not be sufficient to control microscopic disease. Therefore, it remains unclear the extent to which the efficacy and toxicity IMRT+SIB compares to traditionally accepted radiotherapy planning techniques.

Our institution has employed all three techniques for the irradiation of locally advanced HNSCC. To this end, we compared the outcomes in patients treated with concurrent chemoradiation delivered using 3D-CRT, sequential IMRTseq or IMRT+SIB radiotherapy plans.

Patients and Methods

Study Population

We utilized a retrospective database of 803 patients with HNSCC to select 398 patients with Stage III-IVB disease treated with concurrent chemoradiation. 405 of 803 patients were not analyzed due to lower stage, non-concurrent chemotherapy usage or inadequate records. We excluded 19 patients who did not have adequate radiotherapy records and were excluded to give a total of 379 patients for analysis. Patients were treated at the University of Illinois Medical Center at Chicago between 1993 to 2012. This study was specifically approved by the University of Illinois Medical Center Institutional Review Board under protocol 2011-1075 in accordance with the ethical standards of the responsible committee on human experimentation and with the Helsinki Declaration of 1975, as revised in 2000. The University of Illinois at Chicago Institutional Review board waived informed consent given that this study used preexisting medical records and obtaining informed consent on all patients would be impractical given the associated time and cost.

Treatment

All patients were treated with concurrent chemotherapy consisting Platin-containing regimens or paclitaxel, hydroxyurea and 5-flurouracil. Platin-containing regimens consisted of cisplatin or carboplatin given weekly or every three weeks. Of the 379 patients analyzed, 198 patients received concurrent Platin of which 146 patients received cisplatin and 52 patients received carboplatin, 137 patients received paclitaxel, hydroxyurea and 5-flurouracil and 44 patients did not have detailed chemotherapy records. 125 patients received 3D conformal radiotherapy (3D-CRT), 134 patients received IMRT+SIB and 120 patients received IMRTseq. For IMRT planning, the clinical target volumes were typically expanded by 5 mm margins to generate the planning target volumes (PTV). PTVs were shaved at the skin and near critical organs when radiotherapy plans exceeded normal tissue tolerance. In 82% of the patients treated with IMRT+SIB, the fractionation schemes consisted of either: (1) 30 fractions delivering 6600 cGy to the GTV, 6000 to the intermediate risk nodal volumes and 5400 cGy to the low risk nodal volumes or (2) 33 fractions delivering 6996 cGy to the GTV, 5940 cGy to the intermediate risk nodal volumes and 5412 cGy to the low risk nodal volumes. Patients treated with IMRTseq or 3D-CRT were treated with daily fractionation in 200 cGy fractions or twice daily fractionation in 120–150 cGy fractions. Weekly megavoltage portal films were used for localization. No image guided radiotherapy was used in any patients in order to decreased planning margins. During radiotherapy, acute toxicities were recorded during weekly on-treatment visits.

Variables

We approximated comorbidity burden using a modified Charlson Comorbidity Index [16] and performance status using the Karnofsky Performance Status [17]. Staging was categorized using the American Joint Committee staging system at the time of diagnosis. Acute toxicity was scored using RTOG common toxicity criteria. We defined a truncated radiotherapy (RT) course as one shortened by more than 5 treatment fractions due to non-compliance. We defined RT delay as RT courses that were completed 5d or longer than the anticipated. We defined dose modifications during chemoradiation as reducing the drug dosage, switching from chemotherapy delivered every three weeks to weekly, delaying the intended chemotherapy cycle or holding chemotherapy during radiation. We divided the era of RT into three groups: (1) 1993–2000 when all patients were treated with 3D-CRT, (2) 2001–2006 when patients were predominantly treated with IMRTseq and (3) 2007–2012 when patients were predominantly treated with IMRT+SIB. Time to local control (LC), regional control (RC), progression free survival (PFS), and overall survival (OS) were determined from last date of RT. Patterns of local or regional failure were determined as the first failure with any component of local or regional failure, respectively. PFS was calculated as the time to any failure or death from any cause. OS was calculated as the time to death from any cause.

Statistical analysis

Statistical analysis was performed using JMP version 9 (SAS Institute). All tests to determine statistical significance were two-sided and statistical significance was defined as $P<.05$. Discrete variables were compared with chi-square test and continuous variables were compared with the t-test. Differences between medians were assessed using the Wilcoxon test. Survival curves were plotted based on the Kaplan-Meier method. For univariate analysis of toxicity, we selected factors that were significantly different between the 3D-CRT, IMRTseq and IMRT+SIB groups. Multivariate analysis of toxicity was performed using nominal logistic regression analysis to adjust for explanatory confounding prognostic variables with P value<.1 on univariate analysis.

Results

Population and Tumor Characteristics

As shown in Table 1, median follow-up did not differ significantly between groups (25.8 mo 3D-CRT for vs. 17.5 mo for IMRTseq vs. 16.3 mo for IMRT+SIB; $P=.14$). Compared to IMRTseq based techniques, patients treated with 3D-CRT were younger (54.6y for 3D-CRT vs. 58.4y for IMRTseq vs. 59.1y for IMRT+SIB; $P=.003$) and had more alcohol use (70.4% for 3D-CRT vs. 54.2% for IMRTseq vs. 56.7% for IMRT+SIB; $P=.03$). Patients treated with 3D-CRT or IMRT+SIB had a greater smoking history compared to patients treated with IMRTseq (81.6% for 3D-CRT vs. 69.2% for IMRTseq vs. 79.9% for IMRT+SIB; $P=.02$). The three groups did not differ significantly based on gender, performance status, comorbidities, stage or primary site (Table1).

Treatment Characteristics

As shown in Table 2, more patients treated with IMRTseq received induction chemotherapy compared to patients treated with 3D-CRT or IMRT+SIB (32.8% for 3D-CRT vs. 50.8% for IMRTseq vs. 34.2% for IMRT+SIB; $P=.006$). Compared to 3D-CRT, patients treated with either IMRT technique received more platin-based concurrent chemoradiation ($P<.0001$) as well as

Table 1. Patient and Tumor Characteristics (n = 379).

Category	Indicator	3D-CRT[1] (n = 125)	IMRTseq[2] (n = 120)	IMRT+SIB[3] (n = 134)	*P value*
Median age (years)		54.6	58.4	59.1	.003
	(IQR[4])	(45.8–60.6)	(50.0–63.5)	(50.8–65.7)	
Median follow-up (months)		25.8	17.5	16.3	.14
	(IQR)	(6.4–68.6)	(7.4–47.1)	(8.0–39.1)	
Gender	Male	90 (72.0%)	91 (75.8%)	103 (76.9%)	.64
	Female	35 (28.0%)	29 (24.2%)	31 (23.1%)	
KPS[5]	<70	8 (6.4%)	6 (5.0%)	12 (9.0%)	.78
	≥70	102 (81.6%)	101 (84.2%)	106 (79.1%)	
	Not reported	15 (11.3%)	13 (10.8%)	16 (11.9%)	
Comorbidity	Medium	93 (77.4%)	78 (65.0%)	87 (64.9%)	.17
	High	32 (25.6%)	43 (35.0%)	47 (35.1%)	
T stage	Tx	3 (2.4%)	3 (2.5%)	6 (4.5%)	.29
	T1	4 (3.2%)	9 (7.5%)	8 (6.0%)	
	T2	14 (11.2%)	22 (18.3%)	23 (17.2%)	
	T3	34 (27.2%)	32 (26.7%)	41 (30.6%)	
	T4	14 (11.2%)	7 (5.8%)	5 (3.7%)	
	T4a	52 (41.6%)	44 (36.7%)	46 (34.3%)	
	T4b	4 (3.2%)	3 (2.5%)	5 (3.7%)	
N stage	N0	27 (21.6%)	27 (22.5%)	28 (20.9%)	.36
	N1	17 (13.6%)	13 (10.8%)	20 (14.9%)	
	N2	3 (2.4%)	5 (4.2%)	3 (2.2%)	
	N2a	1 (0.8%)	8 (6.7%)	7 (5.2%)	
	N2b	27 (21.6%)	24 (20.0%)	34 (25.4%)	
	N2c	28 (22.4%)	30 (25.0%)	26 (19.4%)	
	N3	22 (17.6%)	12 (10.0%)	15 (11.2%)	
	N.R.	1 (1.9%)	1 (0.8%)	1 (0.7%)	
Stage	III	19 (15.2%)	21 (17.5%)	32 (23.9%)	.12
	IVA	79 (63.2%)	84 (70.0%)	85 (63.4%)	
	IVB	27 (21.6%)	15 (12.5%)	17 (12.7%)	
Primary site	Hypopharynx	17 (14.3%)	7 (5.9%)	8 (6.1%)	.10
	Larynx	18 (15.1%)	24 (20.3%)	26 (19.7%)	
	Nasopharynx	9 (7.7%)	6 (5.1%)	6 (4.6%)	
	Oral cavity	32 (26.9%)	28 (23.7%)	39 (29.6%)	
	Oropharynx	35 (29.4%)	46 (39.0%)	43 (32.6%)	
	Unknown	3 (2.5%)	2 (1.7%)	6 (4.6%)	
	Other	11 (9.2%)	7 (5.9%)	6 (4.6%)	
Alcohol history	≥2 drinks/day	88 (70.4%)	65 (54.2%)	76 (56.7%)	.03
	<2 drinks/day	19 (15.2%)	27 (22.5%)	37 (27.6%)	
	Not reported	18 (14.4%)	28 (23.3%)	21 (15.7%)	
Tobacco history	Yes	102 (81.6%)	83 (69.2%)	107 (79.9%)	.02
	No	18 (14.4%)	32 (26.7%)	20 (14.9%)	
	Not reported	5 (4.2%)	5 (4.2%)	7 (5.2%)	

[1]3D-CRT = Three dimensional conformal radiotherapy.
[2]IMRTseq = Sequential intensity modulated radiotherapy.
[3]IMRT+SIB = Intensity modulated radiotherapy with simultaneous integrated boost.
[4]IQR = interquartile ratio.
[5]KPS = Karnofsky.

experienced more modifications in concurrent chemotherapy. Patients treated with 3D-CRT received higher total radiation doses delivered to the gross tumor (7400 cGy for 3D-CRT vs. 7125cGy for IMRTseq vs. 6600 cGy for IMRT+SIB; $P<.0001$) but received lower total radiation dose to the intermediate and low risk nodal groups. Treatment technique varied according to the

Table 2. Treatment Characteristics (n = 379).

Category	Indicator	3D-CRT[1] (n = 125)	IMRTseq[2] (n = 120)	IMRT+SIB[3] (n = 134)	*P value*
Induction chemotherapy	Yes	41 (32.8%)	61 (50.8%)	46 (34.2%)	.006
	No	84 (67.2%)	59 (49.2%)	88 (65.7%)	
Post-operative RT[4]	Yes	23 (18.4%)	30 (25.0%)	37 (27.6%)	.20
	No	102 (81.6%)	90 (75.0%)	97 (72.4%)	
Post-RT lymphadenectomy	Yes	27 (26.5%)	28 (31.1%)	20 (20.6%)	.26
	No	75 (73.5%)	62 (68.9%)	77 (79.4%)	
CTX[5] dose modification	Yes	33 (26.4%)	52 (43.3%)	75 (56.0%)	<.0001
	No	92 (73.6%)	68 (56.7%)	59 (44.0%)	
Platin-based chemoradiation	Yes	31 (24.8%)	63 (52.5%)	104 (77.6%)	<.0001
	No	94 (75.2%)	57 (47.5%)	30 (22.4%)	
Median dose to gross tumor (cGy)		7400	7125	6600	<.0001
	IQR[6]	(7015–7450)	(6650–7250)	(6600–6996)	
Median dose to intermediate risk lymph nodes (cGy)		5200	5100	5940	<.0001
	IQR	(5045–5450)	(5000–5400)	(5940–6000)	
Median dose to low risk lymph nodes (cGy)		3950	5000	5400	<.0001
	IQR	(3900–5000)	(3650–5000)	(5400–5412)	
Alterations in RT course	No	70 (56.0%)	76 (63.3%)	66 (49.3%)	.06
	Delayed	36 (28.8%)	35 (29.2%)	43 (32.1%)	
	Truncated	19 (15.2%)	9 (7.5%)	25 (18.7%)	
Era of RT	1993–2000	90 (100.0%)	0 (0.0%)	0 (0.0%)	.06
	2001–2006	32 (22.4%)	84 (58.7%)	27 (18.9%)	
	2007–2012	3 (2.4%)	36 (24.7%)	107 (73.3%)	

[1]3D-CRT = Three dimensional conformal radiotherapy.
[2]IMRTseq = Sequential intensity modulated radiotherapy.
[3]IMRT+SIB = Intensity modulated radiotherapy with simultaneous integrated boost.
[4]RT = radiotherapy.
[5]CTX = chemotherapy.
[6]IQR = interquartile ratio.

era of RT as patients treated before 2000 received 3D-CRT and the majority of patients treated after 2000 received IMRTseq or IMRT+SIB ($P<.0001$). Patients did not differ based on rates of post-operative RT or post-RT lymph node dissection.

Outcomes

Compared to 3D-CRT, patients treated with IMRT+SIB had similar LC (HR 1.18; 95% CI 0.72–1.93; $P=.51$), RC (HR 1.41; 95% CI 0.77–2.60; $P=.26$), PFS (HR 1.21; 95% CI 0.87–1.70; $P=.26$) and OS (HR 1.19; 95% CI 0.79–1.79; $P=.41$). Similarly, compared to IMRTseq, patients treated with IMRT+SIB had similar LC (HR 1.15; 95% CI 0.70–1.89; $P=.59$), RC (HR 1.70; 95% CI 0.90–3.31; $P=.10$), PFS (HR 1.26; 95% CI 0.89–1.79; $P=.20$) and OS (HR 1.28; 95% CI 0.84–1.98; $P=.26$). As shown in Figure 1, 3D-CRT, IMRTseq and IMRT+SIB has similar rates of 2y LC ($P=.78$), 2y RC ($P=.24$), 2y PFS ($P=.37$) and 2y OS ($P=.50$).

Toxicity

As shown in Table 3, patients treated with IMRT+SIB had lower rates of Grade ≥3 mucositis, Grade ≥3 dermatitis, feeding tube placement during RT as well as long term use of feeding tubes or tracheostomies ($P<.0001$). On univariate analysis, IMRT+SIB was associated with less mucositis compared to 3D-CRT (HR 0.29; 95% CI 0.16–0.50; $P<.0001$) or IMRTseq (HR 0.40; 95% CI 0.23–0.71; $P=.002$) as well as less dermatitis compared to 3D-CRT (HR 0.08; 95% CI 0.04–0.17; $P<.0001$) or IMRTseq (HR 0.28; 95% CI 0.12–0.60; $P=.001$). Compared to 3D-CRT, IMRT+SIB was associated with less feeding tube during RT (HR 0.26; 95% CI 0.14–0.45; $P<.0001$), long term feeding tube use (HR 0.24; 95% CI 0.14–0.41; $P<.0001$) and long term tracheostomy use (HR 0.26; 95% CI 0.14–0.47; $P<.0001$). By contrast, there was no difference between IMRTseq and IMRT+SIB for feeding tube placement during RT, long term feeding tube use or long term tracheostomy.

On multivariate analysis (Table 4), Grade ≥3 mucositis was inversely associated with IMRT+SIB treatments (HR 0.15; 95% CI 0.04–0.51; $P=.002$), IMRTseq treatments (HR 0.29; 95% CI 0.09–0.87; $P=.03$) and laryngeal primaries (HR 0.33; 95% CI 0.14–0.78; $P=.01$). Grade ≥3 dermatitis was inversely associated with IMRT+SIB (HR 0.11; 95% CI 0.02–0.49; $P=.004$) and Platin-based chemoradiation (HR 0.10; 95% CI 0.03–0.27; $P<.0001$) and was directly associated with hypopharyngeal primaries (HR 4.08; 95% CI 1.20–15.10; $P=.02$). Less short term and long term feeding tube use was associated with IMRTseq as well as IMRT+SIB. Long term tracheostomy use was not significantly associated with any radiotherapy technique. When only patients treated with either IMRT-based planning were analyzed, IMRT+SIB remained predictive for less Grade ≥3 dermatitis (HR 0.23; 95% CI 0.06–0.50; $P=.02$).

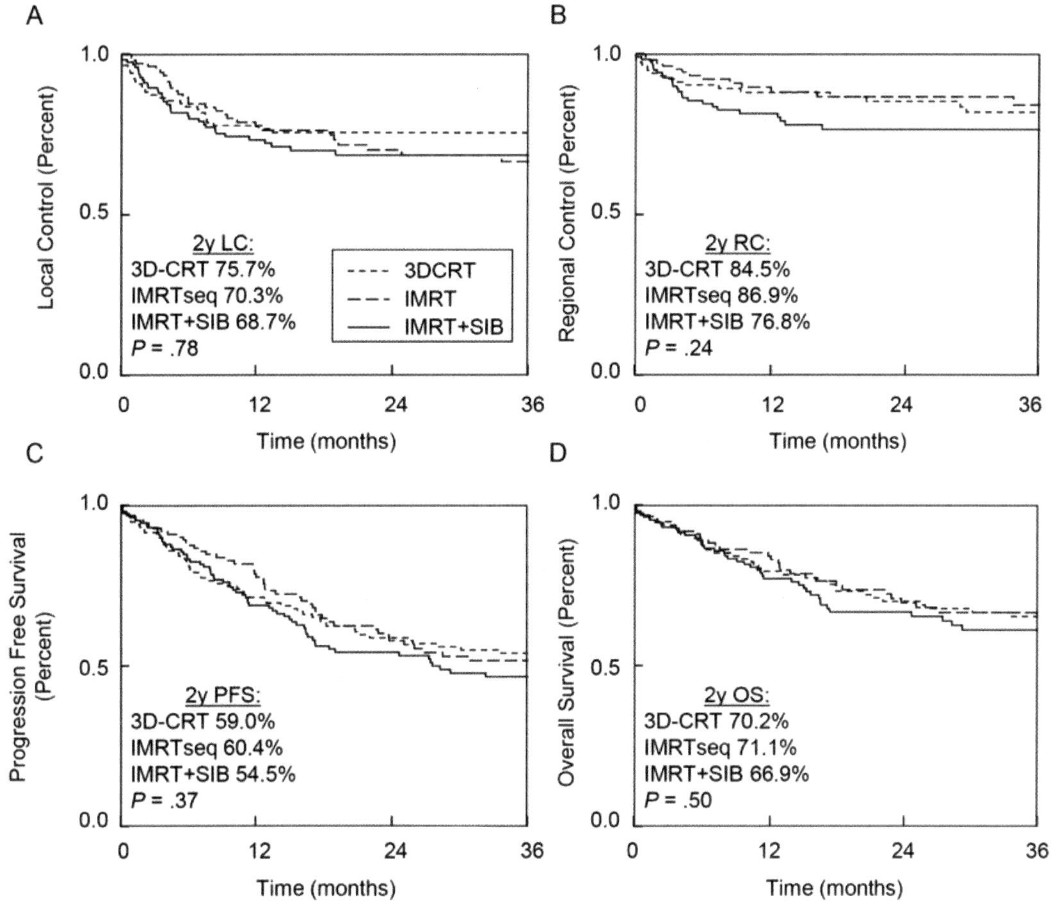

Figure 1. Kaplan-Meier analysis of outcomes in patients treated with 3D-CRT, IMRTseq and IMRT+SIB. (**a**) Local control (**b**) regional control (**c**) progression free survival and (**d**) overall survival for Stage III-IV HNSCC patients treated with chemoradiation using 3D-CRT, IMRTseq and IMRT+SIB. The log rank test was used to assess for differences in outcomes.

Table 3. Toxicity (n = 379).

Category	Indicator	3D-CRT[1] (n = 125)	IMRTseq[2] (n = 120)	IMRT+SIB[3] (n = 134)	*P value*
Feeding tube during RT[4]	Yes	100 (80.0%)	61 (50.8%)	59 (44.0%)	<.0001
	No	25 (20.0%)	59 (49.2%)	75 (56.0%)	
Greater than 10% weight loss during RT	Yes	48 (38.4%)	64 (53.3%)	70 (52.2%)	.10
	No	38 (30.4%)	26 (21.7%)	43 (32.1%)	
	N.S. stated	39 (31.2%)	30 (25.0%)	30 (22.4%)	
Grade ≥3 mucositis	Yes	55 (44.0%)	44 (36.7%)	30 (22.4%)	<.0001
	No	48 (38.4%)	54 (45.0%)	91 (67.9%)	
	N.S. stated	22 (17.6%)	22 (18.3%)	13 (9.7%)	
Grade ≥3 dermatitis	Yes	55 (44.0%)	24 (20.0%)	10 (7.5%)	<.0001
	No	51 (40.8%)	74 (61.7%)	111 (82.8%)	
	N.S. stated	19 (15.2%)	22 (18.3%)	13 (9.7%)	
Feeding tube at failure	Yes	83 (66.4%)	39 (32.5%)	40 (29.9%)	<.0001
	No	42 (33.6%)	81 (67.5%)	94 (70.2%)	
Tracheostomy at failure	Yes	54 (43.2%)	20 (16.7%)	17 (12.7%)	<.0001
	No	71 (56.8%)	100 (83.3%)	117 (87.3%)	

[1]3D-CRT = Three dimensional conformal radiotherapy.
[2]IMRTseq = Sequential intensity modulated radiotherapy.
[3]IMRT+SIB = Intensity modulated radiotherapy with simultaneous integrated boost.
[4]RT = radiotherapy.

Table 4. Multivariate analysis of toxicity (n = 379).

		Odds Ratio				
Timing of toxicity:		**Acute toxicity**			**Late toxicity**	
Category	**Statistic**	**≥ Grade 3 mucositis**	**≥ Grade 3 dermatitis**	**Feeding tube during RT[1]**	**Feeding tube**	**Trach**
IMRTseq[2] (vs. 3D-CRT[3])		0.29	0.47	0.20	0.15	0.66
	(95% CI[4])	(0.09–0.87)	(0.14–1.52)	(0.06–0.60)	(0.04–0.42)	(0.20–2.23)
	P value	.03	.21	.003	.0002	.50
IMR+SIB[5] (vs. 3D-CRT)		0.15	0.11	0.18	0.17	0.78
	(95% CI[4])	(0.04–0.51)	(0.02–0.49)	(0.05–0.58)	(0.05–0.54)	(0.19–3.25)
	P value	.002	.004	.003	.002	.73
Platin-based regimen		0.72	0.10	1.28	0.74	0.47
	(95% CI[4])	(0.36–1.44)	(0.03–0.27)	(0.68–2.46)	(0.40–1.36)	(0.21–1.05)
	P value	.35	<.0001	.45	.33	.07
Primary (OC[6] referant)	Nasopharynx	0.74	2.36	0.33	0.54	2.20×10^{-7}
	(95% CI)	(0.12–3.98)	(0.18–24.68)	(0.06–1.76)	(0.09–2.80)	(0–1.44)
	P value	.73	.50	.19	.47	.09
	Oropharynx	0.77	1.18	1.17	1.33	1.74
	(95% CI)	(0.37–1.62)	(0.46–3.02)	(0.57–2.42)	(0.67–2.67)	(0.72–4.43)
	P value	.49	.73	.66	.42	.22
	Larynx	0.33	1.32	0.57	1.05	8.40
	(95% CI)	(0.14–0.78)	(0.48–3.72)	(0.25–1.27)	(0.48–2.31)	(3.21–23.75)
	P value	.01	.61	.17	.90	<.0001
	Hypopharynx	0.46	4.08	1.26	1.47	7.84
	(95% CI)	(0.16–1.29)	(1.20–15.10)	(0.45–3.75)	(0.57–3.90)	(2.55–25.91)
	P value	.14	.02	.66	.42	.0003
	Unknown	0.30	6.40	0.56	0.37	0.96
	(95% CI)	(0.04–1.58)	(0.92–39.19)	(0.11–2.77)	(0.05–1.96)	(0.04–8.47)
	P value	.16	.06	.48	.25	.97
	Other	0.32	0.25	0.35	0.80	0.47
	(95% CI)	(0.08–1.06)	(0.03–1.36)	(0.10–1.12)	(0.24–2.57)	(0.06–2.41)
	P value	.06	.11	.08	.71	.38
≥2 drinks per day		0.55	1.04	1.71	1.18	1.56
	(95% CI)	(0.28–1.08)	(0.43–2.53)	(0.92–3.17)	(0.64–2.20)	(0.69–3.67)
	P value	.08	.93	.09	.60	.29
>10 pack-years		0.90	1.79	1.29	2.14	0.82
	(95% CI)	(0.37–2.21)	(0.53–6.57)	(0.55–3.04)	(0.89–5.46)	(0.25–2.99)
	P value	.81	.35	.56	.09	.75
Induction CTX[7]		1.53	1.43	1.25	1.23	0.62
	(95% CI)	(0.83–2.83)	(0.66–3.09)	(0.70–2.26)	(0.70–2.16)	(0.30–1.25)
	P value	.18	.36	.45	.48	.18
CTX dose modification		0.74	0.70	0.90	0.76	0.83
	(95% CI)	(0.40–1.39)	(0.30–1.58)	(0.51–1.60)	(0.43–1.33)	(0.40–1.71)
	P value	.35	.39	.73	.33	.62
Altered RT course	Delayed	1.19	0.48	1.23	1.10	1.59
	(95% CI)	(0.61–2.31)	(0.20–1.15)	(0.66–2.30)	(0.61–2.00)	(0.76–3.36)
	P value	.62	.10	.52	0.75	0.22
	Truncated	0.75	0.48	0.54	0.61	0.36
	(95% CI)	(0.31–1.77)	(0.15–1.36)	(0.24–1.20)	(0.27–1.33)	(0.11–1.03)
	P value	.52	.17	.13	.22	.06
Era of RT	2001–2006	2.68	0.96	0.88	2.96	0.41

Table 4. Cont.

		Odds Ratio				
Timing of toxicity:		**Acute toxicity**			**Late toxicity**	
Category	**Statistic**	**≥ Grade 3 mucositis**	**≥ Grade 3 dermatitis**	**Feeding tube during RT[1]**	**Feeding tube**	**Trach**
(vs. 1993–2000)	(95% CI)	(0.87–9.15)	(0.29–3.17)	(0.26–3.27)	(0.99–9.97)	(0.12–1.31)
	P value	.09	.94	.84	0.05	0.13
	2007–2012	2.77	0.34	0.52	1.52	0.10
	(95% CI)	(0.71–11.82)	(0.42–13.11)	(0.13–2.29)	(0.42–6.02)	(0.02–0.48)
	P value	.14	.34	.38	.53	.003

[1]RT = radiotherapy
[2]IMRTseq = Sequential intensity modulated radiotherapy.
[3]3D-CRT = Three dimensional conformal radiotherapy.
[4]CI = Confidence Interval.
[5]IMRT+SIB = Intensity modulated radiotherapy with simultaneous integrated boost.
[6]OC = Oral Cavity.
[7]CTX = Chemotherapy.

Discussion

In our experience, IMRT+SIB provided outcomes similar to the traditional radiotherapy techniques for head and neck cancer. Here, two similar SIB schemes were used to treat 82% of patients indicating that our observations extend to commonly used IMRT+SIB plans. Compared to 3D-CRT and IMRTseq, we report similar disease control and potentially less toxicity in patients treated with IMRT+SIB. These outcomes with IMRT+SIB occurred despite the higher total doses delivered to the gross tumor in patients treated with either IMRTseq or 3D-CRT. In addition, compared to 3D-CRT, IMRT+SIB had lower rates of Grade 3 or greater mucositis and dermatitis as well as less feeding tube use during radiotherapy as well as long term feeding tube use even when the elective nodal areas received lower fractional radiation doses with 3D-CRT. By contrast, IMRTseq-based treatments were associated with lower rates of mucositis mucositis compared to 3D-CRT and higher rates of dermatitis when compared to IMRT+SIB. Therefore, our results suggest that IMRT+SIB may be as effective as other treatment strategies for locally advanced HNSCC.

In our series, we did not observe any differences in local or regional control for IMRT+SIB. These locoregional control rates are similar to other series examining IMRT+SIB where locoregional control ranged from 74–88% [8–11,18]. It is important to note that many of these reports with improved locoregional control that analyzed patients with oropharynx cancers that may be due to HPV-positive disease. Since 2009 when we implemented HPV testing, only 7.8% of the 103 cancers tested were positive for HPV as measured by p16 immunohistochemistry. Therefore, even without a significant proportion of HPV-positive cancers, our outcomes were similar to the outcomes reported for series examining IMRT+SIB, IMRTseq or 3D-CRT. Furthermore, the outcomes for IMRT+SIB, IMRTseq or 3D-CRT were not dependent on the timeframe of radiotherapy as the locoregional control in patients treated between 1993-2000 was similar to patients treated between 2001to 2006 (HR 0.80; 95% CI 0.49–1.28; $P = .35$) and was similar to patients treated between 2007 to 2012 (HR 0.75; 95% CI 0.46–1.20; $P = .23$). Interestingly, we observed that increased dose per fraction using an IMRT+SIB regimen did not improve outcomes with locoregional control. Our data suggest that a slightly increased fraction size and shorter treatment time did not translate into clinically apparent differences between treatment outcomes. These results also parallel those of RTOG 0129 where altered fractionation was not superior to conventional radiotherapy when concomitant chemotherapy was given [19]. Therefore, the benefit of IMRT+SIB may occur with decreasing potential toxicity and efficiency in treatment planning.

In our series, IMRT+SIB lessened acute dermatitis compared to IMRTseq and lessened mucositis, dermatitis and feeding tube use compared to 3D-CRT. These differences in toxicity remained significant for 3D-CRT even when accounting for differences in primary sites, concurrent chemotherapy regimens and distinct timeframes of radiotherapy as well as other factors known to increase toxicity. Our rates of Grade 3 or greater mucositis parallels the 15% to 37.8% mucositis rates observed in other series reporting outcomes with IMRT+SIB [18,20–22]. While IMRT+SIB may deliver higher doses per fraction to mucosal tumors that potentiate mucositis, lower fractional doses to other uninvolved mucosal sites may also minimize this toxicity. In addition, lower fractional doses to at risk nodal areas may also reduce the chances of dermatitis given the proximity of these regions to the skin. Finally, increasing the conformality of high dose regions may also minimize the long term dysphagia and tracheal toxicities as measured by long term feeding tubes and tracheostomy use. Therefore, despite the areas receiving higher fractional doses, IMRT+SIB may minimize both acute and late toxicities compared to IMRTseq and 3D-CRT.

While we observed less acute toxicity as measured by mucositis and dermatitis, we did observe increased higher rates of concurrent chemotherapy dose modifications for patients treated with IMRT+SIB. However, when accounting for other confounding factors such as concurrent-chemoradiation regimens, total doses to the gross tumor and induction chemotherapy use, IMRT+SIB was not associated with increased chemotherapy dose modifications compared to IMRTseq alone (HR 1.49; 95% CI: 0.89–2.51; P = .13). Therefore, IMRT+SIB did not likely impact chemotherapy dose modifications, radiotherapy treatment delays or truncations in the course of radiotherapy.

Our observations are limited due to the retrospective nature of this study. First, we reported on patients possessing heterogeneous clinical and treatment characteristics that may impact our observations of decreased toxicity in the IMRT+SIB cohort. Still, our observations of decreased toxicity with IMRT+SIB remained significant even when these factors were accounted for on multivariate analysis. Furthermore, we observed less acute toxicity with IMRT+SIB despite this group having the most use of concurrent chemotherapy that usually doubles the rates of acute toxicity. Second, our patients were treated with heterogeneous dosing regimens where patients treated with IMRT+SIB generally received lower total doses to the gross tumor and higher total doses to the intermediate and low risk nodal levels. Nevertheless, these dosing strategies are, in part, linked to the treatment technique indicating that doses delivered by an IMRT+SIB technique provided, at worst, similar disease control and toxicity. Given that our treatment deliveries were verified using standard megavoltage portal imaging, our PTV margins remained similar for each treatment technique. Therefore, our observations were not impacted by image guidance techniques that enabled smaller margins. In addition, our patients were treated from 1993 to 2012 during which many changes in the treatment of HNSCC patients occurred. Nevertheless, our conclusions regarding less toxicities with IMRT+SIB hold even when accounting for these distinct eras of treatment on multivariate analysis. Finally, our data likely extrapolates to patients with HPV-positive cancers in terms of efficacy as well as toxicity as only a fraction of our patients tested positive for HPV by p16 IHC. Therefore, when accounting for confounding factors, we observed that IMRT+SIB likely predicted for similar, if not better, outcomes compared to traditional treatment strategies.

Comparing to traditional treatment techniques such as 3D-CRT and IMRTseq, we find that IMRT+SIB was an acceptable alternative as assessed by disease control and toxicity. This technique enables more efficient treatment planning with less uncertainty as well as potentially shorter treatment times. Furthermore, IMRT+SIB may afford even less acute and late toxicity potentially through less fractional doses to the elective nodes. These differences in toxicity await validation in future randomized control trials.

In conclusion, we find that IMRT+SIB provided similar outcomes in terms of disease control and toxicity compared to 3D-CRT and IMRTseq. IMRT+SIB delivered lower fractional doses to the elective nodes and higher fractional doses to the gross disease. Furthermore, it is likely that these results extend to both HPV-positive and HPV-negative patients. These results support the use of IMRT+SIB as an acceptable technique to treat patients in order to more efficiently plan radiotherapy while maintaining similar outcomes as in previous techniques.

Acknowledgments

M.T.S. had full access to all of the data in the study and takes responsibility for the integrity of the data and the accuracy of the data analysis.

Author Contributions

Conceived and designed the experiments: MTS. Performed the experiments: MTS. Analyzed the data: MTS. Contributed reagents/materials/ analysis tools: MTS RRW. Wrote the paper: MTS RRW.

References

1. Mohan R, Wu Q, Manning M, Schmidt-Ullrich R (2000) Radiobiological considerations in the design of fractionation strategies for intensity-modulated radiation therapy of head and neck cancers. Int J Radiat Oncol Biol Phys 46: 619–630.
2. Cozzi L, Fogliata A, Bolsi A, Nicolini G, Bernier J (2004) Three-dimensional conformal vs. intensity-modulated radiotherapy in head-and-neck cancer patients: comparative analysis of dosimetric and technical parameters. Int J Radiat Oncol Biol Phys 58: 617–624.
3. Orlandi E, Palazzi M, Pignoli E, Fallai C, Giostra A, et al. (2010) Radiobiological basis and clinical results of the simultaneous integrated boost (SIB) in intensity modulated radiotherapy (IMRT) for head and neck cancer: A review. Crit Rev Oncol Hematol 73: 111–125.
4. Palazzi M, Orlandi E, Pignoli E, Lualdi M, Zonca G, et al. (2006) Target coverage in head and neck cancer treated with intensity-modulated radiotherapy: a comparison between conventional and conformal techniques. Tumori 92: 503–510.
5. Xia P, Fu KK, Wong GW, Akazawa C, Verhey LJ (2000) Comparison of treatment plans involving intensity-modulated radiotherapy for nasopharyngeal carcinoma. Int J Radiat Oncol Biol Phys 48: 329–337.
6. Nutting CM, Morden JP, Harrington KJ, Urbano TG, Bhide SA, et al. (2011) Parotid-sparing intensity modulated versus conventional radiotherapy in head and neck cancer (PARSPORT): a phase 3 multicentre randomised controlled trial. Lancet Oncol 12: 127–136.
7. Franceschini D, Paiar F, Meattini I, Agresti B, Pasquetti EM, et al. (2013) Simultaneous integrated boost-intensity-modulated radiotherapy in head and neck cancer. Laryngoscope 123: E97–103.
8. Lauve A, Morris M, Schmidt-Ullrich R, Wu Q, Mohan R, et al. (2004) Simultaneous integrated boost intensity-modulated radiotherapy for locally advanced head-and-neck squamous cell carcinomas: II—clinical results. Int J Radiat Oncol Biol Phys 60: 374–387.
9. Leclerc M, Maingon P, Hamoir M, Dalban C, Calais G, et al. (2013) A dose escalation study with intensity modulated radiation therapy (IMRT) in T2N0, T2N1, T3N0 squamous cell carcinomas (SCC) of the oropharynx, larynx and hypopharynx using a simultaneous integrated boost (SIB) approach. Radiother Oncol 106: 333–340.
10. Montejo ME, Shrieve DC, Bentz BG, Hunt JP, Buchman LO, et al. (2011) IMRT with simultaneous integrated boost and concurrent chemotherapy for locoregionally advanced squamous cell carcinoma of the head and neck. Int J Radiat Oncol Biol Phys 81: e845–852.
11. Schwartz M, Vuong T, Ballivy O, Parker W, Patrocinio H (2007) Accelerated radiotherapy with simultaneous integrated boost fractionation and intensity-modulated radiotherapy for advanced head and neck cancer. Otolaryngol Head Neck Surg 136: 549–555.
12. Eisbruch A, Harris J, Garden AS, Chao CK, Straube W, et al. (2010) Multi-institutional trial of accelerated hypofractionated intensity-modulated radiation therapy for early-stage oropharyngeal cancer (RTOG 00-22). Int J Radiat Oncol Biol Phys 76: 1333–1338.
13. Overgaard J, Hansen HS, Specht L, Overgaard M, Grau C, et al. (2003) Five compared with six fractions per week of conventional radiotherapy of squamous-cell carcinoma of head and neck: DAHANCA 6 and 7 randomised controlled trial. Lancet 362: 933–940.
14. Fu KK, Pajak TF, Trotti A, Jones CU, Spencer SA, et al. (2000) A Radiation Therapy Oncology Group (RTOG) phase III randomized study to compare hyperfractionation and two variants of accelerated fractionation to standard fractionation radiotherapy for head and neck squamous cell carcinomas: first report of RTOG 9003. Int J Radiat Oncol Biol Phys 48: 7–16.
15. Brizel DM, Albers ME, Fisher SR, Scher RL, Richtsmeier WJ, et al. (1998) Hyperfractionated irradiation with or without concurrent chemotherapy for locally advanced head and neck cancer. N Engl J Med 338: 1798–1804.
16. Charlson ME, Pompei P, Ales KL, MacKenzie CR (1987) A new method of classifying prognostic comorbidity in longitudinal studies: development and validation. J Chronic Dis 40: 373–383.
17. Karnofsky DA, Burchenal J (1949) The Clinical Evaluation of Chemotherapeutic Agents in Cancer; CM M, editor: Columbia Univ Press.
18. Studer G, Huguenin PU, Davis JB, Kunz G, Lutolf UM, et al. (2006) IMRT using simultaneously integrated boost (SIB) in head and neck cancer patients. Radiat Oncol 1: 7.
19. Ang K, Pajak T, Wheeler R, Rosenthal D, Nguyen-Tan F, et al. (2010) A Phase III Trial to Test Accelerated Versus Standard Fractionation in Combination with Concurrent Cisplatin for Head and Neck Carcinomas (RTOG 0129): Report of Efficacy and Toxicity. International Journal of Radiation Oncology Biology Physics 77: 1–2.
20. Lee NY, O'Meara W, Chan K, Della-Bianca C, Mechalakos JG, et al. (2007) Concurrent chemotherapy and intensity-modulated radiotherapy for locoregionally advanced laryngeal and hypopharyngeal cancers. Int J Radiat Oncol Biol Phys 69: 459–468.
21. Lee SW, Back GM, Yi BY, Choi EK, Ahn SD, et al. (2006) Preliminary results of a phase I/II study of simultaneous modulated accelerated radiotherapy for nondisseminated nasopharyngeal carcinoma. Int J Radiat Oncol Biol Phys 65: 152–160.
22. Chao KS, Ozyigit G, Tran BN, Cengiz M, Dempsey JF, et al. (2003) Patterns of failure in patients receiving definitive and postoperative IMRT for head-and-neck cancer. Int J Radiat Oncol Biol Phys 55: 312–321.

Treatment Outcome of Radiotherapy Alone versus Radiochemotherapy in IE/IIE Extranodal Nasal-Type Natural Killer/T Cell Lymphoma: A Meta-Analysis

Tianxia Deng¶, Cheng Zhang¶, Xi Zhang, Sha Wu, Yaqi Xu, Shanshan Liu, Xinghua Chen*

Department of Hematology, Xinqiao Hospital, Third Military Medical University, Chongqing, China

Abstract

Background: Previous studies have revealed conflicting findings concerning the efficacy of radiotherapy (RT) and radiochemotherapy (RCT) in IE/IIE extranodal nasal-type natural killer/T cell lymphoma (ENKTL). In this study, we conducted a comprehensive meta-analysis to address this issue.

Methods: We systematically searched PubMed, Cochrane Central Register of Controlled Trials (CENTRAL), EmBase, BISOS, Clinical Trials and some Chinese databases for relevant studies, and 2 prospective and 15 retrospective studies involving a total of 1595 patients met our inclusion criteria.

Results: The meta-analysis showed no significant differences in complete remission (CR) [odds ratio (OR) 0.85, 95% confidence interval (CI) 0.42–1.72, p = 0.65], 5-year overall survival (OS) [hazard ratio (HR) 1.11, 95% CI 0.85–1.45, p = 0.43] and 5-year progression free survival (PFS) (HR 1.07, 95% CI 0.75–1.53, p = 0.70) in patients who received RT versus RCT. Furthermore, the addition of CT decreased neither systemic failure (SL) (OR 0.75, 95% CI 0.47–1.21, p = 0.24) nor locoregional failure (LF) (OR 1.17, 95% CI 0.68–2.01, p = 0. 57).

Conclusions: RCT did not have an obvious advantage over RT for treating IE/IIE ENKTL.

Editor: Robert K. Hills, Cardiff University, United Kingdom

Funding: This study was funded by grants from the National Natural Science Foundation (No. 81170467), the Key Discipline of Medical Science of Chongqing and the special foundation for the "1130 Project" of Xinqiao Hospital of Third Military Medical University. The funders had no role in study design, data collection and analysis, decision to publish, or preparation of the manuscript.

Competing Interests: The authors have declared that no competing interests exist.

* Email: xhchen888@aliyun.com

¶ TXD and CZ are co-first authors on this work.

Introduction

Extranodal nasal-type natural killer/T cell lymphoma (ENKTL), which is also referred to as lethal midline granuloma, polymorphic malignant reticulosis, or angiocentric immunoproliferative lesions, accounts for a small fraction of non-Hodgkin lymphomas [1,2]. It has a peculiar geographic distribution: the disease is more prevalent in Asia than it is in Western countries [3–5]. It is usually associated with the Epstein-Barr virus (EBV) [6–8] and often leads to destruction in the upper aero-digestive tract, particularly in the nasal cavity and paranasal areas [9,10]. Additionally, tumors occur in various areas, including the skin, testis, prostate gland and orbit [11–14].

The optimal treatment regimen for IE/IIE ENKTL has not been completely determined. The efficacy of transplantation for IE/IIE ENKTL is still being investigated [9]. Although only a limited number of studies have been conducted, patients with a poor prognosis or advanced disease (stage III/IV) are considered the best candidates for autologous hematopoietic stem cell transplantation (HSCT) or unrelated cord blood transplantation (CBT) [15–18]. Therefore, for early stage (IE/IIE) ENKTL, the most suitable treatment options might be radiotherapy (RT), chemotherapy (CT) or combined therapy. Some studies have demonstrated that this tumor is highly sensitive to RT, suggesting that RT alone is a sufficient treatment regimen [19,20]. However, other studies have suggested that RT alone has a high relapse rate, and the combination of RT and CT has been explored [21,22]. Nevertheless, the efficacy of the additional CT was recently questioned. Numerous studies have revealed no significant differences in the treatment outcomes between RT and radiochemotherapy (RCT) for IE/IIE ENKTL [23–25]. Moreover, G.E. Kim et al. indicated that medical complications (such as sepsis or intractable bleeding) are more severe in patients who received RCT [24].

Although a similar study has been previously published, we used a stricter inclusion criteria and a larger sample size with a total of 1595 patients in our study [26]. Moreover, the subgroup analysis of different types of CT, countries and study designs was performed. The focus of our meta-analysis, which examined parameters including complete remission (CR), 5-year overall survival (OS), 5-year progression free survival (PFS), systemic failure (SF) and locoregional failure (LF), was to compare the effectiveness of RT with that of RCT in IE/IIE ENKTL patients.

Materials and Methods

Search strategy

A literature search of PubMed, Cochrane Central Register of Controlled Trials (CENTRAL), EmBase, BISOS, Clinical Trials, Chinese Biological Medical literature (CBM), Chinese National Knowledge Infrastructure (CNKI) and Chinese science and technology periodical database (VIP) with the keywords ((NK/T cell lymphoma) OR (natural killer/T cell lymphoma)) AND (radiotherapy OR chemotherapy OR treatment OR outcome) was performed. The languages of the published papers were limited to English and Chinese, and only studies conducted before October 2013 were included. To include additional studies, the reference lists from the included studies were also screened. Two independent investigators conducted this search. Figure 1 depicts a flow diagram of the selection procedure.

Inclusion Criteria

The relevant studies were carefully selected based on the following criteria: (1) patients who were confirmed as Ann Arbor stage IE or IIE ENKTL; (2) the disease was not diagnosed as a second primary carcinoma; (3) randomized controlled trials (RCT) were selected as a priori choice; otherwise, other interventional studies were included; (4) the outcomes of RT, RCT and CT were compared; (5) the article measured at least one of the following clinical indicators: CR, 5-year OS, 5-year PFS, SF or LF; (6) the latest paper was preferred if there were affiliated studies; and (7) the paper scored at least 6 based on the Newcastle-Ottawa Quality Assessment Scale (NOS) for retrospective cohort studies and at least 3 based on Jadad scale for RCTs.

Efficacy indicators

CR was defined as the complete disappearance of all detectable clinical and radiographic evidence of disease. OS was defined as the period of time from the date of treatment to the date of death or the date of the last follow-up visit. PFS was calculated from the end date of the initial treatment to the date of the first local or distance relapse or to the date of the last follow-up or death. Any active evidence of clinical, laboratory or radiologic data in extranasal lesions was considered SF. LF was defined as persistence of the primary tumor. The indicators of CR, SF, and LF were measured by odds ratio (OR) and hazard ratio (HR) for OS and PFS.

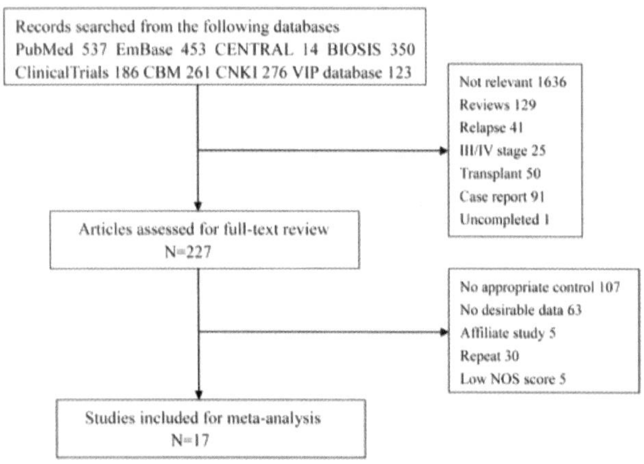

Figure 1. Flow chart of the identification process.

Data extraction

Two independent reviewers extracted the data. Discrepancies were resolved by group discussion. The primary information extracted from the studies included the first author, study design, Eastern Cooperative Oncology Group (ECOG) score and etc. The data from each paper were scrutinized. Table 1 summarizes the primary reported outcomes. Data related to the clinical outcomes, such as CR, OS, PFS, SF and LF, were also extracted.

Statistical analysis

ORs and HRs with 95% confidence intervals (CIs) were used to assess the treatment outcomes. ORs were computed for dichotomous variables by applying the Mantel-Haenszel method. HRs and the 95% CIs were computed using the Engauge Digitizer software and the method of Jayne F Tierney [27]. Statistical heterogeneity in the study was estimated by the χ^2 test and I^2 statistic. Values were considered to display statistically significant heterogeneity when the χ^2 P-value was <0.1 or the I^2 statistic was $> 50\%$. The fixed-effects model was adopted if there was no sign of heterogeneity. Otherwise, the random-effects model was applied. Meta regression was used to locate the source of potential heterogeneity. Then, we applied the subgroup analysis to determine the potential effect on the treatment outcomes. Two-side P values less than 0.05 were considered statistically significant. To examine the publication bias, Egger text was used. All calculations were performed using STATA (version 11.0).

Results

Study selection results

Figure 1 shows the identification process of eligible studies. We retrieved 2,236 potential papers from the electronic databases. Of the initial collection of articles, 2,009 articles were excluded based on the title or abstract. After reading the complete text of the remaining studies, 17 articles met our inclusion criteria [23–25,28–41]. The studies were primarily excluded because the common therapeutic measures were CT, RT or RCT alone. Some studies met the comparison criteria but had no available data. An additional 5 papers were excluded because they were affiliated studies. In addition, 30 duplicate reports and 5 papers with low NOS scores were eliminated.

Characteristics of the final studies

17 studies were finally included. Of these, two were prospective, one was multicenter retrospective, and the remainder was retrospective. All retrospective cohort papers had an NOS score of at least 6 points (Table 2) and all prospective papers had a Jadad scale score of at least 3 points. A total of 1595 patients were enrolled and were classified as Ann Arbor stage IE or IIE ENKTL. The median age of the patients in each study varied from 40 to 53 years. Some clinical manifestations, such as B systems were also recorded. However, regrettably, some papers that included stage IIIE or IVE ENKTL lacked basic information. Based on the different extracted data, we included 3 papers by YX Li et al. that had different publication years [32,33,41]. The basic characteristics of the 17 studies are summarized in Table 1. The details of the CT regimen and combined therapy are listed in Table 3, and the RT information is shown in Table 4.

Table 1. Basic characteristics of the 17 studies used in our meta-analysis.

Studies	Study design	Country	No. of patients (CT/RT/RCT)	Sex (male)	Median age	Stage (IE/IIE)	ECOG score (≤1/≥2)	B symptoms	High LDH	Primary site
HH Ma [23]	retrospective	China	0/23/41	36	44	51/13	62/2	34	9	44 patients: nasal cavity, paranasal sinus
GE Kim [24]	retrospective	Korea	0/104/39	68	46	70/34	NR	18	NR	nasal cavity/paranasal sinuses, larynx/hypopharynx, Waldeyer's ring, oral cavity/soft palate
K Kim [25]	retrospective	Korea	0/33/20	37	45	42/11	44/9	11	NR	nasal cavity, paranasal sinuses, nasopharynx, oropharynx, hypopharynx, oral cavity
A. Avile s [28]	prospective	Mexico	116/109/202	201	NR	247/179	NR	3	40	nasal cavity, nasopharynx, paranasal sinuses, tonsils, hypopharynx, hard palate
SY Li [29]	retrospective	America	2/7/30	NR	NR	NR	NR	NR	NR	NR
JL Luo [30]	retrospective	China	2/30/98	91	NR	116/14	129/1	33	NR	NR
A Chauchet [31]	multicenter retrospective	France	8/0/8	NR	NR	10/6	NR	NR	NR	NR
YX Li [32]	retrospective	China	0/96/118	141	42	182/32	198/16	67	73	nasal cavity
YX Li [33]	retrospective	China	4/13/54	NR	NR	15/56	NR	NR	NR	nasopharynx, tonsil
MJ Huang [34]	retrospective	China	8/9/65	57	45	52/30	66/16	43	31	nasal cavity, paranasal sinuses, other parts of the upper aerodigestive tract, other sites outside nasal cavity of the upper aerodigestive tract
SJ Kim [35]	retrospective	Korea	26/0/17	30	40	24/19	37/6	NR	12	nasal cavity, nasopharynx, tonsil, oropharynx, hypopharynx, palate
K Isobe [36]	prospective	Japan	0/17/18	21	51	32/3	NR	7	7	nasal cavity, paranasal sinuses, pharynx
IWK Tham [37]	retrospective	Singapore	0/5/13	NR	NR	13/5	NR	NR	NR	nasal, Waldeyer's ring, both
CC Li [38]	retrospective	Taiwan	18/11/27	42	45	NR	NR	NR	NR	nasal area, paranasal sinuses, nasopharynx, oropharynx, pharynx, tonsils
MM Cheung [39]	retrospective	Hong Kong	0/18/61	58	53	63/16	72/7	22	20	nasal cavity, nasopharynx
V Ribrag [40]	retrospective	France	12/6/2	14	44	16/4	NR	NR	NR	nasal cavity, oropharynx, palate
YX Li [41]	retrospective	China	3/31/71	69	42	83/22	87/18	37	53	left, right, bilateral nasal cavity

CT: chemotherapy; RT: radiotherapy; RCT: radiochemotherapy; ECOG: Eastern Cooperative Oncology group; LDH: lactic dehydrogenase; NR: not reported; No.: number.

Table 2. Quality assessment of retrospective cohort studies by NOS.

Studies	Representativeness of the exposed cohort	Selection of the non-exposed cohort	Ascertainment of exposure	Outcome of interest was not present at start of study	Comparability of cohorts on the basis of the design or analysis	Assessment of outcome	Was follow-up long enough for outcomes to occur	Adequacy of follow up of cohorts	Total quality scores
HH Ma [23]	1	1	1	1	2	1	1	1	9
GE Kim [24]	1	1	1	1	2	1	1	1	9
K Kim [25]	1	1	1	1	0	1	1	1	7
SY Li [29]	1	1	1	1	0	1	1	1	7
JL Luo [30]	1	1	1	1	0	1	1	0	6
A Chauchet [31]	1	1	1	1	0	1	1	0	6
YX Li [32]	1	0	1	1	0	1	1	1	6
YX Li [33]	1	0	1	1	0	1	1	1	6
MJ Huang [34]	1	1	1	1	0	1	1	1	7
SJ Kim [35]	1	0	1	1	0	1	1	1	6
IWK Tham [37]	1	1	1	1	0	1	1	1	7
CC Li [38]	1	1	1	1	0	1	1	1	7
MM Cheung [39]	1	1	1	1	0	1	1	1	7
V Ribrag [40]	1	1	1	1	0	1	1	0	6
YX Li [41]	1	1	1	1	0	1	1	1	7

Table 3. Information about CT and RCT regimens.

Studies	CT regimens	RCT therapy
HH Ma [23]	CHOP, CHOP-bleo, MCOP, COPB	24 patients: RT followed by 4–6 cycles CT; 17 patients: CT followed by RT with or without CT
GE Kim [24]	CHOP, BACOP, m- BACOP	CT followed by RT
K Kim [25]	CHOP, COPBLAM-V	18 patients: 4–6 cycles CT followed by RT; 1 patients: RT followed by CT; 1 patients: concurrent RCT
A. Avile s [28]	CEMD, ESHAP	RT followed by 6 cycles CT
SY Li [29]	CHOP	NR
JL Luo [30]	CHOP, CHOPE, DICE	73 patients: CT followed by RT; 16 patients: CT +RT(at the same time); 9 patients: RT followed by CT
A Chauchet [31]	ACVBP, CHOP, COPADM, CYVE, ESHAP, DHAP, high-dose methotrexate plus L-ASP	CT followed by RT
YX Li [32]	CHOP, CHOP-like, CEVB, DIMG	RT+4 cycles CT
YX Li [33]	CHOP, CHOP-bleo, COBVP-16, COPP	18 patients: RT followed by CT; 36 patients: CT followed by RT;
MJ Huang [34]	CHOP, ECDVP, IME	22 patients: upfront RT + CT; 43 patients: early RT plus RT+CT
SJ Kim [35]	CEOP-B	6 cycles CT followed by RT
K Isobe [36]	anthracycline-containing combination or not	NR
IWK Tham [37]	ESHAP with or without cisplatin, CHOP-M	RT firstly or after CT
CC Li [38]	CHOP, ESHAP with or without ProMACE-CytaBOM, CHOP with BDCVP, CHOP with ProMACE-CytaBOM plus combined MVP, CVPP	RT+3 cycles CT
MM Cheung [39]	ProMACE-CytaBOM, CEOP, CHOP	3–6 cycles CT followed by RT
V Ribrag [40]	CHOP, CHOP-like, COP, COP-like	CT as first-line therapy or after RT
YX Li [41]	CHOP, CHOP-bleo, COBVP-16, COPP	34 patients: RT followed by CT; 37 patients: CT followed by RT

CEMD cyclophosphamide, methotrexate, etoposide, dexamethasone; ESHAP etoposide, solumedrol, high doses of cytosine arabinoside, platinum; CHOP cyclophosphamide, doxorubicin, vincristine, prednisone; CHOPE CHOP+ etoposide; DICE dexamethasone, ifosfamide, cisplatin, etoposide; ACVBP doxorubicin, cyclophosphamide, vincristine, bleomycin, prednisone; COPADM cyclophosphamide, vincristine, prednisone, doxorubicin, methotrexate; CYVE cyclophosphamide, cytosine arabinoside, etoposide; DHAP etoposide, methylprednisolone, cytosine arabinoside, cisplatin, dexamethasone; CEVB cyclophosphamide, etoposide, vincristine, bleomycin; DIMG dexamethasone, ifosfamide, methotrexate, gemcitabine; CHOP-bleo CHOP+ bleomycin; MCOP mitoxantrone, cyclophosphamide, vincristine, prednisone; COPB cyclophosphamide, vincristine, prednisone, bleomycin; ECDVP etoposide, cyclophosphamide, doxorubicin, vincristine, prednisone; IME ifosfamide, methotrexate, etoposide; CEOP-B cyclophosphamide, epirubicin, vincristine, bleomycin, prednisone;COBVP-16 cisplatin, vincristine, bleomycin, prednisone; COPP cyclophosphamide, vincristine, procarbazine, prednisone; COPBLAM-V cyclophosphamide, vincristine, prednisone, bleomycin, procarbazine, adriamycin; CHOP-M cyclophosphamide, adriamycin, vincristine, prednisone, methotrexate; ProMACE-CytaBOM prednisone, doxorubicin, cyclophosphamide, etoposide, cytarabine, bleomycin, vincristine, methotrexate; BDCVP bleomycin, doxorubicin, cyclophosphamide, vincristine, prednisone; MVP mitoxantrone, vincristine, prednisone; CVPP cyclophosphamide, vincristine, procarbazine, prednisone; CEOP cyclophosphamide, epirubicin, vincristine, prednisone; BACOP bleomycin, doxorubicin, cyclophosphamide, vincristine, prednisone; m- BACOP methotrexate and folinic acid rescue, bleomycin, doxorubicin, cyclophosphamide, doxorubicin, vincristine, prednisone; RT: radiotherapy; CT: chemotherapy; RCT: radiochemotherapy; NR: not reported.

Table 4. Information about RT.

Studies	Source or Technique	Dose	Clinical target volume
HH Ma [23]	^{60}Co-ϒrays, 6-MV X-rays of linear accelerator	median: 54 Gy; per fraction: 1.8–2.0 Gy	bilateral nasal cavities, paranasal sinus
GE Kim [24]	^{60}Co-ϒrays, 4-MV X-rays	total: 20–70 Gy; per fraction: 1.8–2.0 Gy	the involved areas with adequate margins
K Kim [25]	^{60}Co-ϒrays,4/6-MV photo beams; three-field technique or bilateral parallel-opposed fields	median:50 Gy; per fraction: 1.8/2.0 Gy	all gross lesions and sites of potential contiguous spread with adequate margins
A. Avile s [28]	a photo beam of 6.0; IMRT, 3DCRT	a total dose of 55 Gy in 25 fractions ver 5 weeks	limited cases: bilateral nasal cavity, nasopharynx, frontal ethmoid sinus, ipsilateral maxillary; extended cases: paranasal sinus, other adjacent organ structures
SY Li [29]	NR	NR	NR
JL Luo [30]	6-MV X-rays linear accelerator; IMRT, 3DCRT	≥50 Gy: 117 patients; <50 Gy: 11 patients; per fraction: 1.8–2.0 Gy	both nasal cavity, maxillary sinus, ethmoid sinus
A Chauchet [31]	a linear accelerator with 4/6/10-MV photos	median: 40 Gy	all macroscopic lesions, paranasal sinus, nasopharynx, upper gum and palate with adequate margins
YX Li[32]	NR	primary tumor: 50 to 56 Gy; residual disease: 5 to 10 Gy; per fraction: 1.8–2.0 Gy	nasal cavity, ipsilateral maxillary sinus, bilateral ethmoid sinus, anatomically adjacent regions
YX Li[33]	6 MV linear accelerator	median: 50 Gy; per fraction: 2.0 Gy	Waldeyer ring, adjacent organs or structures with disease extension
MJ Huang [34]	^{60}Co-ϒrays, 6-MV photo beams	median: 50 Gy; per fraction: 2.0 Gy	all involved area and sites of potential contiguous spread with adequate margins
SJ Kim [35]	NR	total: 44–60 Gy; per fraction: 1.8–2.0 Gy	involved-field
K Isobe [36]	^{60}Co unit, 4/6/10-MV linear accelerator	median: 50 Gy	all macroscopic lesions, paranasal sinus, nasopharynx, upper gum and palate with adequate margins
IWK Tham [37]	6-MV linear accelerator	median: 50 Gy; per fraction: 1.8–2.0 Gy	gross tumor volume using diagnostic CT scans of the head and neck with a margin of 1.5–2.0 cm
CC Li [38]	6-MV linear accelerator	total: 40–50 Gy; per fraction: 1.8–2.0 Gy	involved primary area with adequate margins
MM Cheung [39]	3 fields with 2 lateral opposing photo fields and an anterior photo or electron field	median: 50 Gy; per fraction:1.5– 2.5 Gy	both nasal cavity and nasopharynx, paranasal sinus, and 1 to 2 cm beyond tumor defined by imaging scans
V Ribrag [40]	NR	total: 35–70 Gy	the initial involved areas
YX Li[41]	6/8-MV linear accelerator	median: 50 Gy; per fraction: 2.0 Gy	Stage I: nasal cavity, ipsilateral maxillary/ethmoid sinus; Stage II: extend to encompass involved paranasal tissues

RT: radiotherapy; IMRT intensity-modulated radiotherapy; 3DCRT three-dimensional conformal radiotherapy; MV megavolt; NR: not reported.

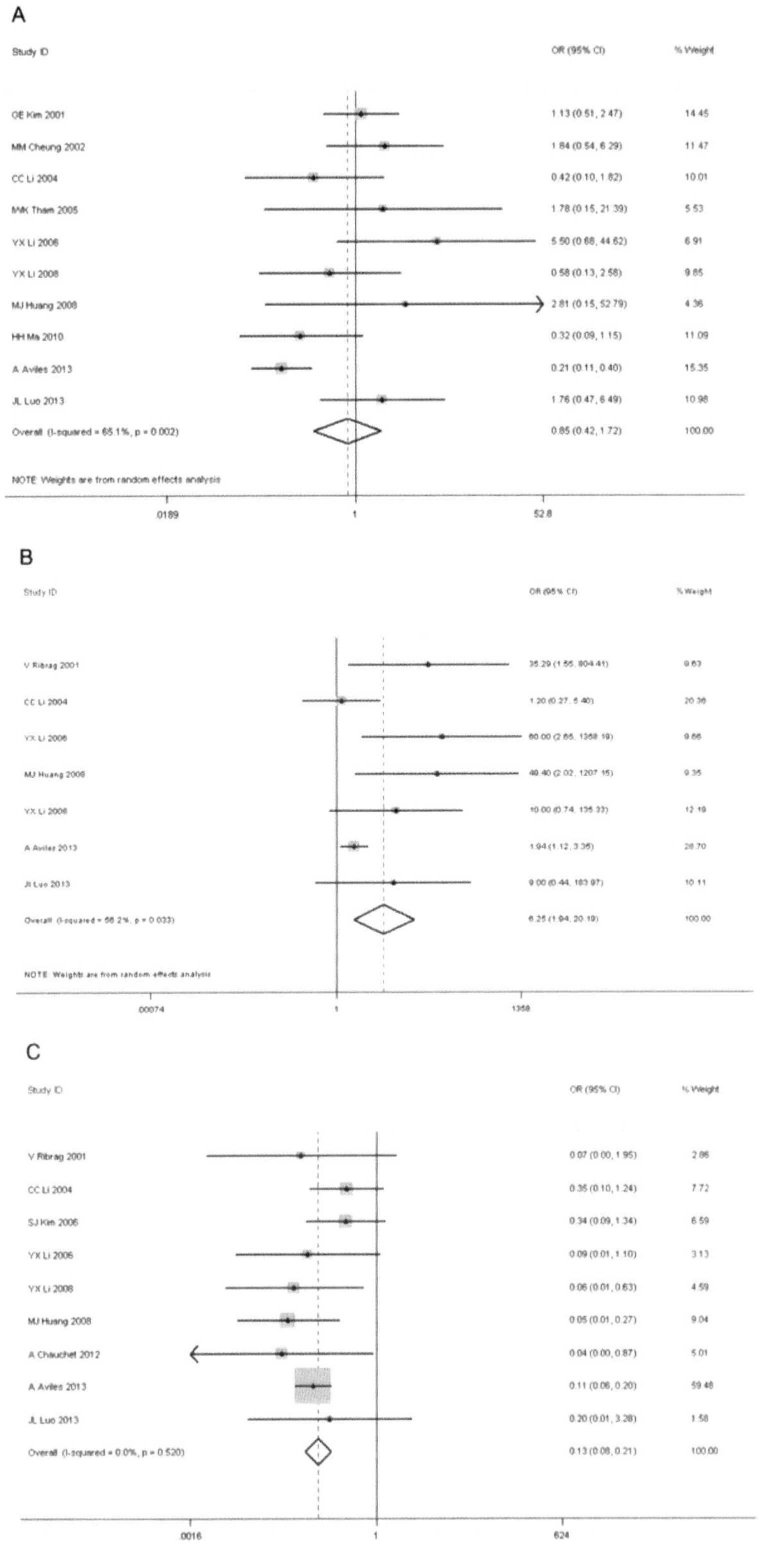

Figure 2. Forest plot of complete remission. A: radiotherapy versus radiochemotherapy; B: radiotherapy versus chemotherapy; C: chemotherapy versus radiochemotherapy.

Response to treatment

CR was used to reflect the tumor's response to treatment for comparisons among RCT, RT and CT. There was no significant difference in CR between RCT and RT (OR 0.85, 95% CI 0.42–1.72, p = 0.65, Figure 2A). A higher pooled CR was found in patients who received RT or RCT compared with that of CT (OR

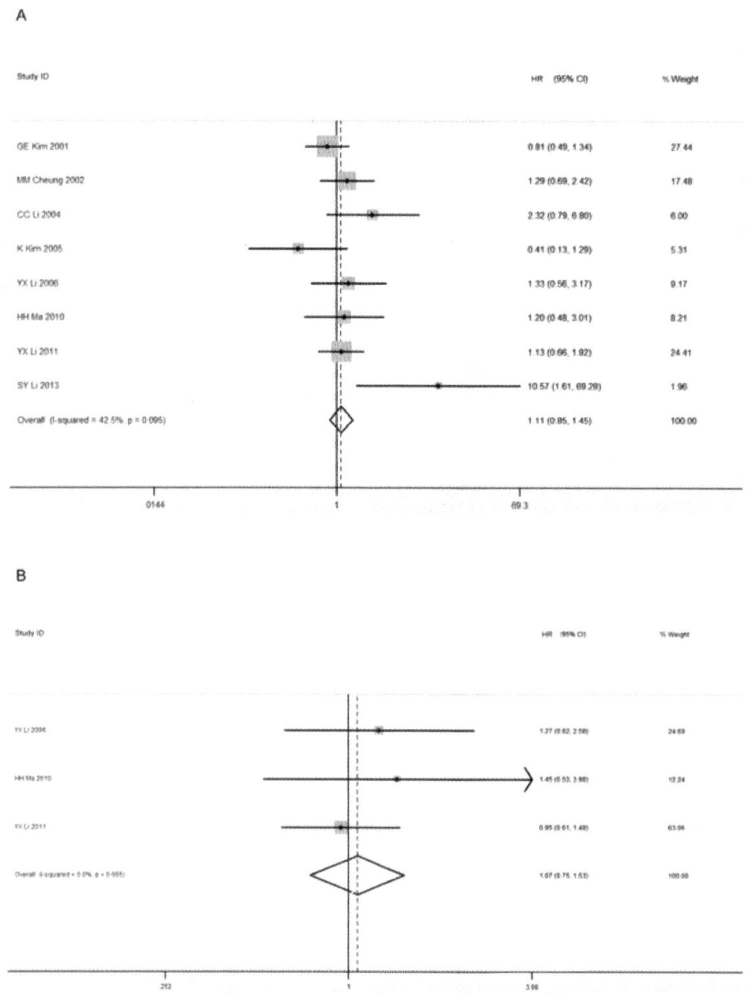

Figure 3. Forest plot of tumor's survival for radiotherapy versus radiochemotherapy. A: 5-year overall survival; B: 5-year progression free survival.

6.25, 95% CI 1.94–20.19, p = 0.002, Figure 2B; OR 0.13, 95% CI 0.08–0.21, p = 0.00, Figure 2C).

Survival

The 5-year OS was reported by 8 studies, in which 323 patients received RT alone and 407 patients received RCT. The addition of CT had no benefit, with a calculated HR value of 1.11 (95% CI 0.85–1.45, p = 0.43, Figure 3A). Only 3 papers were analyzed for 5-year PFS in our meta-analysis, with 150 patients in the RT group and 230 patients in the RCT group. A forest plot revealed that the treatment outcome of the RCT group failed to show any therapeutic advantage over the RT group (HR 1.07, 95% CI 0.75–1.53, p = 0.70, Figure 3B).

Treatment failure

As shown in Figure 4A, no significant difference was observed (OR 0.75, 95% CI 0.47–1.21, p = 0.24) in SF and LF (OR 1.17, 95% CI 0.68–2.01, p = 0.57, Figure 4B).

Meta regression and subgroup analysis

We performed meta regression of different CT plans, countries and study designs for CR and 5-year OS. As shown in Table 5, in the group of CR for RT versus RCT, we noticed that people from Asia or not and different study designs contributed to the heterogeneity. Then, the subgroup analysis was performed. Except for the non-Asian and prospective subgroups, CR and 5-year OS showed no significant differences between RT and RCT. Nevertheless, RT showed a significant improvement in CR compared with CT, except for the non-Asian and non-China subgroups. However, in the CR for CT versus RCT group, all of the subgroups revealed that the efficacy of RCT was better than that of CT. Additionally, for the non-Asian subgroup, RCT produced a significant CR and 5-year OS benefit compared with RT or CT, and RT failed to show any advantage over CT in CR (Table 5).

Toxicity and RT dose

Because toxicity and RT dose were usually reported differently, we cannot determine a pooled estimate. Grade III/IV toxicity was

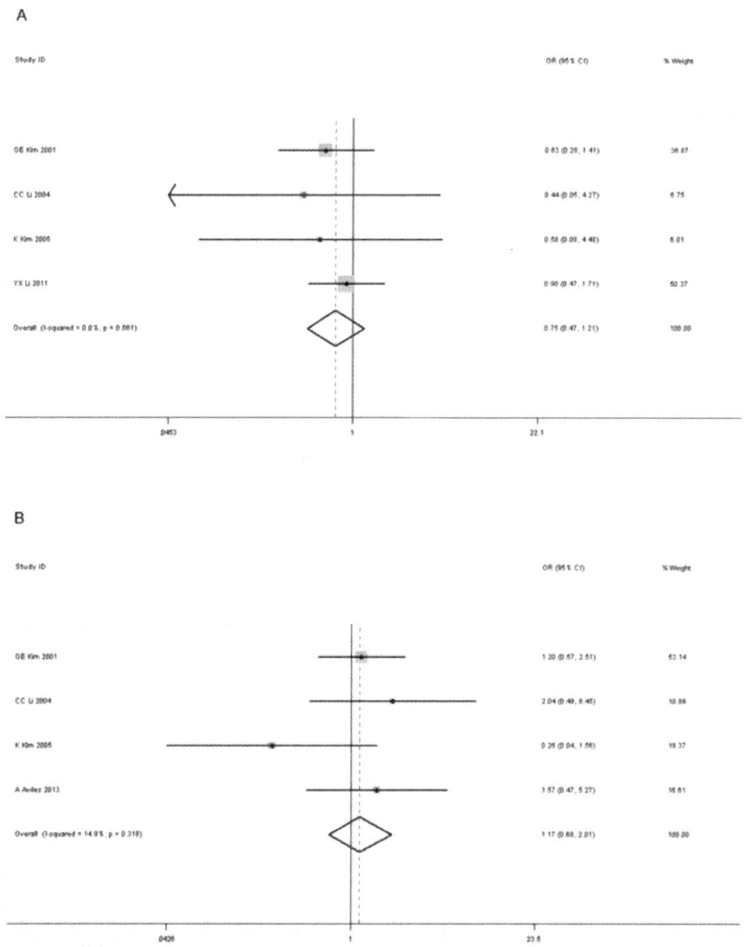

Figure 4. Forest plot of treatment failure for radiotherapy versus radiochemotherapy. A: systemic failure; B: locoregional failure.

more frequent in the CT and RCT groups (Table 6). Controversial viewpoints regarding the appropriate RT dose were observed, as shown in Table 7.

Heterogeneity and publication bias

In the present study, heterogeneity existed in some comparisons. To explore the potential factors, we applied meta regression and subgroup analysis. Then the heterogeneity was decreased in most of these subgroups. Egger text was constructed to assess the publication bias of these studies. There was no evidence of publication bias in OS ($p = 0.19$), PFS ($p = 0.14$), SF ($p = 0.26$) and LF ($p = 0.64$). In the indicator of CR, a potential publication bias was observed in the RT versus CT group ($p = 0.02$), but not in the RT versus RCT group ($p = 0.08$) or the CT versus RCT group ($p = 0.73$).

Discussion

Our results revealed that the clinical outcomes were similar between the RT and RCT groups, as indicated by CR, 5-year OS and 5-year PFS, although treatment of IE/IIE ENKTL with RT alone seemed to be insufficient from a clinical therapeutic standpoint. Patients who received CT alone exhibited lower CR than RT or RCT. Furthermore, RCT decreased the incidence of neither SF nor LF. Some investigations concluded that this lymphoma is sensitive to RT and resistant to CT because of the frequent expression of the multidrug resistance (MDR) genes and P-glycoprotein [23,25,42]. However, W Yong et al. maintained that the addition of CT to RT improved treatment outcomes, concluding that patients with nasal type NK/T cell lymphoma can be primarily treated with the CHOP regimen and local radiotherapy [43]. However, that study had some issues that deserve mention. First, the study did not include the corresponding control group of patients who were treated with RT alone. Second, the study follow-up time was only two years, but a longer observation time is necessary.

Our subgroup analysis suggested that patients from non-Asian and Asian countries usually had the opposite results. The reasons may be as follows: (1) A small number of studies were included in the non-Asian group. (2) The distribution of this disease, which is more commonly observed in Asia, is extraordinary. Thus, differences in the country of origin are the most important. (3) The design of these studies contributed to the differences. One of the non-Asian studies was prospective, while all of the Asian studies were retrospective. However, for the subgroups with different CT plans, the results did not change. Additionally, in the

Table 5. Subgroup analysis of CR and 5-year OS.

Indicators	Subgroup	Meta regression	OR/HR 95% CI	p value	Heterogeneity (I2, %)	p value for heterogeneity
CR for RT versus RCT	**CT regimen**	0.09				
	CHOP*		1.02 (0.57–1.82)	0.94	28.4	0.20
	non-CHOP		0.43 (0.06–3.10)	0.40	62.2	0.10
	Country A	0.02				
	Asia		1.04 (0.61–1.78)	0.87	19.7	0.27
	Non-Asia		0.21 (0.11–0.40)	0.000	-	-
	Country B	0.43				
	China		1.01 (0.48–2.14)	0.98	38.5	0.14
	Non-China		0.61 (0.15–2.54)	0.50	82.9	0.003
	Study design	0.02				
	retrospective		1.04 (0.61–1.78)	0.87	19.7	0.27
	prospective		0.21 (0.11–0.40)	0.000	-	-
CR for RT versus CT	**CT regimen**	0.30				
	CHOP*		10.73 (2.40–47.90)	0.002	48.0	0.09
	non-CHOP		1.94(1.12–3.35)	0.02	-	-
	Country A	0.67				
	Asia		9.03 (1.72–47.41)	0.009	51.7	0.08
	Non-Asia		5.44 (0.35–84.77)	0.27	69.4	0.07
	Country B	0.67				
	China		9.03 (1.72–47.41)	0.009	51.7	0.08
	Non-China		5.44 (0.35–84.77)	0.27	69.4	0.07
	Study design	0.30				
	retrospective		10.73 (2.40–47.90)	0.002	48.0	0.09
	prospective		1.94(1.12–3.35)	0.02	-	-
CR for CT versus RCT	**CT regimen**	0.87				
	CHOP*		0.15 (0.07–0.32)	0.000	0.0	0.50
	non-CHOP		0.13 (0.07–0.22)	0.000	28.3	0.25
	Country A	0.35				
	Asia		0.19 (0.09–0.38)	0.000	5.7	0.38
	Non-Asia		0.10 (0.06–0.19)	0.000	0.0	0.79
	Country B	0.98				
	China		0.15 (0.07–0.35)	0.000	5.0	0.38
	Non-China		0.12 (0.07–0.21)	0.000	0.0	0.41
	Study design	0.67				
	retrospective		0.16(0.08–0.32)	0.000	0.0	0.49
	prospective		0.11(0.06–0.20)	0.000	-	-
5-year OS for RT versus RCT	**CT regimen**	-				
	CHOP*		1.11(0.85–1.45)	0.428	42.5	0.095
	non-CHOP		-	-	-	-
	Country A	0.06				
	Asia		1.06(0.82–1.39)	0.65	8.6	0.36
	Non-Asia		10.57(1.61–69.28)	0.01	-	-
	Country B	0.29				
	China		1.29(0.93–1.79)	0.13	0.0	0.84
	Non-China		0.84(0.54–1.32)	0.45	76.5	0.01
	Study design	-				
	retrospective		1.11(0.85–1.45)	0.428	42.5	0.095
	prospective		-	-	-	-

CR: complete remission; OS: overall survival; CT: chemotherapy; RT: radiotherapy; RCT: radiochemotherapy; CHOP cyclophosphamide, doxorubicin, vincristine, prednisone; CHOP* CHOP, CHOP-like or non-CHOP.

Table 6. Treatment outcomes of grade III/IV toxicity.

Studies	Treatment	Total No.	No. of anemia	No. of granulocytopenia	No. of thrombocytopenia
A. Avile s [28]	CT	116	2	6	3
	RT	109	0	0	1
	RCT	202	2	9	5
JL Luo [30]	CT	2	0	1	0
	RT	30	0	1	0
	RCT	98	5	37	6

No.: number; CT: chemotherapy; RT: radiotherapy; RCT: radiochemotherapy.

subgroups of prospective studies on the CR for RT versus RCT and non-China in the CR for RT versus CT, the results were different compared with those obtained in other studies. The small number of studies may have influenced this observation.

We continued to compare treatment toxicity between the groups. The results revealed that RT alone had a better effect on reducing hematologic toxicity compared with that observed in the CT or RCT groups, and it might be the best treatment option. However, the results were weakened because we were unable to determine the pooled estimates. GE Kim et al. demonstrated that the additional CT may cause medical complications, such as sepsis or intractable bleeding [24]. Additionally, we compared the appropriate RT doses. JL Luo et al. suggested that more than 50 Gy was useful for increasing the rate of 5-year OS and disease free survival (DFS) [30]. MJ Huang et al. indicated that more than 54 Gy was suitable [34]. However, other studies demonstrated that there was no difference in the RT doses regarding 5-year local control probability (LCP), local failure and infield relapse [32,36,39].

Most previous studies on NK/T cell lymphoma were primarily clinical studies or general reviews. To the best of our knowledge, there is only one published meta-analysis of NK/T cell lymphoma [26]. For comparison, we added 3 papers [28,30,36], 2 of which were prospective studies, and we excluded 3 studies with low NOS scores. We employed a more detailed process of identifying studies (Figure 1). Due to the low morbidity of the disease, we had a relatively larger sample size than that used in previous study. Additionally, we applied subgroup analysis based on the CT plans, countries and study designs. Given the uncertainty of the benefit of the additional CT and the optimal mode of therapy, we compared the treatment outcomes of RT and RCT in 17 studies. We analyzed different indicators of treatment outcome to assess the tumor response, long-term survival and treatment failure.

The limitations of our study should be acknowledged. First, most of the included studies were retrospective, though we made every effort to search for relevant studies. Therefore, our analysis may not provide strong evidence for the treatment of IE/IIE ENKTL patients. Second, most of these studies were from Asia, particularly China; therefore, our analysis may only be applicable to people in Asia. Third, due to the lack of treatment guidelines, we did not restrict the RT pattern or CHOP* group, which included the CHOP, CHOP-like, or non-CHOP regimen, and this may weaken our results. Fourth, data on the toxicity and the dose of RT were rarely available in the included studies; as a result, pooled estimates were not determined. Fifth, the limitation of language could decrease the number of included studies. Finally, the heterogeneity and publication bias may strengthen our limitations. Therefore, the results of our meta-analysis should be carefully used in clinical treatment.

Conclusions

Compared with RT, RCT neither prolonged CR, 5-year OS or 5-year PFS nor decreased SF or LF in IE/IIE ENKTL Asian patients. However, our analysis of non-Asian patients was limited, and high quality studies are needed to identify the best therapy for IE/IIE ENKTL.

Table 7. Treatment outcomes for different doses of RT.

Studies	Dose/No.	Clinical indicators/No.	P value
JL Luo [29]	≥50 Gy/<50 Gy:117/11	5-year OS: 69/5	0.023
		5-year DFS: 68/5	0.027
YX Li [31]	≥50 Gy/<50 Gy:201/13	local failure: 15/2	0.592
MJ Huang [33]	≥54 Gy/<54 Gy:28/46	5-year OS: 21/21	0.019
		5-year DFS: 17/15	0.004
K Isobe [35]	≥50 Gy/<50 Gy:/9	5-year LCP: 18/5	0.13
MM Cheung [38]	≥50 Gy/<50 Gy:25/44	infield relapse: 3/12	0.4

No.: number; OS: overall survival; DFS: disease free survival; LCP: local control probability.

Author Contributions

Conceived and designed the experiments: TXD CZ XHC. Performed the experiments: TXD CZ. Analyzed the data: XZ YQX SW SSL. Contributed reagents/materials/analysis tools: XHC. Wrote the paper: TXD CZ.

References

1. Lee J, Cho SG, Chung SM, Ryu MR, Kim SH, et al. (2013) Retrospective analysis of treatment outcomes for extranodal NK/T-cell lymphoma (ENKL), nasal type, stage I-IIE: single institute experience of combined modality treatment for early localized nasal extranodal NK/T-cell lymphoma (ENKL). Annals of hematology 92: 333–343.
2. Liang R (2009) Advances in the management and monitoring of extranodal NK/T-cell lymphoma, nasal type. British journal of haematology 147: 13–21.
3. Aozasa K, Zaki MA (2011) Epidemiology and pathogenesis of nasal NK/T-cell lymphoma: a mini-review. TheScientificWorldJournal 11: 422–428.
4. Aozasa K, Takakuwa T, Hongyo T, Yang WI (2008) Nasal NK/T-cell lymphoma: epidemiology and pathogenesis. International journal of hematology 87: 110–117.
5. Suzuki R, Takeuchi K, Ohshima K, Nakamura S (2008) Extranodal NK/T-cell lymphoma: diagnosis and treatment cues. Hematological oncology: 66–72.
6. Asano N, Kato S, Nakamura S (2013) Epstein-Barr virus-associated natural killer/T-cell lymphomas. Best Pract Res Clin Haematol: 15–21.
7. Motsch N, Alles J, Imig J, Zhu J, Barth S, et al. (2012) MicroRNA profiling of Epstein-Barr virus-associated NK/T-cell lymphomas by deep sequencing. PloS one 7: e42193.
8. Kanemitsu N, Isobe Y, Masuda A, Momose S, Higashi M, et al. (2012) Expression of Epstein-Barr virus-encoded proteins in extranodal NK/T-cell Lymphoma, nasal type (ENKL): differences in biologic and clinical behaviors of LMP1-positive and -negative ENKL. Clinical cancer research: an official journal of the American Association for Cancer Research 18: 2164–2172.
9. Zhang SS, Wei M, Yu L (2011) [Advances of treatment for extranodal NK/T-cell lymphoma --- review]. Zhongguo shi yan xue ye xue za zhi/Zhongguo bing li sheng li xue hui = Journal of experimental hematology/Chinese Association of Pathophysiology 19: 1075–1078.
10. Wang TT, Wang Z (2009) [Recent advances on extranodal NK/T-cell lymphoma of nasal type]. Zhongguo shi yan xue ye xue za zhi/Zhongguo bing li sheng li xue hui = Journal of experimental hematology/Chinese Association of Pathophysiology 17: 1624–1628.
11. Baran AM, Reifenberger J, Helbig D (2012) [NK/T-cell lymphoma, nasal type with cutaneous dissemination]. Hautarzt 63: 272–275.
12. Liang DN, Yang ZR, Wang WY, Zhao S, Yang QP, et al. (2012) Extranodal nasal type natural killer/T-cell lymphoma of testis: report of seven cases with review of literature. Leukemia & lymphoma 53: 1117–1123.
13. Jiang Q, Liu S, Peng J, Xiong H, Xiong Z, et al. (2013) An extraordinary T/NK lymphoma, nasal type, occurring primarily in the prostate gland with unusual CD30 positivity: case report and review of the literature. Diagnostic pathology 8: 94.
14. Pine RR, Clark JD, Sokol JA (2013) CD56 negative extranodal NK/T-cell lymphoma of the orbit mimicking orbital cellulitis. Orbit 32: 45–48.
15. Au WY, Lie AK, Liang R, Kwong YL, Yau CC, et al. (2003) Autologous stem cell transplantation for nasal NK/T-cell lymphoma: a progress report on its value. Annals of oncology: official journal of the European Society for Medical Oncology/ESMO 14: 1673–1676.
16. Cui XZ, Wang HQ, Liu XM, Zhang HL, Li W (2007) [Treatment outcome and prognosis of autologous hematopoietic stem cell transplantation combined with high dose radiotherapy/chemotherapy in 22 patients with nasal NK/T cell lymphoma]. Zhonghua xue ye xue za zhi = Zhonghua xueyexue zazhi 28: 609–611.
17. Kim HJ, Bang SM, Lee J, Kwon HC, Suh C, et al. (2006) High-dose chemotherapy with autologous stem cell transplantation in extranodal NK/T-cell lymphoma: a retrospective comparison with non-transplantation cases. Bone marrow transplantation 37: 819–824.
18. Mori Y, Aoki T, Takenaka K, Yamauchi T, Yamamoto A, et al. (2010) Successful treatment of refractory advanced nasal NK/T cell lymphoma with unrelated cord blood stem cell transplantation incorporating focal irradiation. International journal of hematology 91: 107–111.
19. Li YX, Wang H, Jin J, Wang WH, Liu QF, et al. (2012) Radiotherapy alone with curative intent in patients with stage I extranodal nasal-type NK/T-cell lymphoma. International journal of radiation oncology, biology, physics 82: 1809–1815.
20. Kim TM, Heo DS (2009) Extranodal NK/T-cell lymphoma, nasal type: new staging system and treatment strategies. Cancer science 100: 2242–2248.
21. Yamaguchi M, Tobinai K, Oguchi M, Ishizuka N, Kobayashi Y, et al. (2009) Phase I/II study of concurrent chemoradiotherapy for localized nasal natural killer/T-cell lymphoma: Japan Clinical Oncology Group Study JCOG0211. Journal of clinical oncology: official journal of the American Society of Clinical Oncology 27: 5594–5600.
22. Wu X, Li P, Zhao J, Yang X, Wang F, et al. (2008) A clinical study of 115 patients with extranodal natural killer/T-cell lymphoma, nasal type. Clin Oncol (R Coll Radiol) 20: 619–625.
23. Ma HH, Qian LT, Pan HF, Yang L, Zhang HY, et al. (2010) Treatment outcome of radiotherapy alone versus radiochemotherapy in early stage nasal natural killer/T-cell lymphoma. Med Oncol 27: 798–806.
24. Kim GE, Lee SW, Chang SK, Park HC, Pyo HR, et al. (2001) Combined chemotherapy and radiation versus radiation alone in the management of localized angiocentric lymphoma of the head and neck. Radiotherapy and oncology: journal of the European Society for Therapeutic Radiology and Oncology 61: 1–9.
25. Kim K, Chie EK, Kim CW, Kim IH, Park CI (2005) Treatment outcome of angiocentric T-cell and NK/T-cell lymphoma, nasal type: radiotherapy versus chemoradiotherapy. Japanese journal of clinical oncology 35: 1–5.
26. Jiang L, Li SJ, Jiang YM, Long JX, Wang RS, et al. (2014) The significance of combining radiotherapy with chemotherapy for early stage extranodal natural killer/T-cell lymphoma, nasal type: a systematic review and meta-analysis. Leukemia & lymphoma 55: 1038–1048.
27. Tierney JF, Stewart LA, Ghersi D, Burdett S, Sydes MR (2007) Practical methods for incorporating summary time-to-event data into meta-analysis. Trials 8: 16.
28. Aviles A, Neri N, Fernandez R, Huerta-Guzman J, Nambo MJ (2013) Combined therapy in untreated patients improves outcome in nasal NK/T lymphoma: results of a clinical trial. Med Oncol 30: 637.
29. Li S, Feng X, Li T, Zhang S, Zuo Z, et al. (2013) Extranodal NK/T-cell lymphoma, nasal type: a report of 73 cases at MD Anderson Cancer Center. The American journal of surgical pathology 37: 14–23.
30. Luo J, Liu L, Wu R, Zhu Y (2013) Prognostic analysis of 130 patients with nasal and Waldeyer ring NK/T cell lymphoma treated by radiotherapy and/or chemotherapy. Chinese journal of radiation oncology 22: 180–184.
31. Chauchet A, Michallet AS, Berger F, Bedgedjian I, Deconinck E, et al. (2012) Complete remission after first-line radio-chemotherapy as predictor of survival in extranodal NK/T cell lymphoma. Journal of hematology & oncology 5: 27.
32. Li YX, Liu QF, Wang WH, Jin J, Song YW, et al. (2011) Failure patterns and clinical implications in early stage nasal natural killer/T-cell lymphoma treated with primary radiotherapy. Cancer 117: 5203–5211.
33. Li YX, Fang H, Liu QF, Lu J, Qi SN, et al. (2008) Clinical features and treatment outcome of nasal-type NK/T-cell lymphoma of Waldeyer ring. Blood 112: 3057–3064.
34. Huang MJ, Jiang Y, Liu WP, Li ZP, Li M, et al. (2008) Early or up-front radiotherapy improved survival of localized extranodal NK/T-cell lymphoma, nasal-type in the upper aerodigestive tract. International journal of radiation oncology, biology, physics 70: 166–174.
35. Kim SJ, Kim BS, Choi CW, Seo HY, Seol HR, et al. (2006) Treatment outcome of front-line systemic chemotherapy for localized extranodal NK/T cell lymphoma in nasal and upper aerodigestive tract. Leukemia & lymphoma 47: 15–1273.
36. Isobe K, Uno T, Tamaru J, Kawakami H, Ueno N, et al. (2006) Extranodal natural killer/T-cell lymphoma, nasal type: the significance of radiotherapeutic parameters. Cancer 106: 609–615.
37. Tham IW, Lee KM, Yap SP, Loong SL (2006) Outcome of patients with nasal natural killer (NK)/T-cell lymphoma treated with radiotherapy, with or without chemotherapy. Head & neck 28: 1–134.
38. Li CC, Tien HF, Tang JL, Yao M, Chen YC, et al. (2004) Treatment outcome and pattern of failure in 77 patients with sinonasal natural killer/T-cell or T-cell lymphoma. Cancer 100: 366–375.
39. Cheung MM, Chan JK, Lau WH, Ngan RK, Foo WW (2002) Early stage nasal NK/T-cell lymphoma: clinical outcome, prognostic factors, and the effect of treatment modality. International journal of radiation oncology, biology, physics 54: 182–190.
40. Ribrag V, Ell Hajj M, Janot F, Girinsky T, Domenge C, et al. (2001) Early locoregional high-dose radiotherapy is associated with long-term disease control in localized primary angiocentric lymphoma of the nose and nasopharynx. Leukemia 15: 1123–11.
41. Li YX, Yao B, Jin J, Wang WH, Liu YP, et al. (2006) Radiotherapy as primary treatment for stage IE and IIE nasal natural killer/T-cell lymphoma. Journal of clinical oncology: official journal of the American Society of Clinical Oncology 24: 181–189.
42. Drenou B, Lamy T, Amiot L, Fardel O, Caulet-Maugendre S, et al. (1997) CD3-CD56+ non-Hodgkin's lymphomas with an aggressive behavior related to multidrug resistance. Blood 89: 2966–2974.
43. Yong W, Zheng W, Zhang Y (2001) [Clinical characteristics and treatment of midline nasal and nasal type NK/T cell lymphoma]. Zhonghua yi xue za zhi 81: 773–775.

A Retrospective Review of the Prognostic Value of ALDH-1, Bmi-1 and Nanog Stem Cell Markers in Esophageal Squamous Cell Carcinoma

Cheng-Cheng Hwang[1], Shin Nieh[2], Chien-Hong Lai[3], Chien-Sheng Tsai[4], Liang-Che Chang[1], Chung-Ching Hua[5], Wen-Ying Chi[1], Hui-Ping Chien[1], Chih-Wei Wang[7], Siu-Cheung Chan[6], Tsan-Yu Hsieh[1], Jim-Ray Chen[1]*

1 Department of Pathology, Chang Gung Memorial Hospital, Keelung, Taiwan, **2** Department of Pathology and Graduate Institute of Pathology, National Defense Medical Center & Tri-Service General Hospital, Taipei, Taiwan, **3** Division of Hematology-Oncology, Department of Internal Medicine, Chang Gung Memorial Hospital, Keelung, Taiwan, **4** Department of Radiation Oncology, Chang Gung Memorial Hospital, Keelung, Taiwan, **5** Division of Pulmonary, Critical Care and Sleep Medicine, Chang Gung Memorial Hospital, Keelung, Taiwan, **6** Department of Diagnostic Radiology, Chang Gung Memorial Hospital, Keelung, Taiwan, **7** Department of Anatomic Pathology, Chang Gung Memorial Hospital, Tao-Yuan, Taiwan

Abstract

Stem cell markers are upregulated in various cancers and have potential as prognostic indicators. The objective of this study was to determine the expression of three stem cell markers, aldehyde dehydrogenase 1 (ALDH-1), B cell-specific Moloney murine leukemia virus integration site 1 (Bmi-1), and Nanog, in esophageal squamous cell carcinoma (ESCC) tissues. Immunohistochemistry was used to measure the expression of ALDH-1, Bmi-1, and Nanog in ESCC tissues from 41 patients who received pre-operative chemoradiation. We evaluated the relationship between expression of these markers, and clinicopathological features, tumor regression grade (TRG), and 5-year overall survival (OS). There were no significant associations of ALDH-1 or Bmi-1 expression with age, gender, clinical stage, and treatments ($p>0.05$). However, patients with Nanog-positive tumors were significantly older than those whose tumors were Nanog-negative ($p=0.033$). TRG after treatment was significantly associated with expression of ALDH-1 ($p=0.001$), Bmi-1 ($p=0.004$), and Nanog ($p<0.001$). Although OS was significantly better in patients with low TRGs ($p=0.001$), there were no significant correlations between ALDH-1, Bmi-1, or Nanog with OS. Expression of ALDH-1, Bmi-1, and Nanog correlated with TRG, but not OS. Further large studies are necessary to fully elucidate the prognostic value of these stem cell markers for ESCC patients.

Editor: Anthony W.I. Lo, The Chinese University of Hong Kong, Hong Kong

Funding: This study was supported by grant CMRPG290391 to C.-C. Hwang from Chang Gung Memorial Hospital, Keelung, Taiwan. The funders had no role in study design, data collection and analysis, decision to publish, or preparation of the manuscript.

Competing Interests: The authors have declared that no competing interests exist.

* Email: rrooyyaall@yahoo.com

Introduction

Esopahgeal adenocarcinoma (EAC) and esophageal squamous cell carcinoma (ESCC) are the 2 major histological types of esophageal cancer [1]. EAC is more common in Western countries, but ESCC is more common in East Asia [2]. In China, ESCC is the fourth-leading cause of cancer-associated death [3]. Despite improvements in surgery, chemotherapy, and radiotherapy, the 5-year overall survival remains poor, in part because patients typically have advanced-stage cancer at diagnosis [4]. Thus, in addition to prevention strategies, which focus on modification of risk factors associated with ESCC such as alcohol consumption and cigarette smoking [5], identification of prognostic markers of ESCC may also help to reduce the mortality associated with this cancer.

The levels of serum anti-p53 antibodies and C-reactive protein predict the response to therapy in patients with recurrent esophageal cancer [6]. In addition, the phosphorylation level of mammalian target of rapamycin (mTOR) is associated with response to chemoradiotherapy and overall disease-free survival in ESCC patients [7]. Furthermore, 2 mesenchymal markers of the epithelial mesenchymal transition (EMT), vimentin and fibronectin, are indicators of poor prognosis [4]. The EMT enhances cancer invasion and metastasis, in part because cells develop stem cell-like properties [8].

Cancer stem cells have the capacity of self-renewal, and are thought to be responsible for the generation of multiple cell lineages that are characteristic of many tumors [9–10]. Cancer stem cells have roles in tumorigenesis and resistance to therapy, so the identification of markers for cancer stem cell may provide important information regarding patient prognosis and response to therapy [11–12]. For example, previous research indicated that adenosine triphosphate-binding cassette superfamily G member 2 (ABCG2) expression was associated with ESCC patient survival [13] and Notch1 expression was associated with greater pathological grade and shorter OS in ESCC patients [14].

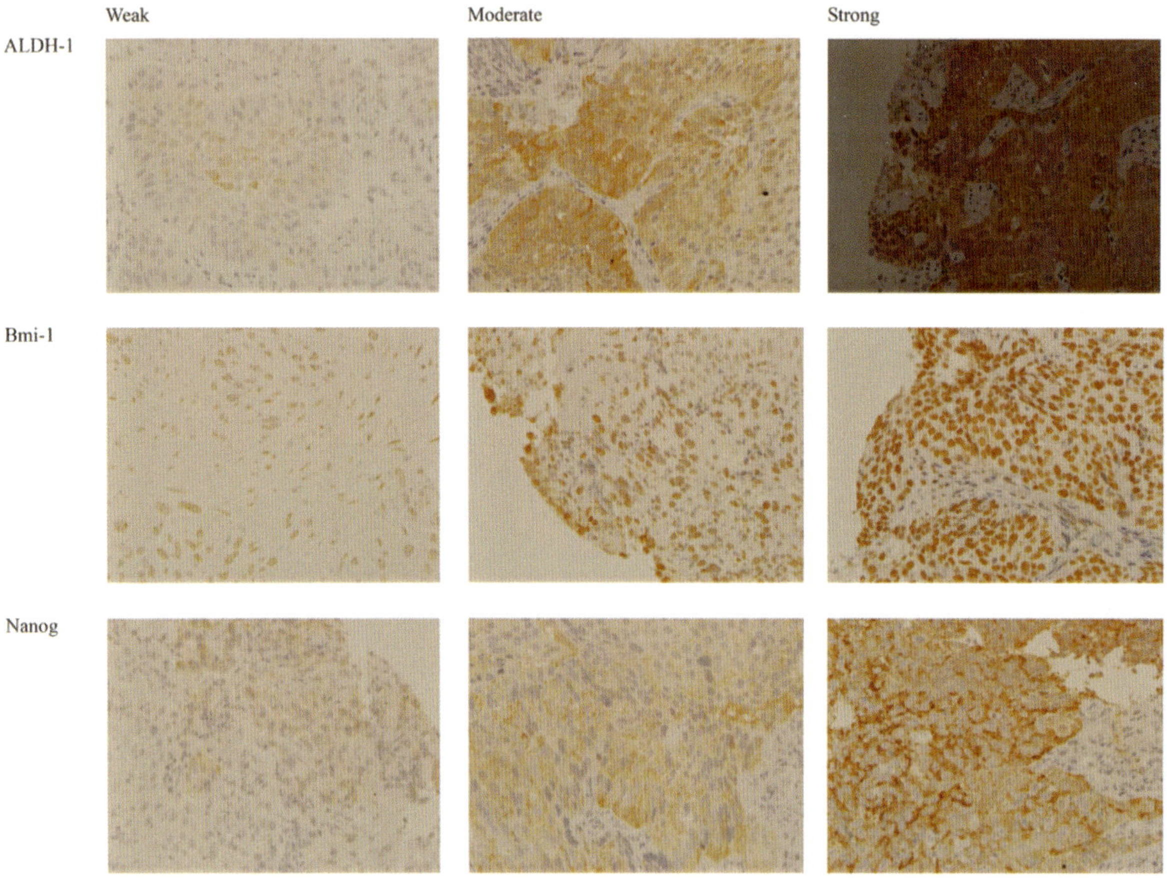

Figure 1. Representative images of cancer stem cell markers (top: ALDH1, middle: Bmi-1, bottom: Nanog) with different stain intensities (weak, moderate, strong).

Identification of markers associated with ESCC may be useful for determining prognosis and response to therapy. Previous research indicated that the expression of 3 cancer stem cell markers, aldehyde dehydrogenase 1 (ALDH-1), B cell-specific Moloney murine leukemia virus integration site 1 (Bmi-1), and Nanog, are associated with esophageal cancer [15–17]. ALDH-1 is one of a family of enzymes that catalyze the oxidation of aldehydes to carboxylic acids; Bmi-1 is a polycomb ring finger oncogene that regulates p16 and p19; and Nanog is a homeobox transcription factor that has elevated expression in stem cells and some solid tumors. The present study used immunohistochemistry to investigate the expression of these 3 genes in human ESCC tissues and examined the relationship of their expression with clinicopathological characteristics and prognosis.

Material and Methods

Sample and data collection

The records of 41 ESCC patients who underwent preoperative chemoradiation therapy and radical esophagectomy/curative surgery from 2000 to 2012 at Keelung Chang Gung Memorial Hospital of Chang Gung Medical Foundation were retrospectively reviewed. Patient information, including gender, age, and clinicopathologic characteristics, was obtained from the Taiwan Cancer Registry, a national database. ESCC tissue samples were obtained from all participants for immunohistochemical analysis. The enrolled patients included 39 males and 2 females, and the median age was 54 years (range, 37–78 years). Histological analysis indicated that 2 patients (4.9%) had well-differentiated tumors, 27 patients (65.9%) had moderately differentiated tumors, and 12 patients (29.3%) had poorly differentiated tumors. The median follow-up time was 13.0 months (range 0.3–57.4 months). The duration of overall survival (OS) began at the day of surgery and ended at last follow-up or death.

Diagnosis was confirmed by pathological examination of hematoxylin and eosin staining results as described previously [18]. There were 5 tumor regression grades (TRGs), ranging from complete tumor response (TRG I) to no regressive changes within the tumor (TRG V) as previously described [19]. Specifically, TRG I was characterized by the absence of residual cancer and fibrosis throughout the esophageal wall; TRG II by the presence of rare residual cancer cells scattered through the fibrosis; TRG III by an increased number of residual cancer cells with predominant fibrosis; TRG IV by residual cancer outgrowing fibrosis; and TRG V by no regressive changes [19]. This study was approved by the institutional review board of the Keelung Chang Gung Memorial Hospital of CGMF, and written informed consent was obtained from all participants.

Immunohistochemical staining

Tissues were embedded in paraffin and sectioned. After deparaffinization, they were hydrated and incubated with an epitope retrieval solution (10 mM citric acid, pH 6.0) at 95°C for 40 min. After incubation with 0.3% H_2O_2 to inactivate endogenous peroxidase, nonspecific binding was inhibited by incubation

Table 1. Relationship between expression of stem cell markers and characteristics of 41 patients with ESCC.

	ALDH-1			Bmi-1			Nanog		
	Positive (n = 24)	Negative (n = 17)	*P*-value	Positive (n = 36)	Negative (n = 5)	*P*-value	Positive (n = 37)	Negative (n = 4)	*P*-value
Age (years)[1]	55 (51, 64)	51 (46, 59)	0.255	54 (47, 62)	56 (53, 61)	0.282	55 (50, 62)	46 (41, 50)	0.033
Gender, n (%)[2]			1.000			1.000			1.000
Male	23 (95.8)	16 (94.1)		34 (94.4)	5 (100)		35 (94.6)	4 (100)	
Female	1 (4.2)	1 (5.9)		2 (5.6)	0 (0.0)		2 (5.4)	0 (0.0)	
Clinical stage, n(%)[2]			0.212			0.435			0.621
II	2 (8.3)	5 (29.4)		6 (16.7)	1 (20.0)		7 (18.9)	0 (0.0)	
III	14 (58.3)	9 (52.9)		19 (52.8)	4 (80.0)		21 (56.8)	2 (50.0)	
IV	8 (33.3)	3 (17.6)		11 (16.7)	0 (0.0)		9 (24.3)	2 (50.0)	

Each number indicates median and interquartile range unless otherwise specified.
P-values are based on [1]Mann-Whitney U test and [2]Fisher's exact test.

with 5% normal serum in PBS at room temperature for 30 min. The sections were next incubated with primary antibodies specific for ALDH-1, Bmi-1, and Nanog (Epitomics, Burlingame CA, USA) at 4°C overnight. The sections were next incubated with biotinylated secondary antibodies (Lab Vision, Kalamazoo, MI, USA) at room temperature for 10 min, and then with streptavidin peroxidase (Lab Vision) at room temperature. Visualization was done with DAB following the manufacturer's instructions (DaKo, Carpinteria, CA, USA). After sections were counterstained with hematoxylin, they were air-dried and observed under a microscope (E600, Nikon, Tokyo, Japan). All cells of each section were observed. The stain intensity was graded as negative (no expression), weak (fewer than one-third positive cells), moderate (one-third to two-thirds positive cells), or strong (more than two-thirds positive cells). Figure 1 shows representative images of the different stain intensities of each marker. Two pathologists who were blinded to the clinical data performed all histological evaluations. Inconsistent results were reviewed and discussed before making a final decision.

Statistical Analysis

Due to the small sample size, continuous data were compared using the Mann-Whitney U test, and categorical variables were compared by Fisher's exact test. Continuous variables are presented as medians and interquartile ranges, and categorical data as numbers and percentages. Correlations between stem cell marker expression and tumor regression grade were performed using Kendall's correlation coefficient. Kaplan-Meier analysis and the log-rank test were used for analysis of cumulative survival curves. All statistical assessments were two-sided, and a p-value less than 0.05 was considered significant. Statistical analyses were performed with SPSS 15.0 Statistics Software (SPSS Inc., Chicago, IL, USA).

Results

Association of stem cell markers with patient characteristics

Table 1 shows that there were no significant correlations between expression of ALDH-1 or Bmi-1 with age, gender, clinical stage ($p>0.05$ for all). However, patients with Nanog-positive tumors were significantly older than those whose tumors were Nanog-negative ($p = 0.033$). Additional analysis and calculation of Kendall's rank correlation coefficients indicated that there were several significant positive correlations in the expression of these markers (ALDH-1 and Bmi-1: $\tau = 0.34$, $p = 0.014$; ALDH-1 and Nanog: $\tau = 0.45$, $p = 0.001$; Bmi-1 and Nanog: $\tau = 0.28$, $p = 0.040$) (Table S1).

Association of stem cell markers with TRG and patient survival

TRG was classified based on complete tumor response to therapy [19]. Figure 2 shows that TRG after treatment was significantly associated with greater expression of ALDH-1 ($p = 0.001$), Bmi-1 ($p = 0.004$), and Nanog ($p<0.001$).

We also analyzed the association between the expression of the 3 stem cell markers with patient survival. By the end of the study, 15 patients had died from ESCC, 9 patients died from complications associated with ESCC, and 2 patients died from unknown causes. The median survival time was 14.8 months (95% CI, 8.8–20.8 months). Kaplan–Meier analysis and the log-rank tests show that there was no significant correlation between expression of any of the stem cell markers with OS ($p>0.05$).

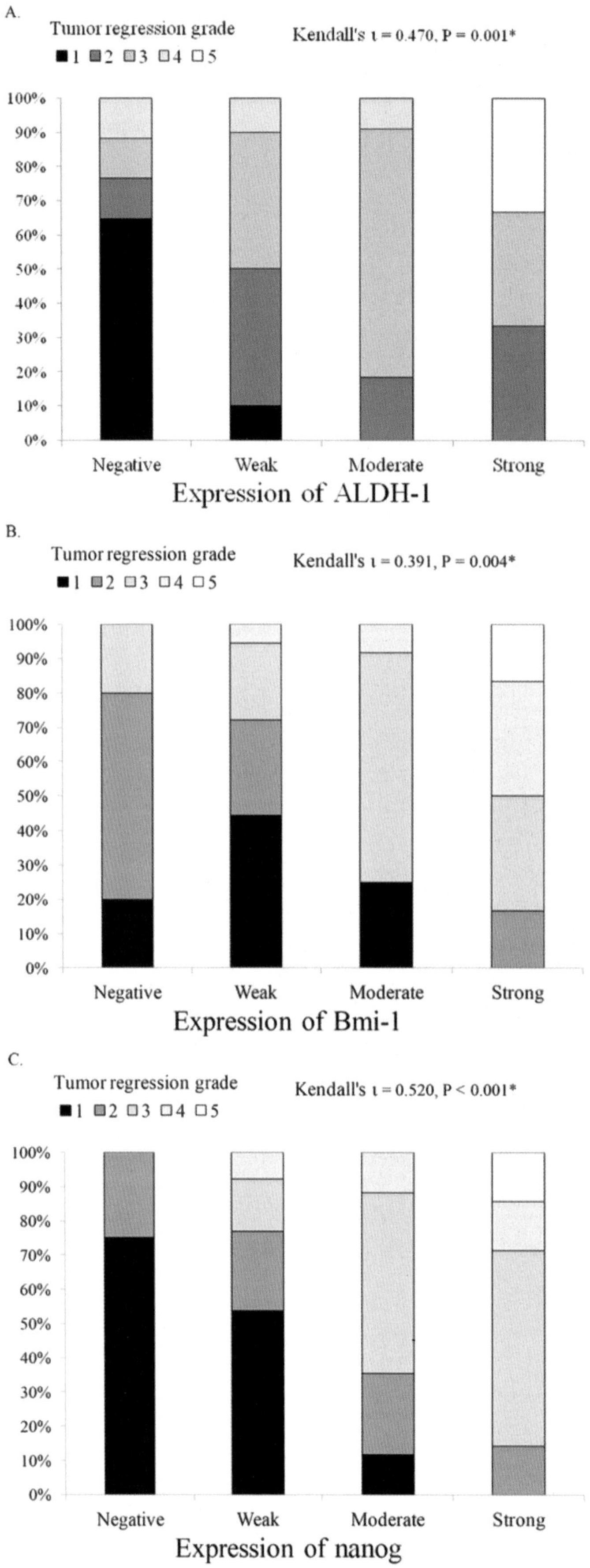

Figure 2. Relationship of expression of cancer stem cell markers (A: ALDH-1, B: Bmi-1, C: Nanog) with tumor regression grade. *$P<0.01$.

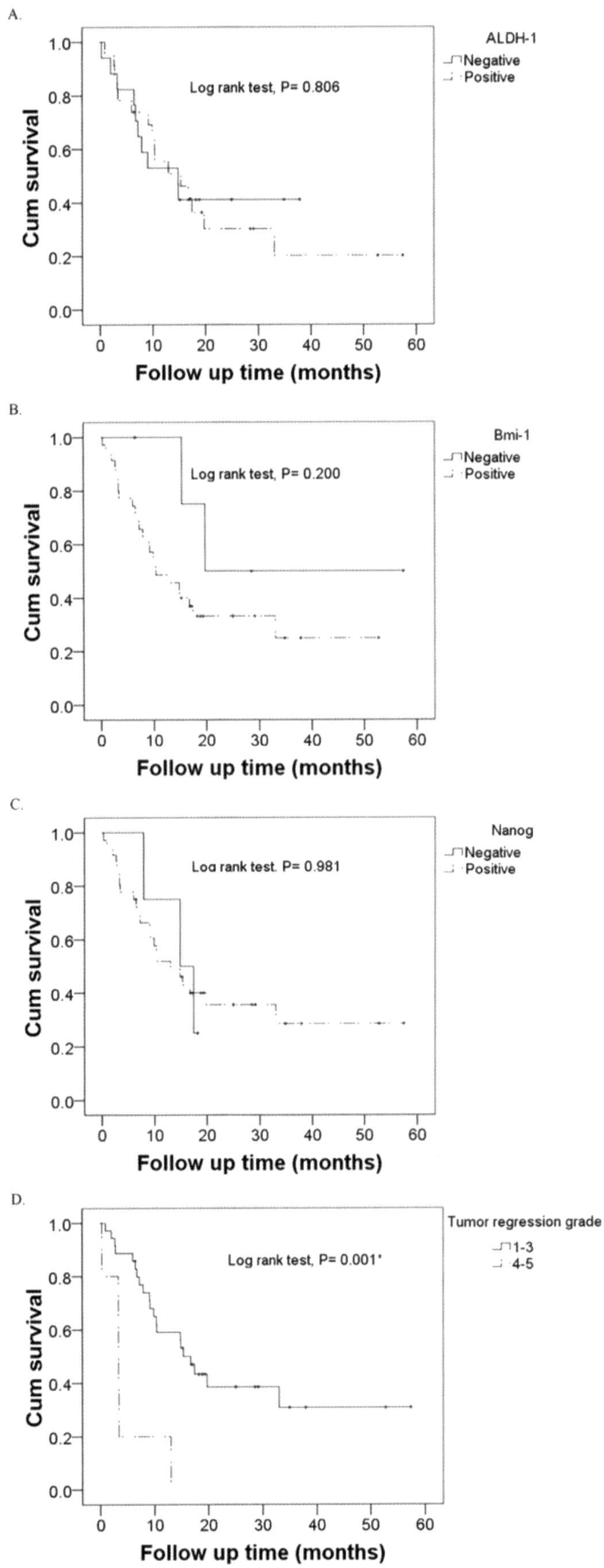
A.
ALDH-1
Negative
Positive
Log rank test, P= 0.806
Cum survival
1.0
0.8
0.6
0.4
0.2
0.0
0
10
20
30
40
50
60
Follow up time (months)
B.
Bmi-1
Negative
Positive
Log rank test, P= 0.200
Cum survival
Follow up time (months)
C.
Nanog
Negative
Positive
Log rank test, P= 0.981
Cum survival
Follow up time (months)
D.
Tumor regression grade
1-3
4-5
Log rank test, P= 0.001*
Cum survival
Follow up time (months)

Figure 3. Kaplan-Meier analysis of the prognostic value of the expression of cancer stem cell markers (A: ALDH-1, B: Bmi-1, C: Nanog) and tumor regression grade (D) in prediction of overall survival. $^*P<0.001$.

However, OS was significantly better in patients TRG 1–3 than in patients with TRG 4–5 ($p = 0.001$, Figure 3).

Discussion

More than 50% of patients with esophageal cancer have metastases or unresectable tumors at diagnosis [20], and this largely explains their poor prognosis [4]. Therefore, identification of early diagnostic markers of esophageal cancer may be useful for improving prognosis and informing treatment decisions. Previous research reported that the expression of ALDH-1, Bmi-1, and Nanog were associated with ESCC and EAC [15–17], and this motivated our examination of the relationship between their expression and the clinicopathological features of patients with ESCC. Although Nanog expression was associated with age, there were no other significant correlations between expression of the 3 examined markers with age, gender, and clinical stage. However, elevated expression of each marker was associated with more advanced TRG after treatment. Although poor OS was associated with more advanced TRG, there were no significant correlations between expression of ALDH-1, Bmi-1, or Nanog with OS.

TNM staging, which considers tumor size, its spread to lymph nodes, and distant metastasis, is the most common staging system but a recent study highlighted several shortcomings of the 7th edition regarding its prognostic value for patients receiving neoadjuvant chemoradiotherapy [21]. Thus, Weider et al. [22] suggested that assessments of early tumor response to chemoradiotherapy predicted esophageal cancer patient survival. Similarly, Mandard et al. [19] observed that tumor regression was a significant predictor of disease-free survival of esophageal cancer patients, consistent with the results of the present study, which indicated that advanced TRG was associated with poor OS. However, identification of prognostic markers that can be detected by noninvasive methods would enable clinicians to continuously monitor response to therapy. Cancer stem cells are important for tumorigenesis and therapy resistance, so analysis of cancer stem cell markers in tumors may provide important information on patient prognosis and response to therapy [11–12].

ALDH-1 has a role in stem cell differentiation by regulating retinal oxidation to retinoic acid [23], and its expression has been used as a marker for normal and cancer stem cells [24]. In Chinese patients with ESCC, nuclear expression of ALDH-1 is associated with poor histological differentiation, lymph node metastasis, TNM stage, and poor 5-year OS [15]. In the present study, ALDH-1 expression was associated with advanced TRG, but not with clinical stage or OS.

Bmi-1, a polycomb-group protein, regulates gene expression by chromatin remodeling, and control of axial patterning, cell proliferation, and senescence [25–26]. Expression of Bmi-1 is upregulated in many solid and hematologic cancers [27]. In addition, previous research reported associations between Bmi-1 expression and ESCC and EAC [17,28–29]. Specifically, He et al. [28] reported an association between Bmi-1 overexpression and advanced pathological stage and poor OS and the presence of Bmi-1 autoantibodies correlated with tumor stage and lymph node metastasis [29]. However, Choy et al. [17] found no association between Bmi-1 expression and OS in patients with EAC or ESCC, consistent with the results of the present study.

The expression of Nanog, a homeobox transcription factor, correlates with cell differentiation [30] and resistance to therapy [31] in patients with breast cancer and with poor survival in patients with oral cancer [32]. Furthermore, a previous study reported that Nanog expression was associated with TNM stage and differentiation of ESCC [16]. The present study indicated that Nanog expression was associated with TRG, but not with clinical stage or OS.

The small sample size of the present study is a limitation. Thus, the findings of no associations between ALDH-1, Bmi-1, or Nanog expression with clinicopathological features or OS cannot be completely ruled out. A larger cohort study would also allow the analysis of the prognostic value of these markers on tumor subpopulations, as in Sudo et al. [4]. Alternatively, it remains possible that the selected stem cell markers may not be suitable for predicting the outcome of patients with ESCC. Therefore, larger studies are necessary. In addition, the present study did not perform survival analysis based on tumor node metastasis stage of ESCC.

Conclusions

Examination of the expression of 3 cancer stem cell markers, ALDH-1, Bmi-1, and Nanog, in patients with ESCC indicated correlations with TRG but not OS. Further large studies are necessary to fully elucidate the prognostic value of these stem cell markers for ESCC patients.

Acknowledgments

We thank Dr. Marjet Heitzer who provided medical writing services on behalf of MedCom Asia, Inc.

Author Contributions

Conceived and designed the experiments: CCH JRC SN. Performed the experiments: CCH JRC. Analyzed the data: CHL CST. Contributed reagents/materials/analysis tools: LCC CCH. Contributed to the writing of the manuscript: WYC SCC. Acquired the data: CHL CST. Contributed to review of slides: HPC CWW TYH.

References

1. Kelsen DP, Daly JM, Kern SE, Levin B, Tepper JE, et al. (2008) Principles and practice of gastrointestinal oncology, 2nd ed. Philadelphia: Lippincott Williams & Wilkins.
2. Lin Y, Totsuka Y, He Y, Kikuchi S, Qiao Y, et al. (2013) Epidemiology of Esophageal Cancer in Japan and China. J Epidemiol 2013 Apr 27. [Epub ahead of print]
3. Jemal A, Bray F, Center MM, Ferlay J, Ward E, et al. (2011) Global cancer statistics. CA Cancer J Clin 61: 69–90.
4. Sudo T, Iwaya T, Nishida N, Sawada G, Takahashi Y, et al. (2012) Expression of mesenchymal markers vimentin and fibronectin: the clinical significance in esophageal squamous cell carcinoma. Ann Surg Oncol 2012 May 30. [Epub ahead of print]

5. Oze I, Matsuo K, Ito H, Wakai K, Nagata C, et al. (2012) Cigarette smoking and esophageal cancer risk: an evaluation based on a systematic review of epidemiologic evidence among the Japanese population. Jpn J Clin Oncol 42: 63–73.
6. Shimada H, Kitabayashi H, Nabeya Y, Okazumi S, Matsubara H, et al. (2003) Treatment response and prognosis of patients after recurrence of esophageal cancer. Surgery 133: 24–31.
7. Li SH, Huang EY, Lu HI, Huang WT, Yen CC, et al. (2012) Phosphorylated mammalian target of rapamycin expression is associated with the response to chemoradiotherapy in patients with esophageal squamous cell carcinoma. J Thorac Cardiovasc Surg 144: 1352–1359.
8. Mani SA, Guo W, Liao MJ, Eaton EN, Ayyanan A, et al. (2008) The epithelial-mesenchymal transition generates cells with properties of stem cells. Cell 133: 704–715.
9. Tu SM, Lin SH, Logothetis CJ (2002) Stem-cell origin of metastasis and heterogeneity in solid tumours. Lancet Oncol 3: 508–513.
10. Stingl J, Caldas C (2007) Molecular heterogeneity of breast carcinomas and the cancer stem cell hypothesis. Nat Rev Cancer 7: 791–799.
11. Clarke MF, Dick JE, Dirks PB, Eaves CJ, Jamieson CH, et al. (2006) Cancer stem cells perspectives on current status and future directions: AACR Workshop on cancer stem cells. Cancer Res 66: 9339–9344.
12. Eyler CE, Rich JN (2008) Survival of the fittest: cancer stem cells in therapeutic resistance and angiogenesis. J Clin Oncol 26: 2839–2845.
13. Hang D, Dong HC, Ning T, Dong B, Hou DL, et al. (2012) Prognostic value of the stem cell markers CD133 and ABCG2 expression in esophageal squamous cell carcinoma. Dis Esophagus 25: 638–644.
14. Liu J, Fan H, Ma Y, Liang D, Huang R, et al. (2013) Notch1 is a 5-fluorouracil resistant and poor survival marker in human esophagus squamous cell carcinomas. PLoS One 8:e56141.
15. Wang Y, Zhe H, Gao P, Zhang N, Li G, et al. (2012) Cancer stem cell marker ALDH1 expression is associated with lymph node metastasis and poor survival in esophageal squamous cell carcinoma: a study from high incidence area of northern China. Dis Esophagus 25: 560–565.
16. Du Y, Shi L, Wang T, Liu Z, Wang Z (2012) Nanog siRNA plus Cisplatin may enhance the sensitivity of chemotherapy in esophageal cancer. J Cancer Res Clin Oncol 138: 1759–1767.
17. Choy B, Bandla S, Xia Y, Tan D, Pennathur A, et al. (2012) Clinicopathologic characteristics of high expression of Bmi-1 in esophageal adenocarcinoma and squamous cell carcinoma. BMC Gastroenterol 12: 146.
18. Gore RM (1997) Esophageal cancer: clinical and pathologic features. Radiol Clin North Am 35: 243–263
19. Mandard AM, Dalibard F, Mandard JC, Marnay J, Henry-Amar M, et al. (1994) Pathologic assessment of tumor regression after preoperative chemoradiotherapy of esophageal carcinoma. Clinicopathologic correlations. Cancer 73: 2680–2686.
20. Enzinger PC, Mayer RJ (2003) Esophageal cancer. N Engl J Med 349: 2241–2252.
21. Nomura M, Shitara K, Kodaira T, Hatooka S, Mizota A, et al. (2012) Prognostic impact of the 6th and 7th American Joint Committee on Cancer TNM staging systems on esophageal cancer patients treated with chemoradiotherapy. Int J Radiat Oncol Biol Phys 82: 946–952.
22. Wieder HA, Brucher BL, Zimmermann F, Becker K, Lordick F, et al. (2004) Time course of tumor metabolic activity during chemoradiotherapy of esophageal squamous cell carcinoma and response to treatment. J Clin Oncol 22: 900–908.
23. Kastan MB, Schlaffer E, Russo JE, Colvin OM, Civin CI, et al. (1990) Direct demonstration of elevated aldehyde dehydrogenase in human hematopoietic progenitor cells. Blood 75: 1947–1950.
24. Ma I, Allan AL (2011) The role of human aldehyde dehydrogenase in normal and cancer stem cells. Stem Cell Rev 7: 292–306.
25. van der Lugt NM, Domen J, Linders K, van Roon M, Robanus-Maandag E, et al. (1994) Posterior transformation, neurological abnormalities, and severe hematopoietic defects in mice with a targeted deletion of the bmi-1 protooncogene. Genes Dev 8: 757–769.
26. Jacobs JJ, Kieboom K, Marino S, DePinho RA, van Lohuizen M (1999) The oncogene and Polycomb-group gene bmi-1 regulates cell proliferation and senescence through the ink4a locus. Nature 397: 164–168.
27. Cao L, Bombard J, Cintron K, Sheedy J, Weetall ML, et al. (2011) BMI1 as a novel target for drug discovery in cancer. J Cell Biochem 112: 2729–2741.
28. He XT, Cao XF, Ji L, Zhu B, Lv J, et al. (2009) Association between Bmi1 and clinicopathological status of esophageal squamous cell carcinoma. World J Gastroenterol 15: 2389–2394.
29. Liu WL, Guo XZ, Zhang LJ, Wang JY, Zhang G, et al. (2010) Prognostic relevance of Bmi-1 expression and autoantibodies in esophageal squamous cell carcinoma. BMC Cancer 10: 467.
30. Ben-Porath I, Thomson MW, Carey VJ, Ge R, Bell GW, et al. (2008) An embryonic stem cell-like gene expression signature in poorly differentiated aggressive human tumors. Nat Genet 40: 499–507.
31. Bourguignon LY, Peyrollier K, Xia W, Gilad E (2008) Hyaluronan-CD44 interaction activates stem cell marker Nanog, Stat-3-mediated MDR1 gene expression, and ankyrin-regulated multidrug efflux in breast and ovarian tumor cells. J Biol Chem 283: 17635–17651.
32. Chiou SH, Yu CC, Huang CY (2008) Positive correlations of Oct-4 and Nanog in oral cancer stem-like cells and high-grade oral squamous cell carcinoma. Clin Cancer Res 14: 4085–4095.

Thymidylate Synthase Genotype-Directed Chemotherapy for Patients with Gastric and Gastroesophageal Junction Cancers

Laura W. Goff[1], Nilay Thakkar[2], Liping Du[1], Emily Chan[1], Benjamin R. Tan[3], Dana B. Cardin[1], Howard L. McLeod[4], Jordan D. Berlin[1], Barbara Zehnbauer[5], Chloe Fournier[3], Joel Picus[3], Andrea Wang-Gillam[3], Wooin Lee[2], A. Craig Lockhart[3]*

1 Department of Medicine, Vanderbilt-Ingram Cancer Center, Nashville, Tennessee, United States of America, **2** Department of Pharmaceutical Sciences, College of Pharmacy, University of Kentucky, Lexington, Kentucky, United States of America, **3** Department of Medicine, Siteman Cancer Center, Washington University School of Medicine, St. Louis, Missouri, United States of America, **4** Moffitt Cancer Center, Tampa, Florida, United States of America, **5** Centers for Disease Control and Prevention, Atlanta, Georgia, United States of America

Abstract

Background: Retrospective studies indicate associations between *TSER* (thymidylate synthase enhancer region) genotypes and clinical outcomes in patients receiving 5-FU based chemotherapy, but well-controlled prospective validation has been lacking.

Methods: In this phase II study (NCT00515216 registered through ClinicalTrials.gov, http://clinicaltrials.gov/show/NCT00515216), patients with "good risk" *TSER* genotypes (at least one *TSER*2* allele) were treated with FOLFOX chemotherapy to determine whether prospective patient selection can improve overall response rates (ORR) in patients with gastric and gastroesophageal junction (GEJ) cancers, compared with historical outcomes in unselected patients (estimated 43%).

Results: The ORR in genotype-selected patients was 39.1% (9 partial responses out of 23 evaluable patients, 95% CI, 22.2 to 59.2), not achieving the primary objective of improving ORR. An encouraging disease control rate (DCR, consisting of partial responses and stable diseases) of 95.7% was noted and patients with homozygous *TSER*2* genotype showed better tumor response.

Conclusions: In this first prospective, multi-institutional study in patients with gastric or GEJ cancers, selecting patients with at least one *TSER*2* allele did not improve the ORR but led to an encouraging DCR. Further studies are needed to investigate the utility of selecting patients homozygous for the *TSER*2* allele and additional genomic markers in improving clinical outcomes for patients with gastric and GEJ cancers.

Editor: Keitaro Matsuo, Kyushu University Faculty of Medical Science, Japan

Funding: This study was supported in part by the grants from the National Cancer Institute, NIH (R21 CA123881, K23 CA098011), the National Center for Research resources, NIH (5 M01 RR-000095). Additional funding was provided by BJC Foundation Cancer Frontier Fund and Sanofi-Aventis. The authors confirm that the funding agencies, with the exception of the NIH, had no role in the study design, data collection and analysis, decision to publish, or preparation of the manuscript.

Competing Interests: The authors confirm no competing interests with regards to the financial support provided by Sanofi-Aventis. Sanofi-Aventis only provided study medications and covered the cost of administering the study medications.

* Email: alockhar@dom.wustl.edu

Introduction

Cancers of the gastric cardia, gastroesophageal junction (GEJ) and distal esophagus have been rapidly increasing in incidence in the past decades, especially in patients younger than 40 years of age [1]. Unfortunately, 80–90% of newly diagnosed patients present with regional or distant metastatic disease and even with optimal therapy, the median survival in these patients is less than 1 year and survival at 5 years is essentially zero [2,3]. Recent advances in our capacity to detect and target specific molecular lesions in cancer cells and to obtain genetic information from tumor tissues and patients allow for selection of optimal therapies, improving the outcomes for these aggressive cancers. For example, targeting HER-2 expressing gastroesophageal tumors with trastuzumab led to an improvement in the survival of patients with advanced disease [4]. However, for the majority of patients selection of initial therapy remains largely empiric as most of the regimens have similar response rates and median survival [3,5]. Thus, there is a clear need for approaches that can guide treatment selection for the most effective regimens.

5-fluorouracil (5-FU) is one of the most commonly prescribed chemotherapy agents. It has demonstrated preclinical synergy with oxaliplatin in a variety of tumor types and this combination has demonstrated clear efficacy in treating patients with gastric and GEJ cancers [6–8]. Thymidylate synthase (TS, encoded by the *TYMS* gene) is the critical enzyme in DNA synthesis and repair and it is the primary target for 5-FU and other folate-based antimetabolites [9]. Overexpression of TS has been linked to clinical resistance to TS-targeted agents including 5-FU [10]. In turn, genetic polymorphisms involving the promoter region of the *TYMS* gene, specifically, the number of tandem repeat sequences in the TS enhancer region (*TSER* - the 28-nucleotide G/C-rich sequence in the 5′-untranslated region) have been shown to be important determinants of tumoral TS expression [11–15]. The two most common *TSER* alleles are the two tandem repeats (*TSER*2*, allelic frequency = 0.2~0.4) and the three tandem repeats (*TSER*3*, allelic frequency = 0.6~0.8) [15].

Retrospective studies in colorectal cancer have demonstrated that individuals with *TSER*3/*3* genotype had a significantly lower response rate and poorer outcomes to 5-FU compared with those with at least one *TSER*2* allele [11,16–18]. Additional retrospective analyses of TS expression or *TSER* genotypes in relation to clinical outcomes in patients with gastric cancers replicated these findings [19,20]. More recently, findings from the first prospective study evaluating the utility of *TSER* genotypes in directing neoadjuvant chemoradiation for patients with rectal carcinoma demonstrated that patients treated with 5-FU-based chemoradiotherapy according to their *TSER* genotypes had improved tumor downstaging [21]. Together, these studies provide ample evidence that TS expression status and/or *TSER* genotyping may be useful in selecting patients who are likely to respond to treatment with 5-FU or its analogues.

This Phase II study was designed to prospectively select patients with "good risk" *TSER* genotypes (i.e. *TSER*2/*2* or **2/*3*) and treat them with a standard 5-FU-based regimen (FOLFOX; 5-FU, leucovorin, oxaliplatin) in order to improve clinical outcomes in patients with gastric and GEJ cancers. The primary end point of this study was to determine whether *TSER* genotype-directed chemotherapy would result in an improved overall response rate (ORR, 60% or higher) compared to historical control response rates in non-genotype selected patients (estimated 43%). The secondary end points were to retrospectively assess whether other genetic variations, in particular, additional polymorphic loci in the *TYMS* gene and other genes involved in the disposition and response to the FOLFOX regimen would influence the response in the treated patients.

Materials and Methods

Ethics Statement

The trial was done in accordance with the Declaration of Helsinki and ICH Good Clinical Practice. The study protocol was approved by the Vanderbilt University and Washington University Institutional Review Boards and all participants provided their written informed consent to participate in this study. The study was registered through ClinicalTrials.gov (Identifier: NCT00515216). The protocol for this trial and supporting TREND checklist are available as supporting information; see Checklist S1 and Protocol S1. The trial started (first patient enrolled) in June 2008 and ended (last patient completed the clinical study) in October 2010.

Eligibility

Adult (≥18 years) patients who had histologically or cytologically confirmed adenocarcinoma of the stomach or GEJ and had received no prior therapy for metastatic disease were eligible. Subjects could have received prior neoadjuvant or adjuvant therapy as long as the disease-free interval was longer than 6 months. Eligible patients had Eastern Cooperative Oncology Group (ECOG) performance status ≤2, adequate organ and bone marrow function, and an ability to understand and willingness to sign written informed consent. Patients with known active brain metastases, HIV on anti-retroviral therapy or other uncontrolled intercurrent illnesses were excluded.

Study Design and Treatment

This was an open-label, non-randomized, investigator-initiated multi-center study involving prospective genotyping (study flow chart shown in Figure 1). Potentially eligible patients underwent a blood draw for *TSER* genotyping. Patients with *TSER*3/*3* genotype were not included in study treatment. Patients with *TSER*2/*2* or *TSER*2/*3* genotypes received the modified FOLFOX-6 treatment consisting of oxaliplatin 85 mg/m^2 and leucovorin 400 mg/m^2 given over 2 hours along with 5-FU 400 mg/m^2 given as an intravenous push over 5 minutes, followed by 5-FU 2,400 mg/m^2 given as an intravenous infusion of 46 hours. This treatment was repeated every 2 weeks in the absence of unacceptable adverse events or disease progression.

Assessment of Efficacy and Toxicity

The patients were reevaluated for response every 8 weeks. In addition to a baseline scan, confirmatory scans were performed not less than 4 weeks following initial documentation of objective response. Tumor response and progression were evaluated using Response Evaluation Criteria in Solid Tumors (RECIST). Partial

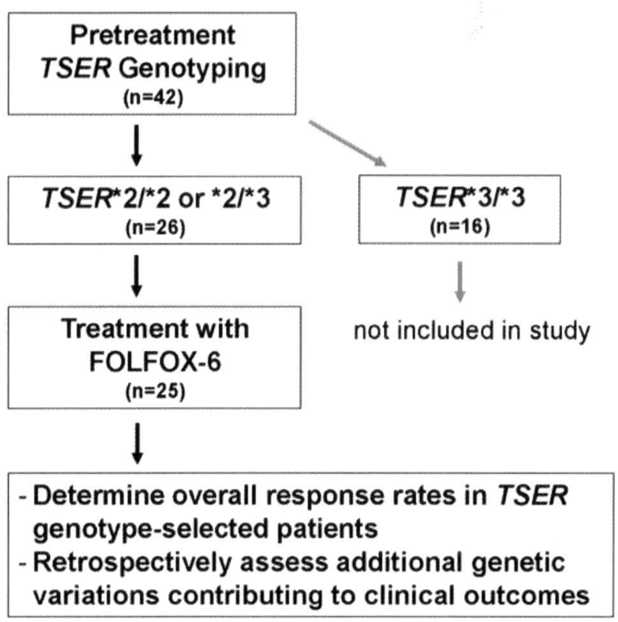

Figure 1. A schematic diagram of the current phase II study design.

response (PR) was defined as at least 30% decrease in the sum of the longest diameter (LD) of target lesions, taking as reference the baseline sum LD. Progressive disease (PD) was defined as at least a 20% increase in the sum of the LD of target lesions, taking as reference the smallest sum LD recorded since the treatment started or the appearance of one or more new lesions. Stable disease (SD) was defined as neither sufficient shrinkage to qualify for PR nor sufficient increase to qualify for PD. Toxicities were graded according to the National Cancer Institute Common Terminology Criteria for Adverse Events (NCI-CTCAE), version 3.0. Dose modifications were made depending on the type and severity of toxicities observed.

Retrospective Genotyping Analyses

Retrospective genotyping analyses by restriction fragment length polymorphism (RFLP) were performed for two additional loci in the *TYMS* gene (G>C SNP within the second 28-bp tandem repeat of the 3R allele, rs34743033; 1494delTTAAAG in the 3′-UTR, rs34489327) and five loci in additional genes reported to be associated with response and toxicity to the FOLFOX regimen (*ERCC1*, c.354C>T, rs11615; *ERCC2*, c.2251A>C, rs13181; *GSTP1*, c.313A>G, rs1695; *XRCC1*, c.1196G>A, rs25487; and *MDR1*, c.3435C>T, rs1045642). Briefly, regions encompassing the respective polymorphisms were PCR amplified (Platinum PCR Supermix, Invitrogen) and subjected to restriction enzyme digest to yield the diagnostic fragmentation patterns (detailed conditions provided in Table S1 in File S1) [13,22–30]. The digested and undigested products from each patient sample were visualized on 3% agarose gel along with positive controls whose genotypes were verified by direct sequencing.

Statistical Analyses

The primary objective of this study was to test whether selection of patients according to *TSER* genotypes would improve treatment response rates compared to the response rates previously reported in an unselected population. Sample size estimation was based on the assumed response rate of 43% with this regimen in an unselected population and improving the response rate to a minimum of 60% based on the retrospective data [19,20]. An Optimum MinMax two-stage accrual design was employed [31]. In the initial step, 45 eligible patients were to be entered into the study, with a final accrual goal of 75 if ≥20 responses were observed in the first group. This design provides 90% statistical power to detect a difference of 17% with a two-sided significance level of <0.05. Unfortunately, the current study had to be terminated earlier than the initial stopping point due to insufficient funding. For 23 patients evaluable for tumor responses, univariate associations between genotypes and tumor response (PR and SD) were evaluated using Fisher's exact test. Overall survival (OS) and progression free survival (PFS) were analyzed using Kaplan-Meier models and associations between genotypes and patient survival were assessed using log-rank tests. No sub-analyses were performed for potential associations between genotypes and toxicities since they were not pre-specified in our analysis plans. All statistical analyses were performed using R package (version 3.0.2).

Results

Patient characteristics

Patient baseline characteristics are listed in Table 1. Between June 2008 and October 2010, 42 patients with gastric and GEJ cancers were screened for their *TSER* genotypes; 26 patients (63.4%) had good risk genotypes (*TSER**2/*2 or *2/*3) and enrolled onto the trial. One patient with a good risk genotype withdrew consent and was not treated on study. The majority of patients had gastric cancer (73%) and good performance status (69% ECOG PS of 1 or better). The median age of the participants was 56 years and a majority (62%) was male.

Treatment and toxicities

Twenty five patients received at least one dose of study treatment with the modified FOLFOX-6 regimen. A total of 128 cycles were administered, with a median of 5.5 cycles per patient (range, 0.5–15 cycles). The occurrence and the incidence of the main toxicities are reported in Table 2. The toxicities experienced by the study participants were within the expected range for patients receiving treatment with FOLFOX. The most common toxicities were hematologic with grade 3 and 4 neutropenia, leukopenia and anemia recorded in 8 out of 25 (32%), 4 out of 25 (16%), and one out of 25 (4%) patients, respectively. Only two out of 25 patients experienced grade 3 gastrointestinal toxicity and no participants had grade 4 gastro-intestinal toxicity. Neurotoxicity was common and was observed in 44% (grade 1 in 20%, grade 2 in 16% and grade 3 in 8%) of the patients. Fatigue was also common and was observed in 52% (grade 1 in 40%, grade 2 in 4% and grade 3 in 8%) of the patients. No treatment-related deaths were reported.

Response to FOLFOX regimen, recurrence and survival and TSER genotypes

Response to the modified FOLFOX-6 regimen in the 23 evaluable patients is shown in Table 3. Nine patients experienced PR and no patient experienced complete response (CR), making the overall response rate (CR+PR) to be 39.1% (95% confidence interval (CI, Wilson), 22.2 to 59.2). When tumor responses are compared between the two *TSER* genotype groups, patients with the *TSER*2/*2* genotype experienced a greater frequency of PR and a less frequency of SD compared to those with the *TSER*2/*3* genotype ($p = 0.02$, Fisher's exact test, Table 3). On the other hand, only one out of 23 patients experienced PD, for an observed disease control rate (CR+PR+SD) of 95.7% (95% CI, 79.0 to 99.2). OS and PFS plots for the enrolled patients are shown in Figure 2. Median values for OS and PFS were 11.4 months (95% CI, 6.3 to 16.3) and 6.2 months (95% CI, 5.2 to 8.6), respectively. For both OS and PFS, patients with the *TSER*2/*2* genotype had a trend towards an improvement in median OS and PFS in comparison to those patients with the *TSER*2/*3* genotype (Figure 3, OS, 20.9 vs 11.4 months; PFS, 10.2 vs 6.0 months).

Potential associations between tumor response and retrospectively analyzed genetic variations

For 21 patients, the retrospective analyses for additional genotypes reported to be associated with treatment responses were completed (the genotypic and allelic frequencies of the interrogated variations are summarized in Table S2 in File S1). Of note, the frequency of *TSER**2 allele is higher in our current study than those reported in the literature since the patients with the *TSER**3/*3 genotype were excluded in this study. When the two additional loci in the *TYMS* genes (rs34743033 and rs34489327) were assessed for their potential association with tumor response (PR vs SD), the results did not indicate any statistically significant association (Table 4). Among the five additional genotypes analyzed, two genetic variations in the *XRCC1* (c.1196G>A, rs25487) and *MDR1* (c.3435C>T, rs1045642) genes displayed a trend supportive of their potential association with tumor response

Table 1. Baseline clinical and demographic characteristics of enrolled patients (n = 26).

Characteristic	Patients (n = 26)	
	No	%
TSER genotypes		
*TSER*2/*2*	5	19
*TSER*2/*3*	21	81
Gender		
Male	16	62
Female	10	38
Age (years)		
median	56	
range	26–81	
Ethnicity		
Caucasians	23	88
African Americans	2	8
Not reported	1	4
ECOG performance status		
0	5	19
1	13	50
2	8	31
Primary tumor type		
Gastric	19	73
Gastroesophageal junction (GEJ)	7	27
Prior neoadjuvant or adjuvant therapy (>6 months)	2	8

($p = 0.050$ and 0.056, respectively, Fisher's exact test, Table 4). However, no apparent association was observed when OS and PFS times were compared among the groups with differing genotypes at the five loci (Table S3 in File S1).

Discussion

This clinical study is unique in that we for the first time applied the strategy of prospectively assessing *TSER* genotypes to improve clinical outcomes in gastric and GEJ cancers. Our initial hypothesis was that selection of patients with good risk *TSER* genotypes would improve the response rate for FOLFOX to 60%, a 17% increase over the historic control response rate of 43% observed in non-genotype selected patients. The observed response rate in this study was 39.1% (9 PR out of 23 patients evaluable for tumor response, 95% CI 22.2 to 59.2), not achieving the primary study endpoint. The median OS and PFS times of 11.3 and 6.2 months in patients with good risk *TSER* genotypes were also comparable to those reported in non-genotype selected populations (Figure 2). Although the observed response rate did not support the utility of *TSER* genotyping as a treatment selection guide, it should also be noted that the enrolled patients experienced a very promising disease control rate of 95.7% (9 PR and 13 SD out of 23 patients), higher than those reported in the literature [32–36]. The high disease control rate in the current study may provide the first prospectively obtained evidence for the utility of *TSER* genotyping in improving clinical outcomes in patients with gastric and GEJ cancers.

The apparent lack of treatment outcome improvement in patients with good risk *TSER* genotypes may be related to the small number of patients enrolled in the current study, therefore necessitating further validation of this approach in a larger clinical trial. It should be however noted that we observed a very encouraging response rate of 83.3% in patients with the homozygous *TSER*2/*2* genotype (5 out of 6 patients experienced PR). This observation was from a very small number of patients, but it suggests that the improvement in clinical outcomes in patients with gastric and GEJ cancers may require selection of patients with two *TSER*2* alleles. Alternatively, the current findings may be related to the presence of multiple molecular/genetic factors contributing to chemotherapy response. Strategies involving more than one host and tumoral markers will likely be more successful in guiding therapeutic decision making. Currently we cannot rule out the possibility that *TSER* genotypes may have prognostic value, independent of therapy, in patients with gastric and GEJ cancers as previously reported in patients with colorectal cancer [37,38]. Consideration of the above-mentioned aspects will be important in the design of future clinical trials which can evaluate multifactorial treatment selection approaches in a larger number of patients.

The findings from another prospective study with selection of patients on the basis of *TSER* genotypes have been recently reported in rectal cancer patients receiving neoadjuvant chemoradiation (n = 135) [21]. In this particular study, patients with good risk *TSER* genotypes (at least one *TSER*2* allele) were treated with standard 5-FU-based chemoradiation. Patients with good risk genotypes had higher rates of downstaging and pathologic complete response than reported in unselected populations. Patients with poor risk TSER genotypes (harboring no *TSER*2* allele) were treated with irinotecan in addition to 5-FU-based

Table 2. Toxicities observed in the treated patients (n = 25).

Toxicity	Grade 1		Grade 2		Grade 3		Grade 4	
	No	%	No	%	No	%	No	%
Leukopenia (total WBC)	4	16	5	20	4	16	0	0
Neutropenia	3	12	2	8	4	16	4	16
Lymphopenia	3	12	4	16	1	4	0	0
Anemia	13	52	6	24	1	4	0	0
Thrombocytopenia	9	36	3	12	0	0	0	0
Nausea	12	48	2	8	1	4	0	0
Vomiting	3	12	3	12	1	4	0	0
Diarrhea	8	32	0	0	0	0	0	0
Mucositis/stomatitis	3	12	1	4	0	0	0	0
Taste alteration (dysgeusia)	8	32	0	0	0	0	0	0
Vision-blurred vision	3	12	0	0	0	0	0	0
Allergic reaction/hypersensitivity	0	0	1	4	0	0	0	0
Rash: hand-foot skin reaction	2	8	0	0	0	0	0	0
AST, SGOT	8	32	2	8	1	4	0	0
ALT, SGPT	10	40	2	8	0	0	0	0
Neuropathy: sensory	5	20	4	16	2	8	0	0
Fatigue (asthenia, lethargy, malaise)	10	40	1	4	2	8	0	0

Table 3. Tumor responses to the FOLFOX regimen in patients of differing *TSER* genotypes.

Tumor response	*TSER* genotypes				*P*-value[a]
	*TSER*2/*2*		*TSER*2/*3*		
	(n = 6)		*(n = 17)*		
	No	%	No	%	
PD (n = 1)	0	0	1	5.9	0.02
PR (n = 9)	5	83.3	4	23.5	
SD (n = 13)	1	16.7	12	70.6	

PD, progressive disease; PR, partial response; SD, stable disease.
[a]Calculated using Fisher's exact test for the association between response (PR and SD) and *TSER* genotype.

chemoradiation. Patients in the poor risk groups receiving additional therapies also showed higher rates of downstaging and pathologic complete response than those for unselected population. This study [21] however did not address whether patients in the poor risk group would have had poorer clinical outcomes if they had not received additional irinotecan therapy. Nevertheless, these findings certainly support the utility of this single genotype-based strategy in improving the clinical outcomes of rectal cancer patients.

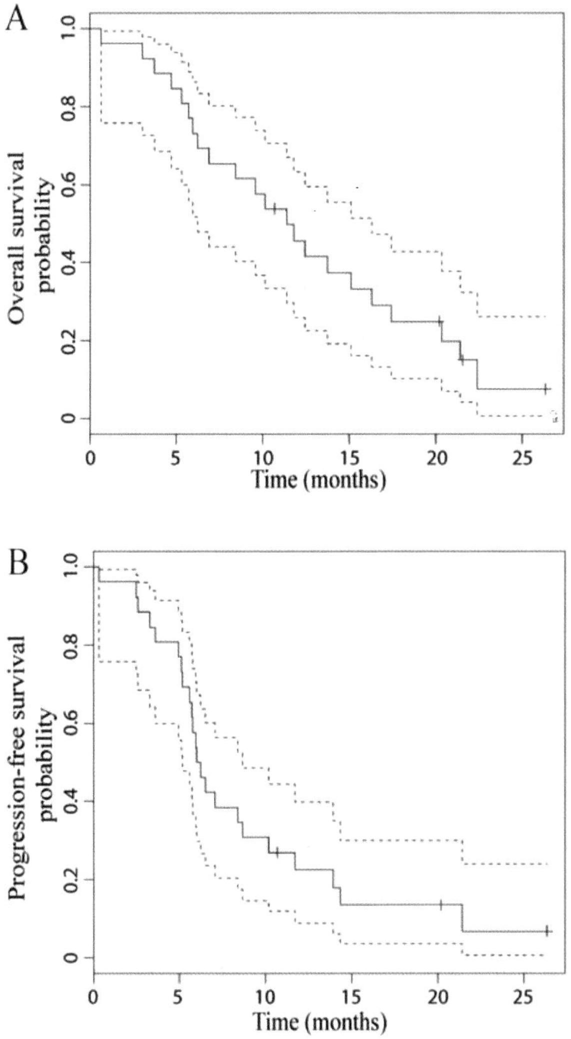

Figure 2. Kaplan-Meier curves showing overall survival (A) and progression free survival (B) with 95% confidence intervals (CI) in the patients enrolled.

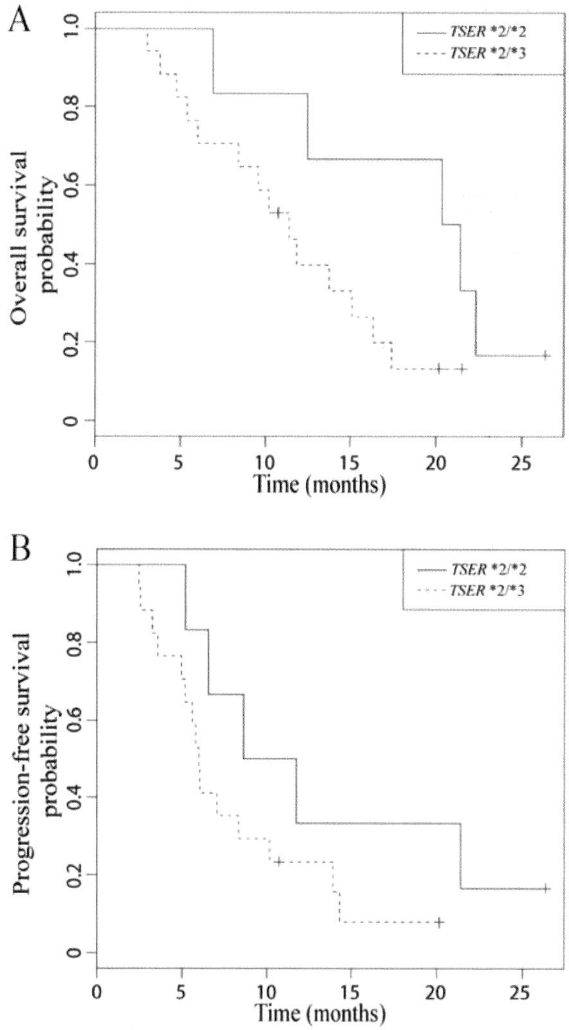

Figure 3. Kaplan-Meier curves showing overall survival (A) and progression free survival (B) according to *TSER* genotypes.

Table 4. Univariate association between additional retrospectively analyzed genotypes and tumor response (PR: partial response and SD: stable disease).

Gene	Genotype	Tumor response				*P*-value[a]
		PR (N = 9)		SD (N = 11)		
		No.	%	No.	%	
TYMS	5′-UTR *TSER* + G>C (rs34743033)					
	*TSER*2/*2*	5	56	1	9	
	*TSER*2/*3(G)*	2	22	4	36	
	*TSER*2/*3(C)*	2	22	6	55	0.137
TYMS	3′-UTR 1494delTTAAAG(6 bp) (rs34489327)					
	+6 bp/+6 bp	5	56	6	55	
	+6 bp/−6 bp	4	44	5	45	1
ERCC1	c.354C>T (rs11615)					
	C/C	2	22	1	9	
	C/T	4	45	8	73	
	T/T	3	33	2	18	0.552
ERCC2	c.2251A>C (rs13181)					
	A/A	5	56	3	27	
	A/C	3	33	6	55	
	C/C	1	11	2	18	0.485
GSTP1	c.313A>G (rs1695)					
	A/A	4	45	8	73	
	A/G	3	33	2	18	
	G/G	2	22	1	9	0.552
XRCC1	c.1196G>A (rs25487)					
	A/A	1	11	6	55	
	G/A	6	67	5	45	
	G/G	2	22	0	-	0.050
MDR1	c.3435C>T (rs1045642)					
	C/C	0	-	1	9	
	C/T	9	100	6	55	
	T/T	0	-	4	36	0.056

[a]Calculated using Fisher's exact test.

No improvement in the overall response rate from this study echo the inconsistent results observed in previous studies utilizing *TSER* genotyping in treating patients with gastric and esophageal cancers [6,39–41]. Less than expected response rates in our current study as well as other previously reported retrospective studies may be explained by the potential effect of oxaliplatin on tumoral TS expression. The clinical synergy of combining 5-FU with oxaliplatin is well documented and is key to the success and frequent use of this combination regimen [42–44]. One proposed explanation for this synergy is oxaliplatin-induced TS downregulation by as yet unexplained mechanisms [45,46]. If oxaliplatin were to cause tumoral TS downregulation or any potential molecular changes influencing tumor response, any benefits from pretreatment *TSER* genotyping may have been obscured in our current study. Interestingly, some *in vitro* studies also indicate that irinotecan may also decrease TS activities and protein levels where irinotecan could overcome 5-FU resistance in tumors [47,48]. These observations could help to explain the favorable response results in the "poor risk" patients who received irinotecan in the Tan *et al.* study [21]. However, our current study design of a single arm (patients with the favorable *TSER* genotypes only) does not allow us to gather treatment outcome for patients with the unfavorable *TSER* genotypes. Our initial study design was indeed two-armed (favorable vs. unfavorable *TSER* genotypes). But, the reviewers in the NIH study section recommended that we revise our study to be single armed for patients with favorable *TSER* genotypes given the patient numbers and other resources available. In future clinical trials, it would be certainly interesting to prospectively compare treatment outcomes of patients with favorable and unfavorable *TSER* genotypes.

Retrospective analyses for two additional *TYMS* genotypes showed no significant association with tumor response (Table 4). For additional non-*TYMS* genes analyzed, *XRCC1* (c.1196G>A, rs25487) and *MDR1* (c.3435C>T, rs1045642) showed a potential association to tumor response (Table 4). We performed these analyses based on the previous findings on the potential association between these genotypes and clinical outcomes in colorectal cancer patients treated with FOLFOX [24,29,40]. However, we did not observe any strong association between the tested genotypes and tumor response, except a trend reflective of potential associations for *XRCC1* and *MDR1*. Similar negative results have been reported from retrospective analyses of *TYMS* and non-*TYMS* genotypes in relation to the histopathological tumor responses in patients with gastric and esophageal cancers [39,41,49]. Interestingly, the polymorphisms in *XRCC1* and *MDR1* have been associated with clinical outcomes in gastric and colorectal cancer [24,50]. Further investigation in larger clinical trials is warranted to determine whether our current findings are indicative of varying impact of the tested genotypes in different tumor types.

In summary, our strategy to improve response rates in patients with gastric and GEJ cancers by pretreatment *TSER* genotyping was unsuccessful, but even in the setting of some limitations of our current study the high disease control rate was encouraging. The future applicability of a single polymorphism strategy to guide therapy selection, while feasible and attractive, does not appear to yield results of sufficient impact to be generally applicable. Our approach may aid in selecting patients who require chemotherapy intensification to achieve favorable results by adding oxaliplatin or irinotecan and avoid chemotherapy toxicities in those who may have a favorable outcome with 5-FU alone. The contemporary confluence of our capacity to molecularly target cancers and the advancement of our ability to characterize patients and their cancers using molecular genetics will allow for multiple variables to be considered and applied towards improvements in cancer care. *TYMS* polymorphism status does not appear to be a singularly important treatment selection factor, but it may be a key contributor to favorable outcomes in a multivariable genomically based therapeutic approach.

Acknowledgments

The Vanderbilt University CHGR/CRC DNA Resources Core provided technical assistance for this work.

Author Contributions

Conceived and designed the experiments: ACL WL HLM. Performed the experiments: LWG BRT ACL EC DBC JDB JP AWG NT BZ WL CF. Analyzed the data: LD WL LWG ACL. Contributed reagents/materials/ analysis tools: LD. Contributed to the writing of the manuscript: LWG NT EC BRT DBC HLM JDB BZ AWG WL ACL.

References

1. Brown LM, Devesa SS (2002) Epidemiologic trends in esophageal and gastric cancer in the United States. Surg Oncol Clin N Am 11: 235–256.
2. Polednak AP (2003) Trends in survival for both histologic types of esophageal cancer in US surveillance, epidemiology and end results areas. Int J Cancer 105: 98–100.
3. Cunningham D, Starling N, Rao S, Iveson T, Nicolson M, et al. (2008) Capecitabine and oxaliplatin for advanced esophagogastric cancer. N Engl J Med 358: 36–46.
4. Bang YJ, Van Cutsem E, Feyereislova A, Chung HC, Shen L, et al. (2010) Trastuzumab in combination with chemotherapy versus chemotherapy alone for treatment of HER2-positive advanced gastric or gastro-oesophageal junction cancer (ToGA): a phase 3, open-label, randomised controlled trial. Lancet 376: 687–697.
5. Van Cutsem E, Moiseyenko VM, Tjulandin S, Majlis A, Constenla M, et al. (2006) Phase III study of docetaxel and cisplatin plus fluorouracil compared with cisplatin and fluorouracil as first-line therapy for advanced gastric cancer: a report of the V325 Study Group. J Clin Oncol 24: 4991–4997.
6. Keam B, Im SA, Han SW, Ham HS, Kim MA, et al. (2008) Modified FOLFOX-6 chemotherapy in advanced gastric cancer: Results of phase II study and comprehensive analysis of polymorphisms as a predictive and prognostic marker. BMC Cancer 8: 148.
7. Oh SY, Kwon HC, Seo BG, Kim SH, Kim JS, et al. (2007) A phase II study of oxaliplatin with low dose leucovorin and bolus and continuous infusion 5-fluorouracil (modified FOLFOX-4) as first line therapy for patients with advanced gastric cancer. Acta Oncol 46: 336–341.
8. De Vita F, Orditura M, Matano E, Bianco R, Carlomagno C, et al. (2005) A phase II study of biweekly oxaliplatin plus infusional 5-fluorouracil and folinic acid (FOLFOX-4) as first-line treatment of advanced gastric cancer patients. Br J Cancer 92: 1644–1649.
9. Chu E, Moto AC, Fogarasi MC (2001) Cancer: Principles & Practice of Oncology; De Vita JVT, Hellman S, Rosenberg SA, editors. Philadelphia: Lippincott Williams & Wilkins. 388–415 p.
10. Marsh S, McLeod HL (2001) Thymidylate synthase pharmacogenetics in colorectal cancer. [see comment]. Clin Colorectal Cancer 1: 175–178; discussion 179–181.
11. Horie N, Aiba H, Oguro K, Hojo H, Takeishi K (1995) Functional analysis and DNA polymorphism of the tandemly repeated sequences in the 5′-terminal regulatory region of the human gene for thymidylate synthase. Cell Struct Funct 20: 191–197.
12. Kawakami K, Omura K, Kanehira E, Watanabe Y (1999) Polymorphic tandem repeats in the thymidylate synthase gene is associated with its protein expression in human gastrointestinal cancers. Anticancer Res 19: 3249–3252.
13. Ulrich CM, Bigler J, Velicer CM, Greene EA, Farin FM, et al. (2000) Searching expressed sequence tag databases: discovery and confirmation of a common polymorphism in the thymidylate synthase gene. Cancer Epidemiol Biomarkers Prev 9: 1381–1385.
14. Kawakami K, Salonga D, Park JM, Danenberg KD, Uetake H, et al. (2001) Different lengths of a polymorphic repeat sequence in the thymidylate synthase gene affect translational efficiency but not its gene expression. Clin Cancer Res 7: 4096–4101.
15. Marsh S, Collie-Duguid ES, Li T, Liu X, McLeod HL (1999) Ethnic variation in the thymidylate synthase enhancer region polymorphism among Caucasian and Asian populations. Genomics 58: 310–312.
16. Iacopetta B, Grieu F, Joseph D, Elsaleh H (2001) A polymorphism in the enhancer region of the thymidylate synthase promoter influences the survival of colorectal cancer patients treated with 5-fluorouracil. Br J Cancer 85: 827–830.
17. Pullarkat ST, Stoehlmacher J, Ghaderi V, Xiong YP, Ingles SA, et al. (2001) Thymidylate synthase gene polymorphism determines response and toxicity of 5-FU chemotherapy. Pharmacogenomics J 1: 65–70.
18. Villafranca E, Okruzhnov Y, Dominguez MA, Garcia-Foncillas J, Azinovic I, et al. (2001) Polymorphisms of the repeated sequences in the enhancer region of the thymidylate synthase gene promoter may predict downstaging after preoperative chemoradiation in rectal cancer. J Clin Oncol 19: 1779–1786.
19. Metzger R, Leichman CG, Danenberg KD, Danenberg PV, Lenz HJ, et al. (1998) ERCC1 mRNA levels complement thymidylate synthase mRNA levels in predicting response and survival for gastric cancer patients receiving combination cisplatin and fluorouracil chemotherapy. J Clin Oncol 16: 309–316.
20. Yeh KH, Shun CT, Chen CL, Lin JT, Lee WJ, et al. (1998) High expression of thymidylate synthase is associated with the drug resistance of gastric carcinoma to high dose 5-fluorouracil-based systemic chemotherapy. Cancer 82: 1626–1631.
21. Tan BR, Thomas F, Myerson RJ, Zehnbauer B, Trinkaus K, et al. (2011) Thymidylate synthase genotype-directed neoadjuvant chemoradiation for patients with rectal adenocarcinoma. J Clin Oncol 29: 875–883.
22. Henriquez-Hernandez LA, Murias-Rosales A, Hernandez Gonzalez A, Cabrera De Leon A, Diaz-Chico BN, et al. (2009) Gene polymorphisms in TYMS, MTHFR, p53 and MDR1 as risk factors for breast cancer: a case-control study. Oncol Rep 22: 1425–1433.
23. Lincz LF, Scorgie FE, Garg MB, Ackland SP (2007) Identification of a novel single nucleotide polymorphism in the first tandem repeat sequence of the thymidylate synthase 2R allele. Int J Cancer 120: 1930–1934.
24. Huang MY, Huang ML, Chen MJ, Lu CY, Chen CF, et al. (2011) Multiple genetic polymorphisms in the prediction of clinical outcome of metastatic colorectal cancer patients treated with first-line FOLFOX-4 chemotherapy. Pharmacogenet Genomics 21: 18–25.
25. Huang MY, Fang WY, Lee SC, Cheng TL, Wang JY, et al. (2008) ERCC2 2251A>C genetic polymorphism was highly correlated with early relapse in high-risk stage II and stage III colorectal cancer patients: a preliminary study. BMC Cancer 8: 50.
26. Zhang XH, Zhang X, Zhang L, Chen Q, Yang Z, et al. (2012) XRCC1 Arg399Gln was associated with repair capacity for DNA damage induced by occupational chromium exposure. BMC Res Notes 5: 263.

27. Lunn RM, Langlois RG, Hsieh LL, Thompson CL, Bell DA (1999) XRCC1 polymorphisms: effects on aflatoxin B1-DNA adducts and glycophorin A variant frequency. Cancer Res 59: 2557–2561.
28. Zhang Z, Wan J, Jin X, Jin T, Shen H, et al. (2005) Genetic polymorphisms in XRCC1, APE1, ADPRT, XRCC2, and XRCC3 and risk of chronic benzene poisoning in a Chinese occupational population. Cancer Epidemiol Biomarkers Prev 14: 2614–2619.
29. Mandola MV, Stoehlmacher J, Muller-Weeks S, Cesarone G, Yu MC, et al. (2003) A novel single nucleotide polymorphism within the 5′ tandem repeat polymorphism of the thymidylate synthase gene abolishes USF-1 binding and alters transcriptional activity. Cancer Res 63: 2898–2904.
30. Kawakami K, Watanabe G (2003) Identification and functional analysis of single nucleotide polymorphism in the tandem repeat sequence of thymidylate synthase gene. Cancer Res 63: 6004–6007.
31. Simon R (1989) Optimal two-stage designs for phase II clinical trials. Control Clin Trials 10: 1–10.
32. Ocvirk J, Rebersek M, Skof E, Hlebanja Z, Boc M (2012) Randomized prospective phase II study to compare the combination chemotherapy regimen epirubicin, cisplatin, and 5-fluorouracil with epirubicin, cisplatin, and capecitabine in patients with advanced or metastatic gastric cancer. Am J Clin Oncol 35: 237–241.
33. Moon YW, Rha SY, Jeung HC, Kim C, Hong MH, et al. (2010) Outcomes of multiple salvage chemotherapy for advanced gastric cancer: implications for clinical practice and trial design. Cancer Chemother Pharmacol 66: 797–805.
34. Moehler M, Mueller A, Trarbach T, Lordick F, Seufferlein T, et al. (2011) Cetuximab with irinotecan, folinic acid and 5-fluorouracil as first-line treatment in advanced gastroesophageal cancer: a prospective multi-center biomarker-oriented phase II study. Ann Oncol 22: 1358–1366.
35. Koizumi W, Takiuchi H, Yamada Y, Boku N, Fuse N, et al. (2010) Phase II study of oxaliplatin plus S-1 as first-line treatment for advanced gastric cancer (G-SOX study). Ann Oncol 21: 1001–1005.
36. Amarantidis K, Xenidis N, Chelis L, Chamalidou E, Dimopoulos P, et al. (2011) Docetaxel plus oxaliplatin in combination with capecitabine as first-line treatment for advanced gastric cancer. Oncology 80: 359–365.
37. Edler D, Hallstrom M, Johnston PG, Magnusson I, Ragnhammar P, et al. (2000) Thymidylate synthase expression: an independent prognostic factor for local recurrence, distant metastasis, disease-free and overall survival in rectal cancer. Clin Cancer Res 6: 1378–1384.
38. Popat S, Matakidou A, Houlston RS (2004) Thymidylate synthase expression and prognosis in colorectal cancer: a systematic review and meta-analysis. J Clin Oncol 22: 529–536.
39. Ott K, Vogelsang H, Marton N, Becker K, Lordick F, et al. (2006) The thymidylate synthase tandem repeat promoter polymorphism: A predictor for tumor-related survival in neoadjuvant treated locally advanced gastric cancer. Int J Cancer 119: 2885–2894.
40. Kawakami K, Graziano F, Watanabe G, Ruzzo A, Santini D, et al. (2005) Prognostic role of thymidylate synthase polymorphisms in gastric cancer patients treated with surgery and adjuvant chemotherapy. Clin Cancer Res 11: 3778–3783.
41. Okuno T, Tamura T, Yamamori M, Chayahara N, Yamada T, et al. (2007) Favorable genetic polymorphisms predictive of clinical outcome of chemoradiotherapy for stage II/III esophageal squamous cell carcinoma in Japanese. Am J Clin Oncol 30: 252–257.
42. Lordick F, Lorenzen S, Stollfuss J, Vehling-Kaiser U, Kullmann F, et al. (2005) Phase II study of weekly oxaliplatin plus infusional fluorouracil and folinic acid (FUFOX regimen) as first-line treatment in metastatic gastric cancer. Br J Cancer 93: 190–194.
43. Chao Y, Yeh KH, Chang CJ, Chen LT, Chao TY, et al. (2004) Phase II study of weekly oxaliplatin and 24-h infusion of high-dose 5-fluorouracil and folinic acid in the treatment of advanced gastric cancer. Br J Cancer 91: 453–458.
44. Rothenberg ML, Oza AM, Bigelow RH, Berlin JD, Marshall JL, et al. (2003) Superiority of oxaliplatin and fluorouracil-leucovorin compared with either therapy alone in patients with progressive colorectal cancer after irinotecan and fluorouracil-leucovorin: interim results of a phase III trial. J Clin Oncol 21: 2059–2069.
45. Yeh KH, Cheng AL, Wan JP, Lin CS, Liu CC (2004) Down-regulation of thymidylate synthase expression and its steady-state mRNA by oxaliplatin in colon cancer cells. Anticancer Drugs 15: 371–376.
46. Chen CC, Chen LT, Tsou TC, Pan WY, Kuo CC, et al. (2007) Combined modalities of resistance in an oxaliplatin-resistant human gastric cancer cell line with enhanced sensitivity to 5-fluorouracil. Br J Cancer 97: 334–344.
47. Fukushima M, Sakamoto K, Ohshimo H, Nakagawa F, Taguchi T (2010) Irinotecan overcomes the resistance to 5-fluorouracil in human colon cancer xenografts by down-regulation of intratumoral thymidylate synthase. Oncol Rep 24: 835–842.
48. Torigoe S, Ogata Y, Matono K, Shirouzu K (2009) Molecular mechanisms of sequence-dependent antitumor effects of SN-38 and 5-fluorouracil combination therapy against colon cancer cells. Anticancer Res 29: 2083–2089.
49. Toriumi F, Kubota T, Saikawa Y, Yoshida M, Otani Y, et al. (2004) Thymidylate synthetase (TS) genotype and TS/dihydropyrimidine dehydrogenase mRNA level as an indicator in determining chemosensitivity to 5-fluorouracil in advanced gastric carcinoma. Anticancer Res 24: 2455–2463.
50. Li Y, Yan PW, Huang XE, Li CG (2011) MDR1 gene C3435 T polymorphism is associated with clinical outcomes in gastric cancer patients treated with postoperative adjuvant chemotherapy. Asian Pac J Cancer Prev 12: 2405–2409.

Effect of Amifostine in Head and Neck Cancer Patients Treated with Radiotherapy: A Systematic Review and Meta-Analysis Based on Randomized Controlled Trials

Jundong Gu[1,2]⁹, Siwei Zhu[2]⁹, Xuebing Li[1], Hua Wu[3], Yang Li[4], Feng Hua[5]*

1 Tianjin Key Laboratory of Lung Cancer Metastasis and Tumor Microenvironment, Tianjin Lung Cancer Institute, Tianjin Medical University General Hospital, Tianjin, China, **2** Department of Oncology, Tianjin Union Medical Center, Tianjin, China, **3** Department of Human resources, Tianjin Union Medical Center, Tianjin, China, **4** Department of obstetrics and gynecology, Tianjin Hospital of Tianjin City, Tianjin, China, **5** Department of surgery oncology, Shandong cancer hospital, Jinan, China

Abstract

Background: Amifostine is the most clinical used chemical radioprotector, but its effect in patients treated with radiation is not consistent.

Methods: By searching Medline, CENTRAL, EMBASE, ASCO, ESMO, and CNKI databases, the published randomized controlled trials (RCTs) about the efficacy of amifostine in HNSCC patients treated with radiotherapy were collected. The pooled efficacy and side effects of this drug were calculated by RevMan software.

Results: Seventeen trials including a total of 1167 patients (604 and 563 each arm) were analyzed in the meta-analysis. The pooled data showed that the use of amifostine significantly reduce the risk of developing Grade3–4 mucositis (relative risk [RR],0.72; 95% confidence interval [CI],0.54–0.95; $p<0.00001$), Grade 2–4 acute xerostomia (RR,0.70; 95%CI,0.52–0.96; $p=0.02$), or late xerostomia (RR,0.60; 95%CI,0.49–0.74; $p<0.00001$) and Grade 3–4 dysphagia (RR,0.39; 95%CI,0.17–0.92; $p=0.03$). However, subgroup analysis demonstrated that no statistically significant reduction of Grade3–4 mucositis (RR,0.97; 95% CI,0.74–1.26; $p=0.80$), Grade 2–4 acute xerostomia (RR,0.35; 95%CI,0.02–5.44; $p=0.45$), or late xerostomia (RR,0.40; 95%CI,0.13–1.24; $p=0.11$) and Grade 3–4 dysphagia (RR,0.23; 95%CI,0.01–4.78; $p=0.35$) was observed in patients treated with concomitant chemoradiotherapy. Compared with placebo or observation, amifostine does not show tumor protective effect in complete response (RR,1.02; 95%CI,0.89–1.17; $p=0.76$) and partial response (RR,0.90; 95%CI, 0.56–1.44; $p=0.66$). For the hematologic side effect, no statistical difference of Grade 3–4 leucopenia (RR,0.60; 95%CI,0.35–1.05; $p=0.07$), anemia (RR,0.80; 95%CI, 0.42–1.53; $p=0.50$) and thrombocytopenia (RR,0.43; 95%CI,0.16–1.15; $p=0.09$) were found between amifostine and control groups. The most common amifostine related side effects were nausea, emesis, hypotension and allergic with an average incidence rate (Grade 3–4) of 5%, 6%, 4% and 4% respectively.

Conclusion: This systematic review showed that amifostine significantly reduce the serious mucositis, acute/late xerastomia and dysphagia without protection of the tumor in HNSCC patients treated with radiotherapy. And the toxicities of amifostine were generally acceptable.

Editor: Olivier Gires, Ludwig-Maximilians University, Germany

Funding: This project was supported by the grants from National Natural Science Foundation of China (to Xuebing Li) (No 81302002). Science and technology foundation of Tianjin Municipal Health Bureau(to Jundong Gu) (2010KZ040). The funders had no role in study design, data collection and analysis, decision to publish, or preparation of the manuscript.

Competing Interests: The authors have declared that no competing interests exist.

* E-mail: kmhf2013@163.com

⁹ These authors contributed equally to this work.

Introduction

Radiotherapy plays a significant role in the management of head and neck squamous cell carcinoma (HNSCC), either for the definitive radiotherapy or for the post-surgical adjuvant radiation[1,2]. The mucositis, acute or late xerostomia caused by radiation are the most common toxic effects, which usually interrupt the planned course of treatment[3]. Mucositis is an acute non-hematologic toxicity that occurs during the treatment; xerostomia usually develops acutely during chemoradiotherapy and persists for a long period of time. The late side effect always disrupts normal activities such as speaking, eating and may also cause sequelae, including tooth loss and dental caries, which could compromise the quality of patients' life.

For the past several decades, researchers have been investigating use of drugs to decrease the side effects during radiotherapy, so as to increase the amount of radiation that can be safely administered to the patients. The most clinical used radioprotective drug is amifostine that was initially developed as part of the nuclear warfare program[4]. Based on some randomized controlled rials (RCTs), it showed that amifostine could reduce acute and chronic xerostomia in HNSCC patients treated with radiation or

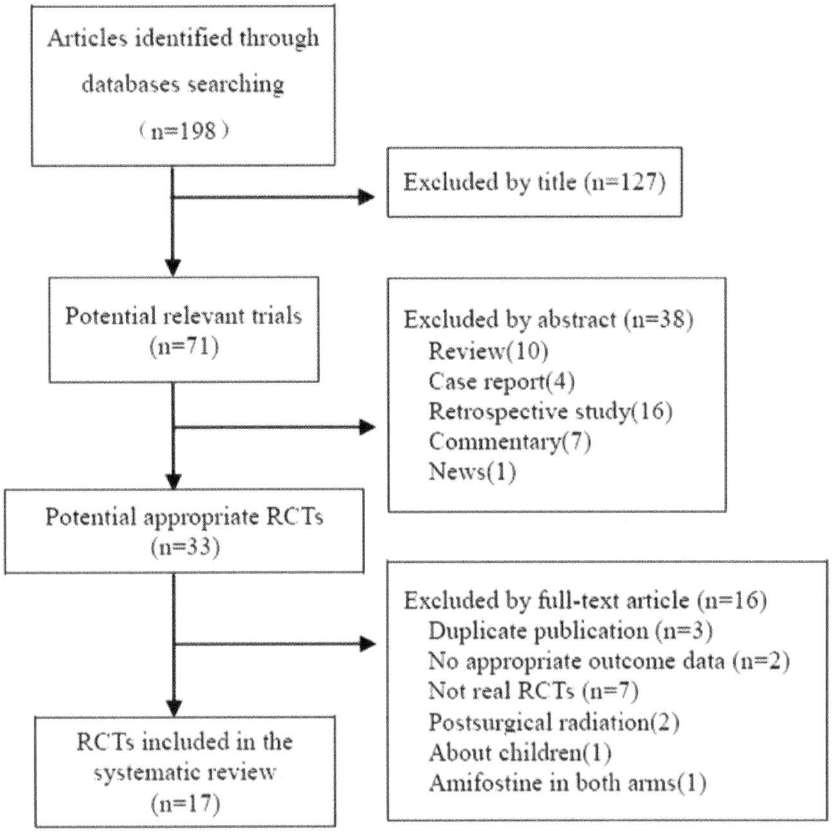

Figure 1. PRISMA Flowchart of the meta-analysis.

concomitant chemoradiotherapy[3,5]. Hower, some other trials did not demonstrate toxicities reduction effects in course of radiation by adding amifostine to the patients[6,7]. And another controversy about the use of this drug is the tumor protective effect. Some researchers worried that amifostine may stop tumor tissue responding to radiation and therefore reduce treatment effectiveness[8]. Unfortunately, even after almost 30 years of its development and clinical use, there is still great controversy about its application. Although some reviews state that evidence is not enough to support the tumor protection efficacy of amifostine, the statistical confirmation of those facts has yet to be achieved. In order to answer this question we performed this systematic review and meta-analysis.

Methods

Search Strategy

The selection procedure of studies was depicted in the PRISMA (Preferred Reporting Items for Systematic Reviews and Meta-Analyses) statement flow chart (Figure 1). Randomized controlled trials comparing radiotherapy vs. radiotherapy plus amifostine for head and neck squamous cell carcinoma, published before January 2012, were identified through an electronic sensitive search of Medline, the Cochrane central register of controlled trials, EMBASE and CNKI databases. The European Society of Medical Oncology (ESMO) and the conference proceedings of the American Society of Clinical Oncology (ASCO) were also searched. The following search terms were used: "Head and neck cancer", "head and neck carcinoma", "amifostine", "Ethyol" "WR-1065", "WR2721","WR1065" or "WR33278". Searches were limited to human trials, with the language restriction of English and Chinese. All references of relevant articles were scanned for additional analysis.

Selection Criteria

Details regarding the patients' eligibility criteria, treatment methods and outcomes of the relevant trials were extracted by two reviewer (JG and YW) and then checked by the third reviewer (FH) as described in the Cochrane Handbook for systematic reviews[9]. The patients were limited to locally advanced (Stage III–IV, or inoperable Stage II) head and neck squamous cell carcinoma. The intervention was radiotherapy or chemoradiotherapy plus amifostine and the control was radiotherapy or chemoradiotherapy with placebo or observation. The outcomes were restricted to about the non-hematological toxicity, response rate, hematological toxicity and side effects of amifostine. No surgical excision or neck dissection was performed before the radiation. The RCTs including patients with both HNSCC and other kinds of tumors were also included in the meta-analysis, but data were extracted only for the HNSCC patients.

Data Extraction and Quality assessment

Data were extracted by two reviewers (JG and HZ) independently from all included RCTs. Any disagreement was consulted to another investigator (YW) for consensus. The general characteristics (name of the first author, year of publication, number of patients, stages, chemoradiation regimens and amifostine dosage), outcomes (non-hematological toxicity: mucositis, acute and late xerostomia, dysphagia; hematological toxicity: leucopenia, anemia and thrombocytopenia; treatment response), and amifostine

Table 1. General characteristics of included randomized controlled trials.

Trials	No.of patiens Ami/Control	Stages included	Daily ami (dose)	Administration	Concomitant Chemotherapy	Radiotherapy
Antonadou[32] (2002)	22/23	III, IV	300 mg/m^2	IV, 30 minutes before RT, q.d	C (90 mg/m^2) once per week before RT	60–74Gy, 2 Gy/fraction, 5 fractions weekly
Bourhis[47] (2000)	13/13	IV	300 mg/m^2	IV, 15–30 minutes before RT, b.i.d	—	62–64 Gy, 2 Gy/fraction, b.i.d with a 8–9 hours interval
Brizel[3] (2000)	143/153	II, III	200 mg/m^2	IV, 15–30 minutes before RT, q.d	—	50–70Gy, 1.8–2.0 Gy/fraction. q.d
Koukourakis[39] (2000)	19/20	II–IV	500 mg	IH, 20 minutes before RT, q.d	—	44–70Gy,2 Gy/fraction, 5 fractions/week
Fan[38] (2011)	30/26	II–IV	200 mg/m^2	IV, 15–30 minutes before RT, q.d	—	70–76Gy, 2Gy/fraction, q.d
Peng[37] (2006)	18/19	III, IV	400 mg	IV, 15 minutes before RT, q.d	5-FU(750 mg/m^2) days:1–3; DDP (50 mg/m^2) day:5; D (75 mg/m^2),day:6	74Gy,1.2 Gy/fraction, 2 fractions daily with a 6 hours interval
Yu[42] (2009)	15/15	III, IV	200 mg/m^2	IV, 20 minutes before RT, q.d	—	70Gy, 2Gy/fraction, q.d
Jiang[41] (2009)	30/30	III, IV	400 mg	IH, 30 minutes before RT.qd	Nedaplatin (100 mg/m^2) day:1,22 and 43	74Gy, 2Gy/fraction, 5 fractions weekly
He[43] (2004)	17/15	III, IV	200 mg/m^2	IV, 15–30 minutes before RT, q.d	—	65–74Gy, 2Gy/fraction, q.d
Zhang[40] (2010)	40/40	III, IV	500 mg	IV, 30 minutes before RT, q.d	—	70Gy, 2Gy/fraction, q.d 5 fractions weekly
Braaksma[34] (2005)	27/27	II–IV	500 mg	IH, 15–30 minutes before RT, q.d	P (60 mg/m2) days: 1,8, 15, and 22	72Gy,12Gy/week
Buntzel[35] (1998)	14/14	II–IV	500 mg	IV, 30 minutes before RT. qd	C (70 mg/m2) days:1–5 and days 21–26	60 Gy, 2 Gy/fraction, 5 fractions weekly
Veerasarn[5] (2006)	32/35	II–IV	200 mg/m^2	IV, 30 minutes before RT, q.d	—	66–70Gy, 2Gy/fraction, q.d
Buentzel[6] (2006)	67/65	II–IV	300 mg/m^2	IV, 30 minutes before RT, q.d	C(70 mg/m2) Days: 1–5 and 21–25	60–66 Gy, 2 Gy/fraction, 5 fractions weekly
Amrein[31] (2005)	28/8	III, IV	400 mg/m2	IV, 30 minutes before RT, q.d	P (60 mg/m2) days: 1, 8, 15, and 22	70.4 Gy, 1.6 Gy/fraction,2 fractions daily with a 4–6 hour interval
Jellema[7] (2006)	60/31	III, IV	200 mg/m^2	IV, 30 minutes before RT, 3/5 times weekly	—	63.5–70Gy,2 Gy/fraction, 5 fractions weekly.
Haddad[36] (2009)	29/29	III,IV	500 mg	IH, 30–60 minutes before RT, q.d	C(AUC 1.5) and P (45 mg/m2), weekly for the first 4 weeks of RT	72 Gy, 1.5–1.8Gy/fraction over 6 weeks

Abbreviations:Ami = amifostine; IV = intravenous injection; IH = Subcutaneously injection; RT = radiotherapy; C = carboplatin; 5-FU = 5-fluorouracil; DDP = Cisplatin; P = Paclitaxel;
D = Docetaxel; AUC = area under the curve; qd = daily; bid = twice daily.

induced side effects were extracted. The methodological qualities of the trials were assessed by the same investigators (JG and HZ) according to the Cochrane Reviews Handbook 5.0. We pay special attention on the generation and concealment of the sequence of randomization, blinding, incomplete outcome date addresse and selective reports, which generally represent the quality of the RCT[9] in the procedure of trials inclusion.

Toxicity Assessment

The toxicities caused by radiation were graded according to "Radiation therapy Oncology Group (RTOG) Acute/Late Radiation Morbidity Scoring Criteria" [10]. Acute mucositis and xerostomia were defined as those that occurred up to 90 days after the start of protocol therapy, and late xerostomia was defined as those that occurred 90 days through 12 months after the start of protocol therapy. The treatment response (complete response and partial response) was assessed at about six weeks after the completion of the treatment regimen according to the World Health Organization guidelines.

Statistical Analysis

Review Manager(RevMan 5.0 provided by The Cochrane Collaboration) was used to do the statistical analysis. Dichotomous data are calculated as the risk ratio (RR) with the 95% confidence interval (CI). The null hypothesis test was considered as no association (RR = 1) between amifostine use and the incidence of radiation toxicity and the tumor response rate. A RR<1 indicates a positive effect of amifostine on the outcome. Statistical heterogeneity of the results across trials was assessed by chi-square (χ^2) test [11], and the inconsistency was calculated by I^2[12]. If heterogeneity was found (χ^2, $p<0.05$ or $I^2>50\%$), the random-effect method (Dersimonian-Laird method) was used to pool the data and subgroups analysis was done for further evaluation. Inversely, without significant heterogeneity, fixed-effect method

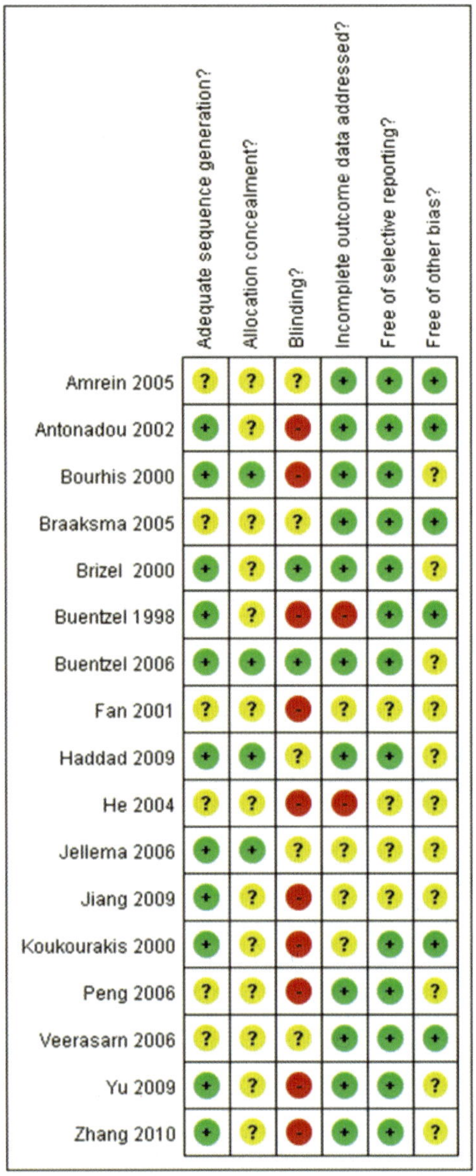

Figure 2. Risk of bias summary. The authors' judgments for each risk of bias item. + is "low risk"; - is "high risk";? is "moderate risk."

was purchased. The Egger's tests were used for each effect size to evaluate possible publication bias as described by Egger[13].

Results

Included Trials and Characteristics

A total of one hundred twelve articles were initially identified by searching the electronic databases. 33 potential applicable studies, published between 1998 and 2010, were retrieved. Of those, sixteen publications were excluded for the reasons: duplicated publication[14–16], not real RCT[17–23], without appropriate outcome data[24,25], postsurgical radiation[26–28], amifostine in both arms comparing different administration[29], about children[30]. Finally, seventeen trials that included a total of 1167 patients (604 and 563 in each arms) were analyzed in the meta-analysis[3,5–7,31–43]. Eight[6,31,32,34–37,41] of the 17 trials evaluated patients treated with concomitant chemoradiation and the other nine trials [3,5,7,33,38–40,42,43] focused on radiation only. Amifostine was delivered intravenously in 13 articles[3,5–7,31–33,35,37,38,40,42,43] and subcutaneously in 4[34,36,39,41]. One trial was a three-arm study that compared different administration schedule of amifostine to observation[7]. The dose of daily amifostine delivered ranged from 200 mg/m^2 to 400 mg/m^2. The general characteristics of included trials were outlined in Table 1.

The summary of methodological quality was evaluated with a five-question instrument described in the Cochrane Reviews Handbook 5.0. Generally, the qualities of seventeen included trials were considered to be of moderate risk of bias. Randomization was performed in all the 17 trials, but only 4 studies mentioned the allocation concealment[6,7,33,36]. And the adequate sequence generation for randomization was delivered in 11 trials[3,6,7,32,33,35,36,39–42]. For the blinding item, only two trials[3,6] describe the blindness on evaluators but not on patients and physicians. The outcome of methodological quality for each trial was demonstrated in Figure 2.

Mucositis

Of the seventeen trials, 16[3,5,6,31–43] evaluated the mucositis with evident heterogeneity between studies($I^2 = 85\%$) (Figure 3). The meta-analysis was performed in the random-effect model (Dersimonian-Laird method). Pooled analysis showed that amifostine reduced 28% of Grade 3–4 mucositis (RR,0.72; 95% CI,0.54–0.95; $p<0.00001$) indicating it can significantly decrease the risk of developing serious mucositis in patients treat with radiation. The publication bias was not detected in this subset analysis by Egger's test ($p = 0.20$). Subgroup analysis was performed cording to different treatment regimens (concomitant chemoradiotherapy or radiotherapy only) and admifostine administration (intravenously in or subcutaneously). In the subgroup analysis, statistically significant reduction of mucositis by using of amifostine was observed in patients treat with radiation only (RR,0.49; 95%CI,0.30–0.78; $p = 0.03$) and delivered intravenously(RR,0.52; 95%CI,0.34–0.78; $p = 0.002$) but not in patients treated with concurrent chemoradiation (RR,0.97; 95%CI,0.74–1.26; $p = 0.80$) and administered subcutaneously (RR,1.09; 95%CI,0.94–1.27; $p = 0.24$) (Table 2).

Acute xerostomia

Eight trials[3,5–7,35,37–39] report the number of patients developed acute xerostomia in both arms. The heterogeneity between the trials was obvious. Pooled analysis with the random-effect model demonstrated that significant reduction of Grade 2–4 acute xerostomia was achieved suing amifostine in patients with HNSCC (RR,0.71; 95%CI,0.52–0.96; $p = 0.02$) (Figure 4). No publication bias was found in the acute xerostomia analysis (Egger's test, $p = 0.76$). But in the subgroup analysis, use of amifostine does not reduce the risk of developing acute xerostomia in patients receiving concomitant radiation (RR,0.35; 95%CI,0.02–5.44; $p = 0.45$) (Table 2).

Late xerostomia

Late xerostomia were reported in six trials[3,5–7,32,37] without the heterogeneity between the studies ($I^2 = 38\%$). Meta-analysis showed amifostine significant reduced 40% risk (RR,0.60; 95%CI,0.49–0.74; $p<0.00001$) of Grade 2–4 late xerostomia compared with placebo or observation (Figure 5). Subgroup analysis also showed that amifostine does not reduce the risk of developing late xerostomia in HNSCC patients treated with radiotherapy plus chemotherapy ($p = 0.11$) (Table2).

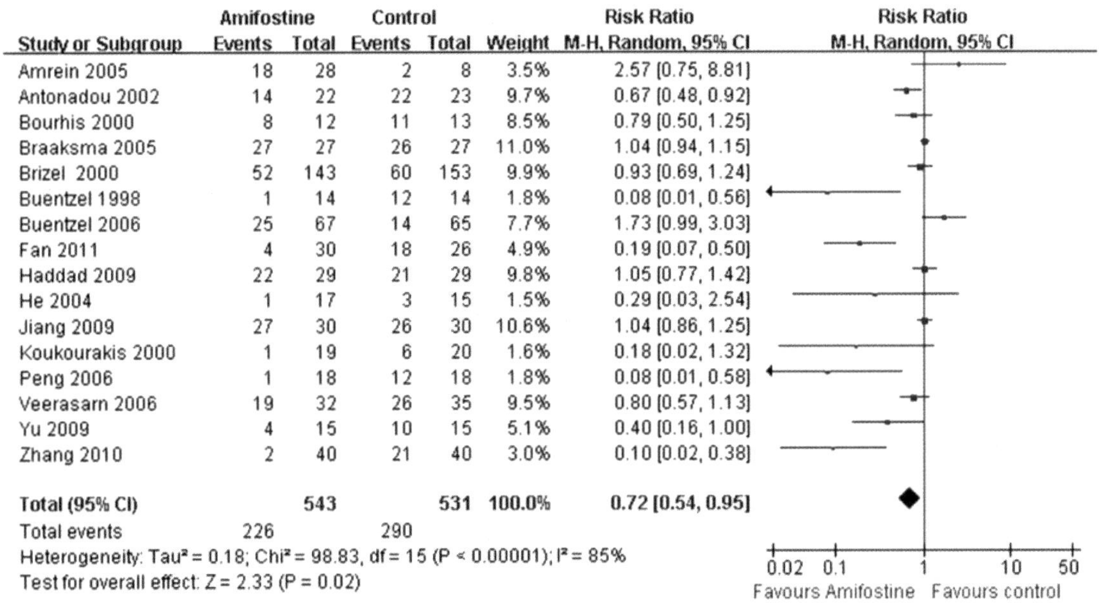

Figure 3. Forest plot of mucositis in HNSCC patients treated with radiotherapy/concomitant chemoradiation. The squares and horizontal lines demonstrate the study-specific OR and 95% CI. The area of the squares reflects the study specific weight (inverse of the variance). The diamond represents the pooled OR and 95% CI.

Dysphagia

Data of dysphagia was pooled from five [5,32–35] of the 17 included trials. Compared with the control, use of amifostine significant decrease the risk of developing Grade 3–4 dysphagia (RR,0.39; 95%CI,0.17–0.92; $p=0.03$). Extreme heterogeneity between the studies was found ($I^2=94\%$). However, all the trials included in the analysis of dysphagia had an estimate point that favored amifostine, and three of them reached statistical significance. We preferred that amifostine significant decrease the risk of developing Grade 3–4 dysphagia.

Treatment response

Response rates were available from six trials[31,32,34,35,37,42]. No statistical heterogeneity between studies was found by Egger's test in both complete ($I^2=21\%$) and partial ($I^2=0\%$) response analysis. The pooled RR estimate for the complete and partial response was 1.02 (95%CI, 0.89–1.17; $p=0.76$) and 0.90 (95%CI,0.56–1.44; $p=0.66$) respectively (Figure 6). Neither of the them reached statistical significance (Figure 6).

Hematological toxicity

Hematological toxicity, including leucopenia, anemia and thrombocytopenia were extracted in five trials[5,6,32,35,37] without heterogeneity between the studies ($I^2=38\%$). Meta-analysis showed that no statistical difference of Grade 3–4 leucopenia (RR, 0.60; 95%CI,0.35–1.05; $p=0.07$), anemia (RR,0.80; 95%CI,0.42–1.53; $p=0.50$) and thrombocytopenia (RR, 0.43; 95%CI, 0.16–1.15; $p=0.09$) were found between amifostine and control groups. Publication bias was not observed by Egger's test ($p=0.63$) (Figure 7).

Side effects of Amifostine

Eight trials[3,5–7,32–35] describe the amifostine toxicity. The most common amifostine related side effects were nausea, emesis, transient hypotension and allergic. The average incidence rate of them (Grade 3–4) was 5%, 6%, 4% and 4% respectively (Figure 8). Of the eight trials reported the amifostine-induced toxic effects, seven studies[3,5–7,32,33,35] delivered the this drug by intravenous injection and only one [34] by subcutaneous injection,

Table 2. Subgroup analysis of radiation induced side effects according to treatment strategy.

Subgroups	Mucositis		*p*	Acute xerostomia		*p*	Late xerostomia		*p*	Dysphagia		*p*
	RR	95%CI		RR	95%CI		RR	95%CI		RR	95%CI	
Treatment												
Chemradiation	0.97	0.74–1.26	0.80	0.35	0.02–5.44	0.45	0.40	0.13–1.24	0.11	0.23	0.01–4.78	0.35
Radiation only	0.49	0.30–0.78	0.03	0.69	0.52–0.93	0.02	0.64	0.45–0.91	0.01	0.32	0.17–0.61	0.0004
Administration												
IV	0.52	0.34–0.78	0.002	0,73	0.54–0.97	0.03	0.60	0.49–0.74	0.00001	0.39	0.17–0.92	0.03
IH	1.09	0.94–1.27	0.24	0.08	0–1.34	0.08						

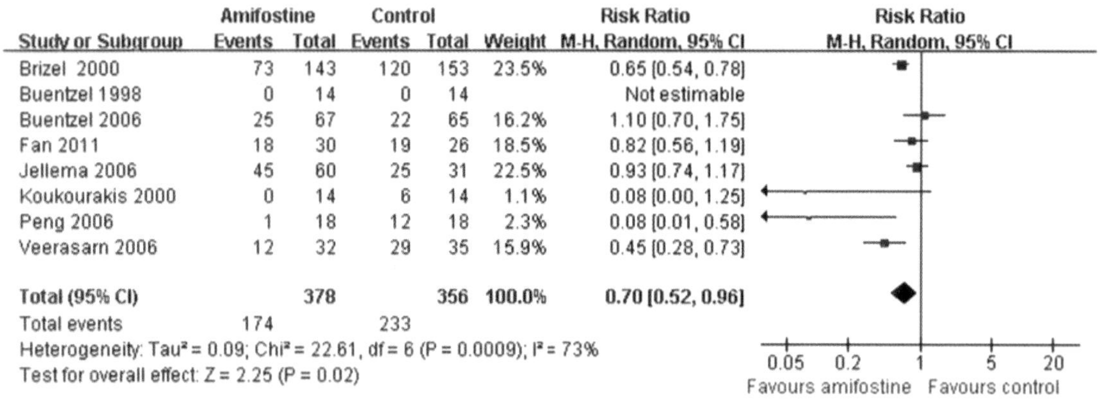

Figure 4. Forest plot of acute xerostomia in HNSCC patients treated with radiotherapy/concomitant chemoradiation. The squares and horizontal lines demonstrate the study-specific OR and 95% CI. The area of the squares reflects the study specific weight (inverse of the variance). The diamond represents the pooled OR and 95% CI.

indicating that hypodermic administration of the drug may substantially reduce these side-effects[44].

Discussion

About half a million cases of head and neck squamous cell carcinomas are diagnosed yearly around the world[45]. The majority of the new cases of head and neck cancer have locally advanced disease. Management of these patients is complex because the vital structures in this area. Radiotherapy or chemoradiation is the most common used strategy at this stage. However, the radiation-related toxicities are inevitable and sometimes vital with the increase of radiotherapy dose. In the past several decades, researchers have been investigating use of drugs to decrease the side effects during radiotherapy, in order to increase the amount of radiation that can be safely administered to the patients. Amifostine is one of the radioprotector initially developed as part of the nuclear warfare program. Some randomized controlled trials demonstrated that this drug reduced some of severity radiation-related toxic effects (acute or late xerostomia) without tumor protection. However, some other trials do not support this. So, we performed this systematic review and meta-analysis to compile the inconsistent evidence together to evaluate the true clinical efficacy of this drug.

In this meta-analysis, we generally find that use of amifostine significantly reduced the radiation-induced toxicities of serious mucositis($p<0.00001$), acute or late xerostomia($p=0.02$), and dysphagia($p<0.00001$). However, the subgroup analysis, according to the treatment regimen (radiation only or concurrent chemoradiotherapy), demonstrate that patients receiving concomitant chemoradiation can not benefit reduction of side effects from use of amifostine. Heterogeneity between trials in this subgroup analysis set was found. And the trials included in this subset had inconsistent estimate points that statistically significant favored the amifostine or placebo/observation. So, the definitive efficacy of this drug in HNSCC patients receiving concomitant chemoradiation is conservative.

Two major controversy for clinical use of amifostine is tumor protection and its toxicity. Some oncologists argued that amifostine may reduce treatment effectiveness by stopping tumor tissue responding to radiation[8]. Morever, some opponents point out that there are not enough evidence to justify the conservative tumor protective effects of this drug[46]. However, considering the realities of randomized controlled trials and practice, absolute rejection the tumor protective effects compromised by amifostine is difficult. To demonstrate a hypothetical 40%–45% reduction of survival odds ($\alpha = 0.05$; 80% power), 2492 patients would require in the trial, which was highly impractical[46].Under this situation, meta-analysis was conducted where possible to gain an objective consensus from repeatedly inconsistent trials. In this systematic review, we did not found statistical significant difference in

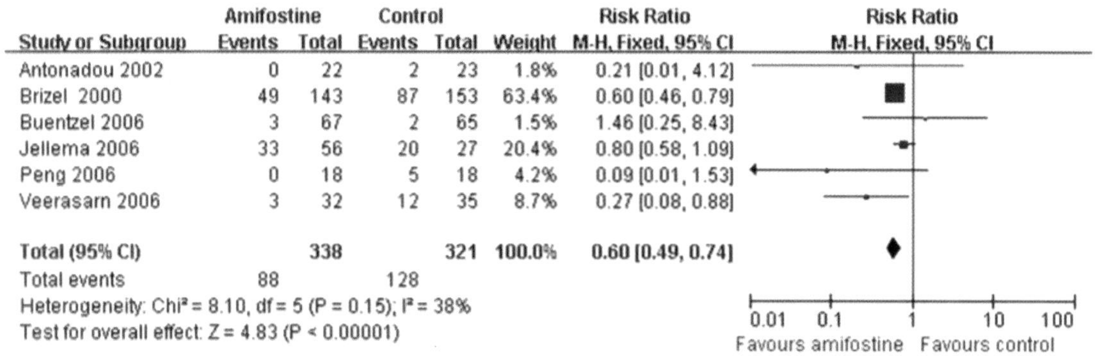

Figure 5. Forest plot of late xerostomia in HNSCC patients treated with radiotherapy/concomitant chemoradiation. The squares and horizontal lines demonstrate the study-specific OR and 95% CI. The area of the squares reflects the study specific weight (inverse of the variance). The diamond represents the pooled OR and 95% CI.

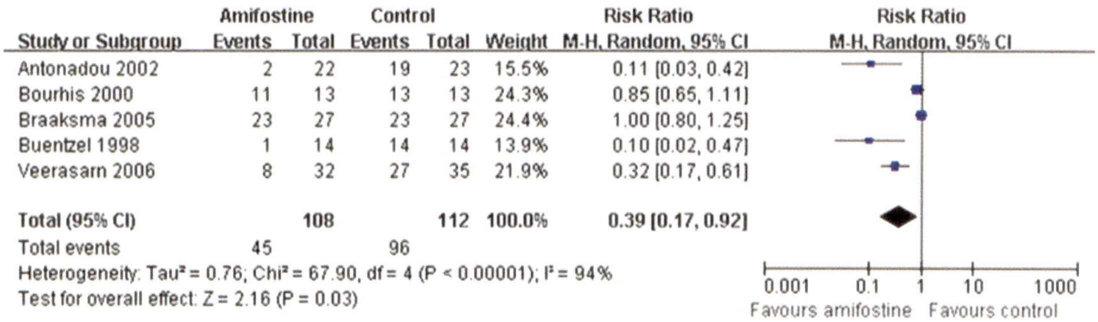

Figure 6. Forest plot of dysphagia in HNSCC patients treated with radiotherapy/concomitant chemoradiation. The squares and horizontal lines demonstrate the study-specific OR and 95% CI. The area of the squares reflects the study specific weight (inverse of the variance). The diamond represents the pooled OR and 95% CI.

complete response (RR,1.02; 95%CI,0.89–1.17; $p=0.76$) and partial response (RR,0.90; 95%CI,0.56–1.44; $p=0.66$) between the groups. However, without enough individual data, the disease-free survival (DFS) and overall survival (OS) were not pooled in this meta-analysis. However, Bourish *et al* [47] published a meta-analysis about effect of amifostine on survival among patients treated by radiotherapy with individual patients data recently. In that meta-analysis, twelve randomized trials consisted of 1119 patients were analyzed in the study and the result showed that amifostine did not reduce OS and DFS in patients treated with radiotherapy or concomitant chemoradiotherapy. So, we concluded that amifostine does not protect the tumor during radiation.

Another controversial issue about amifostine is toxicities induced by itself. The most common side effects of this drug were nausea, vomiting or transient hypotension, ranging from 5% to 30% according to the literatures[7,32,33]. Our study showed that the average incidence of Grade 3–4 nausea, emesis, hypotension and allergic were 5%, 6%, 4% and 4% respectively. Of the nine trials that reported the amifostine-induced toxic effects, 8 delivered the drug by intravenous injection and only one by subcutaneously, indicating that subcutaneous administration of this drug may substantially reduce these side-effects. However, we also find, in the subgroup analysis, that significant reduction of Grade 3–4 mucositis can not be reached in patients receive amifostine subcutaneously($p=0.24$).

The results of this meta-analysis were based on published randomized controlled trials not on individual patients' data. The results should therefore be interpreted cautiously. Although no evident of publication bias was found in this study by Egger's test,

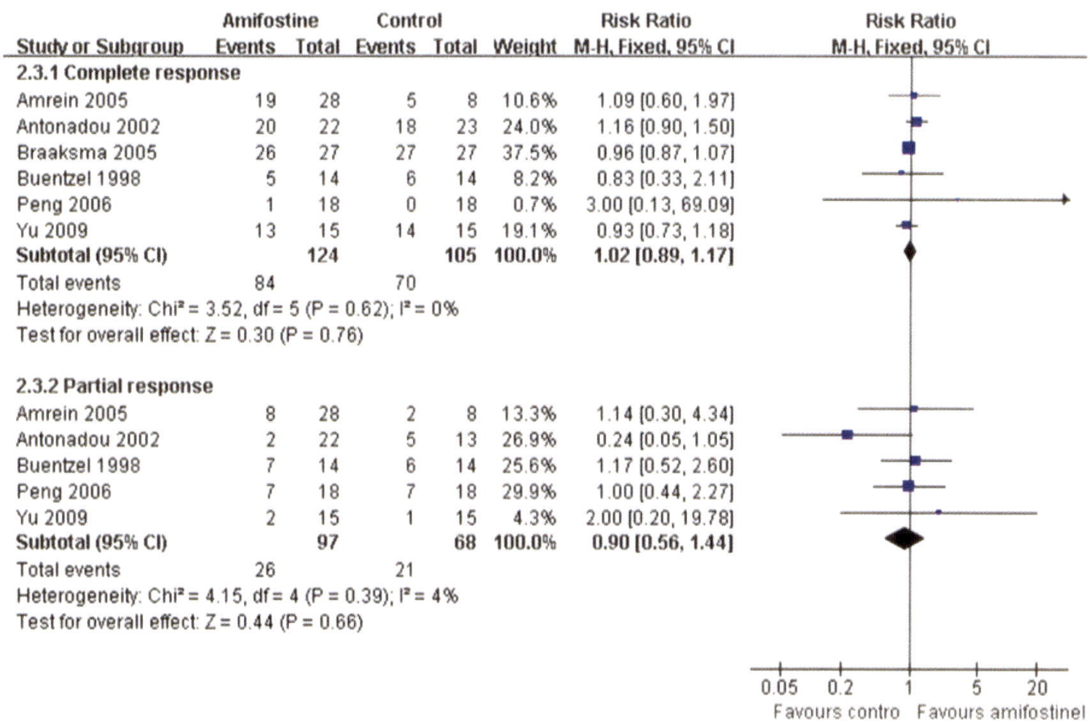

Figure 7. Forest plot of acute response rate in HNSCC patients treated with radiotherapy/concomitant chemoradiation. The squares and horizontal lines demonstrate the study-specific OR and 95% CI. The area of the squares reflects the study specific weight (inverse of the variance). The diamond represents the pooled OR and 95% CI.

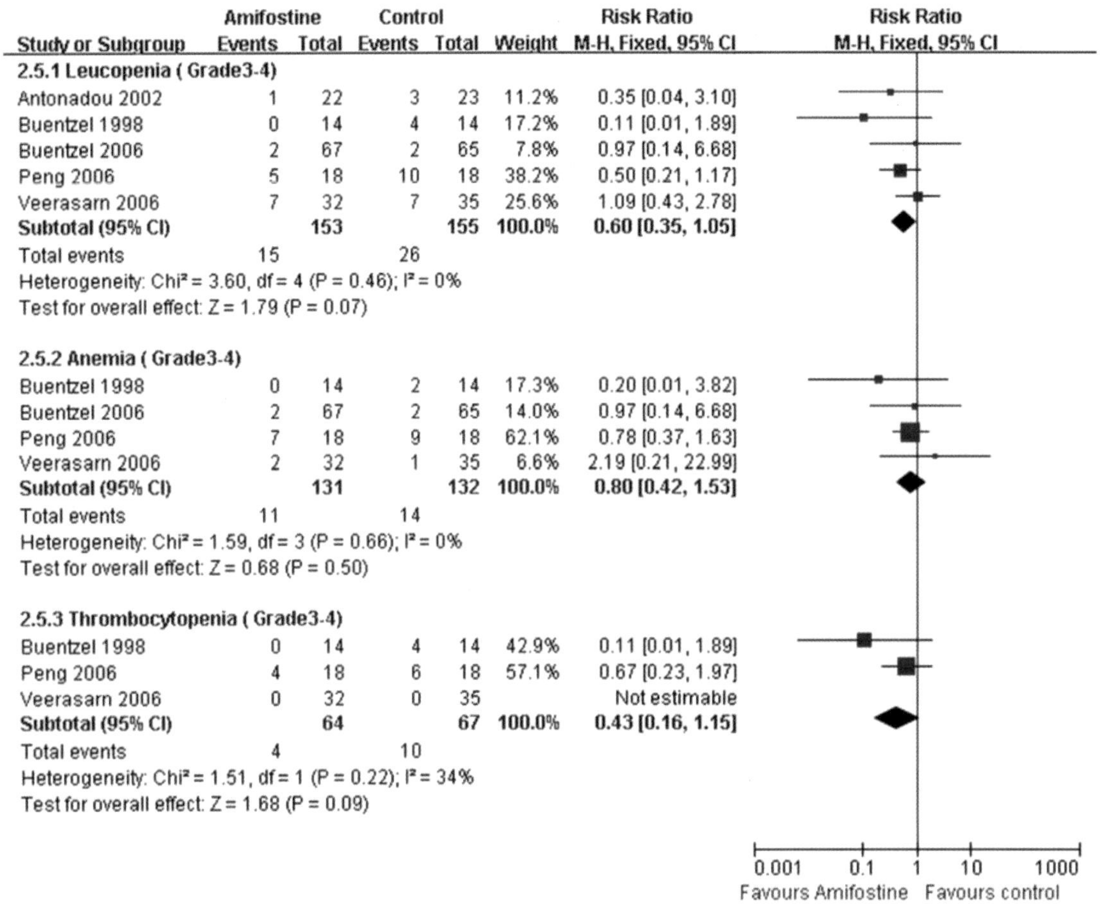

Figure 8. Forest plot of hematological toxicity in HNSCC patients treated with radiotherapy/concomitant chemoradiation. The squares and horizontal lines demonstrate the study-specific OR and 95% CI. The area of the squares reflects the study specific weight (inverse of the variance). The diamond represents the pooled OR and 95% CI.

the small number of trials and possible existence of unpublished studies are inevitable and completely ruling out this possibility in all aspects is difficult[48].

In conclusion, this systematic review demonstrates that amifostine concurrently with RT significantly reduced the side effects of serious mucositis, acute/late xerastomia and dysphagia without protection of the tumor in HNSCC patients. The reduction of radiation-induced toxicities by amifostine should be weighed against the toxicities of amifostine itself according to the individual treatment strategy. Therefore, amifostine does have a role during radiation, a role that is still evolving. Well-designed RCTs are the necessary investments that will further explore the potential benefits of amifostine.

Author Contributions

Conceived and designed the experiments: FH J-DG. Performed the experiments: S-WZ J-DG HW. Analyzed the data: J-DG FH YL. Contributed reagents/materials/analysis tools: J-DG FH. Wrote the paper: J-DG X-BL.

References

1. Toledano I, Graff P, Serre A, Boisselier P, Bensadoun RJ, et al. (2012) Intensity-modulated radiotherapy in head and neck cancer: results of the prospective study GORTEC 2004-03. Radiother Oncol 103(1): 57–62.
2. Cvek J, Kubes J, Skacelikova E, Otahal B, Kominek P, et al. (2012) Hyperfractionated accelerated radiotherapy with concomitant integrated boost of 70–75 Gy in 5 weeks for advanced head and neck cancer: A phase I does escalation study. Strahlenther Onkol 188(8): 666–670.
3. Brizel DM, Wasserman TH, Henke M, Strnad V, Rudat V, et al. (2000) Phase III randomized trial of amifostine as a radioprotector in head and neck cancer. J Clin Oncol 18(19): 3339–3345.
4. Koukourakis MI (2002) Amifostine in clinical oncology: current use and future applications. Anticancer Drugs 13(3): 181–209.
5. Veerasarn V, Phromratanapongse P, Suntornpong N, Lorvidhaya V, Sukthomya V, et al. (2006) Effect of Amifostine to prevent radiotherapy-induced acute and late toxicity in head and neck cancer patients who had normal or mild impaired salivary gland function. J Med Assoc Thai 89(12): 2056–2067.
6. Buentzel J, Micke O, Adamietz IA, Monnier A, Glatzel M, et al. (2006) Intravenous amifostine during chemoradiotherapy for head-and-neck cancer: Arandomized placebo-controlled phase III study. Int J Radiat Oncol Biol Phys 64(3): 684–691.
7. Jellema AP, Slotman BJ, Muller MJ, Leemans CR, Smeele LE, et al. (2006) Radiotherapy alone, versus radiotherapy with amifostine 3 times weekly, versus radiotherapy with amifostine 5 times weekly: A prospective randomized study in squamous cell head and neck cancer. Cancer 107(3): 544–553.
8. Koukourakis MI (2003) Amifostine: is there evidence of tumor protection? Semin Oncol 30(6 Suppl 18): 18–30.

9. Higgins JP, Green S (2008) Cochrane Handbook for Systematic Reviews of Interventions updated March 2011 John Wiley & Sons, Available: http://www.cochrane-handbook.org/.Accessed: 2011 DEC 12.
10. Cox JD, Stetz J, Pajak TF (1995) Toxicity criteria of the Radiation Therapy Oncology Group (RTOG) and the EuropeanOrganization for Research and Treatment of Cancer (EORTC). Int J Radiat Oncol Biol Phys 31(5): 1341–1346.
11. DerSimonian R, Laird N (1986) Meta-analysis in clinical trials. Control Clin Trials 7(3): 177–188.
12. Higgins JP, Thompson SG, Deeks JJ, Altman DG (2003) Measuring inconsistency in meta-analyses. BMJ 327(7414): 557–560.
13. Egger M, Davey SG, Schneider M, Minder C (1997) Bias in meta-analysis detected by a simple, graphical test. BMJ 315(7109): 629–634.
14. Wasserman TH, Brizel DM, Henke M, Monnier A, Eschwege F, et al. (2005) Influence of intravenous amifostine on xerostomia, tumor control, and survival after radiotherapy for head-and- neck cancer: 2-year follow-up of a prospective, randomized, phase III trial. Int J Radiat Oncol Biol Phys 63(4): 985–990.
15. Bennett CL, Lane D, Stinson T, Glatzel M, Buntzel J (2001) Economic analysis of amifostine as adjunctive support for patients with advanced head and neck cancer: preliminary results from a randomized phase II clinical trial from Germany. Cancer Invest 19(2): 107–113.
16. Buntzel J, Schuth J, Kuttner K, Glatzel M (1998) Radiochemotherapy with amifostine cytoprotection for head and neck cancer. Support Care Cancer 6(2): 155-160.
17. Anne PR, Machtay M, Rosenthal DI, Brizel DM, Morrison WH, et al. (2007) A Phase II trial of subcutaneous amifostine and radiation therapy in patients with head-and-neck cancer. Int J Radiat Oncol Biol Phys 67(2): 445–452.
18. Abitbol A, Abdel-Wahab M, Harvey M, Lewin A, Troner M, et al. (2005) Phase II study of tolerance and efficacy of hyperfractionated radiation therapy and 5-fluorouracil, cisplatin, and paclitaxel (taxol) and amifostine (ethyol) in head and neck squamous cell carcinomas: A-3 protocol. Am J Clin Oncol 28(5): 449–455.
19. Trog D, Bank P, Wendt TG, Koscielny S, Beleites E (1999) Daily amifostine given concomitantly to chemoradiation in head and neck cancer. Apilot study. Strahlenther Onkol 175(9): 444–449.
20. Rosenthal DI, Chambers MS, Weber RS, Eisbruch A (2004) A phase II study to assess the efficacy of amifostine for submandibular/sublingual salivary sparing during the treatment of head and neck cancer with intensity modulated radiation therapy for parotid salivary sparing. Semin Oncol 31(6 Suppl 18): 25–28.
21. Zoberi I, Wasserman TH, Chao KS (2002) A prospective, nonrandomized study of the impact of amifostine on subsequent hypothyroidism in irradiated patients with head and neck cancers. Semin Radiat Oncol 12(1 Suppl 1): 14–17.
22. Suntharalingam M, Jaboin J, Taylor R, Wolf J, Banglore M, et al. (2004) The evaluation of amifostine for mucosal protection in patients with advanced loco-regional squamous cell carcinomas of the head and neck (SCCHN) treated with concurrent weekly carboplatin, paclitaxel, and daily radiotherapy (RT). Semin Oncol 31(6 Suppl 18): 2–7.
23. Thorstad WL, Haughey B, Chao KS (2003) Pilot study of subcutaneous amifostine in patients undergoing postoperative intensity modulated radiation therapy for head and neck cancer: preliminary data. Semin Oncol 30(6 Suppl 18): 96–100.
24. Vacha P, Fehlauer F, Mahlmann B, Marx M, Hinke A, et al. (2003) Randomized phase III trial of postoperative radiochemotherapy +/− amifostine in head and neck cancer. Is there evidence for radioprotection. Strahlenther Onkol 179(6): 385–389.
25. Wasserman T, Mackowiak JI, Brizel DM, Oster W, Zhang J, et al. (2000) Effect of amifostine on patient assessed clinical benefit in irradiated head and neck cancer. Int J Radiat Oncol Biol Phys 48(4): 1035–1039.
26. Thorstad WL, Chao KS, Haughey B (2004) Toxicity and compliance of subcutaneous amifostine in patients undergoing postoperative intensity-modulated radiation therapy for head and neck cancer. Semin Oncol 31 (6 Suppl 18): 8–12.
27. Chao KS, Ozyigit G, Thorsdad WL (2003) Toxicity profile of intensity-modulated radiation therapy for head and neck carcinoma and potential role of amifostine. Semin Oncol 30 (6 Suppl 18): 101–108.
28. Machtay M, Rosenthal DI, Chalian AA, Lustig R, Hershock D, et al. (2004) Pilot study of postoperative reirradiation, chemotherapy, and amifostine after surgical salvage for recurrent head-and-neck cancer. Int J Radiat Oncol Biol Phys 59(1): 72–77.
29. Bardet E, Martin L, Calais G, Tuchais C, Bourhis J, et al. (2002) Preliminary data of the GORTEC 2000-02 phase III trial comparing intravenous and subcutaneous administration of amifostine for head and neck tumors treated by external radiotherapy. Semin Oncol 29 (6 Suppl 19): 57–60.
30. Anacak Y, Kamer S, Haydaroglu A (2005) Daily subcutaneous amifostine administration during irradiation of pediatric head and neck cancers. Pediatr Blood Cancer 48(5): 579–581.
31. Amrein PC, Clark JR, Supko JG, Fabian RL, Wang CC, et al. (2005) Phase I trial and pharmacokinetics of escalating doses of paclitaxel and concurrent hyperfractionated radiotherapy with or without amifostine in patients with advanced head and neck carcinoma. Cancer 104(7): 1418–1827.
32. Antonadou D, Pepelassi M, Synodinou M, Puglisi M, Throuvalas N (2002) Prophylactic use of amifostine to prevent radiochemotherapy-induced mucositis and xerostomia in head-and-neck cancer. Int J Radiat Oncol Biol Phys 52(3): 739–747.
33. Bourhis J, De Crevoisier R, Abdulkarim B, Deutsch E, Lusinchi A, et al. (2000) A randomized study of very accelerated radiotherapy with and without amifostine in head and neck squamous cell carcinoma. Int J Radiat Oncol Biol Phys 46(5): 1105–1108.
34. Braaksma M, van Agthoven M, Nijdam W, Uyl-de GC, Levendag P (2005) Costs of treatment intensification for head and neck cancer: concomitant chemoradiation randomised for radioprotection with amifostine. Eur J Cancer 41(14): 2102–2111.
35. Buntzel J, Kuttner K, Frohlich D, Glatzel M (1998) Selective cytoprotection with amifostine in concurrent radiochemotherapy for head and neck cancer. Ann Oncol 9(5): 505–509.
36. Haddad R, Sonis S, Posner M, Wirth L, Costello R, et al. (2009) Randomized phase 2 study of concomitant chemoradiotherapy using weeklycarboplatin/paclitaxel carboplatin/paclitaxel with or without daily subcutaneous amifostine in patients with locally advanced head and neck cancer. Cancer 115(19): 4514–4523.
37. Peng LH, Sun Y, Zhang XL, Zhang Q, Fu S (2006) Efficacy of Amifostine on Patients with Head and Neck Squamous Cell Carcinomas Undergoing Radiation Therapy and Chemotherapy. China Pharmacy 17(5): 1166–1168.
38. Fan ZG, Lin HX, Liu ZQ, He QH, Zhang SL, et al. (2011) Protective effect of amifostine for mucositis and xerostomia in nasopharyngeal carcinoma patients treated with irradiation. Military Medical Journal of Southeast China 13(2): 146–148.
39. Koukourakis MI, Kyrias G, Kakolyris S, Kouroussis C, Frangiadaki C (2000) Subcutaneous administration of amifostine during fractionated radiotherapy: a randomized phase II study. J Clin Oncol 18(11): 2226–2233.
40. Zhang N, Xu LJ, Ding JY (2010) Protection effect of amifostine on oral mucosa in patients treated with concurrent chemoradiation. Chin J Prim Med Pharm 17(5): 668–669.
41. Jiang F, Chen XZ, Wang FZ (2009) Effects of amifostine on nasopharyngeal patients treated with chemoradiotherapy. Chin J Radiol Med Prot 29(6): 612–613.
42. Yu DS, Zhao W, Wu XL, Huang ZQ, Huang RB (2009) Amifostine in Prevention of Radiation induced Xerostomia. Journal of Sun Yatsen University(Medical Sciences) 30(4S): 86–87;95.
43. He XY, Hu CS, Wu YR (2004) Radioprotective Effect of Amifostine in Nasopharyngeal Carcinoma. Fudan Univ J Med Sci 31(1): 53–58.
44. Anne PR, Curran WJ Jr (2002) A phase II trial of subcutaneous amifostine and radiation therapy in patients with head and neck cancer. Semin Radiat Oncol 12 (1 Suppl 1): 18–19.
45. Jemal A, Bray F, Center MM, Ferlay J, Ward E, et al. (2011) Global cancer statistics. CA Cancer J Clin 61(2): 69–90.
46. Brizel DM, Overgaard J (2003) Does amifostine have a role in chemoradiation treatment. Lancet Oncol 4(6): 378–381.
47. Bourhis J, Blanchard P, Maillard E, Brizel DM, Movsas B, et al. (2011) Effect of amifostine on survival among patients treated with radiotherapy: meta-analysis of individual patient data. J Clin Oncol 29(18): 2590–2597.
48. Trinquart L, Abbe A, Ravaud P (2012) Impact of reporting bias in network meta-analysis of antidepressant placebo-controlled trials. PLOS ONE 7(4): e35219.

26

AKT Inhibitors Promote Cell Death in Cervical Cancer through Disruption of mTOR Signaling and Glucose Uptake

Ramachandran Rashmi[1], Carl DeSelm[1], Cynthia Helms[2], Anne Bowcock[2,5], Buck E. Rogers[1,6], Janet Rader[7], Perry W. Grigsby[1,4,5,6], Julie K. Schwarz[1,3,6]*

1 Department of Radiation Oncology, Washington University School of Medicine, St. Louis, Missouri, United States of America, **2** Department of Genetics, Washington University School of Medicine, St. Louis, Missouri, United States of America, **3** Department of Cell Biology and Physiology, Washington University School of Medicine, St. Louis, Missouri, United States of America, **4** Division of Nuclear Medicine, Mallinckrodt Institute of Radiology, Washington University School of Medicine, St. Louis, Missouri, United States of America, **5** Division of Gynecologic Oncology, Washington University School of Medicine, St. Louis, Missouri, United States of America, **6** Alvin J. Siteman Cancer Center, Washington University School of Medicine, St. Louis, Missouri, United States of America, **7** Dept of Obstetrics and Gynecology, Medical College of Wisconsin, Milwaukee, Wisconsin, United States of America

Abstract

Background: PI3K/AKT pathway alterations are associated with incomplete response to chemoradiation in human cervical cancer. This study was performed to test for mutations in the PI3K pathway and to evaluate the effects of AKT inhibitors on glucose uptake and cell viability.

Experimental Design: Mutational analysis of DNA from 140 pretreatment tumor biopsies and 8 human cervical cancer cell lines was performed. C33A cells (*PIK3CAR88Q* and *PTENR233**) were treated with increasing concentrations of two allosteric AKT inhibitors (SC-66 and MK-2206) with or without the glucose analogue 2-deoxyglucose (2-DG). Cell viability and activation status of the AKT/mTOR pathway were determined in response to the treatment. Glucose uptake was evaluated by incubation with ^{18}F-fluorodeoxyglucose (FDG). Cell migration was assessed by scratch assay.

Results: Activating *PIK3CA* (E545K, E542K) and inactivating *PTEN* (R233*) mutations were identified in human cervical cancer. SC-66 effectively inhibited AKT, mTOR and mTOR substrates in C33A cells. SC-66 inhibited glucose uptake via reduced delivery of Glut1 and Glut4 to the cell membrane. SC-66 (1 µg/ml-56%) and MK-2206 (30 µM-49%) treatment decreased cell viability through a non-apoptotic mechanism. Decreases in cell viability were enhanced when AKT inhibitors were combined with 2-DG. The scratch assay showed a substantial reduction in cell migration upon SC-66 treatment.

Conclusions: The mutational spectrum of the PI3K/AKT pathway in cervical cancer is complex. AKT inhibitors effectively block mTORC1/2, decrease glucose uptake, glycolysis, and decrease cell viability *in vitro*. These results suggest that AKT inhibitors may improve response to chemoradiation in cervical cancer.

Editor: Jin Q. Cheng, H.Lee Moffitt Cancer Center & Research Institute, United States of America

Funding: This work was supported by grant funding from the NIH (US NIH 5K12HD00145910) to Julie K. Schwarz, MD, PhD. CD was supported by Research Medical Student Grant (#RMS113) from the Radiological Society of North America (Julie K. Schwarz mentor). The Siteman Cancer Center is supported by NCI Cancer Center Support Grant #P30 CA91842. The funders had no role in study design, data collection and analysis, decision to publish, or preparation of the manuscript.

Competing Interests: The authors have declared that no competing interests exist.

* E-mail: jschwarz@radonc.wustl.edu

Introduction

Globally, cervical cancer is the third most common female cancer, and it ranks fourth in terms of mortality [1]. Concurrent chemoradiation (pelvic irradiation with the concurrent administration of cisplatin chemotherapy) is the standard of care for patients with locally advanced cervical cancer. We have previously demonstrated that the results of post-therapy [^{18}F]-fluoro-deoxy-glucose-positron emission tomography (FDG-PET) are predictive of progression-free and overall survival outcomes after chemoradiation [2–4]. Presently there are no effective treatment options available for patients whose tumors fail to respond to traditional chemoradiation.

Recently, we identified PI3K/AKT pathway alterations in tumors from patients with a positive post-therapy FDG-PET. We also observed high p-AKT expression in pre-treatment biopsy samples, and patients whose tumors expressed high levels of p-AKT had decreased survival outcomes and increased metastatic disease after standard chemoradiation [5]. Genetic alterations leading to activation of the PI3K/AKT/mTOR pathway are associated with treatment resistance in variety of solid tumors [6]. Several PI3K/AKT inhibitors have been evaluated in clinical trials for breast and other cancers with positive responses in patients with PI3K/AKT alterations [7]. There are reports suggesting that cancers with *PIK3CA* mutations are more sensitive to AKT or PI3K/mTOR inhibitors [8,9].

We hypothesized that PI3K/AKT inhibitors will improve response to chemoradiation in cervical tumors with PI3K/AKT pathway alterations. To test for mutations in the PI3K/AKT pathway, we analyzed 140 pretreatment cervical tumor biopsies and 8 human cervical cancer cell lines [10]. We then selected the cervical cancer cell line C33A, which is mutated for both *PIK3CA* and *PTEN* (*PIK3CA* R88Q, *PTEN* R233*) and expresses high levels of p-AKT at baseline, to assess the response to two allosteric AKT inhibitors, SC-66 and MK-2206.

Materials and Methods

Patients

The study population included 140 patients prospectively enrolled into tumor banking studies at the time of diagnosis of cervical cancer (March 1998 through July 2011). Approval from the institutional Human Research Protection Office was obtained for this study, and all patients signed informed consent. Clinical follow-up including FDG-PET imaging was performed for each patient according to institutional guidelines as previously described [3]. At the time of last follow up, 76 patients had no evidence of disease, and 8 patients were alive with disease; 7 patients had died due to intercurrent illness; 2 patients had died due to treatment-related toxicity, and 47 patients had died due to cervical cancer. Median follow up for patients alive at the time of last follow up was 41 months (range 4 to 161 months).

Statistical analysis

Survival and tumor recurrence were measured from the completion of treatment. The Kaplan-Meier (product-limit) method was used to derive estimates of survival [11]. Tests of the equivalence of estimates of survival between patient groups were performed by the generalized Wilcoxon log-rank test. Statview version 5.0.1 software (SAS Institute Inc., Cary, NC) was used for the analysis.

Mutational analysis using MALDI-TOF

Tumor biopsies were sectioned and reviewed for tumor cell content as previously described [5]. Tumor DNA was prepared using standard methods by the Washington University Tissue Procurement Core Facility. Assays for a subset of 32 selected oncogenic mutations (*AKT1*, *AKT2*, *PIK3CA* and *PTEN*) from [10] were redesigned into three genotyping multiplexes, using Sequenom's Assay Designer software, version 3.1.2.2. (Sequenom Inc, San Diego, CA). The multiplexes were designed to use the iPLEX chemistry. The Sequenom MassARRAY system (http://www.sequenom.com) employs MALDI-TOF (Matrix-Assisted Laser Desorption/Ionization – Time of Flight) mass spectrometry to measure mass differences following single-base additions to extension primers. Spectral peaks corresponding to expected masses for each extended primer are transformed into sample genotype calls. Using the standard iPLEX protocol, the Genotyping core at Washington University (St. Louis, MO, USA) processed 15 ng sample DNA per multiplex through the MassARRAY system. Peak areas representing normal and mutant base additions were obtained from each sample's mass spectrum. A mutation was considered present in a sample when the mutant peak was responsible for 25% or more of the combined peak areas, and absent when the mutant peak area was less than 25% of the total. List of OncoMap mutations that were tested in our multiplexes are OM_00970-AKT1-E17K, OM_00032-AKT2-S302G,OM_00033-AKT2-R371H, OM_00241-PIK3CA-R88Q,OM_00242-PIK3CA-N345K,OM_00243-PIK3CA-C420R, OM_00246A-PIK3CA-E545K, OM_00248-PIK3CA-H701P, OM_00249-PIK3CA-H1047L, OM_00250A-PIK3CA-H1047R, OM_00250B-PIK3CA-H1047R,OM_00251-PIK3CA-H1047Y,OM_01017-PIK3CA-E545A, OM_01018B-PIK3CA-N1068fs*4,OM_0102-PIK3CA-Y1021C,OM_00839-PTEN-R173C,OM_00840-PTEN-R173H,OM_00841-PTEN-R233*,OM_00842-PTEN-R335*, OM_01038-PTEN-K267fs*9 OM_01039-PTEN-V317fs*3, OM_01069-PTEN-K6fs*4.

Cell culture and Reagents

Cervical cancer cell lines were maintained in IMDM media (Life Technologies, CA) with 10% heat inactivated FBS and incubated at 37°C in 5% CO_2. SC-66 was purchased from Biovision (Milpitas, CA) and MK-2206 from Selleck Chemicals (Houston, TX). 2-Deoxy glucose, protease and phosphatase inhibitor cocktails were purchased from Sigma (Saint Louis, MO). All drugs for cell culture were dissolved in dimethyl sulfoxide (DMSO, Sigma). siRNA oligos against *AKT1*, *AKT2* and *RICTOR* were purchased from Sigma (Saint Louis, MO).

Western blotting and membrane isolation

Phosphorylation of AKT and downstream targets of AKT and mTOR pathway with or without SC-66 (6–10 µg/ml) and MK-2206 (0–2.5 µM) were determined by western blotting with primary antibodies against phosphorylated and total forms of mTOR, p70s6k, 4E-BP1, S6, GSK3-β, FOXO $pAKT^{Thr308}$, $pAKT^{Thr450}$ and $pAKT^{Ser473}$ (1:1000; Cell Signaling Technology, MA), total forms of AKT, mTOR and 4-EBP1 (1:1000, Cell Signaling Technology, MA), total forms of p70s6k and β-Actin HRP from Santa Cruz Biotechnology, CA and total forms of PRAS40 and FOXO from millipore (1:5000, Santa Cruz Biotechnology,CA). β-Actin was used as the internal control. Blots were probed with HRP-conjugated anti-rabbit (Cell Signaling Technology, Beverly, MA) or anti-mouse polyclonal IgG secondary antibodies (Santa Cruz Biotechnology, CA) for 1 h at RT. For detection Pierce West Dura substrate (Pierce Biotechnology) was used according to manufacturer's protocol and exposed on X-ray film.

Cell viability and Annexin staining

For the cell viability assay C33A cells were treated with the allosteric AKT inhibitors SC-66 (0.0001 µg/ml–5 µg/ml) and MK-2206 (125 nM-30 µM) with or without the glucose analogue 2-deoxyglucose (2-DG) (5–20 mM) using dose titration and time courses. For siRNA experiments, C33A cells were transiently transfected and assessed for protein expression after 48 hours. Cell viability was tested using Alamar Blue from Life Technologies, according to manufacturer's instructions. Annexin/7-AAD staining was performed 24 h post-treatment, using a kit from BD, Biosciences following manufacturer's instructions, and cells were analyzed by flow cytometry.

FDG uptake assays

The FDG uptake assay was performed as described previously [5]. Briefly, cells were seeded and pretreated with the block (Cytochalasin B) for 30 min followed by AKT inhibitors for an additional 30 min. After this, ^{18}FDG was added to glucose free medium for 1 h. Cells were washed, harvested and counted on a gamma counter.

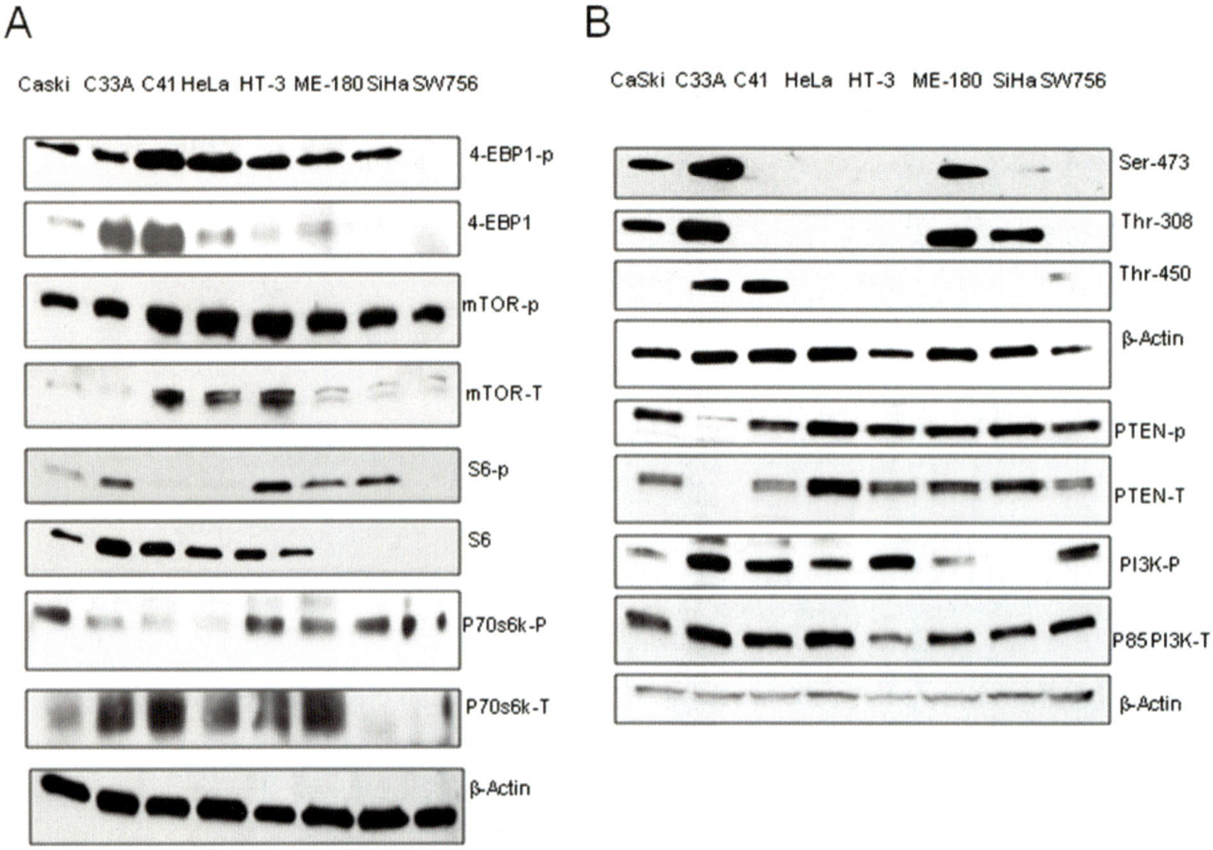

C

Mutational Analysis Cell lines

SAMPLE	AKT2 S302G	AKT2 R371H	PIK3CA R88Q	PIK3CA N345K	PIK3CA C420R	PIK3CA E545K	PIK3CA H701P	AKT1 E17K	PIK3CA Y1021C	PTEN R173C	PTEN R233'
C33a	AGT	CGC	CAA	AAT	TGT	GAG	CAC	GAG	TAC	CGC	TGA
C41	AGT	CGC	CGA	AAT	TGT	GAG	CAC	GAG	TAC	CGC	CGA
Hela	AGT	CGC	CGA	AAT	TGT	GAG	CAC	GAG	TAC	CGC	CGA
HT3	AGT	CGC	CGA	AAT	TGT	GAG	CAC	GAG	TAC	CGC	CGA
ME180	AGT	CGC	CGA	AAT	TGT	AAG	CAC	GAG	TAC	CGC	CGA
SiHa	AGT	CGC	CGA	AAT	TGT	GAG	CAC	GAG	TAC	CGC	CGA
SW756	AGT	CGC	CGA	AAT	TGT	GAG	CAC	GAG	TAC	CGC	CGA
CaSKi	AGT	CGC	CGA	AAT	TGT	AAG	CAC	GAG	TAC	TGC	CGA
Normal	AGT	CGC	CGA	AAT	TGT	GAG	CAC	GAG	TAC	CGC	CGA

Figure 1. PI3K/AKT pathway analysis in cervical cancer cell lines. (A–B) mTOR pathway components and phosphorylated forms of AKT were tested using commercially available antibodies on eight cervical cancer cell lysates prepared without any treatment. (C) *PIK3CA*, *AKT*, and *PTEN* gene mutational status of 8 human cervical cancer cell lines.

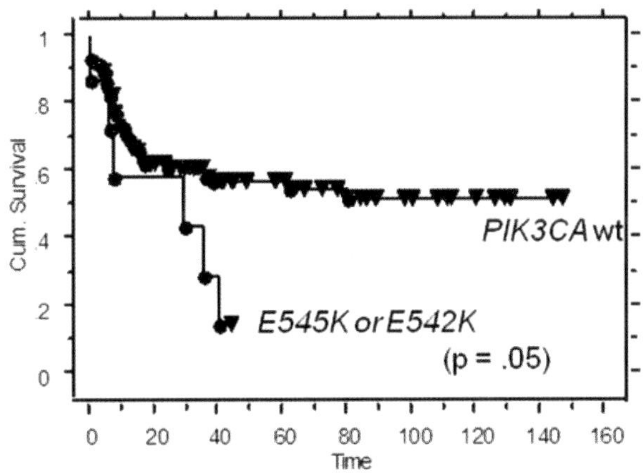

Figure 2. Cervical cancer patients with E545K or E542K mutant tumors have inferior survival outcomes after standard chemoradiation (cisplatin plus pelvic RT). Kaplan Meier curve for progression-free survival for cervical cancer patients with wild type PIK3CA versus E545K or E542K mutant tumors (p = .05).

Immunofluorescence

In a chamber slide (8-well) 25,000 cells were seeded and treated with SC-66 1 μg/ml for 3 h and fixed using 4% p-formaldehyde from Electron Microscopy Sciences (Hatfield, PA) for 10 minutes. The slides were then blocked in 5% normal goat serum (Jackson ImmumoResearch, West Grove, PA) for 1 h, followed by extensive PBS washes. Then primary antibodies Glut1 and Glut4 (Abcam, Cambridge, MA) were added followed by secondary antibody conjugate with Alexa Fluor 488 (Life Technologies, Inc., Grand Island, NY). The slides were finally mounted using Prolong Gold anti-fade (Life technologies, Inc. Grand Island, NY).

Metabolic assays

Lactate assay was performed using a kit from (Sigma, Saint Louis, MO) according to manufacturer's instructions using culture media collected after deproteinization using 10 kDa spin column filters. ATP and NADP/NADPH assays were performed using the commercially available fluorometric kits from (Abcam, Cambridge, MA) according to the manufacturer's instructions using cell lysates.

Wound healing assay

One million C33A cells were plated in a 35 mm tissue culture dish and grown to confluence. Two parallel scratches were made with a 200 μL pipette tip per dish and the scratch width was measured to be the baseline [12]. The wound width was measured at a minimum of six different points for each wound. SC-66 (1 and 2.5 μg/ml) and MK-2206 (2.5 and 5 μM) were added for 24 hr. The width of the scratches was measured using Qcapture Pro software and viewed using OLYMPUS 1×70 microscope. Percent wound healing was calculated by dividing the scratch width after drug addition by the control width minus 100%. The results presented are mean ± SEM.

Results

PI3K/AKT/mTOR pathway is active in cervical cancer cell lines

A panel of human cervical cancer cell lines was tested for the expression pattern and activation status of PI3K/AKT/mTOR pathway molecules. Cell lysates were prepared without any treatment and baseline western blots were performed. P70S6K, the marker for activation of the mTOR pathway, was phosphorylated in majority of the cell lines except for HeLa, C41 and C33A where it was found to be weakly phosphorylated (Fig. 1A). Phosphorylation of 4E-BP1 and S6 were found to be low in the majority of the cell lines studied. In SiHa and SW756, the expression levels of non-phosphorylated forms of mTOR, p70s6k, 4E-BP1 and S6 were low compared to the other cell lines. On the other hand, phosphorylation of mTOR was found to be similar across the cell lines (Fig. 1A). Baseline expression of phosphorylated forms of AKT such as Ser473, Thr308 and Thr450 were determined. C33A expressed all the three forms of p-AKT. To determine the status of upstream regulators of AKT such as PI3K and PTEN, baseline p-PI3K and p-PTEN levels were examined. Phosphorylated PTEN level was similar across the cell lines, except for C33A where the level of total PTEN band was minimal. PI3K was activated in the majority of cell lines studied here. SiHa exhibited very low PI3K activation (Fig. 1B). All these results suggest that cervical cancer cell lines have activated mTOR pathway under basal conditions and wide variations existed in p-AKT levels.

Sequenom mutational analysis of PIK3CA, PTEN and AKT genes in cervical cancer

To test for mutations in the PI3K/AKT pathway, we carried out a Sequenom mutational analysis for oncogenic mutations in genes *PIK3CA*, *PTEN* and *AKT*. We did not detect any *AKT1*or *AKT2* mutations in the cervical cancer cell lines. C33A harbored an R88Q *PIK3CA* mutation. R88Q is an activating mutation found in the ABD domain of the p110α subunit of the *PIK3CA* gene. This defect is associated with enhanced enzymatic activation of PI3K protein and AKT activity *in vitro* [13,14]. We found that the E545K *PIK3CA* mutation was present in ME-180 and CaSki cells (Fig. 1C). The *PIK3CA* E545K mutation is an activating mutation in the helical domain of p110α subunit of PI3K protein. This mutation is known to confer enhanced kinase activity and to constitutively activate AKT [15]. We also found an R173C *PTEN* gene mutation in CaSki and a *PTEN* R233* mutation in C33A cells (Fig. 1C). The *PTEN* R173C mutation is associated with decreased phosphatase activity against PIP_3 [16]. The *PTEN* R233* mutation in exon 7 induces a premature stop codon into the gene, which explains the absence of *PTEN* protein expression in C33A cells [17] (Fig. 1B).

Using the Sequenom assay, we then tested for mutations in *PIK3CA*, *AKT* and *PTEN* genes in 140 pretreatment biopsies collected at our tumor bank. We did not detect any assayed mutation in the *AKT* gene in our patient population. We found that tumors in 7 out of 140 patients harbored a *PIK3CA* E545K mutation and 1 out of 140 had a *PIK3CA* E542K mutation. We also found that 1 tumor harbored a *PTEN* R233* mutation. Patients with E545K and E542K mutations in *PIK3CA* were found to display poor prognosis and shorter disease free survival after standard chemoradiation (pelvic irradiation and concurrent cisplatin chemotherapy) (p = 0.05, Fig. 2).

AKT inhibitors SC-66 and MK-2206 induce non-apoptotic cell death in PIK3CA and PTEN mutant C33A cells

Using C33A cells as a model for PI3K/AKT mutant cervical cancer, we determined whether tumor cell survival was dependent on AKT signaling. C33A cells were incubated with increasing doses of SC-66 and MK-2206 and the viability was determined after 24 and 48 hrs. Cell viability decreased starting from 1 μg/ml of SC-66 after 24 and 48 hrs, to 55% and 43% respectively. The

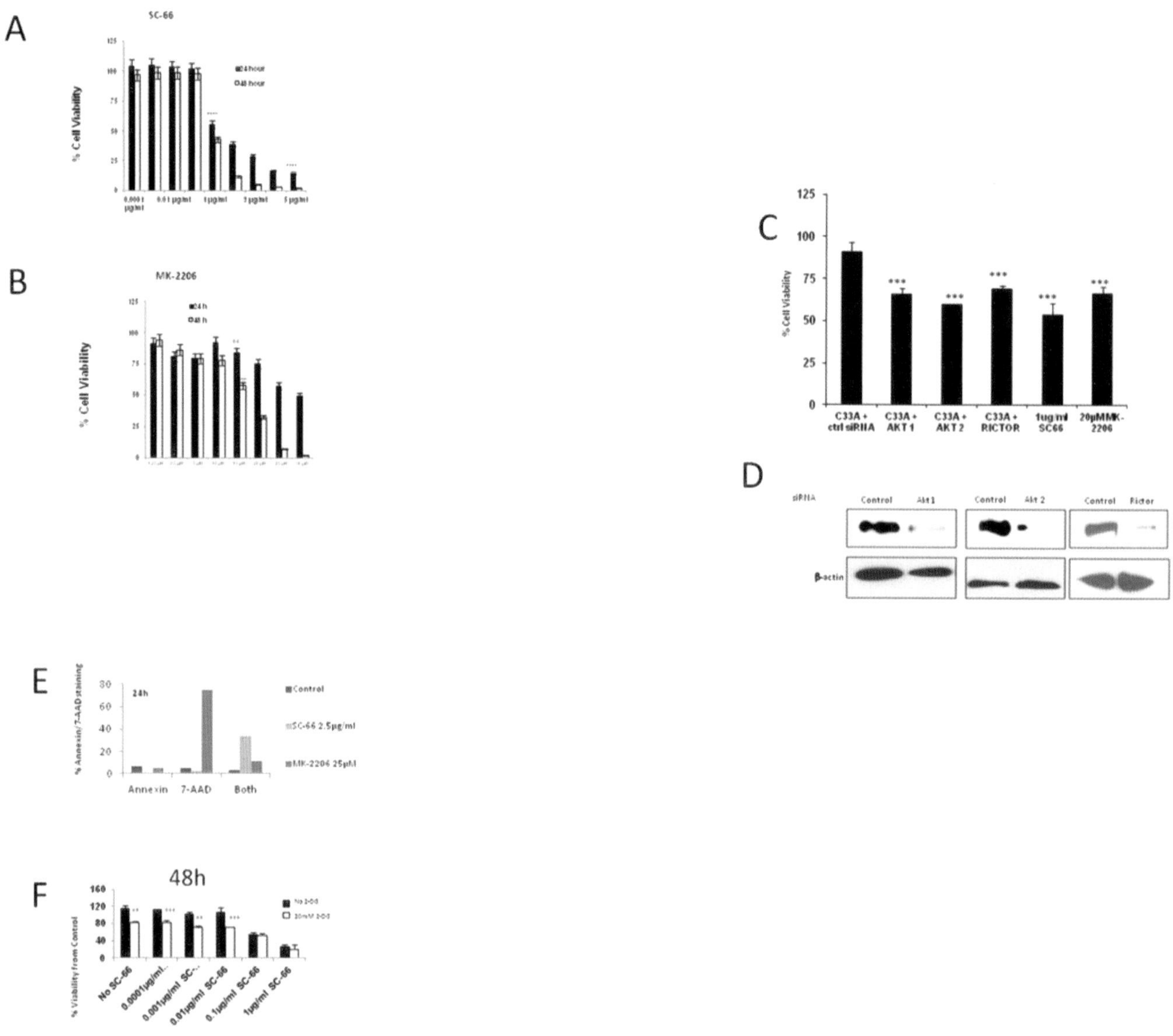

Figure 3. Effects of AKT inhibitors on cell viability. (A–B) C33A cells were seeded on to 48 well plates and treated with increasing doses of SC-66 (0.0001–5 µg/ml) and MK-2206 (1.25–30 µM) in triplicates for 24 and 48 hrs. Viability was measured using Alamar Blue. Percent viability was calculated based on vehicle treated controls. (C) C33A cells were seeded on to 48 well plates and transfected with oligos against *AKT1*, *AKT2* and *RICTOR* and treated with SC-66 (1 µg/ml) and MK-2206 (20 µM) in triplicates for 24. Viability was measured using Alamar Blue. Percent viability was calculated based on vehicle treated controls and control siRNA transfected controls, $p<0.001$ for the comparison of control siRNA versus siRNA for *AKT1*, *AKT2* and *RICTOR*, SC-661 µg/ml, MK-2206 20 µM. (D) C33A cells were seeded on to 48 well plates and transfected with oligos against *AKT1*, *AKT2* and *RICTOR* and lysates were prepared after 48 h and western blots were performed. (E) C33A cells were treated with SC-66 (2.5 µg/ml) and MK-2206 25 µM for 24 h then stained with Annexin/7-AAD and analyzed by flow cytometry. The graph represents % cell viability. (F) C33A cells were treated with SC-66 (0.0001 µg/ml–0.1 µg/ml) with or without 20 mM 2-DG for 48 h.

viability at 5 µg/ml of SC-66 was found to be 15% after 24 h (Fig. 3A). C33A cells were also sensitive to another allosteric AKT inhibitor, MK-2206. Cell viability was found to decrease starting with the concentration of 15 µM (58%) and decreasing to 2% by 48 h (Fig. 3B). To confirm that affects on cell viability were due to AKT inhibition rather than off target effects of SC-66 and MK-2206, siRNA experiments were performed. As shown in Figure 3C, C33A cell viability decreased to a similar extent when cells were transfected with siRNAs resulting in knockdown of *AKT1*, *AKT2*, and *RICTOR* (Fig. 3D).

To explore the mechanism through which AKT inhibitors induce cell death, we performed Annexin/7-AAD staining. Upon SC-66 (2.5 µg/ml) and MK-2206 (25 µM) treatment there were very few cells with Annexin only staining and the fraction of cells with both staining was 35% and less than 20%, respectively. 7-AAD only staining was close to 80% in MK-2206 treated cells (Fig. 3E). To further link effects of SC-66 through glucose uptake inhibition, we combined SC-66 with 2-deoxy glucose (2-DG), a competitive inhibitor of glucose uptake. By 48 hr after treatment with SC-66 (0.01 µg/ml) the viability was at 107%, but with the addition of 2-DG, cell viability decreased to 72% $p<0.001$ (Fig. 3F). MK-2206 exhibited synergistic effects with 2-DG. After 24 hr, the viability of MK-2206 treated cells was 78% which decreased up to 40% after addition of 20 mM 2-DG ($p<0.001$, Data A in File S1).

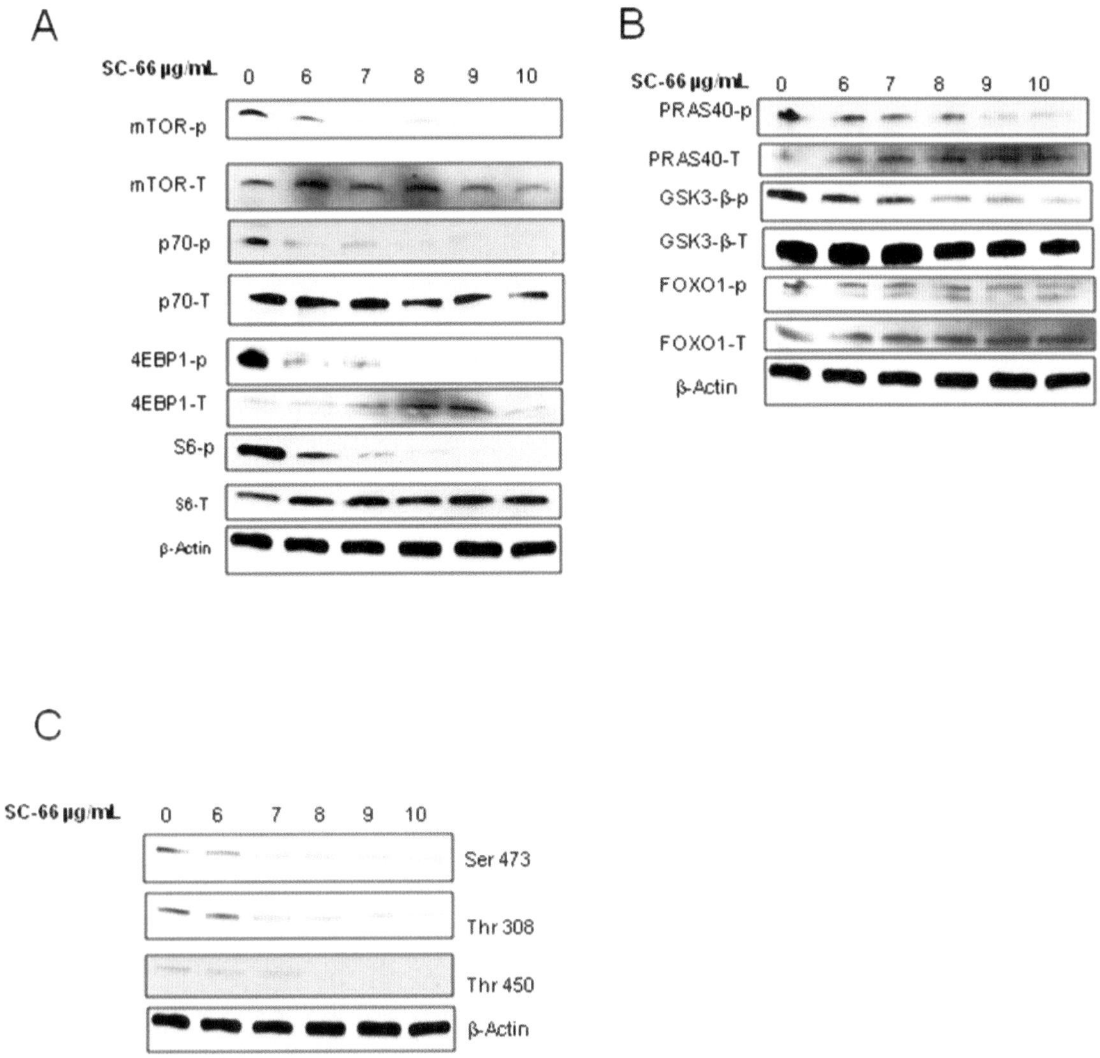

Figure 4. Effect of SC-66 on mTOR signaling. (A–C) C33A cells were treated with increasing concentrations of SC-66(6–10 µg/ml) for 3 h and lysates were prepared for western blot.

SC-66 and MK-2206 inhibited mTOR/AKT pathway effectively in C33A cells

To explore the effects of AKT inhibition on mTOR and its downstream targets in C33A cells, we examined the phosphorylation status of mTOR pathway components by Western blot and used p70S6K as a marker for mTOR activation [18]. SC-66 completely inhibited p70S6K phosphorylation by 3 hours (Fig. 4A). MK-2206 inhibited p70S6K activation but there was slight reactivation by 4 h. MK-2206 inhibited mTOR pathway components such as mTOR, 4E-BP1 and S6 effectively by 2 hours. MK-2206 inhibition of mTOR pathway appears to be transient as p70s6k was still active after 4 h (Data D in File S3). SC-66 and MK-2206 effectively inhibited all the three phosphorylated forms of AKT (Thr308, Thr450 and Ser 473) in a dose dependant manner suggesting that MK-2206 acts primarily through mTORC1 (Fig. 4C and Data F in File S3). This is supported by the observation that SC-66 was more effective in inhibiting AKT substrates such as PRAS 40, GSK3-β and FOXO1(Fig. 4B) compared to MK-2206, particularly PRAS40 which is in mTORC1 complex [19] (Data E in File S3). P70S6K was phosphorylated after 4 h of MK-2206 treatment suggesting the mTOR pathway inhibition was transient (Supplemental data).

Rapamycin, an mTOR inhibitor, relieves feedback inhibitions and induces AKT Ser473 phosphorylation in an mTORC2-dependent manner leading to further AKT activation [20]. To test for this effect using our inhibitors we performed a longer incubation of the cells with SC-66 for 18–24 h. We found that p70S6K, the marker of mTOR activation, was decreased even after 18 and 24 hrs treatment. SC-66 treatment decreased activation of AKT substrates, Thr308 and Thr450 by18 and 24 hours. Thr308 levels did go up compared to 3 h sample but still displayed a decreasing trend at 18–24 h (data not shown). All these results suggest that SC-66 effectively inhibited both mTORC1/2 and AKT. MK-2206 was found to be acting mainly through mTORC1 pathway with slight reactivation of the pathway after 4 hours.

SC-66 inhibited glucose uptake and membrane translocation of glucose transporters

Glucose uptake was tested by performing *in vitro* FDG uptake assays in the presence and absence of the SC-66 (35 µg/ml). We

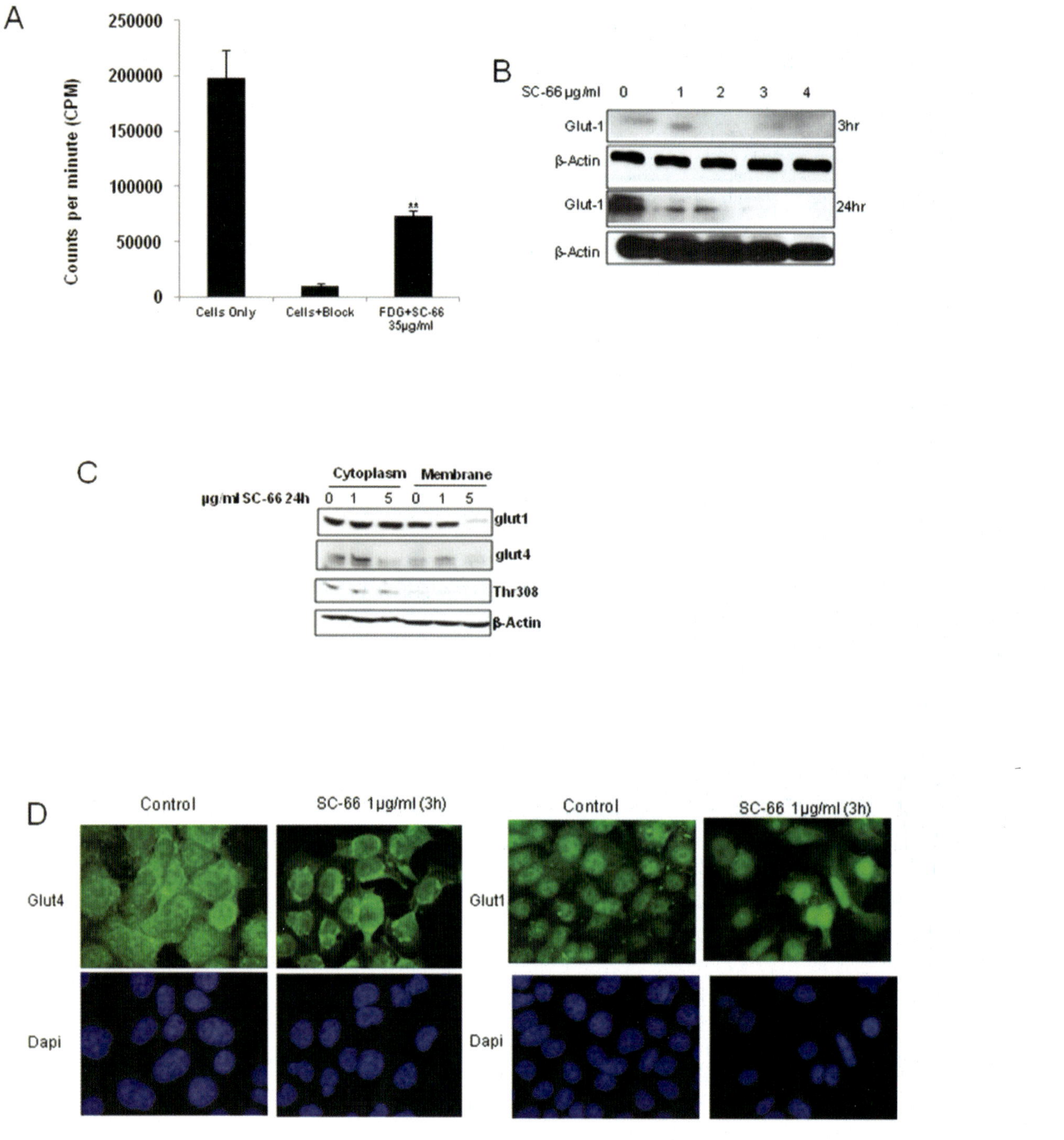

Figure 5. Effects of SC-66 on glucose transport. A) C33A cells were treated with SC-66 (35 µg/ml) or block (cytochalasin B) for 30 minutes prior to incubation with ^{18}F-fluorodeoxyglucose as described in the methods section. The graph represents counts per minute values, $p<0.01$ for the comparison of FDG alone (cells only) versus FDG + SC-66. B) C33A cells were treated with SC-66 (0–5 µg/ml) for 3 and 24 h and Glut1 levels were analyzed by western blot. C) C33A cells were treated with SC-66 (0, 1 and 5 µg/ml) for 24 h. Membrane and cytosol fractions were prepared using a kit (MemPER) from Peirce Biotechnology. These subcellular fractions were then mixed with sample buffer and incubated at 65°C for 20 mins before loading onto the gels for western blot for Glut1 and Glut4. D) Immunofluorescence was performed on C33A cells after treating them with SC-66 (1 µg/ml) for 3 hours in a chamber slide.

found that SC-66 inhibited glucose uptake significantly as evidenced by reduced counts per minute (Fig. 5A). Further we determined the effect of SC-66 on Glut1 and Glut4 translocation to the membrane. For this a membrane cytoplasm fractionation was carried out after treating cells with SC-66 (5 µg/ml) for 24 h. SC-66 inhibited Glut1 and Glut4 translocation from the cytoplasm to the membrane as determined by Western blot (Fig. 5C). We confirmed this with immunofluorescent staining (Fig. 5D). All these results suggest that mTOR inhibition by SC-66 resulted in decreased glucose uptake through Glut1 and Glut4 retention within cytoplasm.

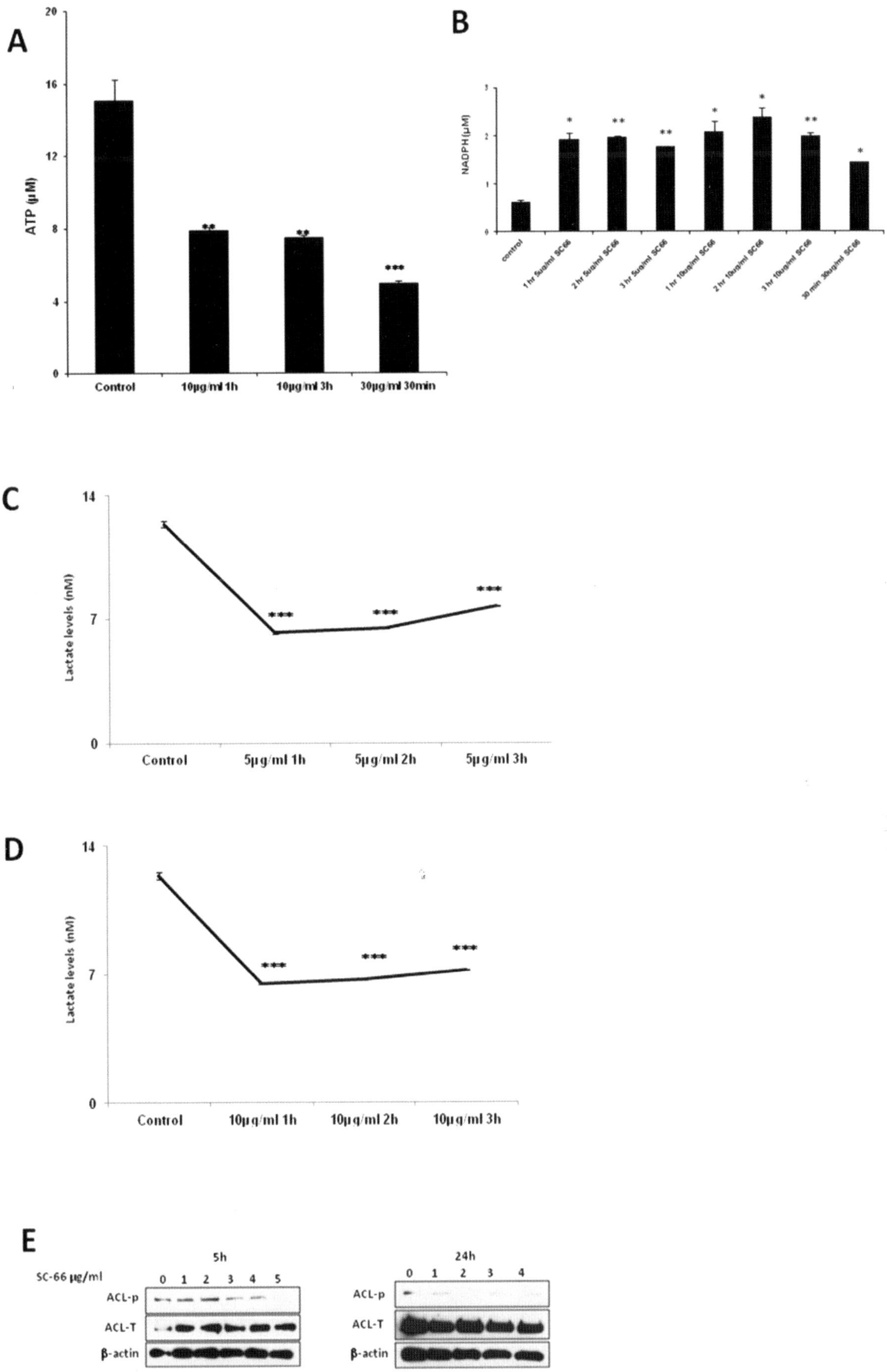
A
ATP (μM)
Control
10μg/ml 1h
10μg/ml 3h
30μg/ml 30min
B
NADPH (μM)
C
Lactate levels (nM)
Control
5μg/ml 1h
5μg/ml 2h
5μg/ml 3h
D
Lactate levels (nM)
Control
10μg/ml 1h
10μg/ml 2h
10μg/ml 3h
E
5h
24h
SC-66 μg/ml
ACL-p
ACL-T
β-actin

Figure 6. Effects of SC-66 on glucose metabolism. (A–B) C33A cells were seeded in T 25 cm^2 tissue culture flasks, treated with SC-66 and intracellular NADPH levels and ATP were determined. The graph represents ATP and NADPH μM levels based on standard curve, p<0.01 for the comparison of control versus SC-66 10 μg/ml 1 and 3 h and p<0.001 for control versus 30 μg/ml for ATP levels; p<0.01 for the comparison of control versus SC-66 5 μg/ml 3 h and p<0.01 control versus 10 μg/ml 3 h for NADPH levels. (C–D) C33A cells were seeded in T 25 cm^2 tissue culture flasks, treated with SC-66 and excreted lactate levels were measured in nM concentrations using a standard curve, p<0.001 for the comparison of control versus SC-66 5 and10 μg/ml. (E) C33A cells were treated with increasing concentrations of SC-66 (0–5 μg/ml) for 5 h and 24 h and lysates were prepared for western blot.

AKT inhibitor SC-66 inhibits glycolysis

To determine whether AKT inhibition resulted in reduced glycolysis, we measured ATP and NADPH levels after SC-66 treatment. We found that ATP levels were decreased significantly after SC-66 treatment, and NADPH levels were increased, suggesting that alternative pathways of glucose metabolism, such as the pentose phosphate shunt, may be more active in C33A cells when AKT signaling is suppressed (Fig. 6A and 6B). Total lactate levels were also decreased in C33A cells after treatment with SC-66 (Fig. 6C and 6D). All these results indicate that inhibition of AKT suppresses glycolysis in C33A cells. To evaluate for downstream effects on tumor cell metabolism, we monitored the activation status of a substrate of AKT, ATP-citrate lyase (ACL) after SC-66 treatment. C33A cells were incubated with increasing doses of SC-66 and western blots were performed. SC-66 inhibited ACL phosphorylation by 5 and 24 hours, suggesting that inhibition of AKT may also influence other aspects of tumor cell metabolism, including lipid synthesis (Fig. 6E).

SC-66 reduces migration of C33A cells in vitro

There are reports showing the role of AKT in the metastatic process including cell migration and invasion [21]. To study the effects of SC-66 and MK-2206 on cell migration we treated cells with 1 μg/ml SC-66 and 2.5 μM MK-2206 for 24 h and performed a scratch assay. We found that SC-66 inhibited the migration of cells about 50% compared to control whereas MK-2206 did not have any effect (Fig. 7).

Discussion

In this study, we performed mutational analysis of 140 pretreatment tumor biopsies and 8 human cervical cancer cell lines to screen for mutations in the PI3K/AKT pathway. This is the first study, to our knowledge, to comprehensively analyze mutations in the PI3K/AKT pathway in human cervical cancer. We identified multiple mutations in the PI3K/AKT pathway in human cervical cancer specimens, including activating mutations in *PIK3CA* (E545K, E542K) and inactivating mutations in *PTEN* (R233*). Mutational analysis of cervical cancer cell lines revealed additional defects. C33A cells have both an R233* *PTEN* mutation and an R88Q *PIK3CA* mutation [22].

The present study was also designed to test the hypothesis that cervical cancer cells with altered AKT activation would be sensitive to AKT inhibitors. SC-66 and MK-2206 effectively induced cell death in C33A cells through a non-apoptotic mechanism. SC-66 was found to be a potent mTORC1/2 inhibitor. SC-66 effectively inhibited p70s6k and 4E-BP1 mTORC1 substrates, in addition to inhibiting Ser473 and Thr308 phosphorylation of AKT, and activation of AKT substrates such as PRAS40, GSK3-β and FOXO. SC-66 displayed synergistic effects with 2-DG, and SC-66 inhibited further downstream events such as translocation of glucose transporters to the membrane which resulted in decreased glucose uptake. In addition, inhibition of AKT reduced glycolysis as evidenced by decreased ATP and lactate levels, and increased activity of alternative metabolic pathways resulting in increased cellular NADPH. These results suggest that AKT inhibitors decrease cervical cancer viability by interfering with cellular glucose metabolism. We hypothesize that cervical cancers with PI3K/AKT pathway alterations are dependent upon high rates of glucose uptake and glycolysis for survival. It should be noted that activation of Akt by *PTEN* loss and/or *PIK3CA* mutations would bypass the need for the activation of growth factor receptors (i.e. IGF-1R) to initiate the PI3K/Akt/mTOR signaling cascade. In this manner, cervical cancer cells are able to upregulate glucose import and metabolism even in the absence of the appropriate external signals.

Previously it has been shown that inhibition of mTORC2 leads to rapid inhibition of AKT Ser473 phosphorylation, which accelerates the destabilization process of Thr308 site phosphorylation [23]. In accordance with this, we also observed that SC-66 mediated a concomitant reduction in phosphorylation of Ser473 and Thr308 in C33A cells. Earlier work from others suggested that dephosphorylation of AKT at Thr308 site leads to more profound inhibition of AKT function than would be seen from dephosphorylation of AKT at Ser473 alone [23]. Thr308 is a residue in a key T-loop of the AKT protein and considered as a better indicator of AKT kinase activity. There are discordant data on the Ser473 phosphorylation and AKT kinase activity [24,25]. Our results show that SC-66 inhibits all of the three phosphorylated forms of AKT.

There are reports that mTORC2 is required for development of certain cancers with *PTEN* loss [26]. C33A cells are *PTEN* defective, and we found that SC-66 is a potent mTORC2 inhibitor. The *PTEN* R233* mutation found in C33A cells can lead to greater intracellular accumulation of PIP_3 resulting in enhanced PI3K signaling and PDK-1-mediated AKT Thr308 phosphorylation [25,27,28]. We speculate that SC-66 exerts its inhibitory effect on AKT Thr308 phosphorylation indirectly by acting as a PDK-1 inhibitor. SC-66 might not be as efficient as an inhibitor of PDK-1 as it is for mTOR and AKT, and this explains the slightly higher Thr308 levels observed after longer incubation. Moreover, we observed that SC-66 is a potent cell death inducer by 24 h, thus reactivation of AKT may not be an issue *in vivo*. In concordance with this notion, we found that in mice treated with a combination of cisplatin and SC-66, all p-AKT forms were inhibited compared to the monotherapy counterparts. This is true for the mTOR pathway components such as p70s6k, 4E-BP1 and S6 as well (data not shown).

AKT2 stimulates glucose uptake through the glucose transporter 4 (Glut4) translocation to membrane via a substrate called Syntaxin interacting protein (Synip) [29]. Membrane localization of AKT2 is a pre-requisite for Glut4 translocation in response to glucose uptake [30]. SC-66 effectively inhibited Glut1 and Glut4 membrane translocation, a key step mediated by AKT for glucose uptake. AKT activation leads to increased Glut1 expression and translocation to the membrane resulting in greater glucose uptake [31]. Our results indicate that SC-66 also inhibited Glut1 protein expression, suggesting that in C33A cells Glut1 expression is AKT-dependent.

In our study we also show that 2-DG enhanced MK-2206- and SC-66-induced cell death. It is known that glucose deprivation mimicked by glycolytic inhibitors causes cytotoxicity by inducing oxidative stress in human cancer cells [32], and cisplatin is known

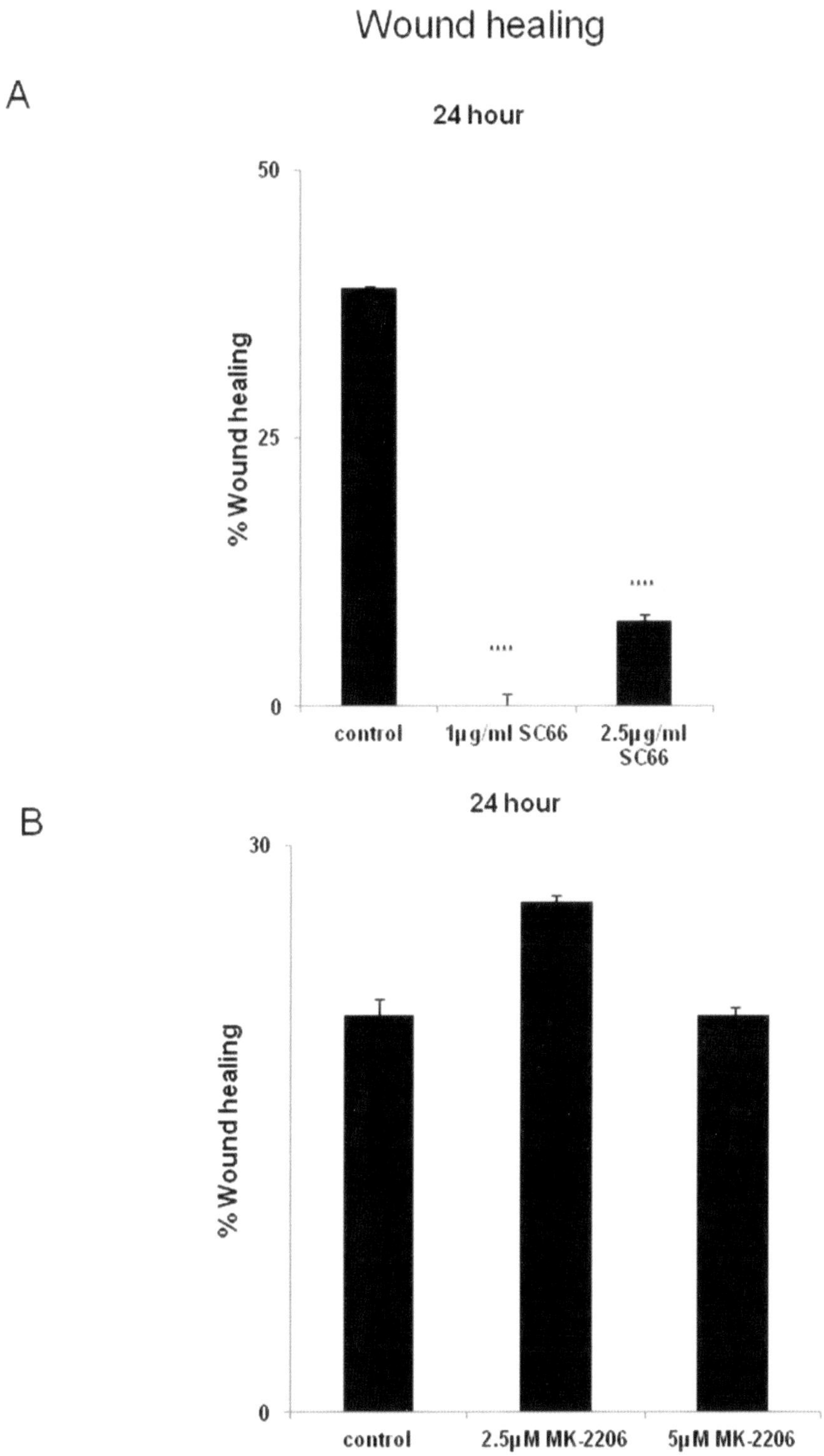

Figure 7. Effects of SC-66 and MK-2206 on cell migration. C33A cells were treated with A) SC-66 (1 and 2.5 μg/ml) and B) MK-2206 (2.5 and 5 μM) for 24 h. Percent wound healing was calculated as described in methods section, $p<0.0001$ for the comparison of control versus 1 ug SC-66 and $p<0.0001$ for control versus 2.5 ug SC-66.

to disrupt thiol metabolism and to enhance oxidative stress [33]. We hypothesize that combining cisplatin, SC-66/MK-2206 and 2-DG will display synergistic effects (Data B in File S1 and Data C in File S2). This synergy could be explained as disruption of cellular thiol pools and enhancement of oxidative stress by cisplatin and 2-DG respectively. Interestingly, treatment with Akt inhibitors does not render C33A cells resistant to death associated with glucose withdrawal, and we have observed induction of autophagy in response to MK2206 treatment. Additional studies will be needed to further characterize the role of autophagy in C33A cell survival.

Our preliminary studies based on Sequenom assays confirm that *PIK3CA* and *PTEN* genes are mutated in cervical cancer patients with poor progression free survival after standard chemoradiation. Frequency of the PI3K/AKT pathway mutations in human tumors widely vary in different types of cancer [10]. Recently, McIntyre *et al* described that *PIK3CA* E545K mutational status was associated with response to chemoradiation in cervical cancer patients [34]. A more comprehensive analysis of mutations in a larger cohort of patients is required to establish the link between PI3K/AKT pathway mutations and treatment outcome. If these results are validated, PI3K/AKT pathway mutations may be used in the future to select tumors at risk for treatment failure using standard chemoradiation (pelvic irradiation and concurrent administration of cisplatin chemotherapy).Our results suggest that AKT inhibitors could improve response to chemoradiation in cervical cancer for appropriately selected patients. It is possible that the mutations reported here (PIK3CAE545K, PIK3-CAE542K and PTEN R233*) may used in the future to select patients for targeted treatment with PI3K/AKT pathway inhibitors. Experiments are ongoing to determine the appropriate timing of AKT inhibition in the context of pelvic irradiation on chemotherapy.

Acknowledgments

We would like to thank Michael Zahner and Stephanie Krieger for technical assistance.

Statement of Translational Relevance

Alterations in expression of genes from the PI3K/AKT pathway are associated with incomplete response to chemoradiation in human cervical cancer. The objective of this study was to test for mutations in the PI3K/AKT pathway and to determine whether PI3K/AKT mutant cancers are sensitive to AKT inhibition. Using 140 pretreatment tumor biopsies and 8 human cervical cancer cell lines, we identified multiple defects in PI3K/AKT pathway genes, including both activating mutations in *PIK3CA* (E545K) and inactivating mutations in *PTEN* (R233*). Using C33A cells as a model for PI3K/AKT mutant cervical cancer, we found that AKT inhibitors effectively block mTORC1/2 signaling, resulting in decreased glucose uptake, glycolysis and cell viability *in vitro*. AKT inhibition also reduced cervical cancer cell migration. These results suggest that AKT inhibitors may improve response to chemoradiation in PI3K/AKT mutant cervical cancer, and emphasize the need for a personalized approach in the management of this disease.

Author Contributions

Conceived and designed the experiments: RR JKS CD AB. Performed the experiments: RR CD. Analyzed the data: RR CD CH AB BR JR PWG JKS. Contributed reagents/materials/analysis tools: JKS RR. Wrote the paper: RR CD JR PWG JKS. Review and approval of manuscript: RR CD CH AB BR JR PWG JKS.

References

1. Jemal A, Bray F, Center MM, Ferlay J, Ward E, et al. (2011) Global cancer statistics. CA Cancer J Clin 61: 69–90.
2. Grigsby PW, Siegel BA, Dehdashti F (2001) Lymph node staging by positron emission tomography in patients with carcinoma of the cervix. J Clin Oncol 19: 3745–3749.
3. Schwarz JK, Siegel BA, Dehdashti F, Grigsby PW (2007) Association of posttherapy positron emission tomography with tumor response and survival in cervical carcinoma. JAMA 298: 2289–2295.
4. Schwarz JK, Grigsby PW, Dehdashti F, Delbeke D (2009) The role of 18F-FDG PET in assessing therapy response in cancer of the cervix and ovaries. J Nucl Med 50 Suppl 1: 64S–73S.
5. Schwarz JK, Payton JE, Rashmi R, Xiang T, Jia Y, et al. (2012) Pathway-specific analysis of gene expression data identifies the PI3K/Akt pathway as a novel therapeutic target in cervical cancer. Clin Cancer Res 18: 1464–1471.
6. Engelman JA (2009) Targeting PI3K signalling in cancer: opportunities, challenges and limitations. Nat Rev Cancer 9: 550–562.
7. Liu P, Cheng H, Roberts TM, Zhao JJ (2009) Targeting the phosphoinositide 3-kinase pathway in cancer. Nat Rev Drug Discov 8: 627–644.
8. She QB, Chandarlapaty S, Ye Q, Lobo J, Haskell KM, et al. (2008) Breast tumor cells with PI3K mutation or HER2 amplification are selectively addicted to Akt signaling. PLoS One 3: e3065.
9. Serra V, Markman B, Scaltriti M, Eichhorn PJ, Valero V, et al. (2008) NVP-BEZ235, a dual PI3K/mTOR inhibitor, prevents PI3K signaling and inhibits the growth of cancer cells with activating PI3K mutations. Cancer Res 68: 8022–8030.
10. MacConaill LE, Campbell CD, Kehoe SM, Bass AJ, Hatton C, et al. (2009) Profiling critical cancer gene mutations in clinical tumor samples. PLoS One 4: e7887.
11. Kaplan EL, Meier P (1958) Nonparametric Estimation from Incomplete Observations. Journal of the American Statistical Association 53: 457–481.
12. Pang H, Flinn R, Patsialou A, Wyckoff J, Roussos ET, et al. (2009) Differential enhancement of breast cancer cell motility and metastasis by helical and kinase domain mutations of class IA phosphoinositide 3-kinase. Cancer Res 69: 8868–8876.
13. Huang CH, Mandelker D, Schmidt-Kittler O, Samuels Y, Velculescu VE, et al. (2007) The structure of a human p110alpha/p85alpha complex elucidates the effects of oncogenic PI3Kalpha mutations. Science 318: 1744–1748.
14. Oda K, Okada J, Timmerman L, Rodriguez-Viciana P, Stokoe D, et al. (2008) PIK3CA cooperates with other phosphatidylinositol 3′-kinase pathway mutations to effect oncogenic transformation. Cancer Res 68: 8127–8136.
15. Isakoff SJ, Engelman JA, Irie HY, Luo J, Brachmann SM, et al. (2005) Breast cancer-associated PIK3CA mutations are oncogenic in mammary epithelial cells. Cancer Res 65: 10992–11000.
16. Han SY, Kato H, Kato S, Suzuki T, Shibata H, et al. (2000) Functional evaluation of PTEN missense mutations using in vitro phosphoinositide phosphatase assay. Cancer Res 60: 3147–3151.
17. Lee JO, Yang H, Georgescu MM, Di Cristofano A, Maehama T, et al. (1999) Crystal structure of the PTEN tumor suppressor: implications for its phosphoinositide phosphatase activity and membrane association. Cell 99: 323–334.
18. Zeng Z, Sarbassov dos D, Samudio IJ, Yee KW, Munsell MF, et al. (2007) Rapamycin derivatives reduce mTORC2 signaling and inhibit AKT activation in AML. Blood 109: 3509–3512.
19. Proud CG (2009) mTORC1 signalling and mRNA translation. Biochem Soc Trans 37: 227–231.
20. Courtois-Cox S, Genther Williams SM, Reczek EE, Johnson BW, McGillicuddy LT, et al. (2006) A negative feedback signaling network underlies oncogene-induced senescence. Cancer Cell 10: 459–472.
21. Larue L, Bellacosa A (2005) Epithelial-mesenchymal transition in development and cancer: role of phosphatidylinositol 3′ kinase/AKT pathways. Oncogene 24: 7443–7454.
22. Cui B, Zheng B, Zhang X, Stendahl U, Andersson S, et al. (2009) Mutation of PIK3CA: possible risk factor for cervical carcinogenesis in older women. Int J Oncol 34: 409–416.
23. Rodrik-Outmezguine VS, Chandarlapaty S, Pagano NC, Poulikakos PI, Scaltriti M, et al. (2011) mTOR kinase inhibition causes feedback-dependent biphasic regulation of AKT signaling. Cancer Discov 1: 248–259.
24. Yang J, Cron P, Thompson V, Good VM, Hess D, et al. (2002) Molecular mechanism for the regulation of protein kinase B/Akt by hydrophobic motif phosphorylation. Mol Cell 9: 1227–1240.
25. Alessi DR, Deak M, Casamayor A, Caudwell FB, Morrice N, et al. (1997) 3-Phosphoinositide-dependent protein kinase-1 (PDK1): structural and functional homology with the Drosophila DSTPK61 kinase. Curr Biol 7: 776–789.
26. Guertin DA, Stevens DM, Saitoh M, Kinkel S, Crosby K, et al. (2009) mTOR complex 2 is required for the development of prostate cancer induced by Pten loss in mice. Cancer Cell 15: 148–159.
27. Currie RA, Walker KS, Gray A, Deak M, Casamayor A, et al. (1999) Role of phosphatidylinositol 3,4,5-trisphosphate in regulating the activity and localization of 3-phosphoinositide-dependent protein kinase-1. Biochem J 337 (Pt 3): 575–583.
28. Majumder PK, Sellers WR (2005) Akt-regulated pathways in prostate cancer. Oncogene 24: 7465–7474.
29. Manning BD, Cantley LC (2007) AKT/PKB signaling: navigating downstream. Cell 129: 1261–1274.

30. Gonzalez E, McGraw TE (2009) The Akt kinases: isoform specificity in metabolism and cancer. Cell Cycle 8: 2502–2508.
31. Wofford JA, Wieman HL, Jacobs SR, Zhao Y, Rathmell JC (2008) IL-7 promotes Glut1 trafficking and glucose uptake via STAT5-mediated activation of Akt to support T-cell survival. Blood 111: 2101–2111.
32. Spitz DR, Sim JE, Ridnour LA, Galoforo SS, Lee YJ (2000) Glucose deprivation-induced oxidative stress in human tumor cells. A fundamental defect in metabolism? Ann N Y Acad Sci 899: 349–362.
33. Simons AL, Ahmad IM, Mattson DM, Dornfeld KJ, Spitz DR (2007) 2-Deoxy-D-glucose combined with cisplatin enhances cytotoxicity via metabolic oxidative stress in human head and neck cancer cells. Cancer Res 67: 3364–3370.
34. McIntyre JB, Wu JS, Craighead PS, Phan T, Kobel M, et al. (2013) PIK3CA mutational status and overall survival in patients with cervical cancer treated with radical chemoradiotherapy. Gynecol Oncol 128: 409–414.

Permissions

All chapters in this book were first published in PLOS ONE, by The Public Library of Science; hereby published with permission under the Creative Commons Attribution License or equivalent. Every chapter published in this book has been scrutinized by our experts. Their significance has been extensively debated. The topics covered herein carry significant findings which will fuel the growth of the discipline. They may even be implemented as practical applications or may be referred to as a beginning point for another development.

The contributors of this book come from diverse backgrounds, making this book a truly international effort. This book will bring forth new frontiers with its revolutionizing research information and detailed analysis of the nascent developments around the world.

We would like to thank all the contributing authors for lending their expertise to make the book truly unique. They have played a crucial role in the development of this book. Without their invaluable contributions this book wouldn't have been possible. They have made vital efforts to compile up to date information on the varied aspects of this subject to make this book a valuable addition to the collection of many professionals and students.

This book was conceptualized with the vision of imparting up-to-date information and advanced data in this field. To ensure the same, a matchless editorial board was set up. Every individual on the board went through rigorous rounds of assessment to prove their worth. After which they invested a large part of their time researching and compiling the most relevant data for our readers.

The editorial board has been involved in producing this book since its inception. They have spent rigorous hours researching and exploring the diverse topics which have resulted in the successful publishing of this book. They have passed on their knowledge of decades through this book. To expedite this challenging task, the publisher supported the team at every step. A small team of assistant editors was also appointed to further simplify the editing procedure and attain best results for the readers.

Apart from the editorial board, the designing team has also invested a significant amount of their time in understanding the subject and creating the most relevant covers. They scrutinized every image to scout for the most suitable representation of the subject and create an appropriate cover for the book.

The publishing team has been an ardent support to the editorial, designing and production team. Their endless efforts to recruit the best for this project, has resulted in the accomplishment of this book. They are a veteran in the field of academics and their pool of knowledge is as vast as their experience in printing. Their expertise and guidance has proved useful at every step. Their uncompromising quality standards have made this book an exceptional effort. Their encouragement from time to time has been an inspiration for everyone.

The publisher and the editorial board hope that this book will prove to be a valuable piece of knowledge for researchers, students, practitioners and scholars across the globe.

List of Contributors

Gene-Fu F. Liu, Ryan J. Bair and Stanley L. Liauw
Department of Radiation and Cellular Oncology, University of Chicago Medical Center, Chicago, Illinois, United States of America

Matthew Koshy
Department of Radiation and Cellular Oncology, University of Chicago Medical Center, Chicago, Illinois, United States of America
Department of Radiation Oncology, University of Illinois Hospital, Chicago, Illinois, United States of America

Eric Bair
Departments of Endodontics and Biostatistics, University of North Carolina-Chapel Hill, Chapel Hill, North Carolina, United States of America

Yong Gao, Jing Zhu, Xiaohui Zhang, Yangqing Liu and Xiaofei Chen
Department of Medical Oncology, Huai'an First People's Hospital, Nanjing Medical University, Huai'an, China

Qingquan Wu
Department of Thoracic Surgery, Huai'an First People's Hospital, Nanjing Medical University, Huai'an, China

Shaoning Jiang
Department of Medicine, University of Alabama at Birmingham, Birmingham, Alabama, United States of America

Zhibin Hu
Department of Epidemiology and Biostatistics, Nanjing Medical University, Nanjing, China

Baorui Liu
The Comprehensive Cancer Center, Gulou School of Clinical Medicine, Nanjing Medical University, Nanjing, China

Nam P. Nguyen, Lexie Smith-Raymond, Rick Davis, Dave Abraham, Michelle Stevie, Beng-Hoey Jo and Misty Ceizyk
Department of Radiation Oncology, University of Arizona, Tucson, Arizona, United States of America

Vincent Vinh-Hung
Department of Radiation Oncology, University Hospitals of Geneva, Geneva, Switzerland

Paul Vos
Biostatistics, East Carolina University, Greenville, North Carolina, United States of America

Anand Desai and Shane P. Krafft
Department of Radiation Oncology, University of Texas at M. D. Anderson, Houston, Texas, United States of America

Thomas Sroka
Department of Radiation Oncology, Darmouth College, Hanover, New Hampshire, United States of America

Homayoun Modarresifar
Department of Radiology University of Arizona, Tucson, Arizona, United States of America

Andreas Deistung, Ferdinand Schweser and Jürgen Rainer Reichenbach
Medical Physics Group, Institute of Diagnostic and Interventional Radiology I, Jena University Hospital - Friedrich Schiller University Jena, Philosophenweg 3, Jena, Germany

Benedikt Wiestler and Wolfgang Wick
Department of Neurooncology, University of Heidelberg, INF 400, Heidelberg, Germany

Matthias Roethke and Heinz-Peter Schlemmer
Department of Radiology, German Cancer Research Center (DKFZ), INF 280, Heidelberg, Germany

Felix Sahm
Department of Neuropathology, University of Heidelberg, INF 220/221, Heidelberg, Germany

Armin Michael Nagel
Institute for Medical Physics, German Cancer Research Center (DKFZ), INF 280, Heidelberg, Germany

Mario Abello, Sabine Heiland and Martin Bendszus
Department of Neuroradiology, University of Heidelberg, INF 400, Heidelberg, Germany

Alexander Radbruch
Department of Neuroradiology, University of Heidelberg, INF 400, Heidelberg, Germany
Section Neurooncologic Imaging (E 012), German Cancer Research Center, INF 280, Heidelberg, Germany

Fumitaka Koga, Soichiro Yoshida, Manabu Tatokoro, Satoru Kawakami, Yasuhisa Fujii and Kazunori Kihara
Department of Urology, Tokyo Medical and Dental University Graduate School, Tokyo, Japan

Jiro Kumagai
Department of Surgical Pathology, Tokyo Medical and Dental University Graduate School, Tokyo, Japan

Len Neckers
Urologic Oncology Branch, National Cancer Institute, Bethesda, Maryland, United States of America

Yousun Chong, Jae-Hun Kim, Ho Yun Lee and Kyung Soo Lee
Department of Radiology and Center for Imaging Science, Sungkyunkwan University School of Medicine, Seoul, Korea

Yong Chan Ahn
Department of Radiation Oncology, Sungkyunkwan University School of Medicine, Seoul, Korea

Myung-Ju Ahn
Division of Hemato-Oncology, Department of Internal Medicine, Sungkyunkwan University School of Medicine, Seoul, Korea

Jhingook Kim and Young Mog Shim
Department of Thoracic Surgery, Sungkyunkwan University School of Medicine, Seoul, Korea

Joungho Han and Yoon-La Choi
Department of Pathology, Samsung Medical Center, Sungkyunkwan University School of Medicine, Seoul, Korea

Christopher H. Chapman, Mohammad Nazem-Zadeh, Matthew J. Schipper, Christina I. Tsien and Theodore S. Lawrence
Department of Radiation Oncology, University of Michigan, Ann Arbor, Michigan, United States of America

Yue Cao
Department of Radiation Oncology, University of Michigan, Ann Arbor, Michigan, United States of America
Department of Radiology, University of Michigan, Ann Arbor, Michigan, United States of America
Department of Biomedical Engineering, University of Michigan, Ann Arbor, Michigan, United States of America

Oliver E. Lee
Department of Biostatistics, University of Michigan, Ann Arbor, Michigan, United States of America

Goutham Hassan Venkatesh, Kamalesh Dattaram Mumbrekar and Satish Rao Bola Sadashiva
Division of Radiobiology and Toxicology, School of Life Sciences, Manipal University, Manipal, Karnataka, India

Hitendra Negi
Division of Biotechnology, School of Life Sciences, Manipal University, Manipal, Karnataka, India

Vadhiraja Bejadi Manjunath
Manipal Hospital, Bangalore, Karnataka, India

Sourjya Banerjee
Department of Radiotherapy and Oncology, Kasturba Medical College and Hospital, Mangalore, Karnataka, India

Donald Jerard Fernandes and Krishna Sharan
Department of Radiotherapy and Oncology, Shiridi SaiBaba Cancer Hospital and Research Centre, Kasturba Hospital, Manipal, Karnataka, India

Wei F. Chen
Division of Plastic and Reconstructive Surgery, Department of Surgery, University of Iowa Hospitals and Clinics, Iowa City, Iowa, United States of America

Kai-Ping Chang
Department of Otolaryngology - Head and Neck Surgery, Chang Gung Memorial Hospital and Chang Gung University College of Medicine, Taoyuan, Taiwan

Chih-Hao Chen, Victor Bong-Hang Shyu and Huang-Kai Kao
Department of Plastic and Reconstructive Surgery, Chang Gung Memorial Hospital and Chang Gung University College of Medicine, Taoyuan, Taiwan

Christiane Jakob, Daniela E. Aust, Birgit Liebscher, Gustavo B. Baretton and Michael H. Muders
Institute of Pathology, University Hospital Carl Gustav Carus, University of Technology, Dresden, Germany

Kaustubh Datta
Institute of Pathology, University Hospital Carl Gustav Carus, University of Technology, Dresden, Germany
Department of Biochemistry, University of Nebraska Medical Center, Omaha, Nebraska, United States of America

Jeeyun Lee, Se Hoon Park, Joon Oh Park, Young Suk Park, Ho Yeong Lim and Won Ki Kang
Division of Hematology-Oncology, Department of Medicine, Samsung Medical Center Sungkyunkwan University School of Medicine, Seoul, Korea

Insuk Sohn and Sin Ho Jung
Samsung Cancer Research Institute, Samsung Medical Center, Seoul, Korea

In-Gu Do
Samsung Cancer Research Institute, Samsung Medical Center, Seoul, Korea

Department of Pathology, Samsung Medical Center Sungkyunkwan University School of Medicine, Seoul, Korea

Kyoung-Mee Kim
Department of Pathology, Samsung Medical Center Sungkyunkwan University School of Medicine, Seoul, Korea

Tae Sung Sohn, Jae Moon Bae, Min Gew Choi and Sung Kim
Department of Surgery, Samsung Medical Center, Sungkyunkwan University School of Medicine, Seoul, Korea

Do Hoon Lim
Department of Radiation Oncology, Samsung Medical Center, Sungkyunkwan University School of Medicine, Seoul, Korea

Byung Hoon Min, Joon Haeng Lee, Poong Lyul Rhee and Jae J. Kim
Department of Gastroenterology, Samsung Medical Center, Sungkyunkwan University School of Medicine, Seoul, Korea

Dong Il Choi
Department of Radiology, Samsung Medical Center, Sungkyunkwan University School of Medicine, Seoul, Korea

Iain Beehuat Tan
Cancer and Stem Cell Biology, Duke-NUS Graduate Medical School Singapore, Singapore

Patrick Tan
Cancer and Stem Cell Biology, Duke-NUS Graduate Medical School Singapore, Singapore
Genome Institute of Singapore, Singapore, Singapore
Cancer Science Institute of Singapore, Singapore, Singapore

Kakoli Das
Genome Institute of Singapore, Singapore, Singapore

Yingjie Zheng1
Department of Radiation Oncology, Beijing Chaoyang Hospital, Capital Medical University, Beijing, China

Xuemei Ji
Department of Radiation Oncology, Beijing Chaoyang Hospital, Capital Medical University, Beijing, China
Department of Radiation and Medical Oncology, Zhongnan Hospital, Wuhan University, Wuhan, China

Conghua Xie and Xia Fan
Department of Radiation and Medical Oncology, Zhongnan Hospital, Wuhan University, Wuhan, China

Desheng Hu and Yajuan Zhou
Department of Radiation Oncology, Tumor Hosptal of Hubei Province, Wuhan, China

Nam P. Nguyen, Rick Davis, Benjamin Slane, Misty Ceizyk, Dave Abraham, Lexie Smith-Raymond, Michelle Stevie and Steven Gelumbauskas
Department of Radiation Oncology, University of Arizona, Tucson, Arizona, United States of America

Alexander Chi
Department of Radiation Oncology, University of West Virginia, Morgantown, West Virginia, United States of America

Michael Betz and Vincent Vinh-Hung
Department of Radiation Oncology, University Hospitals of Geneva, Geneva, Switzerland

Fabio Almeida
Southwest PET/CT Institute, Tucson, Arizona, United States of America

Paul Vos
Department of Biostatistics, East Carolina University, Greenville, North Carolina, United States of America

Siyoung Jang
Department of Radiation Oncology, University of Pittsburgh, Pittsburgh, Pennsylvania, United States of America

Nam P. Nguyen, Misty Ceizyk, Rick Davis, Benjamin Slane, Steven Gelumbauskas, Lexie Smith-Raymond, Dave Abraham, Michelle Stevie and Siyoung Jang
Department of Radiation Oncology, University of Arizona, Tucson, Arizona, United States of America

Paul Vos
Department of Biostatistics, East Carolina University, Greenville, North Carolina, United States of America

Michael Betz
Hirslanden Radiation Oncology Institute, Lausanne, Switzerland

Alexander Chi
Department of Radiation Oncology, West Virginia University, Morgantown, West Virginia, United States of America

Fabio Almeida
Southwest PET-CT Institute, Tucson, Arizona, United States of America

Vincent Vinh-Hung
Department of Radiation Oncology, University Hospitals of Geneva, Geneva, Switzerland

Alisa Talianski
Oncology Institute, Sheba Medical Center, Ramat-Gan, Israel

Leor Zach
Oncology Institute, Sheba Medical Center, Ramat-Gan, Israel
Sackler Faculty of Medicine, Tel-Aviv University, Tel-Aviv, Israel

David Guez and David Last
Advanced Technology Center, Sheba Medical Center, Ramat-Gan, Israel

Dianne Daniels and Yael Mardor
Advanced Technology Center, Sheba Medical Center, Ramat-Gan, Israel
Sackler Faculty of Medicine, Tel-Aviv University, Tel-Aviv, Israel

Yuval Grober and Ouzi Nissim
Neurosurgery Department, Sheba Medical Center, Ramat-Gan, Israel

Roberto Spiegelmann and Zvi R. Cohen
Neurosurgery Department, Sheba Medical Center, Ramat-Gan, Israel
Sackler Faculty of Medicine, Tel-Aviv University, Tel-Aviv, Israel

Chen Hoffmann
Radiology Institute, Sheba Medical Center, Ramat-Gan, Israel
Sackler Faculty of Medicine, Tel-Aviv University, Tel-Aviv, Israel

Dvora Nass
Pathology Institute, Sheba Medical Center, Ramat-Gan, Israel

Alexander K. Dik, Sander Sassen and Roy F. A. Vliegen
Department of Radiology, Atrium Medical Center Parkstad, Heerlen, The Netherlands

Robert M. Kwee
Department of Radiology, Atrium Medical Center Parkstad, Heerlen, The Netherlands
Department of Radiology, Maastricht University Medical Center, Maastricht, The Netherlands

Meindert N. Sosef
Department of Surgery, Atrium Medical Center Parkstad, Heerlen, The Netherlands
Surgical Collaborative Network Limburg, Limburg, The Netherlands

Ralph C. M. Berendsen
Department of Medical Physics, Atrium Medical Center Parkstad, Heerlen, The Netherlands

Guido Lammering
Department of Radiation Oncology, MediClin Robert-Janker-Clinic, Bonn, Germany

Ruud Clarijs
Department of Pathology, Atrium Medical Center Parkstad, Heerlen, The Netherlands

Liekele E. Oostenbrug
Department of Internal Medicine and Gastroenterology, Atrium Medical Center Parkstad, Heerlen, The Netherlands

Rachel L. G. M. Blom
Department of Surgery, Academic Medical Center, Amsterdam, The Netherlands

Junjie Peng, Debing Shi, Xinxiang Li, Hongbin Wu and Sanjun Cai
Department of Colorectal Surgery, Fudan University Shanghai Cancer Center, Shanghai, China
Department of Oncology, Shanghai Medical College, Fudan University, Shanghai, China

Ying Ding
Department of Biostatistics, University of Pittsburgh, Pittsburgh, Pennsylvania, United States of America

Shanshan Tu
Department of Statistics, University of Pittsburgh, Pittsburgh, Pennsylvania, United States of America

Liang Sun
School of Science and Technology, Georgia Gwinnett College, Atlanta, Georgia, United States of America

Kim Wopken, Hendrik P. Bijl, Arjen van der Schaaf, Miranda E. Christianen, Olga Chouvalova, Roel J. H. M. Steenbakkers and Johannes A. Langendijk
Department of Radiation Oncology, University of Groningen, University Medical Center Groningen, Groningen, the Netherlands

Ben J. Slotman and Patricia Doornaert
Department of Radiation Oncology, VU University Medical Center, Amsterdam, the Netherlands

Sjoukje F. Oosting
Department of Medical Oncology, University of Groningen, University Medical Center Groningen, Groningen, the Netherlands

Bernard F. A. M. van der Laan
Department of Otolaryngology/Head and Neck Surgery, University of Groningen, University Medical Center Groningen, Groningen, the Netherlands

Jan L. N. Roodenburg
Department of Oral and Maxillofacial Surgery, University of Groningen, University Medical Center Groningen, Groningen, the Netherlands

C. René Leemans and Irma M. Verdonck-de Leeuw
Department of Otolaryngology-Head and Neck Surgery, VU University Medical Center, Amsterdam, the Netherlands

Peng Zhang, Mian Xi, Lei Zhao, Qiao-Qiao Li, Li-Ru He, Shi-Liang Liu and Meng-Zhong Liu
Sun Yat-sen University Cancer Center, State Key Laboratory of Oncology in South China, Collaborative Innovation Center for Cancer Medicine, Department of Radiation Oncology, Cancer Center, Sun Yat-sen University, Guangzhou, People's Republic of China

Jing-Xian Shen
Sun Yat-sen University Cancer Center, State Key Laboratory of Oncology in South China, Collaborative Innovation Center for Cancer Medicine, Imaging Diagnosis and Interventional Center, Cancer Center, Sun Yat-sen University, Guangzhou, People's Republic of China

Meng Su, Lu-Cheng Zhu, Hang-Ping Wei, Wen-Hua Luo, Rui-Fang Lin and Chang-Lin Zou
Department of Radiation Oncology and Chemotherapy, The First Affiliated Hospital of Wenzhou Medical University, Wenzhou, China

Michael T. Spiotto and Ralph R. Weichselbaum
Department of Radiation and Cellular Oncology, University of Chicago Medical Center, Chicago, Illinois, United States of America
Department of Radiation Oncology, University of Illinois Hospital and Health Sciences System, Chicago, Illinois, United States of America

Tianxia Deng, Cheng Zhang, Xi Zhang, Sha Wu, Yaqi Xu, Shanshan Liu and Xinghua Chen
Department of Hematology, Xinqiao Hospital, Third Military Medical University, Chongqing, China

Cheng-Cheng Hwang, Liang-Che Chang, Wen-Ying Chi, Hui-Ping Chien, Tsan-Yu Hsieh and Jim-Ray Chen
Department of Pathology, Chang Gung Memorial Hospital, Keelung, Taiwan

Shin Nieh
Department of Pathology and Graduate Institute of Pathology, National Defense Medical Center and Tri-Service General Hospital, Taipei, Taiwan

Chien-Hong Lai
Division of Hematology-Oncology, Department of Internal Medicine, Chang Gung Memorial Hospital, Keelung, Taiwan

Chien-Sheng Tsai
Department of Radiation Oncology, Chang Gung Memorial Hospital, Keelung, Taiwan

Chung-Ching Hua
Division of Pulmonary, Critical Care and Sleep Medicine, Chang Gung Memorial Hospital, Keelung, Taiwan

Siu-Cheung Chan
Department of Diagnostic Radiology, Chang Gung Memorial Hospital, Keelung, Taiwan

Chih-Wei Wang
Department of Anatomic Pathology, Chang Gung Memorial Hospital, Tao-Yuan, Taiwan

Laura W. Goff, Liping Du, Emily Chan, Dana B. Cardin and Jordan D. Berlin
Department of Medicine, Vanderbilt-Ingram Cancer Center, Nashville, Tennessee, United States of America

Nilay Thakkar and Wooin Lee
Department of Pharmaceutical Sciences, College of Pharmacy, University of Kentucky, Lexington, Kentucky, United States of America

Benjamin R. Tan, Chloe Fournier, Joel Picus, Andrea Wang-Gillam and A. Craig Lockhart
Department of Medicine, Siteman Cancer Center, Washington University School of Medicine, St. Louis, Missouri, United States of America

Howard L. McLeod
Moffitt Cancer Center, Tampa, Florida, United States of America

Barbara Zehnbauer
Centers for Disease Control and Prevention, Atlanta, Georgia, United States of America

Xuebing Li
Tianjin Key Laboratory of Lung Cancer Metastasis and Tumor Microenvironment, Tianjin Lung Cancer Institute, Tianjin Medical University General Hospital, Tianjin, China

Jundong Gu
Tianjin Key Laboratory of Lung Cancer Metastasis and Tumor Microenvironment, Tianjin Lung Cancer Institute, Tianjin Medical University General Hospital, Tianjin, China
Department of Oncology, Tianjin Union Medical Center, Tianjin, China

Siwei Zhu
Department of Oncology, Tianjin Union Medical Center, Tianjin, China

Hua Wu
Department of Human resources, Tianjin Union Medical Center, Tianjin, China

Yang Li
Department of obstetrics and gynecology, Tianjin Hospital of Tianjin City, Tianjin, China

Feng Hua
Department of surgery oncology, Shandong cancer hospital, Jinan, China

Ramachandran Rashmi and Carl DeSelm
Department of Radiation Oncology, Washington University School of Medicine, St. Louis, Missouri, United States of America

Buck E. Rogers
Department of Radiation Oncology, Washington University School of Medicine, St. Louis, Missouri, United States of America
Alvin J. Siteman Cancer Center, Washington University School of Medicine, St. Louis, Missouri, United States of America

Julie K. Schwarz
Department of Radiation Oncology, Washington University School of Medicine, St. Louis, Missouri, United States of America
Department of Cell Biology and Physiology, Washington University School of Medicine, St. Louis, Missouri, United States of America
Alvin J. Siteman Cancer Center, Washington University School of Medicine, St. Louis, Missouri, United States of America

Perry W. Grigsby
Department of Radiation Oncology, Washington University School of Medicine, St. Louis, Missouri, United States of America
Division of Nuclear Medicine, Mallinckrodt Institute of Radiology, Washington University School of Medicine, St. Louis, Missouri, United States of America
Division of Gynecologic Oncology, Washington University School of Medicine, St. Louis, Missouri, United States of America
Alvin J. Siteman Cancer Center, Washington University School of Medicine, St. Louis, Missouri, United States of America

Cynthia Helms
Department of Genetics, Washington University School of Medicine, St. Louis, Missouri, United States of America

Anne Bowcock
Department of Genetics, Washington University School of Medicine, St. Louis, Missouri, United States of America
Division of Gynecologic Oncology, Washington University School of Medicine, St. Louis, Missouri, United States of America

Janet Rader
Dept of Obstetrics and Gynecology, Medical College of Wisconsin, Milwaukee, Wisconsin, United States of America

Index

O

P

R

S

T